a LANGE medical book

CURRENT
Practice Guidelines in
Primary Care
2025–2026

T0356723

Jacob A. David, MD, FAAFP
Program Director
Family Medicine Residency Program
Ventura County Medical Center
Adjunct Clinical Assistant Professor of Family Medicine
Keck School of Medicine
Ventura, California

New York   Chicago   San Francisco   Athens   London   Madrid
Mexico City   Milan   New Delhi   Singapore   Sydney   Toronto

CURRENT Practice Guidelines in Primary Care, 2025–2026

Copyright © 2025, 2024, 2023, 2022, 2020, 2019, 2018, 2017, 2016, 2015 by McGraw Hill LLC. All rights reserved. Printed in the United States of America. Except as permitted under the United States Copyright Act of 1976, no part of this publication may be reproduced or distributed in any form or by any means, or stored in a data base or retrieval system, without the prior written permission of the publisher. Copyright © 2000 through 2013 by the McGraw Hill Companies, Inc.

1 2 3 4 5 LBC 28 27 26 25 24

ISBN 978-1-265-02589-2
MHID 1-265-02589-4
ISSN 1528-1612

Notice

Medicine is an ever-changing science. As new research and clinical experience broaden our knowledge, changes in treatment and drug therapy are required. The authors and the publisher of this work have checked with sources believed to be reliable in their efforts to provide information that is complete and generally in accord with the standards accepted at the time of publication. However, in view of the possibility of human error or changes in medical sciences, neither the authors nor the publisher nor any other party who has been involved in the preparation or publication of this work warrants that the information contained herein is in every respect accurate or complete, and they disclaim all responsibility for any errors or omissions or for the results obtained from use of the information contained in this work. Readers are encouraged to confirm the information contained herein with other sources. For example and in particular, readers are advised to check the product information sheet included in the package of each drug they plan to administer to be certain that the information contained in this work is accurate and that changes have not been made in the recommended dose or in the contraindications for administration. This recommendation is of particular importance in connection with new or infrequently used drugs.

This book was set in Minion Pro by MPS Limited.
The editors were Kay Conerly and Jennifer Bernstein.
The production supervisor was Catherine Saggese.
Project management was provided by Poonam Bisht, MPS Limited.

This book is printed on acid-free paper.

McGraw Hill books are available at special quantity discounts to use as premiums and sales promotions, or for use in corporate training programs. To contact a representative, please visit the Contact Us pages at www.mhprofessional.com.

CONTENTS

CONTRIBUTORS

Alex An, MD
Resident Physician, Family Medicine Residency Program, Ventura County Medical Center
Ventura, California
[Chapter 9]

David Araujo, MD FAAFP
Core Faculty and DIO, Family Medicine Residency Program, Ventura County Medical Center
Adjunct Clinical Assistant Professor of Family Medicine, Keck School of Medicine
Ventura, California
[Chapters 6, 13]

Macarena Basañes, DO
Resident Physician, Family Medicine Residency Program, Ventura County Medical Center
Ventura, California
[Chapter 17]

Jacob David, MD FAAFP
Program Director, Family Medicine Residency Program, Ventura County Medical Center
Adjunct Clinical Assistant Professor of Family Medicine, Keck School of Medicine
Ventura, California
[Chapters 2, 3, 4, 14, 15, 17, 18]

Rachel David, MD
Resident Physician, Family Medicine Residency Program, Ventura County Medical Center
Ventura, California
[Chapter 1]

Dorothy DeGuzman, MD MPH FAAFP
Associate Program Director, Family Medicine Residency Program, Ventura County Medical Center
Adjunct Clinical Assistant Professor of Family Medicine, Keck School of Medicine
Ventura, California
[Chapters 11, 16]

Micah Gamble, MD
Resident Physician, Family Medicine Residency Program, Ventura County Medical Center
Ventura, California
[Chapter 8]

Danielle Guyer, MD
Resident Physician, Family Medicine Residency Program, Ventura County Medical Center
Ventura, California
[Chapter 3]

Tipu Khan, MD FAAFP FASAM
Fellowship Director, Primary Care Addiction Medicine Fellowship
Core Faculty, Family Medicine Residency Program, Ventura County Medical Center
Adjunct Clinical Professor of Family Medicine, Keck School of Medicine
Ventura, California
[Chapter 1]

Sina Khaksar, MD
Resident Physician, Family Medicine Residency Program, Ventura County Medical Center
Ventura, California
[Chapter 5]

Matthew Lamon, DO

Core Faculty, Family Medicine Residency Program, Ventura County Medical Center
Adjunct Clinical Assistant Professor of Family Medicine, Keck School of Medicine
Ventura, California
[Chapter 5]

Laura Murphy, DO

Associate Program Director, Family Medicine Residency Program, Ventura County Medical Center
Adjunct Clinical Assistant Professor of Family Medicine, Keck School of Medicine
Ventura, California
[Chapter 9]

John Nuhn, MD

Core Faculty, Family Medicine Residency Program, Ventura County Medical Center
Ventura, California
[Chapter 10]

Carlos O'Bryan-Becerra, MD FAAFP

Core Faculty, Family Medicine Residency Program, Ventura County Medical Center
Adjunct Clinical Assistant Professor of Family Medicine, Keck School of Medicine
Ventura, California
[Chapter 8]

Valentina Sedlacek, MD

Resident Physician, Family Medicine Residency Program, Ventura County Medical Center
Ventura, California
[Chapters 11, 16]

Zachary Zwolak, DO FAAFP FASAM

Associate Program Director, Family Medicine Residency Program, Ventura County Medical Center
Core Faculty, Primary Care Addiction Medicine Fellowship, Ventura County Medical Center
Adjunct Clinical Assistant Professor of Family Medicine, Keck School of Medicine
Ventura, California
[Chapters 7, 12]

PREFACE

CURRENT Practice Guidelines in Primary Care 2025–2026 is written for all clinicians seeking easy access to updated evidence-based guidelines for primary care topics in ambulatory and hospital settings. This handy reference consolidates guideline information from national medical associations and government agencies into concise recommendations covering virtually all primary care topics. This book is organized into topics related to screening and prevention and disease management and further subdivided into organ systems for quick reference to the evaluation and treatment of the most common primary care disorders.

The 2025–2026 edition of *CURRENT Practice Guidelines in Primary Care* contains updates and additions reflecting the review of more than 130 new guidelines. The edition contains new topics including bipolar disorder, stimulant use disorder, eating disorders, anxiety screening, esophageal varices, overactive bladder, thromboembolic disease in COVID-19, cancer-related cachexia, low back pain, chronic hand pain, liver disease in pregnancy, mood disorders in pregnancy, interstitial lung disease, obstructive sleep apnea, acne, atopic dermatitis, premenstrual disorders, and hearing loss.

In addition, there have been significant updates in several sections including chronic kidney disease, atrial fibrillation, diabetes, hypothyroidism, acute pancreatitis, Barrett esophagus, cirrhosis, colorectal cancer screening, alcoholic hepatitis, hepatitis C, COVID-19, diabetic foot infections, hip osteoarthritis, headaches, delirium, chronic pain, vaccines, hepatitis in pregnancy, preeclampsia, labor and delivery, substance use in pregnancy, COPD, skin cancer, dementia, and osteoporosis. Finally, there are updated cancer screening recommendations for breast cancer, colorectal cancer, prostate cancer, testicular cancer, ovarian cancer, and lung cancer.

Residents, medical students, mid-level providers, and practicing physicians in family medicine, internal medicine, pediatrics, and obstetrics and gynecology alike will find it a great resource.

Some guidelines include race as a consideration in clinical decision-making. As efforts to explain racial differences in outcomes can be grounded in biased data, recommendations to vary care by race should be considered with caution. A thoughtful assessment is available at *N Engl J Med.* 2020;383:847–882 (https://www.nejm.org/doi/full/10.1056/NEJMms2004740). Additionally, in this text, 'male' and 'female' refer to biological sex rather than gender identity, as most guidelines do not address the distinction.

Although painstaking efforts have been made to find all errors and omissions, some may remain. If you find an error or wish to suggest a change, please contact McGraw Hill: www.mhprofessional.com/contact-us.

Evidence-based guidelines such as those reviewed in this book are wonderful tools. They enable management strategies to be standardized and disseminated to a broad swath of the medical profession. At their best, they offer immediate access to the wisdom and analytical approach to data-driven medical care employed by the experts, elevating the quality of our care. But, as with any endeavor, they are susceptible to bias and misinterpretation. While evidence-based guidelines increasingly dictate the standards for our clinical practice, the highest quality medical care will always derive from a clinician's experience, curiosity, critical thinking, compassion, and personal relationship with a patient. In that spirit, please use the tools in this book to further hone your craft.

This book is dedicated to all our current and former residents at the Ventura County Medical Center.

Jacob A. David, MD, FAAFP

BEHAVIORAL HEALTH AND SUBSTANCE USE DISORDERS

ACUTE PSYCHOSIS

Management: Children, Adolescents, and Adults

Recommendations from

> ACEP 2017, AAFP 2015, AAP 2022

–Do not obtain routine laboratory testing.[1] Medical history, examination, and previous psychiatric diagnoses should guide testing.

–Do not routinely order neuroimaging studies in the absence of focal neurologic deficits.

–Refer to specialty management as indicated.

–Refer to emergency care if the patient appears manic or expresses suicidal/homicidal ideation or intent.

Practice Pearl

- Use the Pediatric Symptoms Checklist-17 or the Strengths and Difficulties questionnaire as a preliminary screening for any behavioral disorder or mental health disorder.

Sources

–*Ann Emerg Med.* 2017;69(4):480–498.

–*Am Fam Physician.* 2015;91(12):856–863.

–AAP. *Quick Reference Guide to Pediatric Care*, 2nd ed. 2022. ISBN 978-1-61002-111-1

–AAP. *Screening Tools: Mental Health MiniSeries.* https://www.aap.org/en/patient-care/mental-health-minute/screening-tools/

ALCOHOL USE DISORDERS

Screening: Adolescents

Recommendations from

> USPSTF 2018, AAP 2019

–Consider screening children and adolescents.

---

[1] Follow your local institutional policy, as some institutions may require laboratory testing.

Guidelines Alert 1–1 GUIDELINES DISCORDANT: SCREENING CHILDREN AND ADOLESCENTS FOR ALCOHOL USE DISORDERS	
USPSTF	Routine screening not recommended
AAP	Screen with HEADSS, CRAFFT, or other similar tool

Sources
  –AAP. *Pediatrics*. 2019;144(1):2018.
  –USPSTF. *JAMA*. 2018;320(18):1899–1909.

Screening: Adults

Recommendations from

> CDC 2024, USPSTF 2018

  –Screen all adults in primary care settings for alcohol misuse, including pregnant persons.
  –If positive, administer a brief behavioral counseling intervention and offer or refer for diagnostic assessment.

Practice Pearls

- Screen regularly using a validated tool such as the AUDIT, CAGE, or MAST questionnaires.
- The TWEAK, T-ACE, and 4P's Plus are designed to screen pregnant persons for alcohol misuse.

Sources
  –CDC. *Alcohol Screening and Brief Intervention*. 2024.
  –USPSTF. *JAMA*. 2018;320(18):1899–1909.
  –ASAM. *Public Policy Statement on Screening for Addiction in Primary Care Settings*. 1997.

Management: Adults

Recommendations from

> USPSTF 2018, APA 2018, WHO 2023

  –For adults identified with an alcohol use disorder, provide a brief intervention and schedule follow-up via SBIRT (Screening, Brief Intervention, and Referral to Treatment) model.
  –Assess all patients with frequent or heavy alcohol use regularly for risk of developing withdrawals. Treat alcohol withdrawal with benzodiazepines, gabapentin, or phenobarbital.
  –Refer all patients with life-threatening withdrawal such as seizure or delirium tremens to a hospital for admission.
  –Refer patients who are stable to outpatient behavioral therapy such as the IOP (intensive outpatient program), an RTC (residential treatment center), or a sober living facility.
  –Recommend naltrexone or acamprosate as first-line therapy for moderate-to-severe use disorder; consider disulfiram, topiramate, or gabapentin as second-line therapies (APA).
  –Recommend prophylactic thiamine for all harmful alcohol use or alcohol dependence.

–Refer suitable patients with decompensated cirrhosis for consideration of liver transplantation.

–Recommend pancreatic enzyme supplementation for chronic alcoholic pancreatitis with steatorrhea and malnutrition.

Practice Pearls

- Assess all patients for a coexisting psychiatric disorder (dual diagnosis).
- Use disorder-focused psychosocial intervention for patients with alcohol dependence.
- Consider adjunctive pharmacotherapy under close supervision for alcohol dependence.

Sources

–USPSTF. *JAMA*. 2018;320(18):1899–1909.

–ASAM. Clinical practice guideline on alcohol withdrawal management. *J Addict Med.* 2020;14(5):376–392.

–APA. *Am J Psychiatr.* 2018;175(1):86–90.

ALCOHOL WITHDRAWAL

Management: Adults

Recommendations from

➤ ASAM 2020

–Diagnose alcohol use disorder when a person exhibits at least two of the following: difficulty controlling use, spending excessive time obtaining alcohol, cravings, persistent use despite consequences, neglecting responsibilities, giving up activities, using alcohol in dangerous situations, developing tolerance, or experiencing withdrawal symptoms.

–Assess risk for complicated withdrawal using Prediction of Alcohol Withdrawal Severity Scale (PAWWS) or Luebeck Alcohol-Withdrawal Risk Scale (LARS). If elevated risk, arrange for inpatient level of care or a specialized ambulatory facility with extended on-site monitoring.

–Assess for medical comorbidities (complete metabolic panel [CMP], viral hepatitis panel, complete blood count [CBC]), pregnancy, mental disorders, and polysubstance use.

–Offer inpatient treatment for all pregnant patients.

–Arrange for daily check-in with nurse or medical assistant for up to 5 d following cessation or reduction of use.

–Monitor withdrawal severity with a validated instrument. Increase monitoring or transfer to inpatient care for the following: multiple doses of medication do not resolve agitation/tremor, severe signs/symptoms (hallucinations, syncope, or seizure), comorbid conditions worsen, oversedation, return to alcohol use, or unstable vital signs.

–Advise a daily multivitamin and noncaffeinated fluids. Consider oral thiamine 100 mg PO daily for 3–5 d.

–Use benzodiazepines as first-line therapy.

–Use phenobarbital or gabapentin as alternatives or adjuncts to benzodiazepines.

–For patients at high risk for developing severe withdrawals, provide front-loaded preventive therapy preferably with long-acting benzodiazepines such as diazepam or chlordiazepoxide.

–Treat mild withdrawal (Clinical Institute Withdrawal Assessment [CIWA] score < 10) with either supportive care or medication.

–Treat moderate withdrawal (CIWA score 10–18) with benzodiazepines.

–Transfer patients with CIWA scores > 19 to emergency department.

–Consider use of a benzodiazepine-sparing protocol utilizing alpha-agonist agents such as clonidine and other agents such as gabapentin and anti-epileptics to reduce total benzodiazepine usage.

–Offer a symptom-triggered approach using Clinical Institute Withdrawal Assessment of Alcohol Scale, Revised (CIWA-Ar) if patient or caregiver can reliably monitor symptoms and follow guidance. Otherwise offer a front-load dosing under supervision or employ a fixed-dose schedule.

Practice Pearls

- Risk factors associated with complicated withdrawal: alcohol withdrawal delirium, alcohol withdrawal seizure, prior withdrawal episodes, comorbidities (particularly traumatic brain injury), age > 65 y, long duration of heavy and regular alcohol consumption, marked autonomic hyperactivity on presentation, benzodiazepines or barbiturates dependence. There is no universal agreement on which factors associated with increased patient risk are most predictive.
- Sample symptom-triggered schedule with chlordiazepoxide:
  - If front-loading, give 50–100 mg PO q1–2h until CIWA-Ar < 10.
  - 25–100 mg PO q4–6h when CIWA-Ar ≥ 10.
  - Consider additional doses as needed.
- Sample fixed-dose schedule with chlordiazepoxide:
  - If front-loading, give 50–100 mg PO q1–2h for 3 doses then begin schedule.
  - Day 1: 25–100 mg PO q4–6h.
  - Day 2: 25–100 mg PO q6–8h.
  - Day 3: 25–100 mg PO q8–12h.
  - Day 4: 25–100 mg PO qHS.
  - Day 5: optional 25–100 mg PO qHS.
- Do not treat alcohol withdrawal with alcohol, baclofen, or magnesium.

Sources

–ASAM. Clinical practice guideline on alcohol withdrawal management. *J Addict Med.* 2020;14(5):376–392.

–*Outcomes After Implementation of a Benzodiazepine-Sparing Alcohol Withdrawal Order Set in an Integrated Health Care System* (nih.gov). https://doi.org/10.1016/j.ccc.2017.03.012

ANXIETY

Screening: Children and Adolescents

Recommendations from

> USPSTF 2022

–Screen all children and adolescents aged 8–18 for anxiety disorders.
–If positive, confirm diagnosis, offer effective treatment, and ensure appropriate follow-up.

Practice Pearls

- To screen for anxiety, administer Screen for Child Anxiety Related Disorders (SCARED) or a similar instrument.
- Optimal screening interval is unknown.

Source
–USPSTF. *JAMA.* 2022;328(14):1438–1444.

Screening: Adults

Recommendations from

> USPSTF 2023

–Screen all adults for anxiety disorders, including pregnant and postpartum persons.
–If positive, confirm diagnosis, offer effective treatment, and ensure appropriate follow-up.

Practice Pearls

- To screen for anxiety, administer Generalized Anxiety Disorder (GAD) Scale or a similar instrument.
- Optimal screening interval is unknown.
- There is insufficient evidence for screening in adults ages 65+.

Source
–USPSTF. *JAMA.* 2023;329(23):2057–2067.

Management: Children and Adolescents

Recommendations from

> AACAP 2020

–First-line therapies include cognitive behavioral therapy and antidepressants.

Source
–*JAACAP.* 2020;59(10):1107–1124.

Management: Adults

Recommendations from
> NICE 2020, AAFP 2022

  –Arrange cognitive behavioral therapy for GAD.
  –Offer a selective serotonin reuptake inhibitor (SSRI) or selective noradrenergic reuptake
   inhibitor (SNRI) if wanting medication management.
  –Avoid long-term benzodiazepine use or antipsychotic therapy for GAD.

Practice Pearls

- Escitalopram, duloxetine, and venlafaxine may be better first-line choices. Consider patient-specific factors such as cost and side-effect profile when choosing an appropriate medication. (*Lancet.* 2019;393(10173):768–777)
- Antipsychotics are not highly effective and have poor side-effect profiles.
- Benzodiazepines are not recommended for the treatment of anxiety; though effective for symptom control, use can lead to withdrawal, rebound anxiety, and dependence.
- Augmenting antidepressants with benzodiazepines, antipsychotics, or buspirone does not seem to improve outcomes in resistant anxiety.
- Psychotherapy works as well as medication; combination may be more effective.

Sources
  –NICE. *Generalised Anxiety Disorder and Panic Disorder in Adults: Management* (CG113). 2020.
  –AAFP. *Am Fam Physician.* 2022;106(2):157–164.

ATTENTION-DEFICIT HYPERACTIVITY DISORDER (ADHD)

Screening: Children

Recommendations from
> AAP 2019

  –Screen children and adolescents ages 4–18 with behavioral concerns or those struggling
   academically who show hyperactivity, inattention, or impulsivity.
  –Assess for coexisting conditions: emotional, behavioral, developmental, or physical. Rule out
   other conditions which may present similarly.
  –Ensure patients undergo full psychiatric assessments to appropriately diagnose ADHD prior to
   treatment.

Source
  –*AAP Clinical Practice Guideline for the Diagnosis, Evaluation, and Treatment of Attention-Deficit/
   Hyperactivity Disorder in Children and Adolescents.* 2019.

Management: Children and Adolescents

Recommendations from

⧽ **AAP 2019, NICE 2019**

–Stress the value of a balanced diet, good nutrition, and regular exercise.

–For children <6-y-old, parent- or teacher-administered behavior therapy is first line.

–Obtain a second opinion or refer to a tertiary service if ADHD symptoms are not controlled on one or more stimulants and one nonstimulant.

Guidelines Alert 1–2 **ROLE OF DRUG THERAPY FOR ADHD IN CHILDREN**	
AAP	–For children aged 6–18 y, use FDA-approved medications for ADHD along with parent training in behavior management and/or behavioral classroom interventions –Methylphenidate is reserved for severe refractory cases
NICE	–Start interventions with education and support groups for parents and caregivers/educators, and with environmental adjustments to limit the impact of ADHD –Consider drug therapy for those over 5 y of age with severe symptoms and impairment, for those with moderate levels of impairment who have refused nondrug interventions, or for those with persistent impairment after environmental adjustments have been implemented –Where drug treatment is considered appropriate, methylphenidate, atomoxetine, and dexamfetamine are recommended, within their licensed indications, as options for the management of ADHD in children and adolescents

Applying to Clinical Practice
- Stimulant medications reduce impairment from ADHD.
- Environmental modifications and educational interventions can help significantly and can be overlooked when medications are used as the first intervention.
- In the United States, resources for psychosocial therapy may not be as universally available as in the United Kingdom, enhancing the value of medications.

Practice Pearls

- Note that ADHD is thought to be underdiagnosed in female patients at all ages.
- Counsel patients on additional beneficial modifications: reducing distractions, movement breaks, frequent feedback, including written instructions, and long-term focused accommodations.
- For children aged 6–18 y, evidence supports stimulant medications, followed by atomoxetine, ER guanfacine, and ER clonidine for ADHD.

Sources

−AAP. Clinical Practice Guideline for the Diagnosis, Evaluation, and Treatment of Attention-Deficit/ Hyperactivity Disorder in Children and Adolescents. 2019.

−NICE. Attention Deficit Hyperactivity Disorder: Diagnosis and Management (NG87). 2019.

Management: Adults

Recommendations from

> NICE 2018, AAFP 2019

−Treat with stimulant or nonstimulant medication therapy.

- Stimulant therapy includes methylphenidate and amphetamine.
- Atomoxctine is currently the only FDA-approved nonstimulant medication.

−Consider monthly follow-ups until symptom and functional improvement.

−Obtain a second opinion or refer to a tertiary service if ADHD symptoms are not controlled on one or more stimulants and one nonstimulant.

−Do not offer atypical antipsychotics for ADHD without advice from a tertiary ADHD service.

−Ensure adherence using prescription state monitoring programs and urine toxicology testing.

Practice Pearl

- No strong evidence exists guiding the duration of treatment or efficacy of drug "holidays."

Sources

−NICE. Attention Deficit Hyperactivity Disorder: Diagnosis and Management (NG87). 2019.

−AAFP. Treatment and Management of ADHD in Adults. https://www.aafp.org/family-physician/ patient-care/prevention-wellness/emotional-wellbeing/adhd-toolkit/treatment-and-management.html

AUTISM SPECTRUM DISORDERS

Screening: Children and Adolescents

Recommendations from

> AAP, USPFTS 2016

−Screen all children at ages 9, 18, and 30 mo with standardized tools such as the ASQ or M-CHAT.

- If identified as high risk, also screen at 24 mo.
- Consider autism if regression in language or social skills in children <3 y.

−Consider clinical signs of possible autism in the context of a child's overall development and account for cultural variations.

−Refer to a specialist for an autism evaluation if any of the following signs of possible autism:

- Language delay.
- Regression in speech.
- Echolalia.

- Unusual vocalizations or intonations.
- Reduced social smiling.
- Rejection of cuddles by family.
- Reduced response to name being called.
- Intolerance of others entering into their personal space.
- Reduced social interest in people or social play.
- Reduced eye contact.
- Reduced imagination.
- Repetitive movements like body rocking.
- Desire for unchanged routines.
- Immature social and emotional development.

–If positive, confirm diagnosis and refer for diagnostic evaluation.

Sources

–USPSTF. *Autism Spectrum Disorder in Young Children: Screening.* 2016.

–NICE. *Autism Spectrum Disorder in Under 19s: Recognition, Referral and Diagnosis* (CG128). 2017.

–AAP. *Pediatrics.* 2020;145(1):e20193447.

Management: Children

Recommendations from

> NICE 2017, AAP 2020

–Pursue interventions that will minimize core deficits, maximize functional independence, and reduce problem behaviors.

–Two categories of intervention are supported by evidence:

- Comprehensive treatment model (CTM): addresses a broad array of symptoms from a central conceptual framework. May include applied behavior analysis (ABA), developmental approaches, and/or naturalistic approaches. Examples include early intensive behavioral intervention, Treatment and Education of Autistic and Related Communication-Handicapped Children (TEACCH), and the Early Start Denver Model (ESDM).
- Focused interventions: designed to address single or limited range of skills (eg, increase social communication, learn a specific task).

–Screen for and medical manage co-occurring medication conditions, such as seizures or feeding disorders.

–No medications correct the core social or communication symptoms of autism spectrum disorder, but certain psychotropic medications may help with common symptoms in conjunction with fully implemented behavioral approaches.

- Hyperactivity, impulsivity, and inattention: start with a low-dose stimulant (eg, methylphenidate) and increase as needed/tolerated. Consider atomoxetine or alpha-2-agonists if stimulant is not tolerated or effective.
- Irritability, severe disruptive behavior: consider risperidone or aripiprazole, with monitoring for weight gain, dyslipidemia, and extrapyramidal symptoms.

- Repetitive behavior: consider aripiprazole or risperidone as short-term treatment.
- Anxiety: consider citalopram or buspirone for anxiety, though hyperactivation may occur as a side effect.

Source

–AAP. *Pediatrics.* 2020;145(1):e20193447.

BIPOLAR DISORDER

Screening: Adults

Recommendations from

> NICE 2024, VA/DoD 2023

–Evaluate all patients with depression for episodes of disinhibition.
–Do not routinely screen the general population.

Sources

–NICE. *Bipolar Disorder: Assessment and Management.* 2024.
–VA/DoD Clinical Practice Guideline. *Management of Bipolar Disorder Work Group.* Washington, DC: U.S. Government Printing Office, 2023.

Management: Adults

Recommendations from

> NICE 2024, VA/DoD 2023

–Offer psychological interventions like cognitive behavior therapy (CBT) or behavioral couples therapy.
–Offer pharmacotherapy according to Table 1–1.
–Refer to specialty care if patient has a poor response to treatment, functional decline, or intolerance to medications.

Sources

–NICE. *Bipolar Disorder: Assessment and Management.* 2024.
–VA/DoD Clinical Practice Guideline. *Management of Bipolar Disorder Work Group.* Washington, DC: U.S. Government Printing Office, 2023.

DEPRESSION

Screening: Children and Adolescents

Recommendations from

> USPSTF 2022

–Screen all adolescents aged 12–18.
–If positive, confirm diagnosis, offer effective treatment, and ensure appropriate follow-up.
–There is insufficient evidence to screen children younger than 11.

TABLE 1–1 PHARMACOTHERAPY FOR BIPOLAR DISORDER		
Condition	**VA/DoD Guidelines**	**NICE Guidelines**
Acute manic episodes	**First-line:** lithium or quetiapine **Second-line:** olanzapine, paliperidone, or risperidone **Third-line:** aripiprazole, asenapine, carbamazepine, cariprazine, haloperidol, valproate, or ziprasidone **Do not use:** brexpiprazole, topiramate, or lamotrigine monotherapy. Adjunctive aripiprazole, paliperidone, or ziprasidone	**First-line:** haloperidol, olanzapine, quetiapine, or risperidone **Second-line:** combination therapy with lithium or valproate + first-line agent **Do not use:** lamotrigine
Acute manic episode despite maintenance therapy	Lithium or valproate + haloperidol, asenapine, quetiapine, olanzapine, or risperidone	Lithium or valproate + haloperidol, olanzapine, quetiapine, or risperidone
Bipolar depression episode	**First-line:** quetiapine monotherapy or lamotrigine + lithium or quetiapine **Second-line:** cariprazine, lumateperone, lurasidone, olanzapine	**First-line:** quetiapine or fluoxetine + olanzapine **Second-line:** lamotrigine
Maintenance, prevention of recurrent episodes	***Prevention of mania*** **First-line:** lithium or quetiapine, or combination therapy with lithium or valproate + aripiprazole, olanzapine, quetiapine, or ziprasidone **Second-line:** olanzapine, paliperidone, or long-acting injectable risperidone **Do not use:** lamotrigine monotherapy ***Prevention of depressive episodes*** **First-line:** lamotrigine, lithium, or quetiapine monotherapy **Combination therapy:** lithium or valproate + olanzapine, lurasidone, or quetiapine **Second-line:** olanzapine	**First-line:** lithium **Second-line:** asenapine, aripiprazole, olanzapine, quetiapine, or risperidone **Third-line:** combination of valproate with antipsychotic or lithium

Source
  –*JAMA*. 2022;328(15):1534–1542.

Screening: Adults

Recommendations from

> USPSTF 2023

  –Screen all adults for depression, including pregnant and postpartum persons.
  –If positive, confirm diagnosis, offer effective treatment, and ensure appropriate follow-up.

Practice Pearls

- To diagnose depression, follow a positive PHQ-2 with a PHQ-9 or a similar instrument.
- Optimal screening interval is unknown. AAP recommends screening mothers for postpartum depression at the infant's 1-, 2-, 4-, and 6-mo visits.

Source
–USPSTF. *JAMA.* 2023;329(23):2057–2067.

Management: Children and Adolescents

Recommendations from

➢ USPSTF 2016, NICE 2019

–Use SSRIs, psychotherapy, or combined therapy to decrease symptoms of major depressive disorder in adolescents aged 12–18 y. (USPSTF)

–There is insufficient evidence to support screening and treatment of depression in children aged 7–11 y. (USPSTF)

–Use behavioral support and treatment (NICE):
- 5–11 y: consider CBT.
- 12–18 y: CBT.

Practice Pearls

- Good evidence showed that SSRIs may increase the absolute risk of suicidality in adolescents by 1%–2%. Therefore, only use SSRIs if close clinical monitoring is possible.
- Fluoxetine is approved by the FDA for treatment of MDD in children aged 8 y or older, and escitalopram is approved for treatment of MDD in adolescents aged 12–17 y.

Sources
–USPSTF. *Depression in Children and Adolescents: Screening.* 2016.

–NICE. *Depression in Children and Young People: Identification and Management.* 2019.

Management: Adults

Recommendations from

➢ ACP 2023, NICE 2022, VA/DoD 2022

–First-line therapies include cognitive behavioral therapy and second-generation antidepressants.

–If unresponsive to initial therapy, consider switching to a second-generation antidepressant or augmenting with psychotherapy or a second medication.

–Assess response to treatment using PHQ-9 or Hamilton Depression Rating Scale.

–Continue treatment for at least 4–9 mo after remission of symptoms.

–Do not routinely offer antidepressants as first-line treatment for mild depression, unless other factors indicate need.

Guidelines Alert 1–3	
GUIDELINES DISCORDANT: INITIAL THERAPY FOR MODERATE-TO-SEVERE MAJOR DEPRESSIVE DISORDER	
ACP	Offer CBT *or* a second-generation depressant (ie, SSRI, SNRI, bupropion)
NICE, VA/ DOD	Offer CBT *and* an antidepressant

Applying to Clinical Practice
- ACP offers the option of combination therapy with CBT and antidepressants as initial therapy, but with low-certainty evidence.
- Combination therapy has not been established to be superior to CBT or antidepressants alone.
- Patient commitment to therapy modality is a major determinant of outcomes—elect an initial therapy approach that considers available resources and patient's preferences.

Practice Pearl

- No single antidepressant choice is clearly more effective than others. Of the SSRIs/SNRIs, escitalopram, paroxetine, and sertraline may have slightly better balance of efficacy and adverse effects. (*Lancet*. 2018;391(10128):1357–1366)

Sources
–ACP. *Nonpharmacologic and Pharmacologic Treatments of Adults in the Acute Phase of MDD: A Living Clinical Guideline from the ACP.* 2023.
–NICE. *Depression in Adults: Treatment and Management.* 2023.
–VA/DoD. *Clinical Practice Guideline for the Management of MDD.* 2022.

EATING DISORDERS

Screening: Children and Adolescents

Recommendations from

➤ APA 2023, AAP 2021
–Screen patients with risk factors with a detailed history and screening tool such as the HEADSS.
–Risk factors include evaluating patient's height and weight trends and eating pattern.

Sources
–APA. *Practice Guidelines for the Treatment of Patients with Eating Disorders,* 4th ed. 2023.
–NICE. *Eating Disorders: Recognition and Treatment* (NG69). 2017.
–*Pediatrics.* 2021;147(1):e2020040279.

Screening: Adults

Recommendations from

> APA 2023, AAP 2020

–Screen patients with risk factors with screening tools such as the SCOFF Questionnaire or Screen for Disordered Eating.

–Risk factors include evaluating patient's height and weight trends and eating pattern.

Sources

–APA. *Practice Guidelines for the Treatment of Patients with Eating Disorders*, 4th ed. 2023.

–NICE. *Eating Disorders: Recognition and Treatment* (NG69). 2017.

Management: All Patients

Recommendations from

> APA 2023, NICE 2017, AAP 2021

–Establish a therapeutic alliance.

–Use a multidisciplinary approach including dietitian, social worker, and physician.

–Complete in-depth initial evaluation including history and physical exam.

–Assess attitude of eating, exercising, and appearance.

–Screen for concurrent psychiatric disorders and co-occurring health conditions.

–Recommend CBT.

–Provide acute medical care (including emergency admission) for people with an eating disorder who have severe electrolyte imbalance, severe malnutrition, severe dehydration, or signs of incipient organ failure.

–Recommend nutritional rehab for seriously underweight patients to observe for refeeding syndrome.

–Recommend nasogastric tube feeding over parenteral nutrition for patients not meeting caloric requirements with oral feeds alone.

–Recommend psychosocial rehab for patients with both anorexia nervosa and bulimia nervosa.

–In adolescents and adults, consider fluoxetine, which is a preferred agent, to prevent relapse during the maintenance phase of bulimia nervosa.

–Consider the following labs:

  • CBC.

  • Chemistry panel.

  • TSH.

–Consider the following additional testing:

  • Bone mineral densitometry if amenorrhea for more than 6 mo.

  • Dental evaluation for history of purging.

Sources

–APA. *Practice Guidelines for the Treatment of Patients with Eating Disorders*, 4th ed. 2023.

–NICE. *Eating Disorders: Recognition and Treatment* (NG69). 2017.

ILLICIT DRUG USE

Screening: Adolescents and Adults

Recommendations from

 USPSTF 2020, AAP 2020

–Screen patients aged ≥ 18 y by asking questions.
–There is insufficient evidence regarding screening adolescents.

Guidelines Alert 1–4	
GUIDELINES DISCORDANT: CHILD AND ADOLESCENT ILLICIT SUBSTANCE USE SCREENING	
AAP	Screen all adolescents
USPFTS	Insufficient evidence for screening children and adolescents for illicit substance use

Applying to Clinical Practice
• Consider screening children and adolescents based on patient-specific risk factors.

Practice Pearls

• The NIH hosts a collection of screening tools at https://nida.nih.gov/nidamed-medical-health-professionals/screening-tools-resources/chart-screening-tools.
• The recommendation is to ask questions about unhealthy drug use, *not* to screen with lab testing.

Source
–USPSTF. *JAMA*. 2020;323(22):2301–2309.

Prevention: Children and Adolescents

Recommendations from

USPSTF 2020

–Current evidence is insufficient to assess the balance of benefits and harms of primary care-based behavioral counseling interventions to prevent illicit drug use, including nonmedical use of prescription drugs in children, adolescents, and young adults.

Source
–USPSTF. *Primary Care-Based Interventions to Prevent Illicit Drug Use in Children, Adolescents, and Young Adults*. 2020.

OPIOID USE DISORDER

Management: Adolescents and Adults

Recommendations from

> ### ASAM 2020, US Dept Health and Human Services 2004, AAP 2016

–Per AAP, consider the below recommendations for adolescent populations.

–Obtain medical history to assess for concomitant medical conditions including infectious diseases (tuberculosis, HIV, viral hepatitis), acute trauma, and pregnancy. Assess mental health status, possible psychiatric disorders, past and current substance use, and social and environmental factors.

–Include CBC, liver function tests, hepatitis C, HIV, and urine drug testing in initial lab evaluation. Consider testing for sexually transmitted infections and tuberculosis. Offer hepatitis B vaccination if appropriate.

–Consider the use of clinical scales that measure withdrawal symptoms, like the Clinical Opioid Withdrawal Scale (COWS).

–Choose medications to manage opioid withdrawal, including methadone, buprenorphine, and naltrexone, rather than abrupt cessation. Consider non-narcotic medications like clonidine, benzodiazepines, loperamide, acetaminophen or NSAIDs, and ondansetron to target specific opioid withdrawal symptoms.

–Provide psychosocial treatment for patients on opioid agonist treatment.

–Consider patients to be candidates for buprenorphine therapy if they want treatment, have no contraindications, can be expected to be compliant, provide informed consent, and are willing to follow safety precautions.

–Consider alternatives to office-based buprenorphine if patients use high doses of benzodiazepines, alcohol, or other CNS depressants; have significant untreated psychiatric disease; have frequently relapsed despite maintenance therapy previously; have previously had poor response to buprenorphine; have significant medical illness.

–Use buprenorphine/naloxone combination for maintenance in most patients rather than buprenorphine monotherapy.

–For buprenorphine induction, consider office-based, home, or microdosing induction protocols.

–If transitioning from methadone to buprenorphine, taper methadone to 30–40 mg or less per day at least 1 wk prior to induction and wait at least 24 h after last dose of methadone before beginning the induction process.

–Monitor for diversion by testing for buprenorphine and metabolites, counting pills, accessing the Prescription Drug Monitoring Program, and arranging frequent visits (weekly at onset of therapy).

–Provide harm reduction tools such as clean needles, naloxone for reversal of opiate overdose, and HIV pre-exposure prophylaxis.

Sources
- –The ASAM National Practice Guideline for the Treatment of Opioid Use Disorder. https://www. asam.org/Quality-Science/quality/2020-national-practice-guideline
- –McNicholas L. *Clinical Guidelines for the Use of Buprenorphine in the Treatment of Opioid Addiction*. Rockville, MD: U.S. Department of Health and Human Services, 2004. https://www. samhsa.gov/medication-assisted-treatment/training-materials-resources/buprenorphine-waiver
- –AAP. *Pediatrics*. 2016;138(3):e20161893.

POSTTRAUMATIC STRESS DISORDER (PTSD)

Screening: Children and Adolescents

Recommendations from

➢ AACAP 2010, AAP 2023

- –Establish a therapeutic patient–physician relationship through building trusting relationships.
- –Consider screening for PTSD in any child or adolescent when screening for additional mental health disorders. Validated tools include the Juvenile Victimization Questionnaire (ages 2–17) or the UCLA Posttraumatic Disorder Reaction Index (ages 7+).
- –Consider referral to specialist for detailed psychiatric evaluation.

Source
- –*JAACAP*. 2010;49(4):414–430.

Management: Children and Adolescents

Recommendations from

➢ AACAP 2010

- –First-line treatment is trauma-focused psychotherapy, such as CBT.
- –Consider SSRIs or anti-adrenergic agents.
- –Assess for concurrent disorders.

Source
- –*JAACAP*. 2010;49(4):414–430.

Screening: Adults

Recommendations from

➢ VA/DoD 2023, NICE 2018
- –Consider use of the Primary Care PTSD Screen from *DSM-5*.

Sources
- –VA/DoD. *Clinical Practice Guidelines for the Management of PTSD*. 2023.
- –nice.org.uk/guidance/ng116

Prevention: Adults

Recommendations from

➤ VA/DoD 2023

  –Recommend trauma-focused CBT for those diagnosed with acute stress disorder. Consider pharmacotherapy.

Source
  –VA/DoD. *Clinical Practice Guidelines for the Management of PTSD*. 2023.

Management: Adults

Recommendations from

➤ VA/DoD 2023, NICE 2018

  –Assess for acute risk of harm to self or others, functional status, medical history, treatment history, and relevant family history.
  –Establish a risk management and safety plan as part of initial treatment planning if there is a risk of harm to self or others.
  –Consider focused debriefing for the prevention or treatment of PTSD.
  –Treat PTSD initially with individual, manualized trauma-focused psychotherapy.
  –Implement pharmacotherapy or other psychotherapy as second-line therapies. Recommended medications include paroxetine, fluoxetine, or venlafaxine.
  –Do not prescribe benzodiazepines or cannabis for treatment of PTSD.

Sources
  –VA/DoD. *Clinical Practice Guidelines for the Management of PTSD*. 2023.
  –nice.org.uk/guidance/ng116

TOBACCO USE DISORDER

Screening: Adults

Recommendations from

➤ AAFP 2015, USPSTF 2021, NICE 2021

  –Screen all adults for tobacco use, including pregnant persons.

Sources
  –NICE. *Tobacco: Preventing Uptake, Promoting Quitting and Treating Dependence (NG209)*. 2021.
  –USPSTF. *JAMA*. 2021;325(3):265–279.

Practice Pearl

- The "5-A" framework is helpful for smoking cessation counseling:
  - Ask about tobacco use.
  - Advise to quit through clear, individualized messages.

- Assess willingness to quit.
- Assist in quitting.
- Arrange follow-up and support sessions.
• There is insufficient evidence to assess the balance of benefits and harms of pharmacotherapy in pregnant individuals.

Prevention: Children and Adolescents

Recommendations from

➤ USPSTF 2020, AAP 2023

  –Provide interventions, including education or brief counseling, to prevent initiation of tobacco use among school-aged children and adolescents.

Practice Pearl

• The efficacy of counseling to prevent tobacco use in children and adolescents is of moderate net benefit.

Sources

  –USPSTF. *Primary Care Interventions for Prevention and Cessation of Tobacco Use in Children and Adolescents.* 2020.
  –AAP. *Pediatrics.* 2023;151(5):e2023061805.

Management: Adults

Recommendations from

➤ NICE 2021, USPSTF 2021, ACOG 2020

  –Offer nicotine replacement therapy, bupropion, and/or varenicline:
    • Bupropion SR 150 mg daily × 3 d then 150 mg BID. Initiate 1–2 wk prior to quit. Continue for 7–12 wk up to 6 mo.
    • Varenicline 0.5 mg qd for 3 d, then 0.5 mg BID for 4 d, then 1.0 mg PO BID. Continue for 12 or 24 wk.
  –Current evidence is insufficient to recommend electronic nicotine delivery systems for tobacco cessation in adults, including pregnant persons.
  –Current evidence is insufficient to assess the benefits and harms of pharmacotherapy interventions for tobacco cessation in pregnant persons.

Practice Pearls

• The combination of nicotine replacement with varenicline produces no higher cessation rates than either method alone. (*JAMA.* 2016;315(4):371–379. doi:10.1001/jama.2015.19284)
• Tables 1–2 and 1–3 outline steps in assessing patient's readiness to quit and motivation strategies to help them quit tobacco.

TABLE 1–2   TOBACCO CESSATION PLAN

Five As:
1. Ask about tobacco use.
2. Advise to quit through clear, personalized messages.
3. Assess willingness to quit.
4. Assist in quitting,[a] including referral to Quit Lines (eg, 1-800-NO-BUTTS).
5. Arrange follow-up and support.

[a]Physicians can assist patients to quit by devising a quit plan, providing problem-solving counseling, providing intratreatment social support, helping patients obtain social support from their environment/friends, and recommending pharmacotherapy for appropriate patients. Use caution in recommending pharmacotherapy in patients with medical contraindications, those smoking <10 cigarettes per day, pregnant/breast-feeding women, and adolescent smokers. As of March 2005, Medicare covers costs for smoking cessation counseling for those who (1) have a smoking-related illness; (2) have an illness complicated by smoking; or (3) take a medication that is made less effective by smoking (http://www.cms.hhs.gov).

Source: Fiore MC et al. *Treating Tobacco Use and Dependence: Quick Reference Guide for Clinicians*. Rockville, MD: U.S. Department of Health and Human Services. Public Health Service, 2008. http://www.ahrq.gov/legacy/clinic/tobacco/tobaqrg.pdf.

TABLE 1–3   MOTIVATING TOBACCO USERS TO QUIT

Five Rs:
1. Relevance: personal
2. Risks: acute, long term, environmental
3. Rewards: have patient identify (eg, save money, better food taste)
4. Road blocks: help problem-solve
5. Repetition: at every office visit

Sources

–USPSTF. *Tobacco Smoking Cessation in Adults, Including Pregnant Women: Behavioral and Pharmacotherapy Interventions*. 2021;325(3):265–279.

–NICE. *Tobacco: Preventing Uptake, Promoting Quitting and Treating Dependence*. 2021.

–ACOG. *Tobacco and Nicotine Cessation During Pregnancy*. Committee Opinion 807. 2020.

STIMULANT USE DISORDER

Management: Children and Adolescents

Recommendations from

⮞ ASAM/AAAP 2023

–Offer contingency management as the first-line treatment plan. CBT or the Matrix Model are second-line psychotherapies.

–Consider psychostimulant medication therapy only if trained to prescribe them.

–Order routine laboratory testing-based exam findings.

–Refer patients with acute intoxication with acute symptomology to appropriate higher levels of care.

Practice Pearls

- For children and adolescents:
  - Review state laws regarding whether a parent or guardian's consent is required prior to treatment.
  - Assess for concurrent ADHD or eating disorders.
- For pregnant people:
  - Obtain informed consent for drug testing, unless in an emergent situation or consent is unattainable, given possible ramifications.
  - Consider specific impacts of use on maternal and fetal health.

Source

–ASAM/AAAP. *Clinical Practice Guideline on the Management of Stimulant Use Disorder.* 2023.

TRAUMA-INFORMED CARE

Management: All

Recommendations from

➤ CDC 2020, ACOG 2021, SAMHSA 2023

–Recognize the prevalence and effect of trauma on patients and the health care team and incorporate trauma-informed approaches to delivery of care.

–Become familiar with the trauma-informed model of care and strive to universally implement a trauma-informed approach across all levels of practice with close attention to avoiding stigmatization and prioritizing resilience. See Table 1–4 for core concepts.

TABLE 1–4   CORE CONCEPTS IN TRAUMA-INFORMED CARE
The Four "Rs" (SAMHSA)
Realize the widespread effect of trauma and understand potential paths for recovery.
Recognize the signs and symptoms of trauma in clients, families, staff, and others involved with the system.
Respond by fully integrating knowledge about trauma into policies, procedures, and practices.
Seek to actively resist retraumatization.
Four Cs—Skills in Trauma-Informed Care
Calm: Pay attention to how you are feeling while caring for the patient. Breathe and calm yourself to help model and promote calmness for the patient and care for yourself.
Contain: Ask the level of detail of trauma history that will allow patient to maintain emotional and physical safety, respect the time frame of your interaction, and will allow you to offer patients further treatment.
Care: Remember to emphasize, for patient and yourself, good self-care and compassion.
Cope: Remember to emphasize, for patient and yourself, coping skills to build upon strength, resiliency, and hope.
Source: Reproduced with permission from Kimberg L, Wheeler M. Trauma and trauma-informed care. In Gerber MR, ed. *Trauma-Informed Healthcare Approaches: A Guide for Primary Care.* Cham, Switzerland: Springer, 2019.

–Build a trauma-informed workforce by training clinicians and staff on how to be trauma-informed.

–Create a safe, physical, and emotional environment for patients and staff.

–Implement universal screening for current trauma and a history of trauma.

Sources

–ACOG Committee Opinion No. 825. Caring for patients who have experienced trauma. *Obstet Gynecol.* 2021;137(4):e94–e99.

–SAMHSA. *Practical Guide for Implementing a Trauma-Informed Approach.* 2024.

CARDIOVASCULAR DISORDERS

ABDOMINAL AORTIC ANEURYSM

Screening: Adults

Recommendations from

➤ USPSTF 2019, Society for Vascular Surgery (SVS) 2018, Canadian Society for Vascular Surgery (CSVS) 2018, European Society for Vascular Surgery (ESVS) 2018, ACR/AIUM/SRU 2014, NICE 2020, ACC/AHA 2022, ESC 2014

–Screen once with ultrasound if of the recommended age and sex.

Guidelines Alert 2–1 GUIDELINES DISCORDANT: POPULATION TO SCREEN FOR ABDOMINAL AORTIC ANEURYSM		
Organization	**Men**	**Women**
ACC/AHA	Age ≥ 65 y who have ever smoked, or who are first-degree relatives of patients with AAA Age < 65 y who have multiple risk factors (smoking history, HTN, dyslipidemia, White race, inherited vascular connective tissue disorder, ASCVD) or a first-degree relative with AAA	Age ≥ 65 y who have ever smoked, or who are first-degree relatives of patients with AAA Age < 65 y who have multiple risk factors (smoking history, HTN, dyslipidemia, White race, inherited vascular connective tissue disorder, ASCVD) or a first-degree relative with AAA
USPSTF	Age 65–75 y if ever smoked Selectively offer screening if no smoking history	Do not screen if no smoking or family history of AAA Insufficient evidence to assess benefits/harms if smoker or positive family history
SVS	Age 65–75 y if ever smoked or first-degree relative with AAA Consider >75 y if in good health and not yet screened	Screen once age 65–75 y if ever smoked or first-degree relative with AAA Consider screening >75 y if in good health and not yet screened

CSVS	Age 65–80 y regardless of smoking history	Screen once age 65–80 y if ever smoked or has cardiovascular disease
ESVS	Age 65 y regardless of smoking history	Do not screen
ACRa, AIUM, SRU	Age ≥ 65 y regardless of history ≥50 y with family history of aortic and/or peripheral vascular aneurysmal disease or personal history of aneurysmal disease	Screen once age ≥ 65 y if positive cardiovascular risk factors Screen once age ≥ 50 y with personal or family history of aortic and/or peripheral vascular aneurysmal disease
NICE	Age > 65 y with COPD, CAD/CVD/PAD, family history of AAA, dyslipidemia, HTN, smoking (current or former)	Age ≥ 70 y with COPD, CAD/PAD/CVD, family history of AAA, dyslipidemia, HTN, smoking (current or former)
ESC	>65 y regardless of history	Consider >65 y only if smoking history

Applying to Clinical Practice
- Screen male smokers older than age 65.
- Consider screening nonsmoking men with strong family history.
- Women: The prevalence of AAA is 6 times lower in women than men,[a] lessening the potential benefit for population-based screening. Consider screening very high-risk women, since AAA may rupture somewhat more frequently in women than men.
- Older patients may have higher operative morbidity if asymptomatic AAA is found, which accounts for the upper limit of the screening ages.

[a]Scott RA, Bridgewater SG, Ashton HA. Randomized clinical trial of screening for abdominal aortic aneurysm in women. *Br J Surg.* 2002;89(3):283–285.

Practice Pearl

- In asymptomatic men or women >75 y who have had a negative initial ultrasound screen, do not repeat screening for detection of AAA.

Sources
–USPSTF. *JAMA.* 2019;322(22):2211–2218.

–*J Vasc Surg.* 2018;67(1):2–77.

–CSVS. *2018 Screening for Abdominal Aortic Aneurysms in Canada: Review and Position Statement from the Canadian Society of Vascular Surgery.* 2018.

–ESVS. 2019 clinical practice guidelines on the management of abdominal aorto-iliac artery aneurysms. *Eur J Vasc Endovasc Surg.* 2018;1–97.

–ACR-AIUM-SRU. *Practice Parameter for the Performance of Diagnostic and Screening Ultrasound Examinations of the Abdominal Aorta in Adults.* 2015.

–*NICE Guidelines 156.* Abdominal aortic aneurysm: diagnosis and management. 2020.

–*Circulation.* 2022;146(24):e334–e482.

–*Eur Heart J.* 2014;35:2873–2926.

Management: Adults

Recommendations from

➤ ACC/AHA 2022, NICE 2020, ESC 2014

–Offer surveillance without intervention if AAA diameter < 5.5 cm in men and < 5.0 in women.

–In patients with stable small AAA, monitor with imaging at the following frequencies:

- Every 3 y for AAA 3–3.9 cm diameter.
- Every year for AAA 4.0–4.9 cm diameter in men.
- Every year for AAA 4.0–4.4 cm diameter in women.
- Every 6 mo for AAA 4.5–5.0 cm diameter.

–In patients with bicuspid aortic valve (BAV), perform transthoracic echocardiogram (TTE) to evaluate aortic root, ascending aorta. Repeat imaging should be based on the above parameters.

–In patients with Marfan syndrome and Loeys-Diets syndrome, perform TTE at the time of diagnosis and 6 mo afterward to check for diameter stability. Perform TTE annually if stable.

–Target modifiable risk factors. No nonsurgical interventions reliably prevent AAA from growing.

- Smoking is a risk factor for rupture. Provide cessation counseling and medications to all patients with AAA, as cessation slows the growth. Duration of smoking is more significant than quantity smoked.
- HTN is a risk factor for AAA rupture. Use beta-blockers as first-line treatment if HTN is a comorbid condition.
- Treat other modifiable risk factors for expansion (coronary artery disease (CAD), peripheral arterial disease (PAD), dyslipidemia) as usual with guideline-directed medical therapy (GDMT).

–Nonmodifiable risk factors include size of aneurysm, age, female sex, cardiac/renal transplant.

–Consider statins and angiotensin-converting enzyme inhibitors (ACEi) to reduce complications.

–Consider beta-blockers to reduce the rate of growth. (ACC)

Guidelines Alert 2–2 GUIDELINES DISCORDANT: BLOOD PRESSURE GOALS IN AAA	
Organization	**Guidance**
ACC/AHA	<130/80
ESC	<140/90

Applying to Clinical Practice
- In the absence of data comparing BP goals, guidance largely relies on expert opinion and extrapolated data from studies for other conditions.
- The ACC believes that lower BP is likely to be better, and that BP of 120/80 may be a better goal for patients who can tolerate it.
- The ESC has determined 140/90 to be the threshold for "control" for HTN and don't see compelling evidence for a lower target in AAA.

Surgical Therapy

–Indication for repair:

- Symptomatic.
- Asymptomatic > 4.0 cm in diameter growing >1 cm/y.
- Asymptomatic and ≥5.5 cm in diameter.

–Indication for referral urgency:

- If symptomatic but nonruptured, urgently refer to vascular specialist.
- If asymptomatic > 5.5 cm, see vascular specialist within 2 wk.
- If asymptomatic 3.0–5.4 cm, see vascular specialist within 3 mo.

–Repair ruptured AAA emergently. Consider TXA to slow blood loss.

Practice Pearl

- Studies of beta-blockers and rate of expansion have produced contradictory data. 2013 ESC HTN guidelines suggest using them as first-line therapy for HTN and AAA, but data do not strongly support their use outside of HTN.

Risk Factors for Developing AAA

–Age > 60 y. AAA will develop in about 1 of 1000 persons between the ages of 60 and 65.

–Smoking. The risk is directly related to the number of years smoking and decreases in the years following smoking cessation.

–AAA develops in men 4–5 times more often than in women.

–Ethnicity. More common in the White population.

–History of CAD, PAD, HTN, and hypercholesterolemia.

–Family history of AAA. Accentuates the risks associated with age and sex. The risk of developing an aneurysm among brothers of a person with a known aneurysm who are >60 y of age is as high as 18%.

Risk Factors for AAA Expansion

–Age > 70 y, cardiac or renal transplant, previous stroke, severe cardiac disease, tobacco use.

Risk Factors for AAA Rupture

–Aneurysms expand at an average rate of 0.3–0.4 cm/y.

–The annual risk of rupture based upon aneurysm size is estimated as follows:

- <4.0 cm diameter = <0.5%.
- Between 4.0 and 4.9 cm diameter = 0.5%–5%.
- Between 5.0 and 5.9 cm diameter = 3%–15%.
- Between 6.0 and 6.9 cm diameter = 10%–20%.
- Between 7.0 and 7.9 cm diameter = 20%–40%.
- ≥8.0 cm diameter = 30%–50%.

–Aneurysms that expand rapidly (>0.5 cm over 6 mo) are at high risk for rupture.

–Growth tends to be more rapid in smokers and less rapid in patients with peripheral artery disease or diabetes mellitus (DM).

–The risk of rupture of large aneurysms ($\geq$5.0 cm) is significantly greater in women (18%) than in men (12%).

–Other risk factors for rupture: cardiac or renal transplant, decreased forced expiratory volume in 1 s, higher mean BP, larger initial AAA diameter, current tobacco use.

Sources

–*ACC/AHA. Aortic Disease Guideline for the Diagnosis and Management of Aortic Disease.* 2022.

–*NICE Guidelines 156.* Abdominal aortic aneurysm: diagnosis and management. 2020.

–*J Vasc Inter Radiol.* 2006;17:1383–1398.

–*Eur Heart J.* 2014;35:2873–2926.

ANAPHYLAXIS

Management: Children and Adults

Recommendations from

> NICE 2011, EACCI 2014

–Obtain blood samples for mast cell tryptase testing at onset and after 1–2 h.

–Administer epinephrine (1:1000) 0.01 mg/kg (maximum 0.5 mg) SC; repeat as necessary IM every 15 min.

–If circulatory instability, place patient supine with lower extremities raised and give intravenous saline 20 mL/kg bolus.

–Give inhaled beta-2-agonists and glucocorticoids for wheezing or signs of bronchoconstriction.

–Consider H_1- and H_2-blockers for cutaneous signs of anaphylaxis.

–Monitor after the reaction resolves. If $\geq$16 y, monitor at least 6–12 h. If <16 y, admit for observation.

–Refer all patients treated for an anaphylactic reaction to an allergy specialist.

–Prescribe an epinephrine injector (eg, EpiPen).

Practice Pearl

• Anaphylaxis is a severe, life-threatening, generalized hypersensitivity reaction. It is characterized by the rapid development of:
  - Airway edema.
  - Bronchospasm.
  - Circulatory dysfunction.

Sources

–http://www.nice.org.uk/nicemedia/live/13626/57474/57474.pdf

–http://www.guideline.gov/content.aspx?id=48690

ATRIAL FIBRILLATION (AF)

Screening: Adults

Recommendations from

> USPSTF 2022

–Current evidence is insufficient to assess the balance of benefits and harms of screening for atrial fibrillation in patients without symptoms.

Practice Pearls

- Several technologies have been proposed for screening for AF including electrocardiograms (ECGs), automated blood pressure (BP) cuffs or pulse oximeters, and consumer-oriented devices such as smartwatches and smartphone apps.
- Clinicians should use their clinical judgment regarding whether to screen and how to screen for AF. It is important to note that the USPSTF considers palpation of the pulse to be part of routine or usual care.

Source
–*JAMA.* 2022;327(4):360–367.

Management: Stroke Prevention in Adults with AF

Recommendations from

> AHA/ACC 2023

Evaluation
–Assess for risk factors of AF including advancing age, smoking, sedentary lifestyle, extreme/elite exercise, alcohol intake, obesity, taller height, systolic hypertension, diabetes, heart failure (HF), CAD, valvular heart disease, cardiac surgery, OSA, hyperthyroidism, sepsis, and family history.
–Stages of AF on a continuum:
  - At risk for AF: presence of risk factors.
  - Pre-AF: presence of predisposing structural or electrical factors (atrial enlargement, frequent atrial ectopy, short bursts of atrial tachycardia, atrial flutter, or high-risk comorbidities such as HF or valvular disease).
  - Paroxysmal AF: intermittent, terminates within 7 d of onset.
  - Persistent AF: continuous, sustains >7 d and requires intervention.
  - Long-standing persistent AF: continuous, >12 mo duration.
  - Successful AF ablation: freedom from AF s/p intervention.
  - Permanent AF: decision reached to not pursue rhythm control.
–At the time of initial AF diagnosis, evaluate the following:
  - Obtain transthoracic echo.
  - Obtain laboratory studies including CBC, CMP, and TSH.
  - Consider evaluation for other comorbidities if clinical suspicion.
  - Do not routinely evaluate for cardiac ischemia unless clinical suspicion exists otherwise.

Therapies

–Modify risk factors when applicable (see Table 2–1).

–Estimate stroke risk with CHA$_2$DS$_2$-VASc score[1] (see Table 2–2) or other annual risk predictor.

–Treat patients with atrial flutter using the same guidelines for atrial fibrillation.

–Treat with anticoagulation[2] when stroke risk is elevated (see Table 2–3).

–Choose direct oral anticoagulant (DOAC; apixaban, dabigatran, edoxaban, or rivaroxaban) over warfarin, except for select patients with valvular disease.

TABLE 2–1 RISK FACTOR MODIFICATION IN ATRIAL FIBRILLATION	
Risk Factor	**Goal**
Obesity	Target 10% weight loss
Physical inactivity	Target 210 min/wk
Tobacco use	Cessation
Alcohol use	Minimize or eliminate
Hypertension	Optimize blood pressure control
Sleep apnea	Consider screening and treating if found
Caffeine	Only recommend caffeine abstention if patient identifies that it triggers symptoms

TABLE 2–2 STROKE RISK STRATIFICATION WITH THE CHA$_2$DS$_2$-VASc SCORE	
CHA$_2$DS$_2$-VASc Score[a]	**Adjusted Stroke Rate (% per year)**
0	0
1	1.3
2	2.2
3	3.2
4	4.0
5	6.7
6	9.8
7	9.6
8	6.7
9	15.20

[a]C, CHF; H, hypertension (BP > 140/90 or on medication); A, age ≥ 75 y (2 pts), 65–74 y (1 pt); D, diabetes mellitus; S, history of stroke or TIA (2 pts); V, vascular disease (CAD, PAD, MI, aortic plaque); S, female sex.

[1] https://www.mdcalc.com/calc/801/cha2ds2-vasc-scoreatrial-fibrillation-stroke-risk

[2] Start anticoagulation for all patients with AF regardless of the pattern, including paroxysmal, persistent, long-standing persistent, or permanent.

TABLE 2–3 DECISION TO START ANTICOAGULATION IN ATRIAL FIBRILLATION		
Annual CVA Risk	**CHA$_2$DS$_2$-VASc Score**	**Recommendation**
≥2%/y	≥2 men, ≥3 women	Start anticoagulation
≥1%/y	≥1 men, ≥2 women	Consider anticoagulation Incorporate into decision-making any additional risk factors not in risk calculator (duration, persistent vs. paroxysmal, obesity, hypertrophic cardiomyopathy, poorly controlled HTN, eGFR < 45 mL/min/1.73 m², proteinuria > 150 mg/24 h, or left atrial enlargement)
<1%/y	0 men, 0–1 women	Do not start anticoagulation Do not start aspirin monotherapy unless other indication exists

- In patients with mitral stenosis (moderate to severe), anticoagulate with warfarin rather than a DOAC regardless of CHA$_2$DS$_2$-VASc score.
- For patients who are candidates for anticoagulation, do not use antiplatelet therapy as an alternative to anticoagulation unless there is another indication for the antiplatelet therapy.
- For patients with an indication for anticoagulation who have an irreversible contraindication,[1] or who are at high risk for major bleeding, consider a percutaneous left atrial appendage occlusion instead of anticoagulation.
- For patients whose AF was detected via an implantable electronic device, consider anticoagulation when the episode lasts ≥24 h and the CHA$_2$DS$_2$-VASc is ≥2 or when the episode lasts 6 min–24 h and the CHA$_2$DS$_2$-VASc is ≥3. Do not initiate anticoagulation because of an episode lasting <5 m.
- For patients taking an oral anticoagulation for AF undergoing an invasive procedure or surgery, hold the anticoagulant and do not bridge. For timing, see Table 2–4.

TABLE 2–4 DURATION TO HOLD ANTICOAGULATION WHEN INTERRUPTION IS NECESSARY FOR A SURGERY OR INVASIVE PROCEDURE		
Scenario	**Low Bleeding Risk Procedure: Hold for**	**High Bleeding Risk Procedure: Hold for**
DOAC, adequate renal function[a]	1 d	2 d
Dabigatran, CrCl 30–50 mL/min	2 d	4 d
DOAC, impaired renal function[b]	Additional 1–3 d	
Warfarin	5 d; 2–3 d if low-risk and target INR < 2.0	

[a]Apixaban: CrCl > 25 mL/min; Dabigatran: CrCl > 50 mL/min; Edoxaban: CrCl > 15 mL/min; Rivaroxaban: CrCl > 30 mL/min
[b]Apixaban: CrCl ≤ 25 mL/min; Dabigatran: CrCl ≤ 30 mL/min; Edoxaban: CrCl ≤ 15 mL/min; Rivaroxaban: CrCl ≤ 30 mL/min

---

[1] Examples include severe bleeding due to nonreversible cause in the gastrointestinal, pulmonary, or genitourinary systems, spontaneous intracranial or intraspinal bleeding, and serious bleeding related to recurrent falls.

–Approach anticoagulation in patients with concurrent indication for antiplatelet therapy as follows:

- Chronic coronary disease: 1 y after revascularization, or if no revascularization, use oral anticoagulation monotherapy rather than combination anticoagulation and antiplatelet therapy
- Peripheral arterial disease: use oral anticoagulation monotherapy rather than combination anticoagulation and antiplatelet therapy

–In patients who are diagnosed with atrial fibrillation during an acute medical illness or surgery, begin anticoagulation if indicated and arrange for close outpatient follow-up as there is a significant risk of recurrent AF. Monitor rhythm, modify risk factors, revisit risk stratification for anticoagulation, and assess the need for ongoing rate and/or rhythm control.

Surveillance

–When on DOAC therapy, order labs at the following frequencies:

- Hemoglobin/hematocrit:
  ◦ Every 6 mo: low-moderate bleed risk (HAS-BLED score 0–2).
  ◦ Every 3 mo: bleeding risk elevated (HAS-BLED score $\geq$ 3).
- Liver function:
  ◦ Every 12 mo: no liver disease.
  ◦ Every 6 mo: mild liver disease/Child-Pugh A.
  ◦ Every 3 mo: moderate liver disease/Child-Pugh B.
  ◦ Every 1–2 mo: severe liver disease/Child-Pugh C.
- Renal function:
  ◦ Every 6 mo: CrCl > 60 mL/min.
  ◦ Every 3 mo: CrCl 30–59 mL/min.
  ◦ Every 1–2 mo: CrCl < 30 mL/min.

Source
  –*JACC*. 2024;83(1).

Management: Adults with AF and Acute Transient Ischemic Attack (TIA) or Ischemic Stroke

Recommendations from

> ESC 2016

–Start oral anticoagulation after stroke or TIA:

- TIA: 1 d after acute event.
- Mild stroke (NIHSS < 8): 3 d after acute event.
- Moderate stroke (NIHSS 8–15): evaluate hemorrhagic transformation by CT or MRI at day 6, then start DOAC 6 d after acute event.
- Severe stroke (NIHSS > 16): evaluate hemorrhagic transformation.

Source
  –*Eur Heart J*. 2016;37:2893–2962.

Management: Rate and Rhythm Control in Adults with AF

Recommendations from

> ### NICE 2021, AHA/ACC 2023, ESC 2018, ACCP 2018

Therapies—Rate and Rhythm Control

–Reduce resting HR to <100–110.

–For patients with rapid ventricular response (RVR) who are hemodynamically stable (see Tables 2–5 to 2–8 for medication details):

- Use beta-blockers or nondihydropyridine calcium channel blockers (provided that EF > 40%) acutely.
- If beta-blockers and calcium channel blockers are ineffective or contraindicated, use digoxin and/or add IV magnesium sulfate.
- If beta-blockers and calcium channel blockers are ineffective or contraindicated *and* the patient is critically ill and/or in decompensated HF, consider IV amiodarone.
- Do not use calcium channel blockers in patients with known moderate or severe left ventricular (LV) systolic dysfunction.

TABLE 2–5   RATE CONTROL IN ATRIAL FIBRILLATION: BETA-BLOCKERS

Beta-Blocker	Acute Rate Control (IV Therapy)	Long-Term Rate Control (PO Therapy)	Adverse Effects	Contraindications and Cautions
Metoprolol	2.5–10 mg bolus	100–200 mg total daily dose	Bradycardia Atrioventricular block Hypotension	Avoid carvedilol in asthma (though bronchospasm is rare) Avoid class in acute heart failure and prior severe bronchospasm
Esmolol	0.5 mg/kg bolus over 1 min, then 0.05–0.23 mg/kg/min Repeat prn	—		
Carvedilol	—	3.125–50 mg BID		
Bisoprolol	—	1.25–20 mg daily		

BID, twice daily; IV, intravenous; PO, orally; prn, as needed.

TABLE 2–6   RATE CONTROL IN ATRIAL FIBRILLATION: CALCIUM CHANNEL BLOCKERS

Calcium Channel Blocker	Acute Rate Control (IV Therapy)	Long-Term Rate Control (PO Therapy)	Adverse Effects	Contraindications and Cautions
Diltiazem	15–25 mg bolus Repeat prn	180–360 mg total daily dose	Bradycardia Atrioventricular block Hypotension	Avoid in LVEF < 40% or pulmonary edema May have additive effects when used with beta-blockers Adjust dose in liver and kidney impairment
Verapamil	2.5–20 mg bolus Repeat prn	120–360 mg total daily dose		

IV, intravenous; LVEF, left ventricular ejection fraction; PO, orally; prn, as needed.

TABLE 2–7 RATE CONTROL IN ATRIAL FIBRILLATION: CARDIAC GLYCOSIDES

Cardiac Glycosides	Acute Rate Control (IV Therapy)	Long-Term Rate Control (PO Therapy)	Adverse Effects	Contraindications and Cautions
Digoxin	0.5 mg bolus, then 0.75–1.5 mg over 24 h in divided doses 0.4–0.6 mg bolus	0.0625–0.25 mg daily dose 0.05–0.3 mg daily dose	When serum level > 2 ng/mL: proarrhythmic and can aggravate heart failure	Mortality increases when serum levels elevate Adapt dose to GFR Avoid in hypertrophic cardiomyopathy, ventricular tachycardia, and accessory conduction pathways

GFR, glomerular filtration rate; IV, intravenous; PO, orally.

TABLE 2–8 RATE CONTROL IN ATRIAL FIBRILLATION: ANTIARRHYTHMICS

Antiarrhythmics	Acute Rate Control (IV Therapy)	Long-Term Rate Control (PO Therapy)	Adverse Effects	Contraindications and Cautions
Amiodarone	300 mg over 30–60 min, preferably via CVC May follow with 900 mg over 2 h	200 mg daily	Hypotension Bradycardia QT prolongation Pulmonary toxicity Skin discoloration Thyroid dysfunction Corneal deposits	

CVC, central venous catheter; IV, intravenous; PO, orally.

–If RVR with hemodynamic instability, perform direct current cardioversion.

–For long-term rate control:

  • Choose beta-blockers or nondihydropyridine calcium channel blockers for most patients.
  • Do not use calcium channel blockers when left ventricular ejection fraction (LVEF) < 40%.
  • Consider using digoxin as monotherapy or in combination for patients with AF and symptomatic HF. Target digoxin levels < 1.2 ng/mL.
  • Do not use dronedarone.

–In patients with uncontrolled RVR refractory to rate-control medications, consider AV nodal ablation to improve symptoms and quality of life. Implant a pacemaker before the ablation and set minimum HR to 80–90 bpm.

–Offer a rhythm control strategy in the following settings:

  • Symptomatic AF.
  • Reduced LV function with high burden of AF, to determine whether AF is contributing to reduced EF.
  • Diagnosis of AF within past year.

-Other variables that suggest a benefit from rhythm control include younger age, shorter history of AF, higher symptom burden, difficult-to-control HR, smaller left atrium, more LV dysfunction, and more AV regurgitation.
-In patients undergoing cardioversion, observe the following anticoagulation periods:
  • Establish anticoagulation before cardioversion and continue for at least 4 wk afterward.
  • If AF duration ≥ 48 h and cardioversion is elective, anticoagulate for 3 wk or rule out intracardiac thrombus with imaging.
-Select a long-term rhythm control agent according to patient preference and comorbidities (see Table 2–9).
-Refer for catheter ablation to improve symptoms in AF when antiarrhythmic drugs are ineffective, contraindicated, not tolerated, not preferred, and continued rhythm control is desired.
-Refer for catheter ablation in symptomatic atrial flutter.

TABLE 2–9 RHYTHM CONTROL OPTIONS, DOSING, AND MONITORING

Antiarrhythmic	Indication/contraindication	Dosing	Monitoring
Amiodarone	HFrEF. Consider in patients with preserved ejection fraction only if other rhythm control strategies are unavailable	Load 400–800 mg daily in 2–4 divided doses for 1–4 wk, then use 200 mg daily	Baseline TSH, AST, ALT, ECG. Repeat labs after 3 mo then q6mo. Repeat ECG annually
Dofetilide	Baseline QT normal. No hypokalemia or hypomagnesemia	500 mcg BID for CrCl > 60 mL/min; dose-adjust for lower CrCl	Baseline ECG; telemetry during hospitalization for initiation; K+, Mg++, Cr q3–6 mo ECG, K+, Mg++, Cr
Dronedarone	Do not use when HF with NYHA class III–IV or decompensated HF within the last 4 wk	400 mg BID	Baseline 12-lead ECG, AST, ALT Repeat AST/ALT within 6 mo
Flecainide propafenone	No prior history of MI or structural heart disease. Do not use if LVEF < 40%	Flecainide 50–300 mg/d divided q8–12h Propafenone 150–300 mg q8h or ER 225–425 mg q12h	
Sotalol	Consider when QT is normal, there is no hypokalemia, hypomagnesemia, or bradycardia	For CrCl > 60, load 40–80 mg BID × 3 d, then dose 80–160 mg BID. Dose-adjust for lower CrCl	Baseline ECG, K+, Mg++, Cr, and telemetry during hospitalization for initiation. q3–6 mo ECG, K+, Mg++ and Cr

ALT, alanine aminotransferase; AST, aspartate aminotransferase; BID, twice daily; CrCl, creatinine clearance; ER, extended release; HF, heart failure; HFrEF, heart failure with reduced ejection fraction; LVEF, left ventricular ejection fraction; MI, myocardial infarction; NYHA, New York Heart Association; TSH, thyroid-stimulating hormone.

–Consider initial treatment with catheter ablation for symptomatic, paroxysmal AF when patients are younger and have few comorbidities. There may even be value for reducing progression in asymptomatic patients.

–In patients going for catheter ablation, ensure effective anticoagulation before the procedure and continue for at least 3 mo after the procedure. For patients with elevated CHA_2DS_2-VASc, continue anticoagulation indefinitely even after ablation.

Practice Pearls

- Expected ventricular heart rate (HR) in untreated AF is between 110 and 210 beats/min.
  - If HR < 110 beats/min, atrioventricular (AV) node disease is present.
  - If HR > 220 beats/min, preexcitation syndrome (Wolff-Parkinson-White syndrome) is present.
- Holter monitor best measures the adequacy of the chronic HR control. In acute medical conditions when the patient has noncardiac illness (ie, pneumonia), the resting HR may be allowed to increase to simulate physiologic demands (mimic HR if sinus rhythm was present). (ESC recommends HR target < 110 beats/min; CCS recommends <100 beats/min; ACCF/AHA/HRS recommends HR target < 110 beats/min only if EF > 40%.)
- *Choosing Wisely* (American Society of Echocardiography 2013) recommends against transesophageal echocardiography to detect cardiac sources of embolization if a source has been identified and patient management will not change. (http://www.choosingwisely.org/sourcessocieties/american-society-of-echocardiography/)
- Various studies (AFFIRM, RACE, PIAF, STAF, etc.) have failed to show quality of life difference for rhythm control vs. rate control. Rhythm control is more likely to be effective in symptomatic patients who are younger with minimal heart disease, few comorbid conditions, and recent onset of AF.

Source

–*JACC.* 2024;83(1).

Management: Adults with AF and Heart Failure with Reduced Ejection Fraction (HFrEF)

Recommendations from

> AHA/ACC 2023, ESC 2016, NICE 2021

–If new diagnosis of HFrEF is concurrent with AF, suspect arrhythmia-induced cardiomyopathy and aggressively control AF rhythm.

–Acutely, avoid calcium channel blockers in patients with LVEF < 40%. Use only beta-blockers and digoxin as rate controllers in HFrEF because of the negative inotropic potential of verapamil and diltiazem.

–Long term, choose amiodarone over other antiarrhythmics in patients with HFrEF. Do not choose amiodarone for AF without HFrEF for long-term antiarrhythmic because of side-effect profile.

–Pursue catheter ablation to restore LV function in AF with HFrEF on GDMT.

Sources

–*JACC.* 2024;83(1).

–*Eur Heart J.* 2016;37:2893–2962.

–*NICE Guideline 196.* Atrial fibrillation: diagnosis and management. 2021.

Management: Adults with AF and Heart Failure with Preserved Ejection Fraction (HFpEF)

Recommendations from

⯈ AHA/ACC 2023, ESC 2016
  –It may be difficult to separate symptoms that are due to HF from those due to AF.
  –Focus on the control of fluid balance and concomitant conditions such as hypertension and myocardial ischemia.
  –Consider catheter ablation for symptom improvement.

Sources
  –*JACC.* 2024;83(1).
  –*Eur Heart J.* 2016;37:2893–2962.

ATHEROSCLEROTIC CARDIOVASCULAR DISEASE (ASCVD)

Prevention: Aspirin Therapy as Primary Prevention in Adults at Risk for ASCVD

Recommendations from

⯈ USPSTF 2022, FDA 2016, ACC/AHA 2019, NICE 2023
  –Use of low-dose aspirin (75–100 mg/d) for primary prevention is controversial.

Guidelines Alert 2–3
GUIDELINES DISCORDANT: ASPIRIN USE FOR PRIMARY PREVENTION OF ASCVD

Organization	Data Supports Use for This Group	Data Does Not Support Routine Use for This Group
USPSTF	Age 40–59 with 10-y ASCVD risk ≥ 10%, a low risk of bleeding and willing to take daily aspirin, utilize shared decision-making for aspirin initiation as there is a small net benefit	Age < 40 or ≥ 60
FDA	No one	Do not use aspirin in any population as primary prevention of heart attack or strokes, given serious risks including intracerebral and GI bleeding
ACC/AHA	Age 40–70 y: consider for select adults at higher ASCVD risk[a] who are not at increased bleeding risk[b]	Age > 70 y or adults at increased bleeding risk
NICE		"Do not routinely offer aspirin for primary prevention of CVD"

Applying to Clinical Practice

- Avoid the general use of aspirin for primary prevention, especially in patients over 60 y.
- There may be a small potential benefit for a narrow subset of high-risk patients who are able to take aspirin for decades.
- Most patients stand to gain too little benefit to warrant the bleeding risk.
- ASCVD risk can be estimated using the AHA's Pooled Cohort Equation (https://tools.acc.org/ascvd-risk-estimator-plus/) or PREVENT tool (https://professional.heart.org/en/guidelines-and-statements/prevent-calculator).

---

[a]A risk value is no longer given due to recent trials calling into question the value of aspirin for primary prevention. Recommend using all available risk factors when determining higher ASCVD risk.
[b]Examples of increased bleeding risk: history of previous GI or other sites bleeding, peptic ulcer disease, age > 70, thrombocytopenia, coagulopathy, CKD, NSAID/steroid/anticoagulant use.

Practice Pearls

- Aspirin for primary prevention does reduce the incidence of cardiovascular events, does not reduce mortality or nonfatal MI, and does increase bleeding risk. (*Fam Prac.* 2020;37(3):290–296)
- Risks of aspirin therapy: hemorrhagic stroke and GI bleeding (risk factors include age, male sex, GI ulcers, upper GI pain, concurrent NSAID/anticoagulant use, and uncontrolled hypertension).
- Establish risk factors using the ACC/AHA pooled cohort equation (PCE).

Sources

–USPSTF. *JAMA.* 2022:327(16):1577–1584.
–FDA. *Use of Aspirin for Primary Prevention of Heart Attack and Stroke.* 2016.
–*J Am Coll Cardiol.* 2019;74(10):e177–e232.
–www.nice.org.uk/guidance/ng238

Prevention: Lifestyle Interventions in Adults at Risk for ASCVD

This recommendation includes adults with elevated BP or known hypertension, metabolic syndrome, dyslipidemia, or estimated 10-y CVD risk > 7.5%. It does not include those with abnormal blood glucose levels, obesity, or smoking, though all persons benefit from healthy eating and physical activity behaviors.

Recommendations from

> **USPSTF 2022, ESC 2016, AHA/ACC 2019, NICE 2023**

–Offer behavioral counseling, cognitive-behavioral strategies, and multidisciplinary/multimodal interventions to promote healthy diet and physical activity on an individualized basis.
–Avoid use of and exposure to tobacco products.
–*Behavioral counseling:*
  - Intensive counseling with multiple contacts over extended periods of time.
  - Interventions typically take 6–18 mo with an estimated 6 h of contact time over a median of 12 contacts.

–*Dietary guidelines:*
- Balance calorie intake and physical activity to achieve or maintain a healthy body weight.
- Increase the consumption of fruits, vegetables, whole grains, and fat-free or low-fat dairy; consume lean proteins and vegetable oils.
- Decrease the consumption of food and drink that contain high sodium, saturated fat, trans fat, and added sugars; limit alcohol intake.
- Follow these Prevention Recommendations for food consumed/prepared inside *and* outside of the home.

–Recommended diets: Dietary Approaches to Stop Hypertension (DASH), USDA Food Pattern, AHA diet, or Mediterranean diet.

–*Physical activity guidelines*:
- 150 min/wk of moderate or 75 min/wk of vigorous aerobic activity in addition to strengthening activities twice per week. For adults unable to meet these Prevention Recommendations, aim for some moderate- or vigorous-intensity physical activity to reduce ASCVD risk.
- Decrease sedentary behavior.

Practice Pearls

- There is a strong correlation between healthy diet, physical activity, and incidence of CVD.
- Behavioral counseling has shown to have a small benefit in the absence of metabolic disorders. There is better data to support behavioral interventions for patients with obesity and adults with abnormal blood glucose. (USPSTF 2018)
- Those who take more steps every day enjoy lower all-cause mortality. (*JAMA.* 2020;323(12): 1151–1160)

Sources

–*J Am Coll Cardiol.* 2019;74(10):e177–e232.
–*Eur Heart J.* 2016;37:2315–2381.
–*JAMA.* 2017;318:167–174.
–USPSTF. *JAMA.* 2022;328(4):367–374.
–USPSTF. *Ann Int Med.* 2015;163(11):861–869.
–www.nice.org.uk/guidance/ng238

Prevention: Statin Therapy as Primary Prevention in Adults at Risk for ASCVD

Recommendations from

> USPSTF 2022, ACC/AHA 2019, ESC/EAS 2019, CCS 2021, VA-DoD 2020, NICE 2023

–A variety of guidelines exist to guide thresholds to initiate statin therapy.

Guidelines Alert 2-4
GUIDELINES DISCORDANT: ASCVD PREVENTION GUIDELINES USING STATIN THERAPY

Guidance	Organization					
	ACC/AHA	CCS	ESC/EAS	USPSTF	VA-DoD	NICE
Risk estimator	PCE	Framingham	SCORE	PCE	PCE or Framingham	QRISK3
Treatment threshold (10-y risk)	≥7.5% age 40–75 LDL-C ≥ 190 mg/dL age ≥ 21 *See Table 2–10 for detail*	≥20% age 40–75 FRS 10%–19.9% and LDL-C > 3.4 or non-HDL-C > 4.1 or ApoB > 1.04 Statin indicated conditions	ASCVD, DM with end-organ damage, or 3 major risk factors[a]	≥10% and 1 risk factor age 40–75	Higher risk CVD or ≥12% risk for adults > 40 y or LDL-C ≥ 190 mg/dL	≥10%, or lower if pt preference Or DM1 with age > 40 y, duration of DM > 10 y, established nephropathy or other CVD risk factors
Treatment Prevention Recommendations *(see Table 2–11 for statin intensity levels)*	Lifestyle ≥7.5% risk: M or H int. statin 5%–7.5% risk: M int. statin Select patients < 5% risk or age < 40 or ≥75 and LDL-C < 190 mg/dL: consider M int. statin	Lifestyle Maximally tolerated statin for LDL-C < 2.0 mmol/L or ApoB <0.8 g/L or non-HDL-C < 2.6 mmol/L	Lifestyle Very high risk: Statin to reduce LDL-C ≥ 50% and <55 mg/dL High risk: Statin to reduce LDL-C ≥ 50% and <70 mg/dL Moderate risk: Statin to reduce LDL < 100 mg/dL Low risk: Statin to reduce LDL < 116 mg/dL	Lifestyle ≥10% risk: L to M int. statin 7.5%–10% risk: L to M int. statin for select patients	Lifestyle ≥12% risk: M int. statin 6%–12% risk: M int. statin for select patients	Lifestyle ≥10%: atorvastatin 20 mg

Treatment					
Prevention Recommendations for patients with ASCVD (secondary prevention)	≤75 y: H int. statin ≥75 y: M int. statin	Hint. Maximally tolerated dose, consider adjunct if LDL-C > 1.7 mmol/L or ApoB > 0.69 g/L or non-HDL-C > 2.3 mmol/L	Maximally tolerated statin for target Goal of LDL-C ≤ 70 mg/dL or ≥50% reduction reasonable	No recommendation	CVD with M int. statin Higher risk CVD with H or M int. statin at either maximal dose or add ezetimibe +/– PCSK9 inhibitor	Start atorvastatin 80 mg (lower dose if drug-drug interaction, risk of adverse effects or pt preference) For all, goal LDL-C < 2.0 mmol/L

Applying to Clinical Practice

- There is a moderate primary prevention net benefit for statins in higher risk patients.
- Societies have used various tools for assessing risk and have set varying thresholds for starting therapy based on their assessment of risk.
- Assess your patients' tolerance of ASCVD risk vs. the burdens of polypharmacy, medication cost, and the emerging data on the potential for side effects.[b]
- The ACC publishes a helpful risk estimator tool that can guide decision-making: https://tools.acc.org/ascvd-risk-estimator-plus/

[a]Severe CKD, heterozygous familial.
[b]Eckel R, et al. Statin toxicity: mechanistic insights and clinical implications. *Circ Res.* 2019;124:328–350.

TABLE 2–10 ASCVD GROUPS THAT BENEFIT FROM STATIN THERAPY

Risk Group	Statin Prescription
Age ≤ 75 y with clinical ASCVD, particularly individuals at very high risk[a]	High-intensity statin or maximal tolerated statin, with goal of reducing LDL-C by ≥50% If LDL-C on statin is still ≥70 mg/dL, consider adding ezetimibe; if still ≥70 mg/dL, consider adding PCSK9-I
Age > 75 y with clinical ASCVD or already tolerating high-intensity statin	Reasonable to continue moderate- or high-intensity statin after shared decision-making
Heart failure with reduced ejection fraction attributable to ischemic heart disease with life expectancy 3–5 y and not already on a statin	Consider initiation of moderate-intensity statin to reduce occurrence of ASCVD events
Age 40–75 y with diabetes Age 40–75 y with diabetes and multiple ASCVD risk factors Age ≥ 75 y with diabetes on statin Diabetes with 10-y ASCVD risk ≥ 20% Age 20–39 y with diabetes-specific risk factors[b]	Moderate-intensity statin High-intensity statin, with goal of reducing LDL-C by ≥50% Reasonable to continue statin or initiate after shared decision-making Add ezetimibe to reduce LDL-C by ≥50% Reasonable to initiate statin

[a]Very high-risk ASCVD is history of multiple major ASCVD events or 1 major ASCVD event and multiple high-risk conditions. Major ASCVD events are ACS in past year, MI, ischemic stroke, symptomatic PAD. High-risk conditions are age ≥ 65 y, heterozygous familial hypercholesterolemia, prior CABG or PCI, diabetes, hypertension, CKD, eGFR 15–59 mL/min/1.73 m², smoking, LDL-C ≥ 100 mg/dL despite statin and ezetimibe, HF.
[b]Diabetes-specific risk enhancers are duration of diabetes type 2 ≥ 10 y or type 1 ≥ 20 y, albuminuria ≥ 30 mcg/mg Cr, eGFR < 60 mL/min/ 1.73 m², retinopathy, neuropathy, ABI < 0.9.
Source: ACC/AHA. *J Am Coll Cardiol*. 2019;73(24):e285–e350.

TABLE 2–11 STATIN INTENSITY DRUG LEVELS

High intensity (lowers LDL-C ≥ 50%)	Atorvastatin 40–80 mg Rosuvastatin 20–40 mg
Moderate intensity (lowers LDL-C 30%–49%)	Atorvastatin10–20 mg Fluvastatin 40 mg BID Fluvastatin XL 80 mg Lovastatin 40 mg Pitavastatin 1–4 mg Pravastatin 40–80 mg Rosuvastatin 5–10 mg Simvastatin[a] 20–40 mg
Low intensity (lowers LDL-C < 30%)	Fluvastatin 20–40 mg Lovastatin 20 mg Pitavastatin 1 mg Pravastatin 10–20 mg Simvastatin 10 mg

Note: If unable to tolerate moderate- to high-intensity statin therapy, consider the use of low-intensity dosages to reduce ASCVD risk.
[a]Avoid simvastatin 80 mg due to high risk of myopathy.

Sources
  –USPSTF. *JAMA*. 2022;328(8):746–753.
  –ACC/AHA. *J Am Coll Cardiol*. 2019;73(24):e285–e350.
  –*Eur Heart J*. 2020;41(1):111–188.
  –*Canadian J Cardiol*. 2021;37:1129–1150.
  –VA/DoD. *Clinical Practice Guidelines: The Management of Dyslipidemia for Cardiovascular Risk Reduction*. 2020.
  –www.nice.org.uk/guidance/ng238

Practice Pearls

- ACC/AHA: If risk is uncertain, assess coronary artery calcium. Potential candidates for coronary artery calcium measurement include:
  - Patients reluctant to start statin therapy, who want to understand risk/benefits.
  - Patients who may want to know the benefits of statin therapy after discontinuation due to side effects.
  - Older men aged 55–80 or women aged 60–80 with fewer risk factors, who question whether they would benefit from statin therapy.
  - Adults aged 40–55 in borderline risk group (with ASCVD risk 5%–7.5%) with other factors that increase their risk.
- Recommend lifestyle management and drug therapy for high-risk groups.
- In patients intolerant of statin, consider reducing dose or switching to an alternate agent unless reaction is severe. See Table 2–12 for a list of proven adverse effects of statins.
- Consider combination of statin and nonstatin therapy (refer to Table 2–13) in select patients.
- CCS:
  - For Primary Prevention:
- Consider add-on therapy with ezetimibe as first-line treatment if LDL-C > 1.9 mmol/L or ApoB > 0.7 g/L or non-HDL-C > 2.6 mmol/L on maximally tolerated statin.
  - For Secondary Prevention:
    - Recommend adjunct treatment to maximally tolerated statin using PCSK9 inhibitor (in patients with highest benefit or LDL-C > 2.2 mmol/L or ApoB > 0.8 g/L or non-HDL-C > 2.9 mmol/L) +/− ezetimibe.
    - Consider icosapent ethyl 2000 mg BID if triglyceride is >2.4 to <5.6 mmol/L in patients already receiving maximally tolerated statin.
  - Statin Indicated Conditions:
    - LDL > 4.9 mmol/L.
    - Most patients with DM: >39 y or >29 y with >14 y duration or microvascular disease.
    - CKD: >49 y and eGFR < 60 mL/min/1.73 m^2.
- VA/DoD:
  - For higher risk groups, shared decision-making should be used regarding harms and benefits when deciding between moderate- and high-intensity statins.
  - For patients needing intensified therapy, it recommends maximal dosing of statin or ezetimibe prior to PCSK9 inhibitors due to safety profile and efficacy.

- For primary or secondary prevention, it recommends against using niacin or omega-3 fatty acids and against adding fibrates to statins.
- For secondary prevention only, consider icosapent ethyl in patients on statin therapy with persistent fasting triglyceride > 150 mg/dL.

Sources

–ACC/AHA. *J Am Coll Cardiol.* 2019;73(24):e285–e350.
–ACC/AHA. *J Am Coll Cardiol.* 2019;74(10):e177–e232.

Prevention: Adults with HTN

See section "Hypertension" for guidance on management of HTN to prevent ASCVD.

Prevention: Adults with Diabetes Mellitus

Recommendations from

➤ ADA 2019

–Lifestyle interventions:
- Diet: Mediterranean or DASH-style diet; reduce saturated fat, trans fat, and cholesterol intake; increase n-3 fatty acids, viscous fiber, and plant stanols/sterols.
  ○ Weight loss: if overweight or obese.
  ○ Physical activity.
  ○ Smoking cessation.

TABLE 2–12 STATIN-ASSOCIATED SIDE EFFECTS			
Side Effect	**Frequency**	**Predisposing Factors**	**Evidence**
Myalgias (no elevation CK)	1%–10%	Age, female, low BMI, Rx interactions, HIV, renal/liver/thyroid disease, Asian descent, alcohol, exertion, trauma	RCTs, observation
Myositis/Myopathy (↑ CK)	Rare		RCTs, observation
Rhabdomyolysis (↑ CK + renal injury)	Rare		RCTs, observation
Statin-associated autoimmune myopathy	Rare		Case reports
New-onset diabetes mellitus	More frequent if risk factors	BMI ≥ 30, FBG ≥ 100 mg/dL, metabolic syndrome, A1c ≥ 6%	RCTs, meta-analyses
Liver transaminases ≥ 3× ULN	Infrequent		RCTs, observation, case reports
Memory/Cognition	Rare: no increase in 3 RCTs		Case reports
Cancer, renal, cataracts, tendon rupture, hemorrhagic stroke, lung disease, low testosterone	Unfounded		

TABLE 2–13 NONSTATIN CHOLESTEROL-LOWERING AGENTS
• In high-risk patients (clinical ASCVD, age < 75 y; LDL-C ≥ 190 mg/dL; 40- to 75-y-old with DM) who are intolerant to statins, the use of nonstatin cholesterol-lowering drugs may be considered.
• **Niacin:** Indicated for LDL-C elevation or fasting triglyceride ≥ 500 mg/dL; avoid with liver disease, persistent hyperglycemia, acute gout, or new-onset AF.
• **BAS:** Indicated for LDL-C elevation; avoid with triglycerides ≥ 300 mg/dL.
• **Ezetimibe:** Indicated for LDL-C elevation; when combined with statin, monitor transaminase levels.
• **Fibrates:** Indicated for fasting triglycerides ≥ 500 mg/dL. If needed, consider adding fenofibrate only to a low- or moderate-intensity statin. Avoid the addition of gemfibrozil to statin agent due to increased risk of muscle symptoms. Avoid fenofibrate if moderate/severe renal impairment.
• **Omega-3 fatty acids:** Indicated in severe fasting triglycerides ≥ 500 mg/dL.
• **PCSK9** (proprotein convertase subtilisin kexin 9) inhibitors: FDA-approved monoclonal antibodies including alirocumab (Praluent®) and evolocumab (Repatha®). Studies have shown decrease in LDL cholesterol most notably in patients with heterozygous familial hypercholesterolemia. FOURIER trial tested evolocumab in combination with statin therapy against placebo plus statin therapy in patients with elevated cholesterol levels and existing CVD. There was a modest additional reduction in LDL and composite cardiovascular events. (*N Engl J Med.* 2017;376:1713–1722)

Source: Adapted from *J Am Coll Cardiol.* 2018;71:794–799.

–Target BP goals:
- BP < 130/80 mmHg in patients with DM, HTN, and 10-y ASCVD risk > 15%.
- BP < 140/90 mmHg in patients with DM, HTN, and 10-y ASCVD risk < 15%.

–BP interventions:
- BP > 120/80: lifestyle modifications.
- BP ≥ 140/90: initiate/titrate pharmacotherapy.
- BP ≥ 160/100: initiate/titrate 2-drug regimen.

–Antihypertensives should include classes demonstrated to reduce CV events in diabetic patients: ACEi, angiotensin receptor blockers (ARBs), thiazide-like diuretics, dihydropyridine calcium channel blockers (CCBs).

–Urinary albumin/Cr ratio ≥ 30 mg/gCr: first-line agents are ACEi or ARBs at maximum tolerated dose for BP treatment.

–Statin therapy:
- All ages with 10-y ASCVD risk > 20% or multiple ASCVD risk factors, use high-intensity statin. If LDL-C is still ≥70 mg/dL, consider adding ezetimibe (preferred) or PCSK9-I.
- Age < 40 y with ASCVD risk factors, consider moderate-intensity statin.
- Age ≥ 40 y without ASCVD risk factors, consider moderate-intensity statin.

–For patients who do not tolerate intended statin intensity, use maximally tolerated dose.

–Although statin use is associated with increased risk of incident diabetes, the CVD rate reduction with statins outweighed the risk of incident diabetes even for patients with the highest risk for diabetes.

–Aspirin therapy:

- Patients with ASCVD: Use aspirin (75–162 mg/d) for secondary prevention. Use clopidogrel 75 mg/d for patients with documented aspirin allergy. Consider ACEi to reduce risk of CV events. Use sodium-glucose cotransporter-2 inhibitors (SGLT2i) or GLP1 A as part of diabetes regimen to reduce risk.
- Patients at increased ASCVD risk: Consider aspirin for primary prevention.

Practice Pearls

- Avoid intensive glucose lowering in patients with a history of hypoglycemic spells, advanced microvascular or macrovascular complications, long-standing DM, or if extensive comorbid conditions are present.
- Treat DM with BP readings of 130–139/80–89 mmHg that persist after lifestyle and behavioral therapy with ACEi or ARB agents. Multiple agents are often needed. *Administer at least one agent at bedtime.*
- No advantage of combining ACEi and ARB in HTN Rx (ONTARGET Trial). (*N Engl J Med.* 2008;358: 1547–1559)
- Note: Statins are contraindicated in pregnancy.

Source
–ADA. *Diabetes Care.* 2019;42(suppl 1):S103–S123.

Prevention: Women at Risk[1] for ASCVD

Recommendations from

➤ AHA 2011, AHA 2019, CCS 2021

–Limit alcohol consumption to ≤1 drink daily.
–Coronary artery calcium may further define risk in low-risk women (<7.5% 10 y).
–Substantial benefit of smoking cessation in pregnant persons on perinatal outcomes.
–Statin therapy may be indicated for women with prior pregnancy-related conditions based on CV age over 10-y risk calculator.

Practice Pearls

- Estrogen plus progestin hormone therapy should not be used or continued.
- Do not recommend antioxidants (vitamins E and C and beta-carotene), folic acid, and B$_{12}$ supplementation to prevent CHD.
- Women who are of reproductive age with indication for statin therapy should use hydrophilic compounds in conjunction with effective birth control.

Sources
–*J Am Coll Cardiol.* 2011;57(12):1404–1423.
–*J Am Coll Cardiol.* 2019;73(24):e285–e350.

---

[1] This includes women with prior pregnancy complications including hypertensive disorders of pregnancy, gestational diabetes, preterm birth, stillbirth, LBW infant, or placental abruption.

Prevention: Children and Adolescents at Risk for ASCVD

Recommendations from

> NIH/NHLBI 2012

Lifestyle Interventions

–If LDL or triglyceride elevated, refer to a registered dietitian for family medical nutrition therapy:

- 25%–30% of calories from fat.
- ≤7% from saturated fat.
- ~10% from monounsaturated fat.
- <200 mg/d of cholesterol.
- Avoid trans fats as much as possible.

–Consider psyllium can be added to a low-fat, low-saturated-fat diet as cereal enriched with psyllium at a dose of 6 g/d for children 2–12 y and 12 g/d for those >12 y.

–Decrease sugar intake by replacing simple with complex carbohydrates and eliminating sugar-sweetened beverages.

–Increase dietary fish to increase omega-3 fatty acids.

–Recommend physical activity (as in all children). Age 5–10, 1 h/d of moderate-to-vigorous physical activity and <2 h/d of sedentary screen time. Age 11–21, 1 h/d of moderate-to-vigorous activity with vigorous intensity 3 d/wk, with <2 h of screen time with quality programming daily.

Pharmacologic Therapies

–Consider medication therapy if:

- Birth–10 y: only with severe primary hyperlipidemia (homozygous familial hypercholesterolemia, primary hypertriglyceridemia with triglyceride ≥ 500 mg/dL), or a high-risk condition or evident cardiovascular disease; all under the care of a lipid specialist.
- 10–21 y: average 2 LDL measurements 2 wk–3 mo apart and consider statin if
  - ◦ 160–189 mg/dL with positive family history or 1 high-level or 2 moderate-level risk factors.
  - ◦ 130–159 mg/dL with 2 high-level risk factors or 1 high-level and 2 moderate-level risk factors.

Source

–Expert panel on integrated guidelines for cardiovascular health and risk reduction in children and adolescents. *Pediatrics.* 2011;128(5):S213–S258. https://www.nhlbi.nih.gov/files/docs/peds_guidelines_sum.pdf

BRADYCARDIA

Management: Adults

Recommendations from

> ACC/AHA/HRS 2018

–Consider evaluating for and treating sleep apnea if nocturnal bradycardia.

–Consider evaluating for structural heart disease including acute myocardial infarction.

–Evaluate for systemic conditions that may contribute, such as medications (many antihypertensives, antiarrhythmics, and psychoactive medications), rheumatologic conditions and inflammatory disorders, physical conditioning, carotid sinus hypersensitivity, syncope disorders, sleep, increased intracranial pressure, hypothyroidism, and sleep apnea.

–When sinus node disease causes bradycardia with symptoms or hemodynamic instability, give atropine.

–If bradycardia is caused by medication, use a reversal agent (eg, if calcium channel blocker overdose, give 10% calcium chloride or gluconate; if beta-blocker overdose, give glucagon or high-dose insulin if digoxin overdose, give digoxin antibody fragment).

–Use transcutaneous pacing for patients who remain hemodynamically unstable after medical therapy.

–Refer for pacemaker regardless of symptoms for second-degree Mobitz type II, high-grade AV block, or third-degree AV block without reversible etiology.

–Refer for pacemaker if symptomatic from bradycardia with other etiologies that are not reversible.

–There is no minimum duration of pause that indicates the need for pacemaker, but rather the correlation between the pause and symptoms.

Practice Pearl

- Sinus bradycardia occurs in 15%–20% of patients with acute MI, especially if it involves the RCA as it supplies the SA node. (*Circulation.* 1972;45:703)

Source
–*JACC.* 2018;74(4):e51–e156.

CAROTID ARTERY STENOSIS (CAS)

Screening: Adults

Recommendations from

> USPSTF 2021, AHA/ASA 2011, AAFP 2015, Society of Thoracic Surgeons 2013, CCF/ACR/AIUM/ASE/ASN/ICAVL/SCAI/SCCT/SIR/SVM/SVS 2012

–Do not screen asymptomatic adults.

Practice Pearls

- The overall US prevalence of internal CAS of ≥70% varies from 0.5% to 1%, with increased prevalence in older adults, smokers, and individuals with hypertension or heart disease. No clinically useful risk stratification tool has been found to reliably distinguish between individuals with clinically important CAS and those who do not. No evidence suggests that screening for asymptomatic CAS reduces fatal or nonfatal strokes. (*Ann Intern Med.* 2014;161(5):356–362)
- Carotid duplex ultrasonography to detect CAS > 70%: 90% sensitivity, 94% specificity. (*Ann Intern Med.* 2014;161(5):356–362)
- In 2021, USPSTF reviewed evidence since 2014 and did not change the recommendation.

Sources

–USPSTF. *JAMA*. 2021;325(5):476–481.

–ACCF/ACR/AIUM/ASE/ASN/ICAVL/SCAI/SCCT/SIR/SVM/SVS. *J Am Coll Cardiol*. 2012;60(3):242–276.

–ASA/ACCF/AHA/AANN/AANS/ACR/ASNR/CNS/SAIP/SCAI/SIR/SNIS/SVM/SVS. *Circulation*. 2011;124:e54–e130.

–AAFP. *Am Fam Physician*. 2015;91(10):online.

–Society of Thoracic Surgeons. *Choosing Wisely*. 2013.

Management: Adults

Recommendations from

> AHA/ASA 2014, 2021; SVS 2021

–Prescribe daily aspirin and statin.

–Use antihypertensives to maintain BP < 140/90 for patients with hypertension and asymptomatic extracranial carotid and/or vertebral atherosclerosis.

–If ischemic stroke or TIA and moderate (50%–69%) or severe (≥70%) stenosis, refer for revascularization procedure. (AHA/ASA)

- If severe stenosis, choose carotid artery stenting (CAS) or endarterectomy (CEA), provided perioperative morbidity/mortality risk < 6%. If age 70+, consider CEA over CAS. If anatomy increases the risk of CEA, choose CAS.

- If moderate stenosis, refer for CEA, provided perioperative morbidity/mortality risk < 6%.

–For patients undergoing CAS, use dual antiplatelet therapy (aspirin 81–325 mg daily and clopidogrel 75 mg daily) preprocedure and for a minimum of 30 d after.

–For patients undergoing CEA, use aspirin alone preprocedure and continue indefinitely postoperatively.

Guidelines Alert 2–5	
GUIDELINES DISCORDANT: CAROTID ENDARTERECTOMY IN ASYMPTOMATIC PATIENTS WITH SEVERE (≥70%) STENOSIS	
AHA/ASA	Consider referring for carotid endarterectomy (CEA) if risk of perioperative stroke, MI, and death is <3%.
SVS	Choose CEA plus medical management over medical therapy alone for low surgical risk patients.

Applying to Clinical Practice
- CEA in asymptomatic patients is best reserved for people in otherwise good health.
- Data is lacking to compare outcomes between CEA + medical management vs. medical management allow.

Practice Pearl

- Do not recommend CEA for asymptomatic carotid artery stenosis if the complication risk is >3% (https://www.choosingwisely.org/clinician-lists/american-academy-neurology-cea-for-asymptomatic-carotid-stenosis/).

Sources
  –*Stroke*. 2014;45:3754–3832.
  –*Stroke*. 2021;52:e364–e467.
  –*J Vasc Surg*. 2022;75:4S–22S.

CHEST PAIN

Management: Adults

Recommendations from

> ACC/AHA/ASE/CHEST/SAEM/SCCT/SCMR 2021

  –Classify chest pain as cardiac, possibly cardiac, or noncardiac based on suspicion (not as "typical" or "atypical").[1]
  –Obtain resting ECG within 10 min in all symptoms of chest pain (cardiac or noncardiac in nature). Send to emergency department for serial ECGs + troponin if high clinical suspicion.
  –In the emergency department, obtain a cardiac troponin (preferably high-sensitivity) as soon as possible when acute coronary syndrome is suspected, then measure serially.
  –Consider chest X-ray to evaluate for nonischemic causes of pain.
  –Consider transthoracic echocardiogram in intermediate-risk patients.
  –After initial evaluation to rule out STEMI, perform a diagnostic test depending on the likelihood of CAD:
    • Low risk: no testing needed.
    • Intermediate risk: stress testing (preferred age ≥ 65 y or suspected obstructive CAD) or CT coronary angiography (CCTA).
    • High risk (generally: higher risk patient, rising troponin, ongoing cardiac chest pain; high-risk findings on stress test or CCTA): invasive coronary angiography.
  –If known CAD, consider deferring testing and intensifying GDMTs vs. stress testing (if ≥50% stenosis) or CCTA (if <50% stenosis).
  –If diagnosis is made of noncardiac chest pain, consider a broad differential diagnosis:
    • Respiratory: pulmonary embolism, pneumothorax, pneumomediastinum, pneumonia, bronchitis, pleural irritation, malignancy.
    • Gastrointestinal: cholecystitis, pancreatitis, hiatal hernia, GERD/gastritis/esophagitis, peptic ulcer disease, esophageal spasm, dyspepsia.
    • Chest wall: costochondritis, chest wall trauma/inflammation, herpes zoster, cervical radiculopathy, breast disease, rib fracture, musculoskeletal injury, or spasm.

---

[1] Descriptors including central, pressure, squeezing, gripping, heaviness, tightness, exertional/stress-related, and retrosternal carry high probability of ischemia. Descriptors including sharp, fleeting, shifting, pleuritic, and positional are lower probability.

- Psychological: panic disorder, anxiety, clinical depression, somatization disorder, hypochondria.
- Others: hyperventilation syndrome, carbon monoxide poisoning, sarcoidosis, lead poisoning, prolapsed intervertebral disc, thoracic outlet syndrome, adverse effect of certain medications (eg, 5-FU), sickle cell crisis.

Source
  –*JACC.* 2021;78(22):e187–e285.

CHOLESTEROL AND LIPID DISORDERS

Screening: Adults

Recommendations from

➤ **USPSTF 2016, AHA/ACC 2018, Canadian Cardiovascular Society (CCS) 2021, AACE 2017, VA/DoD 2020**
  –Screen all adults within the recommended age range.

Guidelines Alert 2–6	
GUIDELINES DISCORDANT: POPULATION TO SCREEN FOR DYSLIPIDEMIA	
Organization	**Population**
USPSTF	Age 40–75: screen (frequency undetermined)
	Age 20–39: use clinical judgment as evidence is insufficient
CCS	Age 40–75 and postmenopausal persons. Screen every 5 y; add lipoprotein(a) once in lifetime at initial screening
AACE	Age 45 (men) or 55 (women) through 65: screen every 1–2 y
	Age 20 through 45 (men) or 55 (women): screen every 5 y
	Age 65+: screen annually
VA/DoD	Age ≥ 40: no more frequently than every 10 y

Applying to Clinical Practice
- Screen all adults older than 40, unless limited life expectancy.
- Screen younger patients who have significant cardiovascular risk factors.
- Screening frequency is a matter of expert opinion. Consider repeating screening when there are significant changes to patient's weight, diet, exercise, and alcohol intake.

  –Use lipid data to determine risk score (ie, ASCVD risk calculator: https://tools.acc.org/ascvd-risk-estimator-plus) to determine need for primary prevention.
  –Use lipid data, other levels (FPG/HgbA1c, eGFR), with Framingham Risk Score (FRS) or the Cardiovascular Life Expectancy Model (CLEM) to determine need for primary prevention. (CCS)

–Consider screening adults regardless of age with other risk factors (clinical evidence of atherosclerosis, abdominal aortic aneurysm, DM, arterial hypertension, cigarette smoking, stigmata of dyslipidemia-corneal arcus, xanthelasma, xanthoma), family history of premature CVD or dyslipidemia, CKD (eGFR ≤ 60 mL/min/1.73 m²), BMI ≥ 30, inflammatory diseases (RA, SLE, PsA, AS, IBD), HIV infection, erectile dysfunction, COPD, history of hypertensive disorder of pregnancy. (CCS)

Sources

–VA/DoD. *Clinical Practice Guideline for the Management of Dyslipidemia for Cardiovascular Risk Reduction.* 2020.
–*JAMA.* 2016;316(19):1997–2007.
–*Circulation.* 2019;139:e1046–e1081.
–*Can J Cardiol.* 2021;37(8):1129–1150.
–*Endocr Pract.* 2017;23(suppl 2).

Management: Adults

See section on ATHEROSCLEROTIC CARDIOVASCULAR DISEASE (ASCVD) for guidance on lipid-lowering medications for primary prevention of ASCVD.

Recommendations from

> National Lipid Association 2023

–Recommend the following dietary guidelines to lower LDL-C:
  • Decrease saturated fats, trans fats, and dietary cholesterol.
  • Increase unsaturated fat intake.
  • If obese/overweight, reduce body weight by 5%–10%.
  • Increase protein, especially plant protein.
  • Increase viscous fiber intake (5–10 g/d).
  • Increase plant stanols/sterols (2 g/d).
–Recommend the following dietary guidelines to lower triglycerides:
  • Reduce added sugars and refined starches.
  • Reduce alcohol.
  • If obese/overweight, reduce body weight by 5%–10%.
  • Increase protein, especially plant protein.
  • Increase eicosapentaenoic acid and docosahexaenoic acid intake (2–4 g/d).
  • Increase physical activity (≥150 min/wk).

Source
–*J Clin Lipidol.* 2023;17:428–451.

CORONARY ARTERY DISEASE

Screening: Adults

Recommendations from

> ⋗ ACC/AHA 2019, ESC 2012, USPSTF 2018, VA/DoD 2020

–For adults aged 40–75 y, routinely assess cardiovascular risk factors and calculate 10-y risk of ASCVD using PCEs.[1]

–For adults aged 20–39 y, assess traditional ASCVD risk factors at least every 4–6 y.

–For adults at borderline risk (5%–7.5% 10-y ASCVD risk) or intermediate risk (≥10% to <20% 10-y ASCVD risk), consider using additional risk-enhancing factors to guide decision-making about preventive interventions. If decisions remain uncertain, it is "reasonable" to measure a coronary artery calcium score to guide risk discussion.

–For adults aged 20–39 y or adults aged 40–59 y with <7.5% 10-y ASCVD risk, consider estimating lifetime or 30-y ASCVD risk (or HeartScore screening risk score in Europe).[2]

–Insufficient evidence to recommend for or against the addition of Ankle-Brachial Index (ABI), high-sensitivity C-reactive protein (hsCRP), and coronary artery calcium score to traditional risk assessment for CVD in asymptomatic adults with no history of CVD.

–Do not offer a cardiovascular risk assessment more frequently than every 5 y, using 10-y risk calculator.

–Do not use coronary artery calcium, high-sensitivity C-reactive protein, or ABI when assessing cardiovascular risk.

–Do not screen with resting or exercise ECG, exercise treadmill test (ETT), stress echocardiogram, or electron-beam CT for coronary artery calcium.

–Do not screen with stress cardiac imaging or advanced noninvasive imaging in the initial evaluation of asymptomatic patients, unless high-risk markers are present.

–Do not perform annual stress cardiac imaging or advanced noninvasive imaging as part of routine follow-up in asymptomatic patients.

Practice Pearls

- The traditional 10-y ASCVD risk calculator (The Pooled Cohort Equation) can be found at: http://tools.acc.org/ASCVD-Risk-Estimator-Plus/

- The AHA released a new tool for primary prevention assessments, PREVENT, in 2024: https://professional.heart.org/en/guidelines-and-statements/prevent-calculator

- USPSTF recommends against screening asymptomatic individuals because of the high rate of false-positive results, low mortality of asymptomatic disease, and iatrogenic diagnostic and treatment risks.

---

[1] Use Pooled Cohort Equations to replace Framingham Risk Score. The Pooled Cohort Equations incorporate age, sex, race, total cholesterol, HDL cholesterol, systolic BP, use of antihypertensive medication, and history of diabetes and/or tobacco use.
[2] HeartScore Europe incorporates age, sex, systolic BP, total cholesterol, HDL cholesterol, and history of tobacco use.

Sources

–*J Am Coll Cardiol.* 2019;74(10):e177–e232.

–*Eur Heart J.* 2012;33:1635–1701.

–USPSTF. *JAMA.* 2018;320(3):272–280.

–AAFP. *Clinical Preventive Service Recommendation: Cardiovascular Disease Risk.* 2018.

–USPSTF. *JAMA.* 2018;319(22):2308–2314.

–VA/DoD. *Clinical Practice Guideline for the Management of Dyslipidemia for Cardiovascular Risk Reduction.* 2020.

–American College of Physicians. *Choosing Wisely.* 2012. http://www.choosingwisely.org/ societies/american-college-of-physicians/

–AAFP. *Choosing Wisely.* 2013. http://www.choosingwisely.org/societies/american-academy-of-family-physicians/

–American Society of Echocardiography. *Choosing Wisely.* 2012. http://www.choosingwisely.org/ societies/american-society-of-echocardiography/

–American College of Cardiology. *Choosing Wisely.* 2014. http://www.choosingwisely.org/ societies/american-college-of-cardiology/

–*Ann Intern Med.* 2012;157:512–518.

–*J Am Coll Cardiol.* 2019;74(10):e177–e232.

Prevention

See section above on ATHEROSCLEROTIC CARDIOVASCULAR DISEASE.

Management: Adults with CAD

Recommendations from

➤ AHA/ACC/ACCP/ASPC/NLA/PCNA 2023

–Recommend dietary changes:
  • Emphasize vegetables, fruits, legumes, nuts, whole grains, and lean protein.
  • Reduce percentage of calories from saturated fat and replace with monounsaturated and polyunsaturated fat, complex carbohydrates, and dietary fiber.
  • Minimize sodium (ideally <1500 mg/d) and processed meats.
  • Limit refined carbohydrates and sugar-sweetened beverages.
  • Avoid trans fats.
–Recommend lifestyle changes:
  • Tobacco cessation for patients who smoke.
  • Limit alcohol intake (maximum 1 drink/d women, 2 drinks/d men).
  • Recommend 150 min/wk of moderate-intensity aerobic activities or 75 min/wk of higher-intensity aerobic activities, unless contraindications. Include strength training at least twice a week.
–Antiplatelets: Prescribe aspirin 81 mg/d unless contraindicated. See Table 2–14 for antiplatelet guidance for varying clinical scenarios.

TABLE 2–14 ANTIPLATELET THERAPY CHOICE AND DURATION IN CHRONIC CORONARY DISEASE	
Clinical Scenario	**Therapy Choice and Duration**
No PCI ACS > 12 mo prior	Aspirin 81 mg indefinitely
Prior ACS	DAPT × 12 mo, then aspirin 81 mg indefinitely Consider DAPT up to 36 mo if low bleeding risk
After PCI	Drug-eluting stent DAPT × 6 mo, then single antiplatelet agent indefinitely
After PCI, high bleeding risk	Drug-eluting stent DAPT × 1–3 mo, then clopidogrel to complete 12 mo, then single antiplatelet agent indefinitely
On oral anticoagulation, after PCI	DOAC + aspirin + clopidogrel up to 1 mo Then DOAC + clopidogrel to complete 6 mo Then DOAC alone indefinitely without antiplatelet agent
On oral anticoagulation, PCI, high ischemic risk	DOAC + aspirin + clopidogrel for 1 mo Then DOAC + clopidogrel for 1–6 mo Then DOAC alone indefinitely without antiplatelet agent
Oral anticoagulation; no PCI	DOAC without antiplatelet agent

PCI: percutaneous coronary intervention
DAPT: dual antiplatelet therapy with aspirin and clopidogrel
Patients with a separate indication for chronic oral anticoagulation therapy, such as atrial fibrillation with elevated
  stroke risk or prior venous thromboembolism
Adapted from Figure 9 in AHA 2023.

–Lipid management:
  • Prescribe high-intensity statin with the goal of LCL reduction ≥ 50%.
  • In very high-risk patients who are on maximal statin therapy and still have LDL > 70 mg/
    dL, consider sequentially adding ezetimibe and then a PSCK9 monoclonal antibody.
–Beta-blockers:
  • Use if LVEF ≤ 40%. Choose metoprolol succinate, carvedilol, or bisoprolol.
  • If beta-blocker was started for prior MI, consider discontinuing after 1 y if LVEF is >50%
    and there is no angina, arrhythmia, or uncontrolled hypertension.
  • Do not use beta-blockers specifically for CAD unless prior MI or LVEF ≤ 50%.
–Renin-angiotensin-aldosterone inhibitors:
  • Prescribe ACEi or ARB for all patients with HTN, DM, LVEF ≤ 40% or CKD.
  • Consider ACEi or ARBs in all patients.
–Colchicine: consider in all patients with chronic coronary disease.
–Blood pressure control: Pursue BP goal of <130/80. ACEi, ARB, and beta-blockers are first-line
  agents.

–DM: use either SGLT2i or GLP-1 receptor agonist.

–BMI > 25: pursue weight loss, employing GLP-1 receptor agonist (favor semaglutide) or bariatric procedures if lifestyle changes are unsuccessful.

–Do not routinely obtain cardiac catheterization unless patient has new LV systolic dysfunction, HF, chest pain refractory to GDMT, or noninvasive testing suggesting >50% left main disease.

–If change in symptoms or functional capacity, refer for invasive coronary angiograph and obtain stress echo, cardiac MRI, or rest/stress nuclear myocardial perfusion imaging to determine presence and extent of ischemia.

–Refer to cardiac rehabilitation if recent MI/PCI/CABG, stable angina, after heart transplant, or after spontaneous coronary artery dissection.

–Vaccinate with annual influenza vaccine and coronavirus vaccination. Consider pneumococcal vaccine.

Source
–*JACC.* 2023;82(9):833–955.

Management: Adults with CAD Experiencing Angina

Recommendations from

➤ AHA/ACC/ACCP/ASPC/NLA/PCNA 2023, ACC/AHA/ASE/CHEST/SAEM/SCCT/SCMR 2021

–Risk-stratify patients with moderate-to-severe CAD presenting with new chest pain:

- Choose exercise treadmill test if the baseline ECG is normal, the patient can exercise, and the pretest likelihood of CAD is intermediate (10%–90%).
- Choose either a nuclear myocardial perfusion study (MPI) or exercise echocardiogram if unable to perform an exercise treadmill and the pretest likelihood is >10%.
- Repeat studies when there is a change in clinical status or if needed for exercise prescription.
- Consider coronary computed tomography angiogram (CTA) if an intermediate pretest probability of CAD, if symptoms persist despite prior normal testing, if equivocal stress tests, or in patients who cannot be studied otherwise. Do not use coronary CTA if known moderate or severe coronary calcification or in the presence of prior stents.
- Obtain an echocardiogram to assess resting LV function and valve disease in patients with suspected CAD, pathological Q waves, presence of HF, or ventricular arrhythmias.

–Treat chronic angina in CAD with the following medications:

- Beta-blocker, calcium channel blocker, or long-acting nitrate as initial monotherapy.
- Add second agent from the above list if not controlled with monotherapy.
- Add ranolazine if still not controlled.
- Use sublingual nitroglycerin or nitroglycerin spray as needed for immediate short-term relief.
- Do not use ivabradine.

–Refer for revascularization with PCI if lifestyle-limiting angina despite GDMT and significant coronary stenosis.

–Recommend CABG when significant left main disease or multivessel disease and LVEF ≤ 35%.

Sources

–*JACC.* 2021;78(22):e187–e285.
–*Circulation.* 2020;141:e779–e806.
–*JACC.* 2023;82(9):833–955.

Management: Adults Experiencing NSTEMI or Unstable Angina

Recommendations from

> ### ACC/AHA 2014, ESC 2023, ACC/AHA/SCAI 2021

–At presentation, obtain ECG, cardiac troponin [ACC: troponin I or T at 0 h then 3–6 h later; ESC: high-sensitivity troponin at 0 h then 1–2 h later] and assess prognosis with risk scores such as TIMI[1] or GRACE.[2]
–See Table 2–15 for a bundle of interventions to initiate at presentation.
–Refer for cardiac catheterization according to Table 2–16.

TABLE 2–15 INTERVENTIONS FOR ACUTE CORONARY SYNDROME	
Therapy	**Detail**
Nitroglycerin	Sublingual nitrogylcerin q5 min ×3 for ongoing ischemic pain IV nitroglycerin for persistent ischemia, HF, or HTN
Antiplatelet therapy	Dual antiplatelet therapy whenever ACS is suspected – Aspirin 325 mg, nonenteric-coated – Clopiodogrel (300–600 mg loading dose, then maintenance) or ticagrelor (180 mg loading dose, then maintenance) Add PPI if high risk of GI bleed
Anticoagulation	In addition to antiplatelet therapy, choose unfractionated heparin, enoxaparin, or fondaparinux. Strongest evidence supports enoxaparin (1 mg/kg q12h; If CrCl < 30 mL/min, 1 mg/kg q24 h; continued minimum of 48 h until clinically stable)
Beta-blockers	ACC: oral beta-blockers in first 24 h unless signs of HF, low output state, risk factors to cardiogenic shock or other contraindication ESC: give if LVEF < 40% unless signs of acute heart failure, SBP < 120 mmHg or other contraindications. Consider if LVEF ≥ 40% as well If already on beta-blockers, continue home dose unless decompensated heart failure
Opioids	IV opioids (eg, morphine 5–10 mg) to relieve severe chest pain
ACEi	Start or continue home dose of ACE/ARB when LVEF < 40%, DM, HTN, or stable CKD
Statins	Start or continue high intensity statin (atorvastatin 40–80 mg or rosuvastatin 20–40 mg daily)
Oxygen	Supplemental oxygen only if SaO_2 ≤ 90% or respiratory distress
Anxiolytics	In patients with significant anxiety, consider anxiolytics

[1] TIMI Risk Score predicts 30-d and 1-y mortality in ACS (mortality rises at TIMI = 3–4). 1 point each for age ≥ 65, ≥ 3 risk factors for CAD, known CAD, ST changes on ECG (≥ 0.5 mm), active angina (≥ 2 episodes in past 24 h), aspirin in past 7 d, elevated cardiac marker.
[2] The GRACE risk model predicts in-hospital and postdischarge mortality or MI. Downloadable tool: http://www.outcomes-umassmed.org/grace/

TABLE 2–16 TIMING OF CARDIAC CATHETERIZATION	
Timing	**Indication**
Immediate	Cardiogenic shock, refractory angina, hemodynamic, or electrical instability
Within 24 h	High risk of clinical events – GRACE score > 140 – Significant troponin elevation – Significant ECG changes
Prior to hospital discharge	Stabilized patients at lower risk for clinical events

Sources

–*Eur Heart J.* 2023;44:3720–3826. https://academic.oup.com/eurheartj/article/37/3/267/2466099

–*J Am Coll Cardiol.* 2014;64(24):e139–e228. http://content.onlinejacc.org/article.aspx?articleid=1910086

–*J Am Coll Cardiol.* 2016;68(10):1082–1115. http://content.onlinejacc.org/article.aspx?articleid=2507082

Management: Adults Experiencing STEMI

Recommendations from

> ACC/AHA 2013, ESC 2023, NICE 2013, ACC/AHA/SCAI 2021

–Draw serum biomarkers, but do not wait for results to initiate reperfusion therapy.

–Elect PCI rather than fibrinolysis for all patients with STEMI if an experienced team is available within 120 min of first medical contact. Consider PCI up to 12–24 h after presentation if prompt intervention is not available.

–Give aspirin (162–325 mg) and a loading dose of an ADP-receptor inhibitor (clopidogrel 600 mg, prasugrel 60 mg, or ticagrelor 180 mg) as early as possible.

–Anticoagulate with unfractionated heparin (UFH), enoxaparin, or bivalirudin. Consider adding a glycoprotein IIb/IIIa inhibitor (abciximab, eptifibatide, tirofiban) to UFH.

–If hypertensive or with ongoing ischemia, give beta-blocker at presentation.

–If PCI is not available, treat instead with fibrinolytics. Give a loading dose of clopidogrel (300 mg; 75 mg if >75 y of age) with aspirin. Anticoagulate with heparin, enoxaparin, or fondaparinux until hospital discharge (minimum 48 h, up to 8 d) or until revascularization is performed. Give fibrinolytic therapy within 30 min of hospital arrival. It is most useful if ischemic symptoms started within the past 12 h and is a reasonable choice between 12 and 24 h if there is evidence of ongoing ischemia or a large area of myocardium at risk. Transfer to a PCI-capable facility if fibrinolysis fails.

–Give patients who have undergone PCI for STEMI dual antiplatelet therapy for 1 y. Continue aspirin indefinitely. Initiate beta-blockers within 24 h of admission, high-intensity statin, and if LVEF < 40% an ace inhibitor or angiotensin receptor blocker.

Sources

–*J Am Coll Cardiol.* 2022;79(2):e21.

–*J Am Coll Cardiol.* 2013;61(4). https://www.guideline.gov/summaries/summary/39429?

–*Eur Heart J.* 2023;44:3720–3826. https://www.guideline.gov/summaries/summary/39353?

–National Institute for Health and Care Excellence (NICE). 2013:28. https://www.guideline.gov/summaries/summary/47019?

–*J Am Coll Cardiol.* 2016;68(10):1082–1115. http://content.onlinejacc.org/article.aspx?articleid=2507082

Management: Patients with CAD and Type 2 Diabetes Mellitus

Recommendations from

➤ AHA 2020

–Use an A1c goal of <8.0–8.5.

–The use of different medications to attain a glycemic goal can affect CAD-related endpoints. See Table 2–17.

–Antiplatelet therapy: data is insufficient to give a definitive recommendation.

–Hypertension: BP goals based on combination of comorbidities:

- T2DM + HTN + CAD <140/<90.
- T2DM + HTN + CAD + stroke risk <130/<80.
- T2DM + HTN + CAD + CKD/microalbuminuria <130/<80.

–Benefits/risks of antihypertensive classes in T2DM and CAD:

- ACEi/ARBs: first-line option. Reduce first and recurrent cardiovascular events; reduce progression of microalbuminuria.
- Long-acting thiazide-like (chlorthalidone/indapamide): second-line option. Increase serum glucose slightly by decreasing insulin sensitivity but unclear if of clinical significance. Has cardiovascular benefit.
- Dihydropyridine CCBs (amlodipine): second-line option. Has cardiovascular benefits and is antianginal.
- Aldosterone antagonists (spironolactone): third-line option. Important in comorbid LV dysfunction or prior MI.
- Beta-blockers: Do not reduce mortality in CAD after 30 d. Can be used in T2DM if there is concurrent chronic angina or if need another agent. Not all beta-blockers have equal benefit. Use carvedilol, labetalol, or nebivolol for vasodilatory effect and neutrality in T2DM. Instead, metoprolol and atenolol will reduce demand but cause peripheral vasoconstriction, which increases insulin resistance and LDL.

–Lipids: Use statins for all with CAD and DM.

- If LDL is >70 despite high-intensity statin, consider ezetimibe or PCSK9 inhibitors (evolocumab or alirocumab) for additional risk reduction in death, MI, stroke, or hospitalization.
- If triglycerides are >135 despite statins, consider addition of icosapent ethyl 2 g BID which has been shown to decrease cardiovascular death, MI, stroke, CABG, unstable angina.

TABLE 2–17 DIABETES MEDICATIONS WITH CARDIOVASCULAR BENEFITS			
Drug Class	**Specific Drugs and Trials**	**Risk/Benefit for CAD**	**Effect in Diabetes**
SGLT2i	Canagliflozin (CANVAS) Dapagliflozin (DECLARE-TIMI) Empagliflozin (EMPA-REG)	– Decreases major cardiac events – Decreases CHF hospitalizations – Decreases blood pressure slightly – Less CKD progression – Contributes to weight loss	– No hypoglycemia risk – Stop medication if at risk for amputation, Fournier gangrene, bone fractures, and euglycemic DKA
GLP1 agonists	Exenatide (EXCEL) Liraglutide (LEADER) Lixisenatide (ELIXA) Semaglutide (SUSTAIN-6)	– Overall recommended for decreasing major cardiac events – Contributes more to weight loss than SGLT2i – More variety within the class for CAD benefit in recent research – Liraglutide and semaglutide decrease major cardiac events – Exenatide and lixisenatide are neutral	– No hypoglycemia risk – Stop medication if at risk for gastroparesis, pancreatitis, or CrCl < 30 mL/min (use caution if 30–50 mL/min)
Metformin		– Benefit is possible	– No hypoglycemia – Stop in CrCl < 30 mL/min – Monitor for anemia and B_{12} deficiency
DPP4 inhibitors	Alogliptin (EXAMINE) Linagliptin (CAROLINA) Saxagliptin (SAVOR-TIMI) Sitaliptin (TECOS)	– Neutral CAD effect – Weight loss neutral – Saxagliptin and alogliptin may contribute to CHF hospitalization	– No hypoglycemia – Stop in gastroparesis and pancreatitis – Monitor for URI symptoms
Insulin		– Neutral CAD effect – Can cause weight gain	– Can cause hypoglycemia
Sulfonylureas	Glimepiride (CAROLINA)	– Neutral CAD effect – Can cause weight gain	– Can cause hypoglycemia
Thiazolidinediones	Pioglitazone (PROactive, IRIS) Rosiglitazone (RECORD)	– Likely CAD benefit – Need to monitor/stop for CHF, esp. if using with insulin – Can cause weight gain	– No hypoglycemia – Stop if risk for bone fractures

– Smoking: Stop smoking. The weight gain in T2DM from cessation does not undo the drop in risk of major cardiac event.

– Diet: Recommend a Mediterranean diet with extra virgin olive oil or mixed nuts saw benefit for reduction in major cardiac events or stroke.

–Activity: Recommend 150 min/wk of moderate to vigorous physical activity. Refer to cardiac rehabilitation after the first major cardiac event, as the intervention has been shown to be preventative of future cardiac events if tailored to T2DM.

–Weight loss: Diet and exercise have modest benefit in CAD and T2DM. Liraglutide has been shown to decrease weight (see Table 2–17) and improve CAD outcomes. Bariatric surgery has been shown to better control CAD risk factors (glycemic control, LDL, triglycerides, HTN) but not necessarily to improve CAD endpoints.

Practice Pearls

- Intensive glycemic control A1c < 6.0%–7.0% has not been shown to decrease major cardiac events, though glycemic control < 7.0% does show some benefit for microvascular consequences of diabetes such as blindness, microalbuminuria, ESRD, and distal neuropathies.

- T2DM is a generalized prothrombotic state, especially when exacerbated by CKD. Responsiveness to DAPT may be impaired. Clopidogrel alone may be reasonable compared to aspirin alone in T2DM with prior MI, ischemic stroke, or PAD. At this time, large trials have not shown benefit when antithrombotic regimens are adjusted based on platelet function testing.

- Seventy percent to eighty percent of patients with T2DM also have HTN. This increases the risk of MI, stroke, and all-cause mortality. Intensive control of systolic blood pressure in this group <130 decreases risk of stroke, but has no benefit in decreasing coronary events. There are increased risks of adverse events in too much control of HTN in CAD.

- The ACCORD trial demonstrated that 30% of T2DM need 2 antihypertensives, 39% of T2DM need 3 antihypertensives.

- Statins have significant benefit in primary and secondary CAD prevention and patients with T2DM. Studies have shown that statins can cause small increase in incident T2DM, but the risk is lower than with thiazides or nonvasodilating beta-blocker; the protective benefit of statins in T2DM is more substantive and favors administration.

- Stress: patients with T2DM have increased risk for stress and depression. This has been shown to increase risk of stroke. Stress in T2DM has been shown to increase risk of major cardiac event. The mechanisms are unknown. It is unknown if decreasing stress/depression then resolves the increased risk.

Source
–*Circulation.* 2020;141:e779–e806.

HEART FAILURE (HF)

Management: Adults

Recommendations from
➤ ACC/AHA 2022, 2017, NICE 2018

Evaluation

–Obtain CXR, 12-lead ECG, blood tests (renal function, thyroid function, liver function, lipid profile, A1c, complete blood count, troponin I level), urine analysis, and peak flow or spirometry. Identify prior cardiac or noncardiac disease that may lead to HF. For patients at risk for developing HF, natriuretic peptide biomarker–based screening (BNP or NT-pro-BNP) and optimizing GDMT can help prevent the development of LV dysfunction (systolic or diastolic) or new-onset HF. B-type natriuretic peptide can help exclude HF in patients with dyspnea.

–Obtain history to include diet or medicine nonadherence; current or past use of alcohol, illicit drugs, and chemotherapy; or recent viral illness.

–If idiopathic dilated cardiomyopathy, obtain a three-generational family history to exclude familial disease.

–Obtain 2D echocardiogram to determine the systolic function, diastolic function, valvular function, and pulmonary artery pressure.

–In patients with angina or significant ischemia, perform coronary arteriography unless the patient is not eligible for surgery.

–Refer for genetic testing in patients whose first-degree relatives have genetic or inherited cardiomyopathies.

–Classify HF as reduced or preserved ejection fraction:

- Heart failure with reduced ejection fraction (HFrEF): LVEF ≤ 40%.
- Heart failure with mildly reduced ejection fraction (HFmrEF): LVEF 41%–49%.
- Heart failure with preserved ejection fraction (HFpEF): LVEF > 50%.

Therapies

–Diuresis, if volume is overloaded:

- Regardless of classification, initiate diuretic therapy and salt restriction.
- Diuretics do not improve long-term survival but improve symptoms and short-term survival.
- Prefer loop diuretic, but consider thiazide (eg, metolazone) if not responding.
- Once euvolemic and symptoms have resolved, carefully wean dosage as an outpatient to the lowest dose possible to prevent electrolyte disorders and activation of the renin-angiotensin system.

–If HFrEF, initiate GDMT. GDMT includes 4 classes of medication:

- Angiotensin receptor-neprilysin inhibitors (ARNi), ACEi, or angiotensin receptor blocker (ARB). Choose ARNi over ACEi or ARB if available, unless New York Heart Association (NYHA) Class IV (symptoms at rest). If taking an ACEi or ARB and ARNi is an option, switch to ARNi. Titrate dose every 2 wk to target doses as BP allows. Measure renal function and electrolytes 1–2 wk after every change.
- Beta-blocker: choose bisoprolol, carvedilol, or sustained-release metoprolol succinate. Start with low dose; titrate to heart rate 65–70 bpm.
- Mineralocorticoid receptor antagonist (MRA) such as spironolactone. Use if GFR is >30 mL/min/1.73 m^2 and K^+ < 5.0 mEq/L. Monitor renal function and potassium levels. Discontinue if K^+ cannot be maintained <5.5 mEq/L.
- SGLT2i: Use regardless of the presence/absence of diabetes.

–If HFmrEF:

- Consider SGLT2i, as it may reduce hospitalizations and mortality, though data for this class is modest. (COR 2a)
- Consider ACEi/ARB/ARNi, MRA, though their benefit has not been well established in this class. (COR 2b)

–If HFpEF:

- Treat hypertension according to clinical practice guidelines.
- Consider SGLT2i, as it may reduce hospitalizations and mortality, though data for this class is modest. (COR 2a)

–If atrial fibrillation, manage to reduce symptoms.

–Alternative agents to consider in HFrEF:

- Use hydralazine plus isosorbide dinitrate to improve outcomes in Black persons with moderate-to-severe HFrEF, in addition to optimal therapy.[1] Consider using it in lieu of ACEi or ARB if they are contraindicated regardless of race/ethnicity.
- Consider ivabradine in select patients: symptomatic stable chronic HFrEF (EF < 35%) at least 4 wk removed from exacerbation on optimal medical therapy including optimal dosing of ACEi and beta-blocker at maximal tolerated dose in sinus rhythm with resting HR $\geq$ 70.
- Consider digoxin if persistent symptoms from HFrEF despite optimized GDMT.
- Consider vericiguat if LVEF < 45%, recent hospitalization, and elevated BNP.
- Consider omega-3 polyunsaturated fatty acid supplementation as adjunct once optimized GDMT.
- Consider potassium binders if hyperkalemia on MRA to preserve their ability to be used.

–Do not use statins as adjunctive therapy solely for the diagnosis of HF. In all patients with a recent or remote history of CAD, CVA, PAD, or hyperlipidemia, use statins according to guidelines.

–Discontinue anti-inflammatory agents, diltiazem, and verapamil.

–Nutritional supplements are not useful therapy for patients with current or prior symptoms of systolic dysfunction (HFrEF).

–Avoid calcium channel blockers in the routine treatment for patients with HFrEF.

–Do not administer long-term anticoagulation therapy in patients with chronic systolic function while in sinus rhythm unless AF, a prior thromboembolic event, or cardioembolic source.

–Maintain BP < 130/80 mmHg.

Additional Interventions

–Recommend exercise training, which is beneficial in HF patients with decreased ejection fraction (systolic dysfunction) or preserved ejection fraction (diastolic dysfunction) once therapy is optimized.

–Refer for intracardiac cardiac defibrillator in patients who survive cardiac arrest, ventricular fibrillation, or hemodynamically significant ventricular tachycardia.

–Refer for intracardiac cardiac defibrillator in patients with EF $\leq$ 35% with NYHA class II or III. Before referring, ensure at least 40 d post-MI, optimize GDMT, and expect a life expectancy of at least 1 y.

–Refer for cardiac resynchronization therapy with biventricular heart pacemaker when QRS duration $\geq$ 150 ms +/− left bundle branch block and EF $\leq$ 35% with NYHA class II and III or ambulatory class IV on GDMT.

---

[1] Race-based recommendations for specific therapies are controversial, in part because the definition of racial groups is not standardized. This guidance comes from a study that looked at patients identified as Black with NYHA Class III or IV HF. All were given standard therapies, and the groups were randomized to add either placebo or isosorbide dinitrate + hydralazine. Mortality rate, admission rate, and quality of life were significantly worse in the placebo group. (*N Engl J Med.* 2004;351:2049–2057)

–Arrange postdischarge appointment with physician and health care team with attention to information on discharge medications.

–Ensure patients are up to date on influenza, COVID-19, and pneumococcal vaccinations.

Practice Pearls

- Lifetime risk of developing HF for Americans ≥40-y-old is 20%.
- Overall mortality is 50% in 5 y; varies with HF stage:
  - Stage B[1]: 5-y mortality 4%.
  - Stage C[2]: 5-y mortality 25%.
  - Stage D[3]: 5-y mortality 80%.
- SGLT2i were added to the recommendations for all classes of HF in 2022 after a number of trials showed benefit. For HFrEF, the DAPA-HF and EMPEROR-Reduced trials suggest a 25% reduction in the composite end point of cardiovascular death or HF hospitalization. Dapagliflozin (but not empagliflozin) reduced all-cause mortality. For LVEF > 40%, the EMPEROR-Preserved trial suggested a reduction in hospitalization rate but not mortality. (*Circulation*. 2022;145:e895–e1032;146:299–302; *Lancet*. 2022;400(10354):757–767)
- NNT over 3 y for all-cause mortality in HFrEF by GDMT agent. (*Circulation*. 2022;145: e895–e1032)
  - ACEi/ARB: 26.
  - ARNi: 27.
  - Beta-blocker: 9.
  - Mineralocorticoid receptor antagonist: 6.
  - SGLT2i: 22.
  - Hydralazine or nitrate: 7.
  - Cardiac resynchronization therapy: 8.
  - Implantable cardiac defibrillator: 23.

Sources

–*Circulation*. 2022;145:e895–e1032. doi:10.1161/CIR.0000000000001063

–ACCF/AHA. 2017 guidelines. *Circulation*. 2017. doi:10.1161/CIR.0000000000000509

–*N Engl J Med*. 2012.

–*J Am Coll Cardiol*. 2012;59(20):1812–1832.

–*Circulation*. 2013;128:e240–e327.

HYPERLIPIDEMIA

The risk assessment and management of ASCVD risk factors, including hyperlipidemia, is detailed in the ASCVD section above.

---

[1] Previous MI, LV remodeling/LVH and low EF, or asymptomatic valvular disease.

[2] Known structural heart disease; shortness of breath and fatigue, reduced exercise tolerance.

[3] Symptoms at rest despite maximal medical therapy; recurrent hospitalizations.

HYPERTENSION (HTN)

Screening: Adults

Recommendations from

> ACC/AHA 2018, ESH/ESC 2018, USPSTF 2021, NICE 2023

–Screen for hypertension in adults $\geq$ 18-y-old with office BP measurement. Obtain BP measurements outside of clinical setting before starting treatment.

–Screen for HTN using an average BP measurement based on $\geq$2 readings obtained on $\geq$2 occasions.

–Use single-visit BP measurement to diagnose HTN only in cases of severe BP elevation/grade 3 HTN ($\geq$180/110) with clear evidence of hypertension-mediated organ damage (eg, hypertensive retinopathy, LVH, vascular or renal damage). (ESH/ESC)

–Elements of proper measurement include appropriately sized cuff at the level of right atrium, while patient is seated, $\geq$5 min between office entry and BP measurement.

–Screen every 3–5 y for age 18–39 without risk factors.

–Screen annually at age 40+ or if risk factors are found (prior BP $\geq$ 130–139/85–89, obese, overweight, Black).

Practice Pearls

- Blood pressure can be measured with a programmed portable device that automatically takes BP every 20–30 min over 12–24 h, or self-measured at home 1–2 times a day or week with an automated device. (USPSTF)

- Blood pressure measurements should be taken at upper arm, while seated, after resting for 5 min. (USPSTF)

- Corresponding BPs based on site/methods: office/clinic 140/90, home monitoring 135/85, day-time ambulatory monitoring 135/85, night-time ambulatory monitoring 120/70, 24-h ambulatory monitoring 130/80. (*J Am Coll Cardiol.* 2018;71:e127–e248)

- Electronic (oscillometric) measurement methods are preferred to manual measurements. Routine auscultatory Office BP Measurements (OBPMs) are 9/6 mmHg higher than standardized research BPs (primarily using oscillometric devices). (*Can Pharm J.* 2015;148(4):180–186)

- Assess global cardiovascular risk in all hypertensive patients. Informing patients of their global risk ("vascular age") improves the effectiveness of risk factor modification.

Sources

–ACC/AHA. *J Am Coll Cardiol.* 2018;71:e127–e248.

–USPSTF. *JAMA.* 2021;325(5):476–481.

–ESC/ESH. *Eur Heart J.* 2018;39:3021–3104.

–www.nice.org.uk/guidance/ng136

Prevention: Adults

Recommendations from

> **ACC/AHA 2017, ESC/ESH 2018, Hypertension Canada 2018, JNC 8, ICSI 2018**
>
> –Persons at risk for developing HTN—family history of HTN, African ancestry, overweight or obesity, sedentary lifestyle, excess intake of dietary sodium, insufficient intake of fruits, vegetables, and potassium, excess consumption of alcohol—should undergo lifestyle changes (Table 2–18).
>
> –Achieve and maintain normal BMI < 25, restrict sodium intake < 2 g/d, moderate alcohol consumption < 14 drinks/wk for men, <8–9 drinks/wk for women, increase physical exercise 30 min/d 5–7 d/wk, emphasize smoking cessation.
>
> –Consume diet rich in vegetables, fruit, fish, nuts, whole grains, low-fat dairy products, and unsaturated fats.
>
> –Do not supplement calcium or magnesium for the prevention or treatment of HTN.
>
> –For patients not at risk of hyperkalemia, increase dietary potassium intake to reduce BP.
>
> –Recommend stress management including relaxation techniques for patients whose stress might be contributing to high BP.

TABLE 2–18 LIFESTYLE MODIFICATIONS FOR PREVENTION OF HYPERTENSION

Maintain a healthy body weight for adults (BMI 18.5–24.9; waist circumference < 102 cm for men and <88 cm for women).

Reduce dietary sodium intake to no more than 2000 mg sodium/d (approximately 5 g of sodium chloride). Per CHEP 2015: adequate intake 2000 mg daily (all ≥ 19-y-old) (80% in processed foods; 10% at the table or in cooking); 2000 mg sodium (Na) = 87 mmol sodium (Na) = 5 g of salt (NaCl) ~1 teaspoon of table salt.

Engage in regular aerobic physical activity, such as brisk walking, jogging, cycling, or swimming (30–60 min per session, 4–7 d/wk, or 90–150 min/wk), in addition to the routine activities of daily living. Higher intensities of exercise are not more effective. Weight training exercise does not adversely influence BP. Isometric exercise, eg, hand grip 4 × 2 min, 1 min rest between exercises, 3 sessions/wk shown to reduce BP.

Limit alcohol consumption to no more than 2 drinks (eg, 24 oz [720 mL] of beer, 10 oz [300 mL] of wine, or 3 oz [90 mL] of 100-proof whiskey) per day in most men and to no more than one drink per day in women and lighter-weight persons (≤14/wk for men, ≤9/wk for women).

Maintain adequate intake of dietary potassium (≥90 mmol [3500 mg]/d). Above the normal replacement levels, do not supplement potassium, calcium, and magnesium for prevention or treatment of hypertension.

Maintain daily K dietary intake ≥ 80 mmol.

Consume a diet that is rich in fruits and vegetables and in low-fat dairy products with a reduced content of saturated and total fat (DASH eating plan).

Offer advice in combination with pharmacotherapy (varenicline, bupropion, nicotine replacement therapy) to all smokers with a goal of smoking cessation.

Consider stress management as an intervention in hypertensive patients in whom stress may be contributing to BP elevation.

Practice Pearls

- A 10-mmHg reduction in SBP or 5-mmHg reduction in DBP would decrease all major cardiovascular events by 20%, all-cause mortality by 10%–15%, stroke by 35%, coronary events by 20%, and HF by 40%. (ESC/ESH. *Eur Heart J*. 2018;39:3021–3104)
- For overweight patients, expect 1-mmHg reduction in SBP for every 1-kg reduction in body weight. (ACC/AHA. *J Am Coll Cardiol*. 2018;71:e127–e248)

Sources

–ACC/AHA. *J Am Coll Cardiol*. 2018;71:e127–e248.

–USPSTF. *Ann Int Med*. 2015;163(10):778–787.

–ESC/ESH. *Eur Heart J*. 2018;39:3021–3104.

–*Can J Cardiol*. 2018;34:506–525.

–*JAMA*. 2014;311(5):507–520.

–ICSI. Hypertension Work Group: 2018 Commentary.

–CHEP. 2015. http://guidelines.hypertension.ca

–*J Am Coll Cardiol*. 2018;71(19):e127–e248.

Management: Adults Without Comorbidities

Note that management for adults with comorbidities such as DM, CKD, CAD, and HF is covered in subsequent management sections.

Recommendations from

➢ **ACC/AHA 2017, JNC8 2014, ESC/ESH 2018, CHEP 2020, NICE 2023**

–Initiate lifestyle modification including structured exercise and dietary adjustments including lower sodium diet and efforts at weight loss if overweight or obese. Further measures include weight reduction, DASH/Mediterranean diet, dietary sodium restriction, exercise, moderate ETOH, cessation of smoking, and K+ supplementation in diet.

–Consider overall cardiovascular risk in patients with hypertension and evaluate need for primary prevention measures for ASCVD including smoking cessation, aspirin, and statin.

Guidelines Alert 2–7	
GUIDELINES DISCORDANT: WHEN TO INITIATE TREATMENT FOR HYPERTENSION	
Organization	**Guidance**
ACC/AHA	BP 120–129/<80: lifestyle changes, follow-up 3–6 mo BP 130–139/80–89, 10-y ASCVD risk ≥ 10%: lifestyle changes and medications, follow-up 1 mo BP 130–139/80–89, 10-y ASCVD risk < 10%: lifestyle changes and medications, follow-up 3–6 mo BP ≥ 140/90: lifestyle changes and medications, follow-up 1 mo
ACC/AHA	BP ≥ 140/90 mmHg in the general population age < 60-y-old BP ≥ 150/90 mmHg in general population age ≥ 60-y-old

ESC/ESH	BP 130–139/85–89: lifestyle modification (salt restriction < 5 g/d, alcohol intake < 14 drinks/wk for men and <8 drinks/wk for women, increasing fruits/vegetables/fish/nuts/olive oil in diet, controlling BMI, regular physical activity, and smoking cessation) BP 140–159/90–99: lifestyle modification; medications if high cardiovascular risk, hypertension-mediated organ damage, or persistent elevation after 3–6 mo lifestyle changes BP 160+/100+: lifestyle modification and drug therapy
CHEP	BP ≥ 160/100 mmHg in patients without macrovascular target organ damage or any cardiovascular risk factors BP ≥ 140/90 mmHg in patients with macrovascular target organ damage or any cardiovascular risk factors SBP ≥ 130 mmHg in those with high cardiovascular risk, with treatment goal of SBP < 120
NICE	BP ≥ 140/90 ≥135/85 for patients monitored at home

Applying to Clinical Practice
- Emphasize lifestyle changes (salt and alcohol restriction, exercise, weight loss, smoking cessation) at diagnosis and thereafter.
- Ensure close follow-up to adjust/escalate therapy.

Guidelines Alert 2–8	
GUIDELINES DISCORDANT: TREATMENT TARGETS IN HYPERTENSION	
Organization	**Guidance**
ACC/AHA	<130/80 for CVD or 10-y ASCVD risk ≥ 10%; consider <130/80 for all
JNC8	BP < 140/90 mmHg in patients < 60-y-old BP < 150/90 mmHg in patients ≥ 60-y-old If BP cannot be reached within 1 mo, increase the dose of the initial drug or add a second and then third drug from the recommended classes
ESC/ESH	Target < 140/90 in all patients Target SBP < 150 in patients > 65 y If tolerating 140/90, target SBP 120–129 if <65 y and 130–139 if ≥65 y
CHEP	BP < 140/90 mmHg in the general population SBP < 150 mmHg in older adults (≥60 y) SBP < 120 mmHg in adults at high cardiovascular risk Caution in older patients who are frail and in patients with CAD and have low DBP < 60 mmHg

Applying to Clinical Practice
- JNC 8 relaxed BP targets for patients over age 60, based on mixed results from RCTs around BP control in older patients.
- AHA/ACC maintain that the lack of definitive evidence is insufficient to rule out benefit, and point to the strong data in younger patients for stroke prevention with lower BP.
- While SBP target of 150 is acceptable for patients over age 60, push for an SBP closer to 140 if polypharmacy and medication side effects are not significant and there are risk factors for ASCVD.

Guidelines Alert 2–9	
GUIDELINES DISCORDANT: CHOICE OF ANTIHYPERTENSIVE AGENTS	
Organization	**Guidance**
ACC/AHA	First-line therapy: thiazide diuretics, calcium channel blockers, ACEi, and angiotensin receptor blockers Begin therapy with two drugs initially if desired BP reduction is more than 20/10 mmHg In the general Black[a] population, initial treatment should include a thiazide-type diuretic or CCB
JNC8	First-line therapy is any of the following: thiazide diuretics, calcium channel blockers, ACEi, ARBs. Second/third line is high doses or combinations of those classes.
ESC/ESH	Start with combination pill including ACEi or ARBs plus a calcium channel blocker (CCB) or diuretic. Consider using a single agent in older/frailer patients or those with mild elevations If not controlled with initial therapy, switch to a three-drug combination pill including ACEi/ARB + CCB + diuretic If not controlled on three drugs, add spironolactone, diuretic, alpha-blocker, or beta-blockers, and consider further investigation for resistant hypertension
CHEP	Isolated systolic: start monotherapy with a thiazide diuretic, a long-acting CCB or an ARB Isolated diastolic: single-pill combination with ACEi/ARB + CCB, ACEi/ARB + thiazide or monotherapy with thiazide, ACEi (except in Black patients), ARB, long-acting CCB, or beta-blocker (if <60 y)
NICE	Start ACEi, or ARB if ACEi not tolerated, if DM2 or age < 55 y Start CCB if age ≥ 55 y or are of Black African or African-Caribbean family origin and do not have DM2. If CCB not tolerated, use thiazide diuretic If not controlled on ACEi/ARB, add CCB or thiazide If not controlled on CCB, add ACEi/ARB or thiazide

Applying to Clinical Practice
- Comorbidities often drive the choice of antihypertensive.
- ACE/ARB, CCB, and thiazide diuretic are consistently recommended for uncomplicated hypertension.
- In the absence of comorbidities, let patient preferences related to tolerance guide choice (ie, electrolyte monitoring and potential for peripheral edema).

[a]As race is a social rather than scientific construct, and purportedly scientific mechanisms to explain the racial differences in outcomes have their roots in biased data, guidelines that suggest different treatments for different races should be considered with caution. Drs. Vyas, Einstein, and Jones offer a thoughtful assessment in *N Engl J Med*. 2020;383:847–882 (https://www.nejm.org/doi/full/10.1056/NEJMms2004740). A more detailed discussion of the role of race in blood pressure guidelines is available from Drs. Williams, Ravenell, Seyedali, Nayef, and Ogedegbe in *Prog Cardiovasc Dis*. 2016;59(3):282–288 (https://www.ncbi.nlm.nih.gov/pubmed/27693861).

Sources
–ACC/AHA; Whelton PK, et al. *JACC*. 2018;71(19):e127–e248.
–JNC8. *JAMA*. 2014;311(5):507–520.
–ESC/EHA. *Eur Heart J*. 2018;39:3021–3104.
–CHEP. *Can J Cardiol*. 2020;36:596–624.
–www.nice.org.uk/guidance/ng136

Management: Adults with HTN and CAD

Recommendations from

> **ACC/AHA 2017, ESC/ESH 2018, CHEP 2020**

–Prioritize medications indicated by CAD.

–Treatment target (ACC/AHA):

- <130/80 if CAD, prior MI/stroke/TIA/PAD/AAA.
- <140/90 if chronic stable angina.

Guidelines Alert 2–10	
GUIDELINES DISCORDANT: CHOICE OF ANTIHYPERTENSIVE AGENT IN CAD	
Organization	**Guidance**
ACC/AHA	Prioritize medications indicated by CAD – Beta-blocker in patients with a history of prior MI. If not tolerated, use nondihydropyridine CCB if no LV dysfunction – ACEI/ARB if prior MI, LV systolic dysfunction, DM, or CKD – A thiazide or thiazide-like diuretic If angina or uncontrolled BP, add nondihydropyridine CCB to beta-blockers. Consider avoiding combination of beta-blocker and CCB—risk of bradyarrhythmias and HF
ESC/ESH	Initial combination should be ACEI/ARB or diuretic plus beta-blocker or CCB
CHEP	Use ACEI as first-line therapy For patients with stable angina, use beta-blockers as initial therapy Avoid combination of ACEI with ARB In high-risk patients, use combination of ACEI and a dihydropyridine CCB rather than an ACEI and a thiazide Myocardial ischemia may be exacerbated when DBP ≤ 60 mmHg

Applying to Clinical Practice
- Use ACEi as first-line antihypertensive if BP control is still required after guideline-directed therapy for CAD is optimized.

Sources
–ACC/AHA; Whelton PK, et al. *JACC*. 2018;71(19):e127–e248.
–ESC/EHA. *Eur Heart J*. 2018;39:3021–3104.
–CHEP. *Can J Cardiol*. 2020;36:596–624.

Management: Adults with HTN and CKD

Recommendations from

➤ ACC/AHA 2017, ESC/ESH 2018, CHEP 2020, JNC8 2014

–Use ACEi or angiotensin receptor blocker (ARB), particularly if proteinuria.
  • Consider starting with ACEI/ARB plus CCB or diuretic as initial therapy. (ESC)
  • In patients over 75 y, use CCB and thiazide-type diuretic instead of ACE/ARB. (JNC8)

Guidelines Alert 2–11	
GUIDELINES DISCORDANT: BLOOD PRESSURE GOALS IN CKD	
Organization	**Guidance**
ACC/AHA	<130/80, regardless of proteinuria
JNC8, CHEP	<140/90; <130/80 if proteinuria
ESC/ESH	SBP 130–139/80 If DM or high cardiovascular risk, do not reduce <120/70

Applying to Clinical Practice
• Lower BP targets are best supported in preventing progression to ESRD in patients with proteinuria and CKD.
• Mortality benefit comes primarily from the cardiovascular risk reduction of lower blood pressure.

Sources
–ACC/AHA; Whelton PK, et al. *JACC.* 2018;71(19):e127–e248.
–JNC8. *JAMA.* 2014;311(5):507–520. doi:10.1001/jama.2013.284427
–ESC/EHA. *Eur Heart J.* 2018;39:3021–3104.
–CHEP. *Can J Cardiol.* 2020;36:596–624.

Management: Adults with HTN and HF

Recommendations from

➤ ACC/AHA 2017, CHEP 2020

–Target BP of <130/80 mmHg.
–In patients with an elevated DBP who have CAD and HF with evidence of myocardial ischemia, lower the BP slowly. In older hypertensive individuals with wide pulse pressures, lowering SBP may cause very low DBP values (<60 mmHg).
–If stable ischemic heart disease, prioritize medications indicated by CAD/CHF as first drugs: ACEI/ARB, beta-blocker (carvedilol, metoprolol succinate, bisoprolol, or nebivolol), and aldosterone receptor antagonist.
–Use thiazide/thiazide-type diuretic for BP control and to reverse volume overload and associated symptoms. In patients with severe HF (NYHA III or IV), or those with severe renal impairment (eGFR < 30 mL/min/1.73 m²), use loop diuretics for volume control (less effective than thiazide/thiazide-type diuretics in lowering BP). Use diuretics together with an ACE/ARB and a beta-blocker.

–Use aldosterone receptor antagonists spironolactone and eplerenone if there is HF (NYHA III or IV) with reduced EF < 40%. One or the other may be substituted for a thiazide diuretic in patients requiring a K-sparing agent. If used with an ACEI/ARB in the presence of renal insufficiency, monitor serum K level frequently. Do not use if creatinine level ≥ 2.5 mg/dL in men or ≥2.0 mg/dL in women, or if serum K level ≥ 5 mEq/L.

–Add hydralazine plus isosorbide dinitrate to the regimen of diuretic, ACEi, or ARB, and beta-blocker in Black patients with NYHA class III or IV HF with reduced ejection fraction.

–Do not use nondihydropyridine CCBs in the treatment of HTN in adults with HFrEF.

–Preserved ejection fraction: consider beta-adrenergic blocking agents, ACEI/ARBs, or CCB as antihypertensives in patients with HF to minimize symptoms of HF.

–Avoid the following drugs in patients with hypertension and HF with reduced ejection fraction:
  • Nondihydropyridine CCBs (such as verapamil and diltiazem).
  • Clonidine.
  • Moxonidine.
  • Hydralazine, without a nitrate.
  • Alpha-adrenergic blockers such as doxazosin (unless all other drugs for the management of hypertension and HF are inadequate to achieve BP control at maximum tolerated doses).
  • Nonsteroidal anti-inflammatory drugs, given their effects on BP, volume status, and renal function.

Sources
–ACC/AHA; Whelton PK, et al. *JACC.* 2018;71(19):e127–e248.
–CHEP. *Can J Cardiol.* 2020;36:596–624.

Management: Adults with HTN and Diabetes

Recommendations from
➤ ADA 2017, ACC/AHA 2018, JNC8 2014, CHEP 2020

Guidelines Alert 2–12 GUIDELINES DISCORDANT: BLOOD PRESSURE GOALS IN DIABETES	
Organization	**Guidance**
ACC/AHA	<130/80
JNC8	<140/90
ADA	<140/90 <130/80 if younger or "high risk" of cardiovascular disease
CHEP	<130/80
ASH	<140/90 mmHg (without proteinuria) <130/80 mmHg (with proteinuria) or if they are at "high risk" for cardiovascular disease

Applying to Clinical Practice
• Treat HTN early in DM to prevent progression to CKD and retinopathy.
• The guidelines that allow for a higher SBP goal all comment that patients at higher risk for ASCVD may benefit from tighter BP control.

Guidelines Alert 2–13
GUIDELINES DISCORDANT: CHOICE OF ANTIHYPERTENSIVE AGENT IN DIABETES

Organization	Guidance
ACC/AHA	Consider ACEI or ARB if proteinuria
JNC8	Same as non-DM population
ADA	ACEI or ARB: Administer at bedtime
CHEP	ACEI or ARB if renal disease, CV disease, microalbuminuria, or high ASCVD risk. Otherwise, ACEI/ARB, CCB, or thiazide

Applying to Clinical Practice
- ACEIs have a reputation for preventing progression to CKD in patients with DM and proteinuria.
- In the absence of proteinuria or CKD, ACEIs/ARBs remain first-line agents alongside thiazides or CCB.
- Only use beta-blockers in CAD or if refractory to or intolerant of combination of ACEI/ARB + CCB + thiazide.

Sources

–Standards of medical care in diabetes. *Diabetes Care*. 2017;40(suppl 1):S1–S142. www.care.diabetesjournals.org

–ACC/AHA; Whelton PK, et al. *JACC*. 2018;71(19):e127–e248.

–JNC8. *JAMA*. 2014;311(5):507–520.

–CHEP. *Can J Cardiol*. 2020;36:596–624.

Management: Adults with HTN Attempting Lifestyle Changes

–See Table 2–19 for the impacts of behavior changes on blood pressure, and Table 2–20 for impacts of specific lifestyle modifications.

TABLE 2–19 IMPACT OF HEALTH BEHAVIOR MANAGEMENT ON BLOOD PRESSURE

Intervention	Systolic BP (mmHg)	Diastolic BP (mmHg)
Diet and weight control	−6.0	−4.8
Reduced salt/sodium intake < 2000 mg sodium (Na)[a]	−5.4	−2.8
Reduced alcohol intake (<2 drinks/d)	−3.4	−3.4
DASH diet	−11.4	−5.5
Physical activity (30–40 min 5–7× wk)	−3.1	−1.8
Relaxation therapies	−5.5	−3.5

[a]2000 mg sodium (Na) = 87 mmol sodium (Na) = 5 g of salt (NaCl) ~1 teaspoon of table salt.
Source: Adapted from Canadian Hypertension Education Program (CHEP) Recommendations. 2015. www.hypertension.ca/en/chep

TABLE 2–20 LIFESTYLE MODIFICATIONS FOR TREATMENT OF HYPERTENSION

Modification	Recommendation[a]	Approximate SBP Reduction (Range)
Weight reduction	Maintain normal body weight (BMI 18.5–24.9)	5–20 mmHg per 10-kg weight loss
Adopt DASH eating plan	Consume diet rich in fruits, vegetables, and low-fat dairy products with a reduced content of saturated and total fat	8–14 mmHg
Dietary sodium reduction	Reduce dietary sodium intake to less than 100 mmol/d (2.4 g sodium or 6 g sodium chloride)	2–8 mmHg
Physical activity	Engage in regular aerobic physical activity such as brisk walking (at least 30 min/d, most days of the week)	4–9 mmHg
Moderation of alcohol consumption	Limit consumption to no more than 2 drinks (1 oz or 30 mL ethanol; eg, 24 oz beer, 10 oz wine, or 3 oz 80-proof whiskey) per day in most men and to no more than 1 drink per day in women and lighter-weight persons	2–4 mmHg

DASH, dietary approaches to stop hypertension.

[a]The effects of implementing these modifications are dose- and time-dependent and could be greater for some individuals. DASH diet is effective in lowering SBP in adolescents.

Sources: Couch SC, et al. The efficacy of a clinic-based behavioral nutrition intervention emphasizing a DASH-type diet for adolescents with elevated blood pressure. *J Pediatr.* 2008;152:494–501; Aronow WS, et al. ACCF/AHA 2011 expert consensus document on hypertension in the older adults: a report of the American College of Cardiology Foundation Task Force on Clinical Expert Consensus documents developed in collaboration with the American Academy of Neurology, American Geriatrics Society, American Society for Preventive Cardiology, American Society of Hypertension, American Society of Nephrology, Association of Black Cardiologists, and European Society of Hypertension. *J Am Coll Cardiol.* 2011:57:2037–2110.

Management: Adults with Refractory Hypertension

Recommendations from

> **CHEP 2020, NICE 2023, ACC/AHA 2017, ESC 2018**
>> –Confirm with BP measurements from home to rule out white-coat hypertension.
>> –Validate adherence using data such as pill counts, refill data, or direct observation.
>> –Assess for lifestyle contributors such as high sodium intake, alcohol consumption, and obesity. When applicable, recommend weight loss, sodium restriction, increased physical activity, and limited alcohol intake.
>> –Screen for secondary hypertension: primary aldosteronism, CKD, OSA, pheochromocytoma, and renovascular hypertension.
>> –Ensure that patient is on ACEI/ARB + CCB.
>> –If eGFR < 30 mL/min/1.73 m², switch from a thiazide to a loop diuretic.
>> –Add spironolactone. Monitor for hyperkalemia and renal dysfunction.
>> –If spironolactone is not tolerated, consider eplerenone, amiloride, bisoprolol, or doxazosin. Hydralazine or minoxidil are also options but require close monitoring.
>> –Refer to specialty care if these interventions are ineffective.

Sources

–ACC/AHA; Whelton PK, et al. *JACC*. 2018;71(19):e127–e248.

–JNC8. *JAMA*. 2014;311(5):507–520. doi:10.1001/jama.2013.284427

–ESC/EHA. *Eur Heart J*. 2018;39:3021–3104.

–CHEP. *Can J Cardiol*. 2020;36:596–624.

Management: Children and Adolescents

Recommendations from

⮞ AAP 2017

–For children age ≥ 13 y, normal BP is <120/80. Diagnose hypertension when BP is ≥130/80.

–For children age < 13 y, reference normal ranges based on age, sex, and height. Normal is <90th percentile. Diagnose hypertension when ≥95th percentile. One point of care tool is available at https://www.mdcalc.com/calc/4052/aap-pediatric-hypertension-guidelines. Screening values requiring further evaluation are listed in Fig. 2–1.

–Confirm elevated office BP measurements with ambulatory BP measurement.

–If a child is ≥6 y and is overweight or obese, has a positive family history of HTN, and does not have examination findings suggestive of secondary HTN, do not evaluate for secondary causes.

–If considering pharmacologic treatment of hypertension, obtain an echocardiogram to assess for LVH and EF.

FIG. 2–1 SCREENING BP VALUES REQUIRING FURTHER EVALUATION

Screening BP values requiring further evaluation

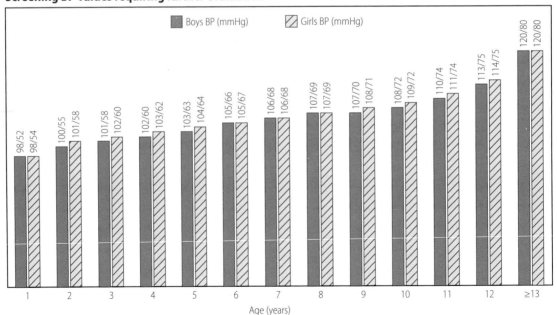

–Obtain Doppler renal ultrasound in normal-weight patients ≥8 y when renovascular hypertension is suspected.

–When starting medication, treat to a goal of <90th percentile, or <130/80 if ≥13 y.

–Initiate treatment with lifestyle modifications:

- Recommend DASH approach: increase fruits/vegetables (4–5 servings/d), low-fat dairy (2+ servings /d), whole grains (6 servings/d), fish, poultry, nuts, lean red meat. Limit sweets (max 1 serving/d) and sodium (<2.3 g/d).
- Recommend 3–5 d/wk with 30 min of moderate to vigorous physical activity.
- For children with obesity, pursue weight loss and recommend 1 h of physical activity 3–5 d/wk.
- Consider mindfulness-based stress reduction.

–If hypertension persists despite lifestyle modifications, start medications:

- Choose ACEI, ARB, calcium channel blocker, or thiazide-type diuretic as initial therapy.
- If comorbid CKD, choose ACEI or ARB.

Source

–*Pediatrics.* 2017;140(3):e20171904.

LEFT VENTRICULAR THROMBUS

Management: Adults

Recommendations from

> AHA 2022

–Consider low-dose anticoagulant (DOAC) for 1–3 mo if poor LV thrombus is due to MI.

–If "specified" dilated cardiomyopathy (due to Takotsubo, hypertrophic cardiomyopathy, peripartum cardiomyopathy, LV noncompaction, amyloidosis, Chagas disease, eosinophilic myocarditis) puts patient at high risk for LV thrombus, employ shared decision-making and consider indefinite anticoagulation.

–If subsequent echo shows resolution of thrombus (and/or a major bleed episode occurs), discontinue anticoagulation.

Practice Pearl

- Highest risk of LV thrombus is 2 wk to 1 mo after STEMI.

Source

–*Circulation.* 2022;146:e205–e223.

PERIPHERAL ARTERY DISEASE (PAD)

Screening: Adults

Recommendations from

> USPSTF 2018, AHA/ACC 2017

–Do not screen the general low-risk population with ankle-brachial index (ABI).

Guidelines Alert 2–14	
GUIDELINES DISCORDANT: WHETHER TO SCREEN	
Organization	**Population**
USPSTF	Insufficient evidence to recommend for or against routine screening with ABI
ACC	Consider screening with resting ABI if increased risk of PAD, despite absence of suggestive history or physical examination findings

Applying to Clinical Practice
- Most ABI testing will be done to evaluate symptoms rather than asymptomatic screening.
- Screening of higher risk patients may allow for early initiation of medication management, so consider performing ABI in asymptomatic high-risk patients who aren't already on antiplatelet and statin therapy.

Practice Pearls

- Patients at increased risk of PAD:
  - Age ≥ 65 y.
  - Age 50–64 y, with atherosclerotic risk factors or family history of PAD.
  - Age < 50 y with DM and 1 additional atherosclerotic risk factor.
  - Known atherosclerotic disease in another vascular bed.
- Suggestive history and physical examination findings: claudication, nonjoint-related exertional lower extremity symptoms, impaired walking function, ischemic rest pain, abnormal lower extremity pulses, vascular bruit, nonhealing lower extremity wound, lower extremity gangrene, elevation pallor, dependent rubor.

Sources
–*JAMA*. 2018;320(2):177–183.
–AHA/ACC. *Circulation*. 2017;135(12):e686–e725.

Management: Adults

Recommendations from

> NICE 2020, ACC/AHA 2016

–If history or physical examination suggest PAD (most common initial symptom: intermittent claudication), use the resting ankle-brachial index (ABI) to establish the diagnosis.
  - Ensure patient is resting and supine while obtaining systolic blood pressures of brachial arteries, posterior tibialis artery, dorsal pedal artery, and peroneal arteries. If a wave exists,

consider using a Doppler probe to determine type of velocity wave form (triphasic, biphasic, or monophasic).

- Report resting ABI results as abnormal (ABI ≤ 0.90), borderline (ABI 0.91–0.99), normal (ABI 1.00–1.40), or noncompressible (ABI > 1.40).

–Measure toe-brachial index (TBI) to diagnose patients with suspected PAD when the ABI > 1.40 (noncompressible).

–As the ABI in longstanding T2DM may be normal or elevated due to systemic hardening of the arteries, consider imaging if clinically concerned.

–Use duplex ultrasound of the lower extremities to diagnose anatomic location and severity of stenosis for patients with symptomatic PAD if revascularization is being considered. If nondiagnostic, use MRA. If MRA is contraindicated, use CTA.

–Counsel patients with PAD and DM about self-foot examination and healthy foot behaviors.

–Use antiplatelet therapy with aspirin alone (range 75–325 mg/d) or clopidogrel alone (75 mg/d), smoking cessation, a statin, and good glycemic control to reduce MI, stroke, and vascular death in patients with symptomatic PAD.

–Use cilostazol to improve symptoms and increase walking distance in patients with claudication.

–Recommend a supervised exercise program for patients with claudication to improve functional status and quality of life and to reduce leg symptoms. A supervised program should involve 120 min of supervised exercise a week for at least 3 mo. The exercise should reach a point of maximal reproduced pain.

–Refer to angioplasty if the exercise program is nonsatisfactory and modifiable risk factors are addressed but nonsatisfactory for symptoms. Endovascular procedures are effective as a revascularization option for patients with lifestyle-limiting claudication and hemodynamically significant aortoiliac occlusive disease.

–Endovascular procedures establish in-line blood flow to the foot in patients with nonhealing wounds or gangrene.

–In patients with critical limb ischemia, perform revascularization when possible and construct bypass to the popliteal or infrapopliteal arteries (ie, tibial, pedal) with suitable autogenous vein. Critical limb ischemia shows diminished circulation, ischemic pain, ulceration, tissue loss, or gangrene. Twenty percent of critical limb ischemia goes onto amputation.

–In patients with acute limb ischemia (ALI), give systemic anticoagulation with heparin immediately unless contraindicated.

–Monitor and treat patients with ALI (eg, fasciotomy) for compartment syndrome after revascularization.

–Perform amputation as the first procedure in patients with a nonsalvageable limb.

Practice Pearls

- Recommend bare metal stents when stenting people with intermittent claudication.
- Prefer autologous vein bypass when possible for infrainguinal bypass surgery.
- Prefer bypass surgery over stenting for aortoiliac or femoropopliteal stenosis causing intermittent claudication or critical limb ischemia.
- Stenting is an option for complete aortoiliac occlusion.

Sources

–*NICE Guidelines CG147*. Peripheral arterial disease: diagnosis and management. Updated 11 December 2020.

–2016 AHA/ACC guideline on the management of patients with lower extremity peripheral artery disease: executive summary. *Circulation*. 2017;135:e686–e725.

–https://guidelines.gov/summaries/summary/38409

PREOPERATIVE EVALUATION

Management: Adults

Recommendations from

> ESC 2022

Preoperative Evaluation

–Do not obtain routine ECG in asymptomatic patients undergoing low-risk[1] surgical procedures.

–Consider ECG in patients with known coronary heart disease, significant arrhythmia, peripheral arterial disease, or other structural heart disease or are >65-y-old.

–Do NOT routinely perform chest X-rays preoperatively.

–Do NOT routinely test for hemoglobin in healthy, asymptomatic patients. Consider in patients with history of anemia or with prior anticoagulation.

–If known or suspected sleep apnea, communicate with the surgical and anesthesia teams.

–Initiate smoking cessation before elective surgery.

–Delay elective noncardiac surgery at least 60 d after myocardial infarction unless coronary intervention.

Perioperative Medications

–If patients have been on beta-blockers, continue, but do not start on the day of surgery to reduce perioperative risk.

–Hold ACEi and ARBs the morning of the surgery (risk for intraoperative hypotension morbidity). No specific recommendation recording calcium channel blockers or diuretic therapies.

–Do not start alpha-2-agonists to prevent cardiac events in noncardiac surgery.

–Continue statins perioperatively.

–If patients require urgent noncardiac surgery in the 4–6 wk after bare metal or drug-eluting stent, continue dual antiplatelets unless relative risk of bleeding exceeds benefit of preventing stent thrombosis.

–If patients on dual antiplatelets for coronary stents require the P2Y12 platelet receptor-inhibitor to be stopped, continue the aspirin if possible and restart the P2Y12 receptor-inhibitor as soon as possible.

---

[1] ACC/AHA: low risk means combined surgical and patient characteristics that predict risk of a major adverse cardiac event (MACE) of death or MI of <1%.

Practice Pearl

- ACC *Choosing Wisely*: Do not obtain stress cardiac imaging or advanced noninvasive imaging as a preoperative assessment in patients scheduled to undergo low-risk noncardiac surgery.

Sources
   –http://www.choosingwisely.org/societies/american-college-of-cardiology/
   –https://www.icsi.org/guideline/perioperative-guideline/

VALVULAR HEART DISEASE (VHD)

Management: Adults Who Require Anticoagulation for Valvular Disease

Recommendations from

➤ AHA/ACC/HRS 2020, ESC 2018, ACCP 2018
   –If mechanical valve present, anticoagulate with warfarin titrated to following INR goals:
   - Mitral valve: INR 2.5–3.5.
   - Aortic valve without increased risk factors for VTE: INR 2.0–3.0.
   - Aortic valve with increased risk factors for VTE (AF, prior VTE, LV dysfunction, hypercoagulable state): INR 2.5–3.5. Bridge with heparin or low-molecular-weight heparin for procedures that require warfarin to be held. Do not use direct thrombin inhibitors (dabigatran/edoxaban) or DOAC (rivaroxaban/apixaban).
   –DOAC may be used in mild to moderate valvular disease. They are also likely acceptable in aortic stenosis (including severe) and >3 mo after mitral valve repair or bioprosthetic valve placement.

Sources
   –*Eur Heart J.* 2018;39(16):1330–1393.
   –*Chest.* 2018;154(4):1121–1201.
   –2019 AHA/ACC/HRS focused update of the 2014 AHA/ACC/HRS. Guideline for the management of patients with atrial fibrillation.
   –*Circulation.* 2021;143:e72–e227.

Management: Adults with Valvular Heart Disease

See the following sections for specific guidance on aortic stenosis, aortic regurgitation, mitral stenosis, mitral regurgitation, and mitral regurgitation as related to infective endocarditis and bicuspid aortic valve.

Recommendations from

➤ ACC/AHA 2020
   –Obtain TTE with 2D or 3D evaluation of chamber volume. Doppler echo gives noninvasive determination of valve dynamics. Each subtype of VHD has different recommendations of follow-up imaging if TTE is discordant with clinical picture.
   –In valvular stenosis, important measurements are maximum velocity across the valve, mean pressure gradient, and valve area.

–In valvular regurgitation, important measurements are regurgitant surface area, volume fraction, and severity grade.

–Patients should be seen at least annually for clinical evaluation. Repeat TTE if there are new symptoms or a change in physical exam.

–Valve replacement replaces a native value disease with a palliated valve disease. If choosing between mechanical and bioprosthetic valves, then patient is choosing between risk of long-term anticoagulation with warfarin vs. a risk of reintervention. Therefore, generally older patients receive bioprosthetic valves and younger patients receive mechanical valves.

–If AF develops in first 3 mo after a bioprosthetic valve replacement, use warfarin. After 3 mo with new bioprosthetic valve, if AF develops, can use a DOAC.

–With a mechanical heart valve, the corresponding INR goals for warfarin depend on the location of the valve. Determine the INR at least weekly during initiation and at least monthly when anticoagulation is stable following these goals:

  • Mitral valve: INR 2.5–3.5.
  • Aortic valve without increased risk factors for VTE: INR 2.0–3.0.
  • Aortic valve with increased risk factors for VTE (AF, prior VTE, LV dysfunction, hypercoagulable state): INR 2.5–3.5.

–Symptoms ongoing after valve replacement may be due to irreversible causes of valve disease such as LV dysfunction, pulmonary HTN, or RV dysfunction. Also, may be due to concurrent noncardiac etiologies or other cardiac etiology.

–After repair, repeat TTE at 1–3 mo. Then patients should be seen at least annually for clinical evaluation.

–Risk calculator for valve replacement surgery: https://riskcalc.sts.org/stswebriskcalc/calculate

Management: Adults with Aortic Stenosis (AS)

Recommendations from

> ACC/AHA 2020

–No medical therapy is available to specifically address AS symptoms or disease progression.

–On TTE, note that velocity and pressure gradients across the valve measured by Doppler may be underestimated if the patient is hypertensive.

–Note that pressure gradients are underestimated if there is LV dysfunction.

–In severe AS with velocity > 4.0 m/s, rate of progression is high.

–Exercise treadmill testing is rarely indicated but helpful to evaluate patients who have discordant echo/clinical findings (ie, moderate or severe stenosis in the absence of expected symptoms). Previously undetected symptoms of chest pain, shortness of breath, exertional dizziness, or syncope may be identified to prevent sudden death.

–GDMT for HF should be continued in AS.

–Statins prevent atherosclerosis in calcific AS but do not prevent progression of AS hyperdynamics.

–Treat hypertension in the presence of significant AS. HTN doubles the risk for mortality in AS and increases the risk for cardiovascular event in AS. However, abruptly lowering the systolic blood pressure should be avoided so start medication at low dose and increase slowly over months. Resolving the HTN will not stop AS progression.

–Strong indications for aortic valve replacement (AVR):
- Symptomatic patient (exertional dyspnea or presyncope, HF, angina, syncope).
- Asymptomatic patients with severe AS and decreased LV function (EF 50%).
- Asymptomatic patient with severe AS already undergoing another cardiac surgery.

–Percutaneous aortic balloon dilation procedure should be considered a "bridging therapy" to surgical AVR or TAVR/TAVI therapy. However, this procedure is used less frequently in adults given increased availability and success of transcatheter intervention. It is now mostly used in children, adolescents, and young adults.

Management: Adults with Aortic Regurgitation (AR)

Recommendations from

> ACC/AHA 2020

–Endocarditis is the most common cause of AR. Other causes include aortic dissection, transcatheter procedure, or blunt chest trauma.

–Acute AR may acutely lead to higher LV volumes contributing to low cardiac output and pulmonary congestion.
- Using beta-blockers for associated ascending aortic dissection or aneurysm may increase the transaortic stroke volume, causing a paradoxical increase in systolic blood pressure. Go slowly.
- Do not use beta-blockers in other causes of AR. Cardiac output may suffer without the compensatory tachycardia.

–Cardiac magnetic resonance (CMR) is an alternative form of evaluation if the TTE is nondiagnostic or suboptimal.

–Treat hypertension to keep SBP < 140 mmHg with nondihydropyridine calcium channel blocker, ACEi, or ARB agent.

–Strong indications for AVR:
- Symptomatic (decrease in exercise capacity) with severe AR.
- Asymptomatic with chronic AR and LVEF < 55%.
- Going for another cardiac surgery and have severe AR.

Management: Adults with Mitral Regurgitation (MR)

Recommendations from

> ACC/AHA 2020, 2017

–Determine etiology of MR: primary (papillary muscle rupture, mitral valve prolapse, etc.) or secondary (dilated LV).

–Treatment options for primary MR:
- Observe with periodic monitoring (TEE q6–12 mo) if nonsevere or severe/asymptomatic but repair/replacement contraindicated.
- Refer for repair if stage C1[1] and likelihood of successful repair is >95% with <1% mortality.
- Refer for replacement if symptomatic, or asymptomatic but LVEF 30%–60% or LVEF > 60% but falling.

[1] Stage C1: Asymptomatic; LVEF > 60% and LVEDS < 40 mm, or new-onset AF or PASP > 50 mmHg.

–Treatment options for secondary MR:
- Refer for replacement if severe MR with persistent class III–IV symptoms.
- Otherwise, optimize therapies for CAD and CHF, consider cardiac resynchronization therapy if indicated, and monitor with TEE q6–12 mo.

Management: Adults with Mitral Regurgitation Related to Infective Endocarditis

Recommendations from

⯈ ACC/AHA 2017

–Valve surgery during initial hospitalization before completion of full course of antibiotics is indicated for infective endocarditis (IE) associated with:
- Valve dysfunction resulting in symptoms of HF.
- Left-sided IE caused by *S. aureus*, fungal, or other highly resistant organisms.
- Complicated by heart block, annular or aortic abscess, or destructive penetrating lesions.

–Evidence of persistent infection as manifested by persistent bacteremia or fevers lasting longer than 5–7 d after onset of appropriate antimicrobial therapy.

–Surgery is recommended for patients with prosthetic valve endocarditis and relapsing infection (defined as recurrence of bacteremia after a complete course of appropriate antibiotics and subsequently negative blood cultures) without other identifiable source for portal of infection.

–Complete removal of pacemaker or defibrillator systems, including all leads and the generator, is indicated as part of the early management plan in patients with IE with documented infection of the device or leads.

Management: Adults with Mitral Stenosis

Recommendations from

⯈ ACC/AHA 2020

–The majority of mitral stenosis is due to rheumatic heart disease. The time between initial rheumatic illness and MS can be decades. In older people, the cause of MS is more often calcific MS. Between age and comorbidities, the prognosis of calcific MS is <50% in 5 y, meaning the indications for intervention are palliative in highly asymptomatic patients.

–Consider transesophageal echocardiogram (TEE) prior to sending the patient for percutaneous mitral balloon commissurotomy (PMBC) to exclude the presence of left atrial thrombus.

–Give warfarin to patients with mitral stenosis and AF, prior embolic event, or intracardiac thrombus. Rheumatic MS patients were excluded from DOAC studies, hence indication for warfarin in Afib.

–Use rate control in Afib and MS to allow optimal diastolic filling time across the stenotic valve. The fibrosis in rheumatic MS may also make it more challenging to rhythm control.

–To increase exercise duration and improve symptoms in younger people, beta-blockers or ivabradine may be beneficial.

–Balloon commissurotomy is indicated in symptomatic patients with severe mitral stenosis (MVA < 1.5 cm^2) with no atrial thrombus and no or minimal mitral insufficiency. In rheumatic disease, delay until NYHA III or IV due to slow course of disease.

–Mitral valve replacement is indicated if balloon commissurotomy is contraindicated in a patient with severe symptoms and severe mitral stenosis.

Management: Adults with Bicuspid Aortic Valve (BAV)

Recommendations from

> ### ACC/AHA 2020

–Aortic aneurysms will affect 20%–40% of adults with BAV. They therefore require lifelong surveillance even in the absence of symptoms.

–Replace the valve if the diameter of the ascending aorta or aortic sinuses is >5.5 cm.

Sources

–*Circulation.* 2021;143:e72–e227.

–*Circulation.* 2017;135:e1159–e1195.

ENDOCRINE AND METABOLIC DISORDERS

ADRENAL INCIDENTALOMAS

Management: Adults

Recommendations from

➤ AACE 2009

–In adults incidentally found to have an adrenal mass, evaluate clinically, biochemically, and radiographically for evidence of hypercortisolism, aldosteronism, the presence of pheochromocytoma, or a malignant tumor.

–Reevaluate patients who will be managed expectantly at 3–6 mo and then annually for 1–2 y.

Practice Pearls

- Use a 1-mg overnight dexamethasone suppression test to screen for hypercortisolism.
- Measure plasma-fractionated metanephrines and normetanephrines to screen for pheochromocytoma.
- Measure plasma renin activity and aldosterone concentration to assess for primary or secondary aldosteronism.

Source

–https://pro.aace.com/files/adrenal-guidelines.pdf

CUSHING SYNDROME

Management: Children and Adults

Recommendations from

➤ Endocrine Society 2015

–Treatment goals:

- • Normalize cortisol levels to eliminate signs and symptoms.
- • Monitor and treat cortisol-dependent comorbidities.

–Vaccinate against influenza, herpes zoster, pneumococcus.

–Use perioperative thromboprophylaxis for venous thromboembolism.

–Refer for surgical resection of primary adrenal or ectopic focus.

–Assess postoperative serum cortisol levels.

Source

–www.endocrine.org/guidelines-and-clinical-practice/clinical-practice-guidelines/treatment-of-cushing-syndrome

DIABETES MELLITUS (DM), TYPE 1 (T1DM)

Management: Children and Adolescents

Recommendations from

> ADA 2023, NICE 2023, Endocrine Society 2022

Evaluation

–Screen for other autoimmune conditions at the time of diagnosis of T1DM:

- Celiac disease: IgA tissue transglutaminase antibodies. If negative, rescreen at 2 and 5 y after DM diagnosis.
- Thyroid disease: check TSH, thyroid peroxidase, and thyroglobulin antibodies; screen q1–2 y thereafter.
- Pernicious anemia: check B_{12} level if anemia or peripheral neuropathy is present. (ADA)
- Hypertension: check BP[1] at diagnosis and each follow-up visit.
- Consider screening for sleep health, including sleep disorders and sleep disruptions due to diabetes symptoms or management needs. Refer to sleep medicine and/or behavioral health professional as indicated. (ADA)

Therapies

–Use insulin therapy with multiple injections daily, either via basal plus prandial insulin or an insulin pump and ensure rotation of injection sites. (NICE)

–Instruct patients using multiple insulin injections to self-monitor blood glucose at least 5 times daily. (NICE)

–Offer diabetes self-management education and support. Consider social determinants of health of the target population to guide design and delivery of diabetes self-management education and support with the ultimate goal of health equity across all populations. (ADA)

–Offer medical nutrition therapy, preferably with a registered dietitian nutritionist.

–Encourage physical activity: 60 min/d of moderate-intensity aerobic activity, 3 d/wk of muscle and bone-strengthening activities.

–Assess psychological and social situation. Screen/refer to specialist for anxiety, depression, disordered eating.

–Encourage at least 4 clinic visits per year. (NICE)

–Advise all patients not to smoke.

–Consider statin therapy if age ≥ 10 y and LDL ≥ 160 mg/dL, or LDL ≥ 130 mg/dL and one or more cardiovascular disease (CVD) risk factors.

---

[1] For patients < 13 y, BP goal is <90th percentile for age, sex, and height. For patients ≥13-y-old, BP goal is <120/80 mmHg. Use lifestyle modifications as first-line intervention and ACEI or ARB as first-line pharmacotherapy.

–Advise on higher risk of periodontitis and recommend regular oral health reviews, as managing periodontitis can improve glycemic control. (NICE)

–Encourage eye exams every 2 y. (NICE)

–Consider continuous glucose monitoring, as it results in lower HbA1c levels.

–Consider referral to government disability for medication and social support. (NICE)

–Encourage annual immunization against influenza at 6-mo-old. (NICE)

–Encourage pneumococcal vaccine if taking insulin or oral hypoglycemic medication. (NICE)

Guidelines Alert 3–1
GUIDELINES DISCORDANT: GLYCEMIC CONTROL TARGETS IN CHILDREN WITH T1DM

Organization	Guidance
ADA	HbA1c goal < 7% appropriate for most, <6.5% if obtainable without hypoglycemia, or 7%–8% if hypoglycemia unawareness
NICE	Glucose targets are: • 72–126 mg/dL fasting • 72–126 mg/dL before meals • 90–162 mg/dL 90 min after meals • >90 mg/dL while driving • HbA1c ≤ 6.5%

Applying to Clinical Practice
• Tight glycemic control in T1DM slows progression to end-organ damage.
• A1c of <6.5% may not be practical or safe for some patients, which is acknowledged explicitly in the ADA guideline.

Guidelines Alert 3–2
GUIDELINES DISCORDANT: SURVEILLANCE FOR END-ORGAN DAMAGE IN CHILDREN WITH T1DM

Organization	Guidance
ADA	Begin screening at age 10, at onset of puberty, or 5 y after diagnosis of T1DM, whichever is earlier: • Albuminuria: albumin-to-creatinine ratio (ACR) annually • Retinopathy: fundoscopic exam every 2–4 y • Comprehensive foot exam and monofilament testing annually • Lipid panel near time of diagnosis, at 9–11 y, and q3 y thereafter • If abnormal, confirm with fasting labs and repeat annually
NICE	Begin screening annually at 12 y of age: • Thyroid disease • Hypertension Albuminuria: urine ACR • Retinopathy: fundoscopic exam • Comprehensive foot examination and monofilament testing

Applying to Clinical Practice
• The subtle differences between the guidelines are unlikely to have patient-oriented significance.

Sources

–https://diabetesjournals.org/care/article/46/Supplement_1/S230/148046/14-Children-and-Adolescents-Standards-of-Care-in

–https://www.nice.org.uk/guidance/ng18

–Endocrine Society. *Management of Individuals with Diabetes at High Risk for Hypoglycemia: An Endocrine Society Clinical Practice Guideline*. 2022. https://doi.org/10.1210/clinem/dgac596

Management: Adults

Recommendations from

> **ADA 2023, NICE 2023, Endocrine Society 2022, KDIGO 2022**

Evaluation

–Do not routinely confirm diagnosis of T1DM by checking C-peptide levels or autoantibody testing. Consider doing so only if diagnosis is uncertain.[1] (NICE)

–Screen for other autoimmune conditions at the time of diagnosis of T1DM (ADA):

- Celiac disease: consider screening with IgA tissue transglutaminase antibodies if suggestive symptoms (eg, diarrhea, malabsorption, abdominal pain) or signs (eg, osteoporosis, vitamin deficiencies, iron deficiency anemia).
- Thyroid dysfunction: check TSH, thyroid peroxidase, and thyroglobulin antibodies initially; routine screening thereafter.
- Pernicious anemia: check B_{12} level if anemia or peripheral neuropathy is present.

–Consider screening for other associated conditions including autoimmune hepatitis, primary adrenal insufficiency (Addison disease), collagen vascular diseases, and myasthenia gravis. T1DM may also occur with other autoimmune diseases in the context of specific genetic disorders or polyglandular autoimmune syndromes.

Therapies

–If using multiple insulin injections, self-monitor blood glucose at least 4 times daily.

–Use basal insulin (NICE: preferably detemir BID) plus at least twice-a-day prandial insulin before meals.

–If available, an insulin pump is a useful alternative. (ADA)

–Consider continuous glucose monitoring, as it results in lower HbA1c levels.

–Consider one of the following as an alternative basal insulin therapy to twice-daily insulin detemir (NICE):

- An insulin regimen that is already being used by patient if it meets their treatment goals (eg, meeting HbA1c targets or time in target glucose range and minimizing hypoglycemia).
- Once-daily glargine if detemir is not tolerated or patient has strong preference for once-daily basal injections.
- Once-daily degludec if concern about nocturnal hypoglycemia.
- Once-daily ultra–long-acting insulin such as degludec if patient needs assistance to administer injections.

---

[1] The false-negative rate of diabetes-specific autoantibody tests is lowest at the time of diagnosis, and the false-negative rate can be reduced by carrying out quantitative tests for 2 different diabetes-specific autoantibodies (with at least 1 being positive).

–Provide all adults with T1DM a structured education program including carbohydrate counting education, benefits of routine exercise, avoidance of smoking, management of hypoglycemia, and peer support groups.

–Advise on higher risk of periodontitis and recommend regular oral health reviews, as managing periodontitis can improve glycemic control. (NICE)

Surveillance

–Measure glycohemoglobin every 3–6 mo. Fructosamine level is an alternative test for anemic patients.

–Surveillance for complications:

- Urine ACR ratio annually.
- Dilated fundoscopic exam upon diagnosis and q2y after initial assessment.
- Monofilament screening for diabetic neuropathy annually.
- Comprehensive foot examination at least annually.

–Fasting lipid panel: repeat annually if results are abnormal or q5y if results are acceptable (LDL < 100 mg/dL).

–TSH annually. (NICE)

–Consider screening for sleep health, including sleep disorders and sleep disruptions due to diabetes symptoms or management needs. Refer to sleep medicine and/or behavioral health professional as indicated. (ADA)

Guidelines Alert 3–3	
GUIDELINES DISCORDANT: GLYCEMIC CONTROL TARGETS IN ADULTS WITH T1DM	
Organization	**Guidance**
ADA	HbA1c goal < 7% appropriate for most, <6.5% if obtainable without hypoglycemia, or 7%–8% if hypoglycemia unawareness
NICE	Glucose targets are: • 90–126 mg/dL fasting • 72–126 mg/dL before meals • 90–162 mg/dL 90 min after meals • HbA1c ≤6.5%

Applying to Clinical Practice
- Tight glycemic control in T1DM slows progression to end-organ damage.
- A1c of <6.5% may not be practical or safe for some patients.

Guidelines Alert 3–4	
GUIDELINES DISCORDANT: ROLE OF STATINS IN T1DM	
Organization	**Guidance**
ADA	Consider the use of moderate-intensity statin therapy in those with T1DM who have one or more ASCVD risk factors

NICE	Consider statin therapy for all with T1DM Prescribe atorvastatin 20 mg for those that are older than 40 y, have had T1DM > 10 y, have nephropathy, or have other CVD risk factors
ESC 2019	Consider starting a statin in all patients >30 y with T1DM, even if asymptomatic or with normal lipid panel

Applying to Clinical Practice
- Statins are well tolerated and effective in preventing ASCVD.
- While not required in all patients with T1DM, those with risk factors are likely to benefit.

Guidelines Alert 3–5
GUIDELINES DISCORDANT: ROLE OF ASPIRIN IN T1DM

Organization	Guidance
ADA	Consider aspirin 75–162 mg/d for adults with a 10-y risk of CVD > 10% Provide aspirin 75–162 mg/d if preexisting CVD is present
NICE	Do *not* offer aspirin for primary prevention of CVD to adults with T1DM

Applying to Clinical Practice
- Aspirin modestly reduces ischemic vascular events. The main adverse effect is an increased risk of gastrointestinal bleeding. For adults with ASCVD risk > 1% per year, the number of ASCVD events prevented will be similar to the number of episodes of bleeding induced, although these complications do not have equal effects on long-term health.
- Avoid routine aspirin use for primary prevention, though it may be considered in the context of shared decision-making in younger patients with higher cardiovascular risk and low bleeding risk.
- Use aspirin routinely for secondary prevention with patients who have documented ASCVD.

Sources
–https://diabetesjournals.org/care/issue/46/Supplement_1

–https://nice.org.uk/guidance/ng17

–https://academic.oup.com/eurheartj/article/41/2/255/5556890

–Endocrine Society. *Management of Individuals with Diabetes at High Risk for Hypoglycemia: An Endocrine Society Clinical Practice Guideline.* 2022. https://doi.org/10.1210/clinem/dgac596

–KDIGO. *Clinical Practice Guideline for Diabetes Management in Chronic Kidney Disease.* 2022.

DIABETES MELLITUS (DM), TYPE 2 (T2DM)

Screening: Adults

Recommendations from

➤ USPSTF 2021, ADA 2023, IDF 2017

See Ch 16 for screening recommendations for children and adolescents.
See Ch 11 for screening recommendations specific to pregnancy.

Guidelines Alert 3–6 GUIDELINES DISCORDANT: WHO TO SCREEN FOR T2DM	
Organization	**Guidance**
ADA	All adults beginning age 35
USPSTF	Asymptomatic adults age 35–70 with (BMI) ≥ 25. Consider screening younger patients from high-prevalence populations[a] and at a lower BMI (≥23) if the patient is Asian American

Applying to Clinical Practice
- While diabetes is much less common in patients without risk factors such as obesity, the harms of screening are few.
- If a patient with a normal BMI is interested in diabetes screening, it is reasonable to offer it after age 35.

[a]Alaska Native, Black, Hawaiian/Pacific Islander, Latino persons.

–Offer patients with prediabetes effective preventative interventions.
–Screen individuals planning pregnancy who are overweight or have one or more risk factors for diabetes.
–Screen individuals with a history of gestational diabetes at least every 3 y for life.
–Screen HIV positive patients with a fasting blood glucose (FBG) before starting antiretroviral therapy, when switching antiretroviral therapy, and 3–6 mo after starting or switching therapy.
–Screen patients with prediabetes annually for the development of diabetes.
–Screen with a fasting blood glucose, 2-h plasma glucose after 75-g oral GTT, or HgbA1c.

Practice Pearls

- Repeat screening at least every 3 y in asymptomatic adults above the age of 35.
- Screen and treat patients with prediabetes for modifiable cardiovascular risk factors such as hypertension and dyslipidemia.
- Risk factors for diabetes and prediabetes in asymptomatic adults:
  - First-degree relative with diabetes.
  - High-risk race/ethnicity (eg, Black, Latino, Alaska Native, Asian, Pacific Islander persons).
  - History of CVD.
  - Hypertension.

  - HDL < 35 and/or triglycerides > 250.
  - Patients with polycystic ovary syndrome (PCOS).
  - Physical inactivity.
  - Increased abdominal waist circumference.
  - Clinical conditions associated with insulin resistance (eg, severe obesity, acanthosis nigricans).
- Risk factors for diabetes and prediabetes in asymptomatic children:
  - Maternal history of diabetes found to have abnormal glucose metabolism.
  - Family history of T2DM in first- or second-degree relatives.
  - High-risk race/ethnicity (eg, Black, Latino, Alaska Native, Asian, Pacific Islander persons).
  - Clinical conditions associated with insulin resistance (eg, acanthosis nigricans, hypertension, dyslipidemia, PCOS, small-for-gestational-age birth weight).
- Criteria for diagnosing diabetes:
  - Fasting plasma glucose ≥ 126 mg/dL (fasting is no caloric intake for at least 8 h)*

                                OR

  - 2-h plasma glucose ≥ 200 mg/dL during OGTT, using the 75-g anhydrous glucose dissolved in water*

                                OR

  - A1c ≥ 6.5% (using a method that is National Glycohemoglobin Standardization Program certified)*

                                OR

  - Classic symptoms of hyperglycemia with a random plasma glucose ≥ 200 mg/dL

  *Diagnosis requires two abnormal test results from either the same sample or two separate test samples unless patient has unequivocal hyperglycemia. Plasma blood glucose criteria ideally should be used instead of A1c for those with sickle cell disease, pregnancy, G6PD, HIV, hemodialysis, recent blood loss or transfusion, or erythropoietin therapy.

Sources

–USPSTF. *Recommendation: Screening for Prediabetes and Type 2 Diabetes*. 2021.

–ADA. Standards of medical care in diabetes—2023. *Diabetes Care*. 2023;46(1):S19–S32.

–International Diabetes Federation. *IDF Clinical Practice Recommendations for Managing Type 2 Diabetes in Primary Care*. 2017. www.idf.org/managing-type2-diabetes

Prevention: Adults with Prediabetes

Recommendations from

➤ ADA 2023, AACE 2023

–A variety of eating patterns are acceptable for persons with prediabetes, impaired glucose tolerance (IGT), or impaired fasting glucose.[1]

–Employ intensive behavioral lifestyle intervention with a goal of sustained 7%–10% weight loss (AACE).

---

[1] *Prediabetes* is the term used for individuals whose glucose levels do not meet the criteria for diabetes yet have impaired fasting glucose and/or impaired glucose tolerance and/or A1c 5.7%–6.4%. Impaired fasting glucose is a fasting glucose of 100–125 mg/dL and impaired glucose tolerance is a 2-h glucose after 75-g anhydrous glucose load of 140–199 mg/dL.

–Recommend regular physical activity including moderate aerobic activity of at least 150 min/week over 2–3 d and resistance exercise 2–3 times per week. (AACE)

–Encourage nonsedentary leisure activities. (AACE)

–Pursue tobacco cessation.

–Obtain 6–8 h of sleep a night; purse OSA evaluation based on STOP-BANG scoring. (AACE)

–Consider metformin for patients at highest risk for developing diabetes (eg, those aged 25–59 y with BMI 35, higher fasting plasma glucose of $\geq$110 mg/dL, A1c of $\geq$6.0%, and individuals with prior GDM). Consider periodic measurement of vitamin B_{12} levels for those on long-term use of metformin, especially in the setting of peripheral neuropathy or anemia.

–Consider pharmacotherapy for weight loss if lifestyle is not sufficient. Options include phentermine, topiramate ER, metformin, pioglitazone, and acarbose. (AACE)

–Based on patient preference, consider technology-assisted diabetes prevention interventions (eg, SBGM) as they may be effective in preventing T2DM.

–Monitor at least annually for the development of T2DM.

–Screen for and treat modifiable cardiovascular risk factors including hypertension and dyslipidemia.

–For those with a history of stroke and evidence of insulin resistance and prediabetes, consider pioglitazone to lower the risk of stroke or myocardial infarction. This should be balanced with the increased risk of weight gain, edema, and fracture.

–For individuals with prediabetes and cardiometabolic risk factors who either have elevated liver enzymes (ALT) or fatty liver on imaging, evaluate for the presence of nonalcoholic steatohepatitis and liver fibrosis.

Practice Pearls

- An integrated lifestyle change program, such as the CDC's National Diabetes Prevention Program,[1] reduces the progression to diabetes by more than 50%. This intervention included 7% weight loss, reducing intake of fat and calories, and exercising 150 min/wk. This is twice the benefit seen with metformin, and the benefit persisted 15 y after the initial intervention (https://www.niddk.nih.gov/about-niddk/research-areas/diabetes/diabetes-prevention-program-dpp).

- Older adults with prediabetes are unlikely to ever develop diabetes. (*JAMA Intern Med.* 2021; 181(4):511–519)

Source
–*Diabetes Care*. Standard of Care in Diabetes. 2023;46(suppl 1):S41–S48.

Management: Adults in the Outpatient Setting

Management of adults with comorbid coronary artery disease and hypertension is discussed in Ch 2.

Management of adults with comorbid coronary kidney disease is discussed in Ch 13.

Management of pregnant people with diabetes is discussed in Ch 11.

[1] https://www.cdc.gov/diabetes/prevention/index.html

Recommendations from

> AACE/ACE 2023, ACP 2017/2018/2024, ADA 2023, ESC 2019, NICE 2022, Endocrine Society 2022, KDIGO 2022, ACSM 2022

Lifestyle Interventions

–Weight loss:
  - Recommend >5% weight loss if overweight or obese; consider adjunctive weight loss medications approved by FDA. (ADA, AACE, IDF)
  - Consider more intensive weight loss goals (ie, 15%) to maximize benefit depending on need, feasibility, and safety.
  - Larger, sustained weight losses (>10%) usually confer greater benefits, including disease-modifying effects and possible remission of T2DM, and may improve long-term cardiovascular outcomes, NAFLD, sleep apnea, osteoarthritis, and mortality. (ADA, AACE)
  - Consider addition of pharmacotherapy for weight loss if BMI > 27. (AACE)
  - Consider bariatric surgery for BMI 27–35 and refer to bariatric surgery for BMI > 35 good surgical candidates. (AACE)

–Exercise:
  - Regular physical activity (150 min/wk moderate aerobic activity), supplemented with 2–3 resistance, flexibility, and/or balance training sessions/wk. (ADA, AACE, IDF, ACSM)
  - Encourage reduced sedentary time and breaking up sitting time with frequent small "doses" of activity throughout the day. (ADA, ACSM)

–Team-based care:
  - Use a multidisciplinary model (including physicians, nurses, dietitians, exercise specialists, dentists, podiatrists, mental health, etc.) to assess barriers to care, including food, housing, and financial insecurity as well as literacy and numeracy. Refer to available community resources.
  - Consider socioeconomic factors that may impact nutrition choices, such as food insecurity and cultural circumstances. (ADA)

–Counsel regarding limited alcohol use to alcohol cessation. (AACE)

–Screen for mood disturbances. (AACE)

–Sleep: (AACE)
  - Screen for sleep disturbances
  - Sleep goal should be 6–8 h
  - If BMI > 27 refer to sleep study

–Provide diabetes self-management education and support at appropriate intervals including education about hypoglycemia management and adjustments during illness. Complement in-person visits with telehealth and other digital solutions to optimize glycemic management and offer self-management education and clinical support. (ADA, Endocrine Society)

–Advise against tobacco use, including e-cigarettes (given evidence of associated deaths), and provide smoking cessation counseling/treatment routinely.

Therapies: Noninsulin Medications

–Individualize medication regimens and blood glucose targets (fasting and postprandial) based on patient-specific factors (likely adherence, safety, efficacy, cost, and comorbidities such as cardiac, cerebrovascular, hepatic, and renal disease). (AACE, NICE, ADA)

–Use metformin as first-line medication.[1]

–Start with metformin monotherapy unless A1c is >9%. (ADA)

–Add SGLT2i or GLP-1 when inadequate control on metformin alone. Do not add DPP-4. (ACP)

–Combination therapy is often necessary. Choose agents with complementary mechanisms of action, especially in patients with comorbidities. See Tables 3–1 and 3–2 for further guidance for patients with specific comorbidities.

–Add either a sulfonylurea, a thiazolidinedione (pioglitazone), an SGLT2i, or a DPP-4 inhibitor to metformin when a second agent is required, based on discussion of benefits, adverse effects, and cost. (ACP, NICE)

TABLE 3–1 RECOMMENDATIONS FOR ADJUNCTIVE DIABETES THERAPIES COMPLEMENTARY TO COMMON COMORBIDITIES			
Comorbidity	**ADA**	**ESC**	**AACE**
ASCVD	Add an SGLT2i or GLP-1 receptor agonist (RA) regardless of A1c unless contraindicated	Prioritize empagliflozin and/or liraglutide (both have mortality benefit and reduce CV events) Then consider canagliflozin, dapagliflozin, semaglutide, and dulaglutide (which reduce CV events)	Add GLP-1 RA (Prefer for ASCVD) or SGLT2i (Prefer for Stroke or TIA)
HF (particularly EF < 45%)	Choose SGLT2i over GLP-1 RA	Further considerations in HF: • Preferentially start sacubitril/valsartan instead of ACEI • Use GLP-1 RAs and DPP4 inhibitors except saxagliptan if additional agents are needed • Avoid thiazolidinediones • Consider device therapy (ICD, CRT, CRT-D) • Pursue CABG if 2 or 3 vessel CAD • Consider ivabradine in symptomatic patients in sinus rhythm with HR ≥ 70 and already on max therapy • Avoid aliskiren	SGLT2i over GLP-1 RA
CKD with albuminuria	Use an SGLT2i over GLP-1 RA	No recommendation	SGLT2i or GLP-1 RA
CKD without albuminuria	Either SGLT2i or GLP-1 RA	No recommendation	

[1] Titrate metformin from 500 to 2000 mg/d to minimize GI side effects.

TABLE 3–2 INTERNATIONAL PANEL GUIDELINE ON SELECTING SGLT2i OR GLP-1 RECEPTOR AGONISTS			
Population	**SGLT2i**	**GLP-1**	**Comments**
Patients with 3 cardiovascular risk factors[a] or fewer	Avoid for most		While there is a small mortality benefit with both agents and small cardiovascular benefit with SGLT2is, there is a large increase in genital infections (vaginitis, balanitis) with SGLT2is and severe GI events (pain, nausea, vomiting, diarrhea) with GLP-1s
Patients with >3 cardiovascular risk factors	Consider for most	Avoid for most	The mortality benefit for SGLT2is becomes more pronounced in higher risk patients
Patients with established cardiovascular or renal disease	Offer one or the other to most		Both agents offer mortality benefit; GLP-1 reduces stroke incidence and SGLT2is reduce nonfatal MI and heart failure exacerbations in this group
Patients with established cardiovascular and renal disease	Offer to all	Offer as alternative	The benefits seen in patients with cardiovascular or renal disease are more pronounced in those with both, but the mortality benefit is larger with SGLT2is

Note: A panel reviewed a meta-analysis of benefits and harms from SGLT2is and GLP-1 agents, incorporated patient focus groups, and assessed practical implications of the recommendations. These recommendations are independent of effect on A1c. Patient-oriented benefits of reducing A1c in T2DM are underwhelming, while SGLT2is and GLP-1 agents have renal- and cardioprotective benefits independent of blood glucose reduction.
[a]Risk factors: age > 60 y, male, family history of CVD or CKD, A1c > 6.5%, BP > 140/90, dyslipidemia, current smoking, or Asian/Latino/African heritage.
Source: BMJ. 2021;373:n1091. https://doi.org/10.1136/bmj.n1091

–Consider starting two agents if the HbA1c is 1%–2% or more above target. Combination therapy should be metformin plus sulfonylurea (SU),[1] DPP4 inhibitor, SGLT2i,[2] or GLP-1 RA.[3] (IDF)

–When selecting a regimen, consider approaches that support weight management goals. Dual GLP-1/glucose-dependent insulinotropic polypeptide RAs are a glucose-lowering option with the potential for weight loss. (ADA)

–Consider combination therapy with metformin and GLP-1 RA or SGL2i for patients with renal or cardiovascular comorbidities. Use of GLP-1 RA or SGLT2i may be appropriate as monotherapy if there is a contraindication to metformin. (ADA, NICE)

–Use SGLT2i for patients with T2DM and comorbidities including CVD, HFpEF/HFrEF, and CKD with eGFR ≥ 20 mL/min/1.73 m² and UACR > 3.0 mg/mmol (> 30 mg/g) independent of use of metformin or baseline HbA1C in patients with these comorbidities. (ADA)

[1] When starting an SU, the patient must learn how to prevent, recognize, and treat hypoglycemia. Avoid SU in patients on insulin therapy because of the hypoglycemia risk. Caution in hepatic impairment.
[2] SGLT2is reduce major cardiovascular events in patients with T2D and are preferred in patients with CVD. Counsel on the increased risk for urinary tract infections. Monitor volume status and BP. Discontinue prior to surgery, during illness, or fasting. Use caution in hepatic impairment.
[3] GLP-1 RA can be used if weight loss is a priority and the drug is affordable. Discontinue if suspected pancreatitis. Evaluate for gallbladder disease if cholelithiasis or cholecystitis is suspected.

–In patients with T2DM and comorbid CVD, HF, CKD, and contraindications or intolerance to SGLT2i use, consider a GLP-1 RA to reduce cardiovascular events until renal replacement therapy is indicated. (ADA)

Therapies: Insulin

–Consider initiating insulin in the following situations: ongoing catabolic weight loss, symptomatic hyperglycemia, A1c > 10%, or BG > 300 mg/dL. (ADA)

–Consider starting insulin after addition of second or third oral agent and HbA1c > 7%. (NICE)
  • Initial insulin therapy: NPH once or twice daily vs. long-acting insulin.
  • Consider basal bolus vs. premixed biphasic regimen if A1c > 9%.

–See Fig. 3–1 for a consolidated insulin initiation strategy.

–When titrating insulin, be cautious of overbasalization (basal dose > 0.5 U/kg, high bedtime–morning glucose differential, or hypoglycemia) and adjust therapy as appropriate. (ADA)

–Prefer GLP-1 RA when combination therapy is needed, as it may address prandial control while minimizing risks of hypoglycemia and weight gain associated with insulin therapy. (ADA)

–If insulin is used, choose combination therapy with a GLP-1 RA[1] as it has greater efficacy, more durable treatment effect, and more weight and hypoglycemia benefit. (ADA)

–Glycemic control recommendations: [ADA]
  • Preprandial glucose: 80–130 mg/dL.
  • Postprandial glucose: <180 mg/dL (1–2 h post meals).

FIG. 3–1 STRATEGIES FOR INSULIN INITIATION AND TITRATION IN T2DM.

(1) INITIAL THERAPY: Start basal insulin (10 U/d or 0.1–0.2 U/kg/d).
Increase q3–14d (↑10–15% or↑2–4 U) until FBG < 130–140

(2) COMBINATION THERAPY: If uncontrolled postprandial BG (>180) or A1c (>7%–8%), escalate therapy using one of the following strategies:

RAPID-ACTING INSULIN AT LARGEST MEAL	BASAL-BOLUS	ADD GLP-1 RA	PRE-MIXED INSULIN TWICE DAILY
Start 4U, 0.1 U/kg, or 10% of basal dose ↑1–2 U or 10%–15% weekly until controlled	Divide total daily insulin (0.3–0.5 U/kg) into 50% basal, 50% prandial	Could also consider SGLT2i or DPP-4i	Replace basal dose with BID dosing divided one-half to two-thirds in morning, one-third to one-half in evening
If necessary add second or third meal	Divide prandial insulin over 3 meals		

RECONSIDER: If control not achieved or therapy not tolerated, switch to a different combination therapy strategy.

HYPOGLYCEMIA: Reduce total daily insulin ↓10%–20% (40% if severe)

Source: Adapted from Figure 9.4 in *Diabetes Care 2023;*46(suppl 1):S140–S157 and Algorithm Figure 8 in *Endocr Pract.* 2023;29:305E340.

[1] Two different once-daily, fixed dual combination products containing basal insulin plus a GLP-1 RA are available: insulin glargine plus lixisenatide (iGlarLixi) and insulin degludec plus liraglutide (IDegLira).

- CGM parameters: TIR ("time-in-range") should be used to assess glucose control (associated with risk of microvascular complications) and "time below/above target" should be used to reevaluate treatment regimen.

Preventing Complications

–Minimize the risks of hypoglycemia, weight gain, and other adverse drug reactions. (AACE)

–Hypoglycemia: assess for symptomatic/asymptomatic hypoglycemia (BG < 70 mg/dL) at each visit. Prescribe IM or intranasal glucagon to patients at high risk of level 2 hypoglycemia (BG < 54 mg/dL). Reevaluate treatment regimen and glycemic targets if hypoglycemia unawareness or level 3 hypoglycemia (altered mental/physical functioning requiring assistance). (ADA)

–Control lipids and BP. (AACE)

–Start statin in patients with T2DM and risk factors of ASCVD (age > 40, HTN, CKD > 3a, smoking, family history of premature ASCVD, low HDL-C, high non-HDL-C. (NICE)

–Optimize BP alongside glycemic control to prevent progression of diabetic kidney disease.

–Instruct patients with T2DM and HTN to monitor their BP at home. (ADA)

–Recommend ACEI or ARB for patients with hypertension and diabetes with urinary ACR ratio > 30 mg/g creatinine or eGFR < 60 mL/min/1.73 m². (ADA, IDF, AACE)

- Start ACEI/ARB if patient has microalbuminuria without high BP. (IDF)

–Additional therapy with calcium channel blocker (CCB) or thiazide diuretic as needed to reach BP goals. (ADA)

–Antiplatelet agents for primary and secondary prevention of CVD are indicated.

–Maintain updated vaccination status (ADA and AACE, NICE) with pneumococcal, influenza, hepatitis B, HPV, Tdap, Zoster, and COVID-19 vaccines. See Appendix for details.

–Refer patients with any evidence of diabetic retinopathy to ophthalmologist. (ADA, NICE)

–Patients who observe Ramadan should interrupt their fast if SMBG is <70 or >300. High-risk patients are advised not to fast at all.

–Advise on higher risk of periodontitis and recommend regular oral health reviews, as managing periodontitis can improve glycemic control. (NICE)

Surveillance

–Monitor therapy q3 mo until stable, then at least twice a year. (AACE, ADA)

–On follow-up, address interval medical history, medication adherence, side effects including hypoglycemia, lab evaluation, nutrition, psychosocial health, routine health maintenance screening. (AACE, ADA)

–Perform foot examination at every visit for high-risk patients, and annually for lower risk patients. (ADA, IDF, NICE)

–Screen for or check annually:

- Lipid panel if on statin therapy (otherwise, q5 y is sufficient). (ADA)
- Dilated fundoscopic exam or retinal photography q1–2 y. (ADA, IDF)
- Monofilament screening for diabetic neuropathy. (ADA, IDF)
- Screen for peripheral vascular disease by checking foot pulses and/or calculating the ankle/brachial index. (ADA)
- Depression with PHQ-2. (IDF)

○ Consider screening for sleep health, including sleep disorders and sleep disruptions due to diabetes symptoms or management needs. Refer to sleep medicine and/or behavioral health professional as indicated. (ADA)

Guidelines Alert 3–7	
GUIDELINES DISCORDANT: A1c TARGET FOR T2DM	
Organization	**Guidance**
ADA	<7%; less (8%) or more stringent (<6.5%) goals may be appropriate for select patients
AACE	6.5%; consider higher targets if older or with comorbidities
ACP	7%–8%; de-intensify therapy if A1c < 6.5% or if life expectancy < 10 y
IDF	<7%; <8% if life expectancy < 10 y
NICE	6.5%; higher (7%) if on a drug known to cause hypoglycemia; higher targets on case-by-case basis

Applying to Clinical Practice
- Mitigation of cardiovascular risk is more important than glycemic control in T2DM.
- Guidelines favoring tight glucose control lean on studies of patients with T1DM and surrogate endpoints (ie, nerve conduction velocities).
- Guidelines favoring higher A1c targets note the failure of large studies to show patient-oriented data supporting lower targets, and the risk for harm from tighter control.
- Choose tighter targets in those patients who select them, who tolerate therapy well, and would not suffer undue burden from extra therapies.

Guidelines Alert 3–8	
GUIDELINES DISCORDANT: LIPID STRATEGY IN T2DM	
Organization	**Guidance**
ADA	High-intensity statin therapy if diabetes plus existing ASCVD or 10-y ASCVD risk > 20%. Consider addition of ezetimibe or PCSK-9 as well Moderate-intensity statin therapy if >40 y and no ASCVD or consider if <40 y with ASCVD risk Add LDL-lowering therapy (ezetimibe or PCSK9 inhibitor) if LDL > 70 mg/dL on max statin with existing CVD
ESC	Titrate lipid therapy to CV risk such that LDL < 100 for moderate risk, < 70 and with ≥50% reduction for high risk, and < 55 with ≥50% reduction for very high risk. PCSK9 is recommended in patients at very high risk of CV with high LDL-C levels on maximum tolerated statin dose. If statin not tolerated consider adding ezetimibe +/− PCSK9 inhibitor
IDF	Prescribe a high-intensity statin for patients with: established CVD (secondary prevention) or without CVD who are >40 y with LDL > 100 mg/dL (primary prevention)

Applying to Clinical Practice
- Patients with elevated ASCVD risk will benefit from statin therapy for primary prevention.

Guidelines Alert 3–9
GUIDELINES DISCORDANT: BP GOALS IN T2DM

Organization	Guidance
ADA	Target BP < 130/80 mmHg if 10-y ASCVD risk > 15% or existing ASCVD, and < 140/90 for lower risk patients. Recommend single-agent pharmacotherapy for BP > 140/90 and two-drug therapy for BP > 160/100
ESC	SBP of 120–130 and DBP of 70–80 unless age ≥ 65 without high risk of cerebrovascular events or diabetic kidney disease, in which case goal is SBP of 130–140
IDF	BP goal is 130–140/80; SBP of 130 is recommended in younger patients and those with CV risk or microvascular disease
JNC-8	<140/90

Applying to Clinical Practice
- Always lower BP below 140/90.
- For patients at higher risk of ASCVD, consider reducing BP < 130/80 if the therapy is tolerable.

Guidelines Alert 3–10
GUIDELINES DISCORDANT: ROLE OF ANTIPLATELET THERAPY IN T2DM

Organization	Guidance
ADA	ASA 75–162 mg/d if primary prevention of ASCVD if 10-y risk of CAD > 10% or for secondary prevention of existing ASCVD. Consider ASA 75–162 mg/d plus low-dose rivaroxaban in patients who have stable CAD/PAD and low risk of bleeding
ESC	Start ASA 81–100 mg daily for primary prevention in high-risk CV patients only. In highest risk patients who can tolerate it, use DAPT for up to 3 y; add PPI if high risk for GIB
IDF	Start low-dose aspirin (75–350 mg/d) in patients with T2DM and CVD

Applying to Clinical Practice
- Assess ASCVD risk and recommend antiplatelet therapy for higher risk patients.
- Adding rivaroxaban to aspirin was better than aspirin alone in preventing cardiovascular events per the VOYAGER and COMPASS-PAD trials, but it also increased bleeding risk.

Guidelines Alert 3–11
GUIDELINES DISCORDANT: WHEN TO REFER TO BARIATRIC SURGERY IN T2DM

Organization	Guidance
ADA	BMI ≥ 40 (≥37.5 in Asian American persons), or ≥35 without durable weight loss and poor diabetes control with nonsurgical methods
IDF	BMI ≥ 35, or BMI 30–35 who have not responded to regular treatment

NICE	Expedited referral for BMI > 35; consider referral for BMI 30–34.9, or those of Asian descent even with lower BMI than 30. All should be receiving concomitant medical therapy

Applying to Clinical Practice
- Patients with obesity who have diabetes benefit from bariatric surgery.
- Those with BMI > 35 are likely to see the most benefit.

Practice Pearls

- Metformin may cause vitamin B_{12} deficiency; consider periodic monitoring of vitamin B_{12} levels especially in patients with anemia or neuropathy. Avoid if eGFR < 30 mL/min/1.73 m^2 or unstable HF.

- Consider GLP-1 RA as first-line injectable medication before insulin.

- ACEIs or ARBs are first-line antihypertensives. Second-line antihypertensives are dihydropyridine CCBs, thiazide diuretic if GFR ≥ 30 mL/min/1.73 m^2 or a loop diuretic if GFR < 30 mL/min/1.73 m^2.

- Metformin, smoking cessation, BP control, and statins consistently improve cardiovascular outcomes.

- Glycemic control is a staple of care, but controversy exists regarding optimal A1c goals for ambulatory adults. Advocates of tighter control (ie, <7) rely on data from several trials (ACCORD, ADVANCE, UKPDS, VADT) that show improvements in surrogate markers (ie, nerve conduction velocity) but not patient-oriented outcomes (ie, painful neuropathy or mortality) with tighter control. The DCCT trial showed 50%–76% reductions in development and progression of microvascular complications. Long-term follow-up demonstrated persistence of microvascular benefit over two decades, independent of persistence of glycemic control. Advocates of more permissive control (ie, <8%) point to potential harm from medication burden and hypoglycemia and the absence of evidence for patient-oriented benefit in tighter control of T2DM. (ADA)

- The largest trials for glycemic control (such as listed above) do not include SGLT2i or GLP-1 RAs, which may provide some cardiovascular benefit apart from glycemic reduction.

- Continuous glucose monitoring is now recommended for anyone on multiple daily insulin injections, regardless of type of diabetes or age.

- Self-monitoring of blood glucose levels in patients not on insulin is controversial. There are no agreed upon frequencies within the guidelines (once/d vs. twice/d vs. twice/wk). It is reasonable to consider self-monitoring when making medication changes, diet changes, or alterations in physical activity. It is also reasonable to prescribe self-monitoring in patients on medications with known side effects of hypoglycemia (such as sulfonylureas).

- The ODYSSEY OUTCOMES trial demonstrated statistically significant absolute risk reduction in primary endpoints (death from CAD, nonfatal MI, nonfatal ischemic stroke, unstable angina) in patients with T2DM with recent ACS who were treated with combination statin and alirocumab (PCSK-9). Consider dual therapy in post-ACS patients with T2DM.

- In patients with ASCVD risk factors with elevated triglycerides (135–499), but controlled LDL cholesterol on a statin, consider treatment with icosapent ethyl.
- Though guidelines suggest NPH and regular insulins are less efficacious and carry increased risk of hypoglycemia, the hypoglycemia risk is small and these formulations are typically less costly than preferred therapy. They may be appropriate for selected patients. (Endocrine Society, ADA).

Sources

–https://pro.aace.com/pdfs/diabetes/algorithm-exec-summary.pdf

–https://academic.oup.com/eurheartj/article/41/2/255/5556890

–https://diabetesjournals.org/care/issue/46/Supplement_1

–*Ann Intern Med.* 2017;166:279–290.

–*Ann Intern Med.* 2018;168:569–576.

–International Diabetes Federation. *Recommendations for Managing Type 2 Diabetes in Primary Care.* 2017. www.idf.org/managing-type2-diabetes

–https://www.nice.org.uk/guidance/ng28

–Endocrine Society. *Management of Individuals with Diabetes at High Risk for Hypoglycemia: An Endocrine Society Clinical Practice Guideline.* 2022. https://doi.org/10.1210/clinem/dgac596

–KDIGO. *Clinical Practice Guideline for Diabetes Management in Chronic Kidney Disease.* 2022.

–ACSM. *Exercise/Physical Activity in Individuals with Type 2 Diabetes: A Consensus Statement from the American College of Sports Medicine.* 2022. doi:10.1249/MSS.0000000000002800

–Management of Hyperglycemia in Type 2 Diabetes. A consensus report by the American Diabetes Association (ADA) and the European Association for the Study of Diabetes (EASD). *Diabetes Care.* 2022;45(11):2753–2786. https://doi.org/10.2337/dci22-0034

–2023 ESC guidelines for the management of cardiovascular disease in patients with diabetes. Developed by the task force on the management of cardiovascular disease in patients with diabetes of the European Society of Cardiology. *Eur Heart J.* 2023; 44 4043–4140. https://doi.org/10.1093/eurheartj/ehad192

–https://doi.org/10.7326/M23-278

Management: Hospitalized Adults

Recommendations from

> AAFP 2017, ADA 2023, Endocrine Society 2022

–Avoid intensive insulin therapy in hospitalized patients (even in ICU).

–Target blood glucose level of 140–180 mg/dL if insulin therapy is used in hospitalized patients, especially those who are critically ill. More stringent goals, such as 110–140 mg/dL (6.1–7.8 mmol/L) or 100–180 mg/dL (5.6–10.0 mmol/L), may be appropriate for selected patients and are acceptable if they can be achieved without significant hypoglycemia. (ADA)

–Use either basal insulin or basal plus bolus correctional insulin in the treatment of hospitalized patients; sliding scale regimens alone are no longer recommended.

–For patients receiving glucocorticoid therapy, consider ordering NPH simultaneously with their steroid to prevent worsening daytime and prandial hyperglycemia. (ADA)

–Support continued use of devices such as insulin pumps and CGM systems during hospitalization if competency is established and proper management/supervision is available. (ADA, Endocrine Society)

Practice Pearl

- Intensive insulin therapy in SICU/MICU patients does not improve mortality but has a 10- to 15-fold increased risk of hypoglycemia.

Sources

–https://www.aafp.org/journalpdfrestricted/afp/2017/1115/p648.pdf

–https://diabetesjournals.org/care/issue/46/Supplement_1

–Endocrine Society. *Management of Individuals with Diabetes at High Risk for Hypoglycemia: An Endocrine Society Clinical Practice Guideline.* 2022. https://doi.org/10.1210/clinem/dgac596

Management: Children and Adolescents

Recommendations from

> AAP 2021, ADA 2023, NICE 2022

Therapies

–Recommend diet, exercise, and lifestyle modification for all those diagnosed.

–Offer diabetes self-management education and support (DSMES). (ADA)

–Limit nonacademic screen time to <2 h/d.

–Assess psychological and social situation.

–Advise all patients not to smoke.

–Recommend annual influenza vaccine. (NICE)

–Recommend immunization against pneumococcal if taking insulin or oral hypoglycemic medication. (NICE)

–Monitor HbA1c every 3 mo.

–Use metformin as first-line therapy.

–Add liraglutide if insufficient control on metformin alone.

–Start insulin therapy if:

- DKA.
- A1c > 8.5% on metformin + liraglutide.
- Random glucose > 250 mg/dL.

Guidelines Alert 3–12 GUIDELINES DISCORDANT: A1c TARGET IN CHILDREN WITH T2DM	
Organization	**Guidance**
AAP	<7%
ADA	<7%; less (7.5%) or more stringent (<6.5%) goals may be appropriate for select patients

NICE	<6.5% if tolerated

Applying to Clinical Practice
- A1c targets of 6.5% or lower are unrealistic for many patients but may provide some benefit to those who can tolerate.
- Most benefits can be realized using an A1c target of <7%.

Surveillance

–BP measurement at every clinical visit. If BP ≥ 95th percentile (confirmed using 24 h ambulatory BP monitoring) despite lifestyle management, start ACEI/ARB. (ADA, NICE)

–Measure height and weight, and calculate BMI at every visit.

–Screening for PCOS at time of diagnosis for adolescent females. (ADA)

–If LDL persistently ≥ 130 after 6 mo of medical nutrition therapy, start statin for goal LDL < 100. (ADA)

–If triglycerides are >400 fasting or >1000 nonfasting, treat with fibrate. (ADA)

–Screen annually for:
  - Albuminuria: urine ACR ratio (use first sample of the day to avoid false positives). (NICE)
  - Dyslipidemia: lipid panel.
  - Neuropathy: comprehensive foot examination and monofilament testing.
  - Retinopathy: retinal exam after 12-y-old. (NICE)
  - NAFLD: LFTs. (ADA)
  - Symptoms of OSA. (ADA)

–Annual dentist appointment for periodontitis screening. (NICE)

Sources

–pediatrics.aappublications.org/content/131/2/364.full.pdf

–https://diabetesjournals.org/care/issue/44/Supplement_1

–https://www.nice.org.uk/guidance/ng18

HYPOGONADISM, MALE

Management: Men

Recommendations from

> Endocrine Society 2018, EAU 2018, AUA 2018, ACP 2020

Evaluation

–Evaluate men who have symptoms and signs of androgen deficiency: lethargy, easy fatigue, lack of stamina or endurance; reduced libido, decreased spontaneous erections; male infertility; mood changes; gynecomastia, loss of body hair, small testes; osteopenia/osteoporosis.

–Consider testing testosterone in men with pituitary masses, obesity, metabolic syndrome, moderate-to-severe COPD, infertility, osteoporosis, HIV, T2DM, or chronic use of corticosteroids and/or opiates. (EAU)

–See Fig. 3–2 for evaluation algorithm for suspected hypogonadism.

FIG. 3-2 EVALUATION OF SUSPECTED MALE HYPOGONADISM.

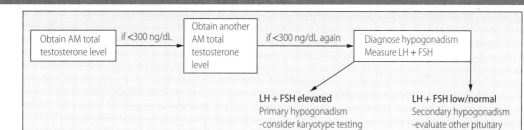

–Discuss risks, benefits, costs, and patient preferences in men with low testosterone and sexual dysfunction who desire to improve sexual function. (ACP)

–Measure serum estradiol in testosterone-deficient patients who present with breast symptoms or gynecomastia prior to the commencement of testosterone therapy. (EAU)

–Obtain a dual-energy X-ray absorptiometry (DEXA) scan for all men with severe androgen deficiency.

Therapies

–Testosterone therapy is indicated for androgen deficiency syndromes (low testosterone with symptoms) unless contraindications exist.[1]

–Do not start treatment for goals of improving energy, vitality, physical function, or cognition. (ACP)

–Consider IM over transdermal therapy, given lower cost with similar risks and efficacy. (ACP)

–Obtain a hemoglobin and hematocrit (and PSA in men over 40 y) prior to initiating testosterone therapy and educate patients about the risk of polycythemia. (EAU)

–Adjust testosterone therapy dosing to achieve a total testosterone level in the middle tertile of the normal reference range. (AUA)

–Monitor clinical response to therapy, testosterone level, PSA, digital prostate exam, and hematocrit 3, 6, and 12 mo after starting therapy, and annually thereafter. (EAU)

–Consider stopping testosterone therapy after 3–6 mo in patients who normalized total testosterone levels but failed to achieve improvement in clinical signs or symptoms. (AUA)

Practice Pearl

- Testosterone therapy options (goal is a total testosterone level in mid-normal range):
  - Testosterone enanthate or cypionate: 150–200 mg IM every 2 wk, or 75–100 mg IM weekly.
  - Testosterone transdermal patch: 4–6 mg daily.
  - Testosterone 1% gel: 50–100 mg daily.
  - Testosterone 2% gel: 10–70 mg daily.

---

[1] Breast cancer, prostate cancer, hematocrit > 50%, PSA > 4 ng/mL, desire for fertility in the near term, MI or CVA within last 6 mo, untreated severe obstructive sleep apnea, severe obstructive urinary symptoms, or uncontrolled heart failure.

- Testosterone 2% solution: 60–120 mg (2–4 pumps or twists) applied to the axillae daily.
- Testosterone buccal bioadhesive tablets: 30 mg to buccal mucosa q12 h.
- Testosterone nasal gel: 11 mg (2 pump actuations, 1 actuation per nostril) TID.

Sources
–https://academic.oup.com/jcem/article/103/5/1715/4939465
–https://uroweb.org/guideline/male-hypogonadism/
–http://www.auanet.org/guidelines/testosterone-deficiency-(2018)#x7697

MENOPAUSE

Management: Women

Recommendations from

> AACE 2017, NICE 2015, Endocrine Society 2015

–Start hormonal therapy for severe vasomotor symptoms or vulvovaginal atrophy.
–Consider avoiding therapy in patients with excess cardiovascular or breast cancer risk.
–Cautions with menopausal hormone therapy:

- Avoid unopposed estrogen use in women with an intact uterus.
- Micronized progesterone is the safer alternative for women needing progesterone.
- Consider transdermal or topical estrogens which may reduce the risk of venous thromboembolism (VTE).
- Use hormonal therapy in the lowest effective dose for the shortest duration possible. (NICE: no more than 5 y)
- Custom-compounded bioidentical hormone therapy is *not* recommended.
- Hormone replacement is *not* appropriate for prevention or treatment of dementia, diabetes, or CVD.
- Avoid if at high risk for VTE.

–Contraindications of menopausal hormone therapy (AACE):

- History of breast CA.
- Suspected estrogen-sensitive malignancy.
- Undiagnosed vaginal bleeding.
- Endometrial hyperplasia.
- History of VTE.
- Untreated hypertension.
- Active liver disease.
- Porphyria cutanea tarda.

–Offer vaginal estrogen cream for urogenital atrophy (even if already on systemic estrogen).
–Consider adjuvant testosterone therapy for decreased libido despite HRT. (NICE)
–Offer nonhormonal remedies for women at high risk of CVD or breast cancer. (ES)

- Options include an SSRI, SNRI, gabapentin, or pregabalin.
- Clonidine is an option for women with severe vasomotor symptoms who do not respond to or tolerate nonhormonal modalities.

–For women at moderate risk of CVD, recommend transdermal estradiol and micronized progesterone for severe vasomotor symptoms. (ES)

Practice Pearls

- Use of hormone therapy should always occur after a thorough discussion of the risks, benefits, and alternatives of this treatment with the patient.
- Risks of HRT:
  - VTE: the risk is greater for oral than transdermal preparations.
  - HRT with estrogen and progesterone may slightly increase risk of breast cancer but declines after stopping HRT.
- Review benefits of HRT: risk of fragility fracture is decreased while taking HRT but this benefit decreases once treatment stops.
- SSRIs or gabapentin may offer relief of menopausal symptoms for women at high risk from hormone replacement therapy.
- Do not use paroxetine or fluoxetine in patients with breast cancer as they inhibit the effect of tamoxifen.

Sources

–www.aace.com/files/position-statements/ep171828ps.pdf
–https://www.nice.org.uk/guidance/ng23/chapter/Recommendations#managing-short-term-menopausal-symptoms
–https://www.endocrine.org/guidelines-and-clinical-practice/clinical-practice-guidelines/treatment-of-menopause

OBESITY

Screening: Adults

Recommendations from

> AAFP 2012, USPSTF 2017, 2021, VA/DoD 2014, NICE 2023

–Screen all adults using BMI and offer intensive counseling and behavioral weight loss interventions to prevent obesity-related morbidity and mortality in adults with BMI ≥ 30.
–Encourage adults with BMI < 35 to utilize waist to height measurement to assess for central adiposity. (NICE)

Practice Pearls

- Intensive counseling involves more than one session per month for at least 3 mo.
- Offer intensive intervention to promote weight loss in:
  - Obese adults (BMI ≥ 30 or waist circumference ≥ 40 in. [men] or ≥ 35 in. [women] or waist-to-height > 0.6).
  - Overweight adults (BMI 25–29.9 or waist to height 0.5 to 0.59) with an obesity-associated condition.[1]

[1] HTN, DM type 2, dyslipidemia, obstructive sleep apnea, degenerative joint disease, or metabolic syndrome.

Sources

–USPSTF. *Obesity in Adults: Screening and Management.* 2021.

–USPSTF. *Obesity in Children and Adolescents: Screening.* 2017.

–VA/DoD. *Clinical Practice Guideline for Screening and Management of Overweight and Obesity,* Version 2.0. 2014.

–NICE. Obesity: identification, assessment, and management. 2023.

Prevention: Adults

Recommendations from

➢ ICSI 2013, CDC 2011, NICE 2023

–Ask permission to discuss weight and weight management. (NICE)

–Provide counseling regarding health risks. (NICE)

–Employ a team approach for weight management in all persons of normal weight (BMI 18.5–24.9) or overweight (BMI 25–29.9), including:

- Nutrition.
  - Physical activity: 150 min of moderate-intensity aerobic exercise/wk.
  - Lifestyle changes: avoid inactivity.
  - Screen for depression.
  - Screen for eating disorders.
  - Review medication list and assess if any medications can interfere with weight loss.

–Ensure regular follow-up to reinforce principles of weight management.

Practice Pearls

- Recommend 30–60 min of moderate physical activity on most days of the week.
- Nutrition education focused on decreased caloric intake, encouraging healthy food choices, and managing restaurant and social eating situations. Eat 5–6 servings of fruits and vegetables daily.
- Check weight weekly.
- Encourage nonfood rewards for positive reinforcement.
- Stress management techniques.
- Five percent to ten percent weight loss can produce a clinically significant reduction in heart disease risk.

Source

–Fitch A, Everling L, Fox C, et al. *Prevention and Management of Obesity for Adults.* Bloomington, MN: ICSI; 2013.

Management: Adults and Mature Adolescents

Recommendations from

➢ JCEM 2015, CMAJ 2020, AGA 2022, NICE 2022

–Approach to obesity management (CMAJ) (Fig. 3–3):

- Assess and acknowledge provider bias regarding obesity.

FIG. 3–3 APPROACH TO OBESITY INTERVENTIONS.

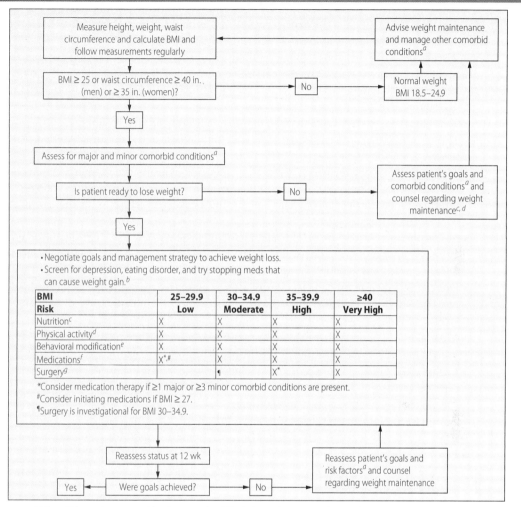

BMI	25–29.9	30–34.9	35–39.9	≥40
Risk	**Low**	**Moderate**	**High**	**Very High**
Nutrition[c]	X	X	X	X
Physical activity[d]	X	X	X	X
Behavioral modification[e]	X	X	X	X
Medications[f]	X*,#	X	X	X
Surgery[g]		¶	X*	X

*Consider medication therapy if ≥1 major or ≥3 minor comorbid conditions are present.
#Consider initiating medications if BMI ≥ 27.
¶Surgery is investigational for BMI 30–34.9.

[a]**Minor comorbid conditions:** cigarette smoking; hypertension; LDL cholesterol > 130 mg/dL; HDL cholesterol < 40 mg/dL (men) or < 50 mg/dL (women); glucose intolerance; family history of premature CAD; age ≥ 65 y (men) or ≥55 y (women).

Major comorbid conditions: waist circumference ≥ 40 in. (men) or ≥35 in. (women); CAD; peripheral vascular disease; abdominal aortic aneurysm; symptomatic carotid artery disease; T2DM; and obstructive sleep apnea.

[b]Sulfonylureas; thiazolidinediones; olanzapine, clozapine; risperidone, quetiapine; lithium; paroxetine, citalopram, sertraline; carbamazepine; pregabalin; corticosteroids; megestrol acetate; cyproheptadine; tricyclic antidepressants; monoamine oxidase inhibitors; mirtazapine; valproic acid; and gabapentin.

[c]Encourage a healthy, balanced diet including daily intake of ≥5 servings of fruits/vegetables; 35 g fiber; <30% calories from fat; eliminate takeout, fast foods, soda, and desserts; dietitian consultation for a calorie reduction between 500 and 1000 kcal/kg/d to achieve a 1–2 lb weight reduction per week.

[d]Recommend 30–60 min of moderate activity at least 5 d/wk.

[e]Identify behaviors that may contribute to weight gain (stress, emotional eating, boredom) and use cognitive behavioral counseling, stimulus control, relapse prevention, and goal setting to decrease caloric intake and increase physical activity.

[f]Medications that are FDA approved for weight loss: phentermine; orlistat; lorcaserin phendimetrazine; diethylpropion; and benzphetamine can be used for up to 3 mo as an adjunct for weight loss. Avoid phentermine and diethylpropion in patients with uncontrolled HTN or a history of heart disease.

[g]Bariatric surgery is indicated for patients at high risk for complications. They should be motivated, psychologically stable, have no surgical contraindications, and must accept the operative risk involved.

- Ask permission to discuss obesity/weight with patient, approach conversations in a nonjudgmental way, and praise success to encourage continued positive behavior.
- Assess their story (subjective experiences as well as objective measures such as BMI, height, waist circumference, BP, lipid panel, A1c, and LFT measurements).
- Discuss and agree on choice of interventions with patient and tailor weight management program to patient's needs/preferences, initial fitness, health status, and lifestyle. Consider factors including weight-related comorbidities, ethnicity, and special education needs and disabilities. (NICE)
- Use clinical judgment to decide when to measure height and weight. Interpret BMI with caution, especially in patients aged 65+, with high muscle mass, and/or of Asian or African descent. (NICE)
- Recognize that surprise, denial, disbelief, or anger about health situation may diminish patient's ability/willingness to change. Offer patients who are not yet ready to change information on the benefits of losing weight, and a chance to return for further consults when ready to discuss again. (NICE)
- Assess possible reasons for weight gain, including patient's view of weight/diagnosis and attitudes about eating and physical activity that may be unhelpful, previous experiences/attempts, readiness to adopt changes. (NICE)
- Exercise (45–60 min moderate-intensity activity on most days of the week), with added resistance training. Consider increasing exercise to 60–90 min daily to avoid regaining weight. (NICE)
- Medical nutrition therapy facilitated by registered dietitian when possible.
- Weight loss of 5%–7% in setting of prediabetes, 7%–15% in diagnosed T2DM.
- Ensure weight management programs include behavior change strategies to increase physical activity levels and improve eating behavior (NICE). Offer multicomponent psychological care in a longitudinal setting.
- Ensure weight loss diet approach is total energy intake is less than energy expenditure. Often, a diet with a calorie deficit of 600 kcal/d is sufficient. (NICE)
- Pharmacotherapy:
    - Use when BMI ≥ 30, or ≥ 27 with adiposity-related complications, in conjunction with intensive lifestyle changes listed above.
    - Choices include semaglutide, liraglutide, naltrexone-bupropion combination, phentermine-topiramate ER.
    - Use semaglutide only for patients with BMI ≥ 35, or ≥ 30 with associated risk factors. Consider stopping if less than 5% of the initial weight has been lost after 6 mo (NICE). Minimize exposure to other medications that carry the side effect of weight gain.
- Bariatric surgery considerations:
    - Indicated when BMI ≥ 40, BMI ≥ 35 with at least 1 adiposity-related disease or diagnosis of T2DM in the last 10 y, BMI between 30 and 35 with presence of poorly controlled T2DM despite maximal medical therapy. (NICE)
    - Do not offer adjustable gastric banding procedure due to long-term treatment failure and rate of complications.

Guidelines Alert 3–13
GUIDELINES DISCORDANT: ORLISTAT FOR WEIGHT LOSS

Organization	Guidance
CMAJ	Use orlistat (or liraglutide or naltrexone-bupropion)
AGA	Generally, avoid orlistat in adults with obesity or weight-related complications. However, a minority of patients who place a higher value on the potential small weight loss benefit and lower value on GI adverse effects may reasonably choose treatment with orlistat
NICE	Use orlistat only for patients with BMI $\geq$ 30, or $\geq$ 28 with associated risk factors. Only continue orlistat therapy beyond 3 mo if the patient has lost at least 5% of initial body weight. Do not coprescribe orlistat with other drugs aimed at weight loss

Applying to Clinical Practice
- While its side-effect profile limits its general use, select patients may elect orlistat as a component of their weight loss regimen.
- Patients taking orlistat should also take a daily multivitamin containing fat-soluble vitamins, taken 2 h apart from orlistat. (AGA)

Practice Pearl

- Bariatric surgery does improve all-cause mortality and comorbidities such as diabetes, hypertension, and sleep apnea. (*PLoS Med.* 2020;17(7):e1003206)

Sources
–*CMAJ.* 2020;192:E875–E891. doi:10.1503/cmaj.191707

–Adapted from the *ICSI Guideline on the Prevention and Management of Obesity.* https://academic.oup.com/jcem/article/100/2/342/2813109/Pharmacological-Management-of-Obesity-An-Endocrine

Management: Children and Adolescents (2–18 y)

Recommendations from

> NICE 2023, AAP 2023

Evaluation
–Ask permission from patient and their families/caregivers before discussing weight, and conduct all discussions in a manner that is supportive, age-appropriate, nonjudgmental, and recognizes cultural values. Understand that these discussions may elicit strong emotional responses such as sadness/anger, and acknowledge and validate these responses, focusing on patient's health.

–Approach to diagnosis (AAP):
  - Screening: Measure height and weight, calculate BMI, and assess BMI percentile/weight classification using age- and sex-specific CDC growth charts or growth charts for children with severe obesity at least annually for all children aged 2[1]–18 y to screen for overweight/obesity.

[1] N.B.: U.S. Preventative Services Task Force recommends screening to begin at 6 y rather than 2.

- Evaluation: If BMI indicates overweight or obese (see Guidelines Alert 3–14), conduct full evaluation for overweight/obesity and obesity-related comorbidities by using a comprehensive patient history, mental and behavioral health screening, SDoH evaluation, physical examination, and diagnostic studies.
- Comorbidities: Evaluate for:
  - Dyslipidemia.
  - Prediabetes and/or DM, with fasting plasma glucose or HbA1c.
  - NAFLD.
  - Hypertension, by measuring BP at every visit starting at age 3 y in children with overweight or obesity.
  - Obstructive Sleep Apnea.
  - PCOS.
  - Depression, and conduct annual evaluation for depression in adolescents 12 y+ with a formal self-report tool.
- Perform a musculoskeletal review of systems and physical examination (eg, internal hip rotation in growing child, gait) as part of their evaluation for obesity.
- Maintain a high degree of suspicion for idiopathic intracranial hypertension with new-onset or progressive headaches in the context of significant weight gain, especially for women.
–Approach to diagnosis (NICE):
- Consider assessment of comorbidity for children with BMI at or above 98th percentile.
- In addition to BMI, also consider using waist-to-height ratio in children and adolescents age 5 y+ to assess and predict health risks associated with central adiposity (such as T2DM, hypertension, or CVD).
–Treat overweight and obesity concurrently with related comorbidities.

Guidelines Alert 3–14 GUIDELINES DISCORDANT: WEIGHT CLASSIFICATION IN CHILDREN AND ADOLESCENTS			
Organization	**Overweight**	**Clinical Obesity**	**Severe Obesity**
AAP	BMI ≥ 85th percentile to < 95th percentile	BMI ≥ 95th percentile	BMI ≥ 120% of the 95th percentile for age and sex
NICE	BMI 91st percentile + 1.34 SDs	BMI 98th percentile + 2.05 SDs	BMI 99.6th percentile + 2.68 SDs
Applying to Clinical Practice • Ensure BMI/growth charts used are appropriate for children/adolescents and adjusted for age/sex.			

Management

–Involve children/adolescents and their families/caregivers in decision-making.

–Provide or refer children with overweight or obesity to intensive health behavior and lifestyle treatment. When an intensive health behavior and lifestyle treatment program is not available, provide the most intensive program possible, given available community resources and other specialty programs. (AAP)

–Aim to create a supportive environment that helps the child and their family make changes to lifestyle, behavioral, and environmental factors. Ensure that interventions address lifestyle within the family and in social settings and encourage parents/caregivers to take main responsibility for lifestyle changes in children, especially those under 12 y. Involve behavioral health specialists when possible.

–Encourage increasing physical activity (60+ min/d) and reducing inactive behaviors. Choose an activity with the child appropriate to ability and confidence (NICE). Exercise specialists can provide counseling and training to engage children and families in noncompetitive, cooperative, and fun activities. (AAP)

–Offer nutritional advice or refer to a dietitian. Dietary recommendations should be part of multicomponent intervention, as a dietary approach alone is not recommended for children and adolescents (NICE). Total energy intake should be below energy expenditure, and changes should be sustainable. Focus on increasing healthful food consumption. (AAP)

–Consider offering patients aged 12 y+ with obesity weight loss pharmacotherapy, according to medication indications, risks, and benefits, as an adjunct to health behavior and lifestyle treatment. Pharmacotherapy is generally appropriate for children with more severe degrees of obesity and/or comorbidities.

–Consider offering referral for adolescents aged 13 y+ with severe obesity for evaluation for metabolic and bariatric surgery to local or regional comprehensive multidisciplinary pediatric metabolic and bariatric surgery centers. (AAP)

–Treat using a family-centered approach that acknowledges obesity's biological, social, and structural drivers. Assess individual and contextual risk factors for obesity, and tailor interventions to the needs and preferences of the child and family, taking into account the child's physical and mental/emotional health status, as well as SDoHs such as ethnicity, socioeconomic status, household and familial influences/complexities, and access to resources. Recognize and address systemic racial and socioeconomic inequities that often result in disparities in obesity risk and outcomes, including systemic disparities in access to resources and quality health care services. (AAP)

–The aim of weight management programs for children/adolescents can vary; focus on weight management or loss depending on age/stage of growth. (NICE)

–Consider whether patient has experienced weight-based stigma or bullying, which may contribute to binge eating, social isolation, avoiding health care services, and decreased physical activity. (NICE)

–Use long-term care strategies and provide ongoing medical monitoring and access to treatment for obesity and associated comorbidities, appropriate reassessments of medical and psychological risks and comorbidities, and appropriate modifications to treatment plans throughout childhood and adolescence into young adulthood. (AAP)

–Surgery is not recommended in children and should only be considered if they have reached or are close to physiological maturity. (NICE)

Practice Pearl

- Drug treatment is currently not recommended for children under 12 y for the sole indication of obesity (AAP, NICE). However, it may be appropriate in exceptional circumstances when severe comorbidities are present. Prescribing should be started and monitored only in specialist pediatric settings (NICE). AAP notes that the use of pharmacotherapy to aid BMI reduction in children is a rapidly evolving field; new evidence may lead to additional options for children under 12 y in the future.

Sources

–NICE. *Obesity: Identification, Assessment and Management.* 2023. www.nice.org.uk/guidance/cg189

–AAP. Clinical practice guideline for the evaluation and treatment of children and adolescents with obesity. 2023;151(2):e2022060640.

THYROID CANCER

Screening: Adults

Recommendations from

> USPSTF 2017, American Cancer Society, NIH/National Cancer Institute 2019

–Do not screen asymptomatic people with ultrasound.

–Genetic testing is recommended for patients with a family history of medullary thyroid cancer, with or without multiple endocrine neoplasia type 2 (MEN2).

–Be aware of higher risk patients: head-and-neck radiation administered in infancy and childhood for benign (thymus enlargement, acne) or malignant conditions, which results in an increased risk beginning 5 y after radiation and continuing until >20 y later; nuclear fallout exposure (eg, Japanese survivors of atomic bombing); history of goiter; family history of thyroid disease or thyroid cancer; multiple endocrine neoplasia type 2; female sex; Asian race.

Practice Pearls

- Neck palpation for nodules in asymptomatic individuals has sensitivity of 15%–38% and specificity of 93%–100%. Only a small proportion of nodular thyroid glands are neoplastic, resulting in a high false-positive rate.
- Fine-needle aspiration (FNA) is the procedure of choice for evaluation of thyroid nodules. (*Otolaryngol Clin North Am.* 2010;43:229–238) (*N Engl J Med.* 2012;367:705)

Sources

–*JAMA.* 2017;317(18):1882–1887.

–*N Engl J Med.* 2015;373:2347.

–PDQ® Screening and Prevention Editorial Board. *PDQ Thyroid Cancer Screening.* Bethesda, MD: National Cancer Institute. https://www.cancer.gov/types/thyroid/hp/thryoid-screening-pdq. Accessed April 16, 2019.

POLYCYSTIC OVARY SYNDROME (PCOS)

Management: Women

Recommendations from

> ## ACOG 2018

Evaluation

–Diagnose if 2 of 3 criteria are met (Rotterdam criteria):
- Androgen excess.
- Ovulatory dysfunction.
- Polycystic ovaries.

Therapies

–Recommend increase in exercise combined with dietary change to reduce diabetes risk and promote weight loss.

–Prescribe combination low-dose hormonal contraceptives for primary treatment of menstrual disorders.

–Screen women with PCOS for cardiovascular risk, metabolic syndrome, and T2DM (fasting glucose followed by 2-h GTT after 75-g glucose load).

–Consider addition of insulin-sensitizing agent (such as metformin) to decrease androgen levels, improve ovulation rate, improve glucose tolerance, and reduce cardiovascular risk.

–Prescribe letrozole as first-line therapy for ovulation induction in women with PCOS who desire to conceive.

Practice Pearls

- Letrozole has shown an increased live birth rate compared with clomiphene citrate.
- There may be higher pregnancy rates with clomiphene citrate in addition to metformin than with clomiphene alone, particularly in obese women with PCOS.
- Second-line intervention for failure of pregnancy with letrozole or clomiphene is exogenous gonadotropins or laparoscopic ovarian surgery.
- Women in ethnic groups at higher risk of nonclassical congenital adrenal hyperplasia should be screened with a fasting 17-hydroxyprogesterone level (normal < 2–4 ng/mL).
- Lower BMI is associated with improved pregnancy rates, decreased hirsutism, and lower risk for metabolic syndrome.
- There is no clear primary treatment for hirsutism in PCOS, but the addition of eflornithine to laser treatment is superior to laser alone.

Source

–https://journals.lww.com/greenjournal/Fulltext/2018/06000/ACOG_Practice_Bulletin_No_194_Polycystic_Ovary.54.aspx

THYROID DISEASE, HYPERTHYROIDISM

Management: Adults

Recommendations from

> NICE 2023, ATA 2016, AACE 2013

–Determine etiology of thyrotoxicosis. If the diagnosis is not apparent, consider obtaining a thyroid receptor antibody level +/− determination of the radioactive iodine uptake (RAIU).

–Consider US evaluation of the thyroid only if palpable thyroid nodules. (NICE)

–Use beta-adrenergic blockade in all patients with symptomatic thyrotoxicosis.

–For overt Graves disease (GD), treat with either radioiodine (RAI) therapy, antithyroid drugs (ATDs), or thyroidectomy. Prefer RAI unless ATD likely to achieve remission (ie, mild or uncomplicated disease) or patient not an RAI/surgery candidate, concern for compression, malignancy, pregnancy, or trying to become pregnant in the next 4–6 mo; treat with total thyroidectomy if concern for compression, malignancy, or patient not an RAI/ATD candidate. (NICE)

–For toxic goiter, use RAI as first line if multinodular, then consider total thyroidectomy or ADT; if single nodule, consider RAI or hemithyroidectomy.

–For RAI therapy:

• Obtain a pregnancy test within 48 h prior to treatment in any woman with childbearing potential who is to be treated with RAI.

• Recheck a T4, T3, and TSH level every 6 wk after RAI therapy for 6 mo until TSH within reference range. Then at 9 and 12 mo post radiation. If 12 mo TSH within reference range, check TSH every 6 mo. (NICE)

• Assess patients 6 wk after ^{131}I therapy with a free T_4 and total triiodothyronine (T_3) level; repeat q4–6 wk if thyrotoxicosis persists and treat with antithyroid drugs if persists. (NICE)

• Consider retreatment with ^{131}I therapy if hyperthyroidism persists 6 mo after ^{131}I treatment.

–For antithyroid drug therapy:

• When using ADTs for hyperthyroidism, check CBC and liver enzymes prior to starting, and use the titration method in young adult vs. either block and replace or the titration method in older adults.

• Choose methimazole as the preferred antithyroid drug except during the first trimester of pregnancy.

• Educate patients on the signs and symptoms of agranulocytosis and hepatic injury.

–Stop ATD and do not restart if agranulocytosis develops in patient: (NICE)

• Monitor free T4 and total T3 every 4–8 wk. Once normal, monitor every 3 mo. Serum TSH will remain suppressed for several months so is not of value to trend. See Table 3–3 for details about dosing and monitoring.

• Continue antithyroid medications at least 12–18 mo, then taper or stop if TSH level is normal.

• Measure TSH receptor antibody level prior to stopping antithyroid drug therapy.

TABLE 3–3 DOSING AND MONITORING OF ANTITHYROID DRUG THERAPY

Initial Dosing	Maintenance Dosing	Duration of Therapy
Methimazole		
fT_4 1–1.5× ULN: 5–10 mg daily fT_4 1.5–2× ULN (or iodine-induced thyrotoxicosis): 10–20 mg daily fT_4 > 2× ULN: 20–40 mg/d. Consider dividing to 2–3 doses to achieve euthyroidism more quickly and reduce GI-related adverse effects, especially with doses > 30 mg/d	5–10 mg once daily Assess fT_4 and total T3 at 4- to 6-wk intervals When normal, reduce dose by 30%–50% and repeat thyroid function tests in 4–6 wk Continue to adjust dose to achieve euthyroid state	For patients undergoing definitive therapy: continue until euthyroid (typically 4–6 wk); discontinue 2–3 d before radioactive iodine therapy or on the day of thyroidectomy Patients with Graves disease: treat for 12–18 mo, then assess for remission Toxic multinodular goiter/toxic adenoma: continue indefinitely
Propylthiouracil (pregnancy, first-trimester)		
50 mg 2–3 times daily; doses up to 300 mg/d may be required in patients with severe hyperthyroidism	Adjust dose based on thyroid function tests obtained every 4 wk to maintain serum fT_4 concentration at or just above the ULN (using a trimester-specific reference range) and serum TSH concentrations below the reference range for pregnancy. Usual maintenance dose: Oral: ≤50 mg twice daily	May switch to methimazole after 16 wk EGA

Source: 2016 American Thyroid Association guidelines for diagnosis and management of hyperthyroidism and other causes of thyrotoxicosis. *Thyroid.* 2016;26(10):1343–1421.

- Thyroidectomy:
  - If near total or total thyroidectomy is chosen as treatment for Graves disease, render patients euthyroid prior to the procedure with ATD pretreatment and beta-adrenergic blockade. Give potassium iodide in the immediate preoperative period.
  - Follow serial calcium or intact PTH levels postoperatively.
  - Start levothyroxine 1.6 mcg/kg/d immediately postoperatively.
  - Check a serum TSH level 6–8 wk postoperatively.
  - Wean beta-blockers following thyroidectomy.
- Treat subclinical hyperthyroidism in all individuals ≥ 65 of age, and in patients with cardiac disease, osteoporosis, or symptoms of hyperthyroidism when the TSH is persistently <0.1 mIU/L. (ATA)
- Treat thyroid storm in the ICU with beta-blockers, antithyroid drugs, inorganic iodide, corticosteroid therapy, volume resuscitation, and aggressive cooling with acetaminophen and cooling blankets. (ATA)

Sources
–https://www.nice.org/uk/guidance/ng145/resources/thyroid-disease-assessment-and-management-pdf-66141781496773
–2016 American Thyroid Association guidelines for diagnosis and management of hyperthyroidism and other causes of thyrotoxicosis. *Thyroid*. 2016;26(10):1343–1421.
–https://www.aace.com/files/hyperguidelinesapril2013.pdf

THYROID DISEASE, HYPOTHYROIDISM

Management: Adults, Nonpregnant

Recommendations from

> NICE 2023, AACE 2012

–Measure thyroid peroxidase antibody (TPO-Ab) once for adults with elevated TSH. (NICE)
–Start therapy if TSH is >10 mIU/L or if <10 mIU/L with symptoms of hypothyroidism.
–Consider treatment for TSH < 10 mIU/L if positive antithyroid peroxidase antibodies (thyroid peroxidase antibody) or high ASCVD risk. (AACE)
–Treat with levothyroxine rather than natural thyroid extract or liothyronine as first-line therapy (no evidence of benefits and long-term outcomes uncertain).
–Start levothyroxine 1.6 mcg/kg/d, with titration if age < 65 y and no history of CVD. (NICE)
–Start levothyroxine at 25 to 50 mcg/d with titration if >65 and in adults with history of CVD. (NICE)
–Check thyroid peroxidase antibody in patients with subclinical hypothyroidism or recurrent miscarriages. (AACE)
–Monitor TSH 4–8 wk after starting levothyroxine or adjusting dose, then q6–12 mo once euthyroid.
–Monitor FT4 and TSH in adults who start levothyroxine but remain symptomatic. (NICE)
–If therapy was initiated for TSH < 10 mIU/L and symptoms persist after 6 mo despite a TSH in the normal range, stop levothyroxine therapy. (NICE)
–Consider a 6-mo trial treatment of subclinical hypothyroidism for TSH above reference range but <10 mIU/L on 2 separate occasions 3 mo apart and symptomatic hypothyroidism. (NICE)
–Avoid overtreatment with levothyroxine to minimize risk of cardiovascular, skeletal, or affective disturbances. (AACE)
–Do *not* use levothyroxine to treat obesity or depression in euthyroid patients. (AACE)

Sources
–https://www.nice.org/uk/guidance/ng145/resources/thyroid-disease-assessment-and-management-pdf-66141781496773
–https://www.aace.com/files/hypothyroidism_guidelines.pdf

THYROID DYSFUNCTION

Screening: Adults

Recommendations from

> AAFP 2015, USPSTF 2015, ATA 2012, AACE 2012, ASRM 2015, CTF 2019

  –Insufficient evidence to recommend for or against routine screening for thyroid disease in asymptomatic adults without risk factors.
  - ATA/AACE: consider screening patients older than 60, those with risk factors, and women planning pregnancy.
  –CTF: do not screen asymptomatic nonpregnant adults for thyroid dysfunction.
  –Evaluate adults with laboratory or radiologic abnormalities that could be caused by thyroid disease using serum TSH.
  –Do not test for thyroid disease in hospitalized patients unless thyroid disease is strongly suspected.

Practice Pearls

- Individuals with symptoms and signs potentially attributable to thyroid dysfunction require TSH testing.
- Less than 1% of adults have subclinical hypothyroidism; outcomes data to support treatment are lacking. Subclinical hyperthyroidism detected during routine screening may be treated in select patients at high risk for cardiovascular or skeletal complications.
- Higher risk individuals are those with autoimmune disorders (eg, T1DM), pernicious anemia, goiter, previous radioactive iodine therapy and/or head-and-neck irradiation or surgery, pituitary or hypothalamic disorders, first-degree relative with a thyroid disorder, use of medications that may impair thyroid function, and those with psychiatric disorders.
- Thyroid function should be measured in patients with the following: substantial hyperlipidemia, hyponatremia, high-serum muscle enzymes, macrocytic anemia, pericardial or pleural effusions.
- Consider TSH screening in infertile women attempting pregnancy.
- Monitor TSH in patients taking thyroid medication or after thyroid surgery.

THYROID NODULES

Management: Adults

Recommendations from

> NICE 2019

  –Assess with US if palpable nodule or generalized enlargement, and then proceed with FNA if suspicious by standard grading system (which is based on echogenicity, microcalcifications, border, shape in transverse plane, internal vascularity, and lymphadenopathy) (Fig. 3–4).
  –If nonmalignant, treat only if airway symptoms or narrowing on imaging; repeat workup if change in symptoms.
  –If cystic, treat with aspiration +/− ethanol ablation.

FIG. 3–4 APPROACH TO THE PATIENT WITH A THYROID NODULE. FNA, FINE-NEEDLE ASPIRATION; LN, LYMPH NODE; PTC, PAPILLARY THYROID CANCER; Rx, THERAPY; TSH, THYROID-STIMULATING HORMONE; US, ULTRASOUND.

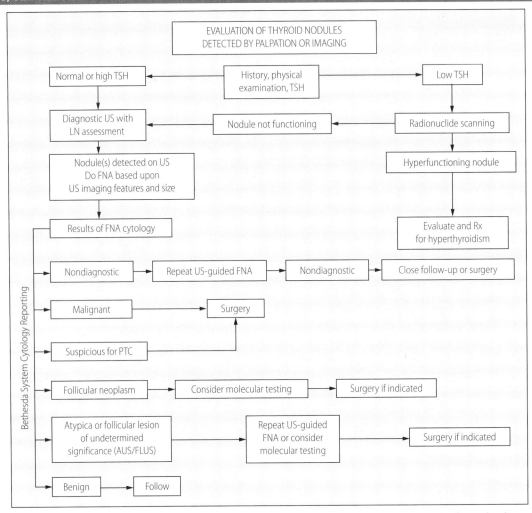

Source: Reproduced with permission from Loscalzo J, Fauci A, Kasper D, Hauser S, Longo D, Jameson JL. *Harrison's Principles of Internal Medicine* (21st ed.). New York, NY: McGraw Hill; 2022.

–If noncystic, multinodular, or diffuse goiter, treat with surgery, RIA, or percutaneous thermal ablation.

Sources
–AACE. 2010. https://www.aace.com/files/thyroid-guidelines.pdf

–ATA. 2015. https://www.ncbi.nlm.nih.gov/pmc/articles/PMC4739132/

–https://www.nice.org/uk/guidance/ng145/resources/thyroid-disease-assessment-and-management-pdf-66141781496773

TRANSGENDER HEALTH CARE

Management: Genderqueer, Gender Nonconforming, and Gender Nonbinary People

Recommendations from

> UCSF 2016, WPATH 2012, Endocrine 2017, ACOG 2021

-Employ cultural humility. Avoid judgment or editorializing. Use gender pronouns consistent with patients' self-identity. Ask for clarification when uncertain.

-Diagnose "Gender Dysphoria" when gender identity is incongruent with assignment and there is clinically significant social impairment. Use the term "gender nonconformity" to represent the broader population with incongruent gender identities.

-Employ informed consent prior to initiating hormone therapy, including effects on fertility; fertility and parenting desires should be discussed early in the process, prior to transition.

-Offer a multidisciplinary team approach including mental health providers and clinicians to inform and guide treatment modalities, especially for younger patients.

-Assess suicide risk. Suicide rates are markedly elevated in this community.

Management: Patients Transitioning to a Female Gender Expression

Recommendations from

> UCSF 2016, WPATH 2012, Endocrine 2017, ACOG 2021

-To develop female secondary sex characteristics, use 17-beta estradiol (typically transdermal patch, oral or sublingual tablet, or injectable). Do not use conjugated equine estrogens because of difficulty. Do not use ethinyl estradiol because of thrombotic risk. Effects include breast development (to Tanner stages 2–3), redistribution of fat, reduction of muscle mass, reduction of body hair, possible arrest/reversal of scalp hair loss, reduced erectile function, and reduced testicular size. There is an increased risk of venous thromboembolism and hypertriglyceridemia, and possibly of hypertension.

-To suppress male secondary sex characteristics, use antiandrogens such as spironolactone (monitor for hyperkalemia; max dose 200 mg BID). If contraindicated or unable to tolerate, use 5-alpha-reductase inhibitors instead. Titrate dose to clinical effect and testosterone levels < 55 ng/dL.

-Screen for breast cancer q2 y if age > 50 and 5–10 y of feminizing hormone use. Prostate and testicular cancer risk is reduced by feminizing hormones but not eliminated; individualize screening.

-Hair removal can be achieved through various methods including laser, electrolysis, waxing, plucking, and shaving.

-Consider referral to speech language pathologist if concerns about incongruent voice pitch are present.

-Patients may consider "tucking" (employ tight-fitting underwear to locate the testicles in the inguinal canal and the penis in the perineal region) and "binding" (tight-fitting bras/shirts/wraps/binders) to disguise male anatomical characteristics.

–If considering breast augmentation ("top surgery"), 24 mo of preoperative hormone therapy is recommended, as breast tissue will continue to develop.

–If considering vaginoplasty ("bottom surgery"), requirements include two assessments by a mental health provider, 12 mo of hormone therapy, and 12 mo of living in a gender role congruent with gender identity.

Management: Patients Transitioning to a Male Gender Expression

Recommendations from

> UCSF 2016, WPATH 2012, Endocrine 2017, ACOG 2021

–To develop male secondary sex characteristics, give testosterone (oral, IM, SQ, or transdermal) and titrate to bioavailable level > 72 ng/dL. Effects include development of facial hair, voice changes, fat redistribution, increase in muscle mass, increase in body hair, hairline recession, increase in libido, clitoral growth, vaginal dryness, and cessation of menses. There is an increased risk of polycythemia and possibly of hyperlipidemia.

–In patients receiving testosterone therapy, monitor testosterone levels and hematocrit every 3 mo for the first year, then every 6–12 mo thereafter.

–Discuss contraceptive options, as hormone therapy does not reliably cause infertility and testosterone is teratogenic.

–Discontinue testosterone prior to pregnancy if possible, or immediately upon discovery of pregnancy; consider that pregnancy may worsen feelings of dysphoria.

–Screen for breast and cervical cancer according to current guidelines for cis-gendered women. Do not routinely screen for endometrial cancer but explore the possibility if unexplained vaginal bleeding.

–Evaluation of abnormal uterine bleeding should follow the same guidelines as for cis-gendered women.

–Patients may consider "packing" (use of a penile prosthesis) to provide a male physical appearance.

–If considering mastectomy ("top surgery"), an assessment by a mental health provider is required.

–If considering gonadectomy or hysterectomy ("bottom surgery"), 12 mo of preoperative hormone therapy is required.

–If considering phalloplasty or metoidioplasty, requirements include two assessments by a mental health provider, 12 mo of hormone therapy, and 12 mo of living in a gender role congruent with gender identity.

Management: Gender Nonconforming Children and Adolescents

Recommendations from

> UCSF 2016, WPATH 2012, Endocrine 2017

–Suppression of endogenous puberty may represent an opportunity to avoid distressing gender dysphoria and the high rate of suicide that accompanies it.

–Adolescents are candidates for puberty suppression if a long-lasting pattern of gender nonconformity or dysphoria exists, dysphoria emerges or worsens with the onset of puberty, their ability to adhere to treatment is intact, and the adolescent and their parents/guardians have consented to the treatment.

–Do not offer hormonal treatment to prepubertal persons.

–If suppression is desired, use GnRH analogs before the patient has reached Tanner stages 2–3 with frequent monitoring of clinical and lab parameters.

Practice Pearls

- Outcomes data are generally lacking for this population, so most guidelines are based on expert opinion from experienced practitioners.

- Terminology may be fluid and highly individualized. Approach conversations with humility and open-ended questions.

- Employ a stepwise approach to therapies. Encourage hormone therapy before surgical intervention for most patients. Informed consent is essential, as every therapy will have reversible and irreversible effects.

- For patients considering surgical options, refer to surgeon comfortable with the treatment of gender dysphoria. While top surgeries are often well tolerated, bottom surgeries are relatively complex with higher complication rates and significant postprocedure care. Informed consent is essential and should include the various techniques available, realistic expectations of outcomes, and inherent risks and complications.

- Dosing of hormones, surveillance regimens, and common adverse effects are detailed in the cited guidelines.

Sources

–AACE. 2010. https://www.aace.com/files/thyroid-guidelines.pdf

–*Guidelines for the Primary and Gender-Affirming Care of Transgender and Gender Nonbinary People*, 2nd ed. University of California, San Francisco Center of Excellence for Transgender Health. 2016. http://www.transhealth.ucsf.edu/guidelines

–*Standards of Care for the Health of Transsexual, Transgender, and Gender-Nonconforming People*, 7th ed. World Professional Association for Transgender Health. 2012. http://wpath.org

–Guidelines on gender-dysphoric/gender-incongruent persons. *J Clin Endocrinol Metab.* 2017;102(11):3869–3903.

–https://www.acog.org/clinical/clinical-guidance/committee-opinion/articles/2021/03/health-care-for-transgender-and-gender-diverse-individuals

VITAMIN DEFICIENCIES, B$_{12}$ AND FOLATE

Management: Adults

Recommendations from

➤ BCSH 2014

Evaluation

–Diagnose cobalamin deficiency when serum cobalamin < 200 ng/L.

–Diagnose folate deficiency if serum folate level < 7 nmol/L (< 3 mcg/L).

–If normal cobalamin level but high suspicion of cobalamin and/or folate deficiency, measure methylmalonic acid (MMA) and total homocysteine (tHC) levels.

–If cobalamin deficiency or unexplained anemia, neuropathy, or glossitis (regardless of cobalamin level), obtain an anti-intrinsic factor antibody test to rule out pernicious anemia.

Therapies

–Treat cobalamin deficiency with vitamin B_{12} 1 mg IM TIW for 2 wk and then maintenance therapy.

–Elect either 1 mg IM every 3 mo (if no neurologic symptoms) or every 2 mo (if neurologic symptoms) or vitamin B_{12} 2 mg PO daily for maintenance therapy.

–Treat folate deficiency with 1–5 mg PO daily for 1–4 mo, or until folate level normalizes.

Practice Pearls

- Do not use antiparietal cell antibody to test for pernicious anemia.
- Both methylmalonic acid and total homocysteine will be elevated in cobalamin deficiency; normal methylmalonic acid and elevated total homocysteine are consistent with folate deficiency.

Source

–onlinelibrary.wiley.com/doi/full/10.1111/bjh.12959

EARS, EYES, NOSE, AND THROAT DISORDERS

CATARACTS

Management: Adults

Recommendations from

➤ **AAO 2021**

–Refer patients with symptomatic cataracts for surgery.

–Do not recommend specific dietary intake or nutritional supplements for the prevention or treatment of cataract.

–Obtain initial history of symptoms, ocular history, systemic history, assessment of visual functional status, and medications currently used (Fig. 4–1).

–Refer for removal of cataracts when visual function no longer meets the patient's needs and cataract surgery provides a reasonable likelihood of quality-of-life improvement.

–Avoid surgery in the following circumstances:

  • Vision with corrective lenses provides acceptable quality of life, surgery is not expected to improve visual function, and no other indication for lens removal exists.

  • The patient cannot safely undergo surgery because of coexisting medical or ocular conditions.

  • Appropriate postoperative care cannot be arranged.

  • Patient or patient's surrogate decision-maker is unable to give informed consent for nonemergent surgery.

Practice Pearls

• Cataracts will cause the red reflex to appear shadowed or absent on physical exam. Postoperative symptoms may include vision impairment, sensitivity to glare, and difficulty with night vision.

• Routine preoperative medical testing does not measurably increase the safety of the surgery. Avoid requiring preoperative clearance for cataract surgeries.

FIG. 4–1 CATARACT IN ADULTS: EVALUATION AND MANAGEMENT ALGORITHM.

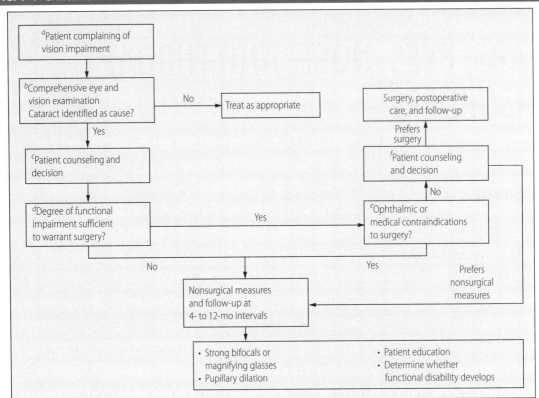

[a]Begin evaluation only when patients complain of a vision problem or impairment.

[b]Essential elements of the comprehensive eye and vision exam:

- Patient history: consider cataract if acute or gradual onset of vision loss; vision problems under special conditions (eg, low contrast, glare); difficulties performing various visual tasks. Ask about refractive history, previous ocular disease, amblyopia, eye surgery, trauma, general health history, medications, and allergies. It is critical to describe the actual impact of the cataract on the person's function and quality of life. There are several instruments available for assessing functional impairment related to cataract, including VF-14, Activities of Daily Vision Scale, and Visual Activities Questionnaire.
- Ocular examination includes Snellen acuity and refraction; measurement of intraocular pressure; assessment of pupillary function; external exam; slit-lamp exam; and dilated exam of fundus.
- Supplemental testing: may be necessary to assess and document the extent of the functional disability and to determine whether other diseases may limit preoperative or postoperative vision. Most elderly patients presenting with visual problems do not have a cataract that causes functional impairment. Refractive error, macular degeneration, and glaucoma are common alternative etiologies for visual impairment.

[c]Once cataract has been identified as the cause of visual disability, patients should be counseled concerning the nature of the problem, its natural history, and the existence of both surgical and nonsurgical approaches to management. The principal factor that should guide decision-making with regard to surgery is the extent to which the cataract impairs the ability to function in daily life. The findings of the physical examination should corroborate that the cataract is the major contributing cause of the functional impairment, and that there is a reasonable expectation that managing the cataract will positively impact the patient's functional activity. Preoperative visual acuity is a poor predictor of postoperative functional improvement: the decision to recommend cataract surgery should not be made solely on the basis of visual acuity.

[d]Patients who report mild-to-moderate limitation in activities due to a visual problem, those whose corrected acuities are near 20/40, and those who do not yet wish to undergo surgery may be offered nonsurgical measures for improving visual function. Treatment with nutritional supplements is not recommended. Smoking cessation retards cataract progression. Indications for surgery: cataract-impaired vision no longer meets the patient's needs; evidence of lens-induced disease (eg, phacomorphic glaucoma, phacolytic glaucoma); necessary to visualize the fundus in an eye that has the potential for sight (eg, diabetic patient at risk for diabetic retinopathy).

FIG. 4–1 CATARACT IN ADULTS: EVALUATION AND MANAGEMENT ALGORITHM.

*Contraindications to surgery: the patient does not desire surgery; glasses or vision aids provide satisfactory functional vision; surgery will not improve visual function; the patient's quality of life is not compromised; the patient is unable to undergo surgery because of coexisting medical or ocular conditions; a legal consent cannot be obtained; or the patient is unable to obtain adequate postoperative care. Routine preoperative medical testing (12-lead ECG, CBC, measurement of serum electrolytes, BUN, creatinine, and glucose), while commonly performed in patients scheduled to undergo cataract surgery, does not appear to measurably increase the safety of the surgery.

†Patients with significant functional and visual impairment due to cataract who have no contraindications to surgery should be counseled regarding the expected risks and benefits of and alternatives to surgery.

Sources: American Academy of Ophthalmology Preferred Practice Pattern: Cataract in the Adult Eye. 2006. http://www.aao.org; American Optometric Association Consensus Panel on Care of the Adult Patient with Cataract. Optometric Clinical Practice Guideline: Care of the Adult Patient with Cataract. 2004. http://www.aoa.org.

Sources

–*American Academy of Ophthalmology Preferred Practice Pattern: Cataract/Anterior Segment Summary Benchmark.* 2021. http://www.aao.org

–American Optometric Association Consensus Panel on Care of the Adult Patient with Cataract. *Optometric Clinical Practice Guideline: Care of the Adult Patient with Cataract.* 2004. http://www.aoa.org

–*Am Fam Physician.* 2016;94(3):219–226.

CERUMEN IMPACTION

Management: Children and Adults

Recommendations from

➤ AAO-HNS 2017

–Treat cerumen impaction when it is symptomatic or prevents a necessary examination.
–Treat with an appropriate intervention:
  • Cerumenolytic agents (water or saline, Cerumenex, Addax, Debrox, or dilute solutions of acetic acid, hydrogen peroxide, or sodium bicarbonate).
  • Irrigation.
  • Manual removal.
–Prevent recurrent impaction by using alcohol or hydrogen peroxide drops, routine irrigation with bulb syringe or irrigation kits, topical cerumen-softening agents, or physical removal by clinician.
–Avoid ear candling, olive oil, and probing ear canal with objects such as cotton swabs.

Practice Pearls

• Removal of cerumen is not necessary if the patient is asymptomatic and adequate clinical exam is possible.
  - Irrigation is contraindicated if TM rupture, tympanostomy tubes are present, or significant anatomic abnormalities exist. While irrigating, pull gentle traction on the external ear, use water that approximates body temperature, and instill gently. Consider instilling a mix of vinegar and isopropyl alcohol after irrigation to prevent infection.

Source

–https://www.entnet.org//content/clinical-practice-guideline-cerumen-impaction

DENTAL CARIES

Screening: Children and Adolescents

Recommendations from

> USPSTF 2023, 2021

   –Insufficient data to assess benefits and harms of routine screenings by primary care physicians for oral health conditions in children and adolescents ages 5–17 y, or in children <5 y.

   Sources
   –*JAMA.* 2023;330(17):1666–1673.
   –*JAMA.* 2021;326(21):2172–2178.

Screening: Adults

Recommendations from

> USPSTF 2023

   –Insufficient data to assess benefits and harms of routine screenings by primary care physicians for oral health conditions in adults.

   Source
   –*JAMA.* 2023;330(17):1666–1673.

Prevention: Infants, Children, and Adolescents

Recommendations from

> USPSTF 2023, 2021, AAP 2014, AAFP 2014, AAP Bright Futures

   –Clean infant gums with a clean, soft, damp cloth once daily.
   –Apply fluoride varnish to the primary teeth of all infants and children starting at the age of primary teeth eruption (see Table 4–1).
   –Start oral fluoride supplementation starting at age 6 mo unless usual water supply contains sufficient fluoride concentrations (see Table 4–2).
   –Insufficient data to assess benefits and harms of routine preventive interventions by primary care physicians in children and adolescents ages 5–17 y. (USPSTF)
   –Prescribe oral fluoride supplementation starting at age 6 mo for children whose water supply is fluoride deficient (≤0.6 mg/L) (see Table 4–2 for dosing).

Practice Pearls

- Fluoride mouthwash used regularly by children under 16 reduces risk of dental caries by >25%. (*Cochrane Database Syst Rev.* 2016;7:CD002284)
- The CDC's My Water's Fluoride resource provides county-level information on content of fluoride in the water system. https://nccd.cdc.gov/DOH_MWF/
- Brush infant teeth with a smear of fluoridated toothpaste at eruption of first tooth twice per day up to age 3. Children aged 3–6 y should brush with a pea-sized amount of fluoridated toothpaste twice daily; parents should be brushing child's teeth once daily until age 7.

- Caries risk assessment tool can be found at: https://www.aapd.org/globalassets/media/policies_guidelines/bp_cariesriskassessment.pdf

TABLE 4–1 CLINICAL RECOMMENDATIONS FOR USE OF PROFESSIONALLY APPLIED OR PRESCRIPTION-STRENGTH, HOME-USE TOPICAL FLUORIDE AGENTS FOR CARIES PREVENTION IN PATIENTS AT ELEVATED RISK OF DEVELOPING CARIES

Age Group or Dentition Affected	Professionally Applied Topical Fluoride Agent	Prescription-Strength, Home-Use Topical Fluoride Agent
Younger than 6 y	2.26% fluoride varnish at least every 3 to 6 mo (In Favor)	
6–18 y	2.26% fluoride varnish at least every 3 to 6 mo (In Favor) or 1.23% fluoride (acidulated phosphate fluoride [APF]) gel for 4 min at least every 3 to 6 mo (In Favor)	0.09% fluoride mouthrinse at least weekly (In Favor) or 0.5% fluoride gel or paste twice daily (Expert Opinion For)
Older than 18 y	2.26% fluoride varnish at least every 3 to 6 mo (Expert Opinion For) or 1.23% fluoride (APF) gel for at least 4 min every 3 to 6 mo (Expert Opinion For)	0.09% fluoride mouthrinse at least weekly (Expert Opinion For) or 0.5% fluoride gel or paste twice daily (Expert Opinion For)
Adult root caries	2.26% fluoride varnish at least every 3 to 6 mo (Expert Opinion For) or 1.23% fluoride (APF) gel for 4 min at least every 3 to 6 mo (Expert Opinion For)	0.09% fluoride mouthrinse daily (Expert Opinion For) or 0.5% fluoride gel or paste twice daily (Expert Opinion For)

Additional Information:

Patients at low risk for developing caries may not need additional topical fluorides other than over-the-counter fluoridated toothpaste and fluoridated water.

Source: Reproduced with permission from Weyant RJ, Tracy SL, Anselmo T (Tracy), et al. Topical fluoride for caries prevention. *J Am Dent Assoc.* 2013;144(11):1279–1291.

TABLE 4–2 RECOMMENDED FLUORIDE SUPPLEMENTATION BY AGE AND FLUORIDE LEVEL IN COMMUNITY WATER SUPPLY

Age	Fluoride Level in Drinking Water < 0.3 ppm	Fluoride Level in Drinking Water 0.3–0.6 ppm
6 mo–3 y	0.25 mg/d	None
3–6 y	0.5 mg/d	0.25 mg/d
6–16 y	1.0 mg/d	0.5 mg/d

Source: Adapted from Table 1 in CDC MMWR. 2001;50(RR14):1–42. https://www.cdc.gov/mmwr/preview/mmwrhtml/rr5014a1.htm

Sources
–USPSTF. *Screening and Interventions to Prevent Dental Caries in Children Younger than 5 Years.* 2021.
–*JAMA.* 2023;330(17):1666–1673.
–AAFP. *Clinical Recommendation.* 2014.
–*Pediatrics.* 2014;133(5):s1–s10.
–*JAMA.* 2021;326(21):2172–2178.

Prevention: Adults

Recommendations from
➢ USPSTF 2023
–Insufficient data to assess benefits and harms of routine screenings by primary care physicians for oral health conditions in adults.

Practice Pearls
- Ninety percent of adults will be affected by dental caries, and about 26% of adults have untreated caries, which can lead to infections and loss of teeth.
- Forty-two percent of adults (60% over age 65) have periodontal disease, which can lead to tooth loss.
- Xerostomia, whether due to medical conditions or medication side effects, can lead to oral health problems. So, can dietary sugar intake, inadequate fluoride exposure, lack of brushing and flossing, and use of tobacco, alcohol, and amphetamines.
- Little evidence exists to support preventative interventions, though it may be wise for patients to modify their risk factors when possible.

Source
–*JAMA.* 2023;330(17):1666–1673.

EPISTAXIS

Management: Adults and Children over Age 3

Recommendations from
➢ AAO-HNS 2020

Evaluation
–Identify the acuity and severity of bleeding to appropriately triage and treat the patient. Bleeding is severe if:
  - Bleeding for greater than 30 min in a 24-h period.
  - History of hospitalization or prior transfusion.
  - Comorbid conditions: uncontrolled HTN, anemia, clotting disorders, etc.
–Remove any blood clot, then perform anterior rhinoscopy to identify a source of bleeding.

–Document factors that increase the frequency or severity of bleeding including personal or family history of bleeding disorders, use of anticoagulant or antiplatelet medications, or intranasal drug use.

Therapies

–First-line interventions:

- Compression: Treat active bleeding with firm sustained compression to the lower third of the nose, with or without the assistance of the patient or caregiver, for 5 min or longer.
- Topical agents (vasoconstrictors).
- Cautery.
- Packing.
- Include patient education and follow-up recommendations for timing of removal.

–Use second-line interventions for refractory bleeding:

- Perform, or refer to a clinician who can perform, nasal endoscopy to identify the site of bleeding and guide further management in patients with recurrent nasal bleeding, despite prior treatment with packing or cautery, or with recurrent unilateral nasal bleeding.

–If further treatment is required, invasive options include surgical ligation and/or cautery and endovascular embolization.

Source

–https://www.entnet.org/quality-practice/quality-products/clinical-practice-guidelines/nosebleed-epistaxis/

HEARING LOSS, SUDDEN

Management: Adults

Recommendations from

> **AAO-HNS 2019**

–Distinguish between sensorineural and conductive hearing loss (ie, impacted wax, acute otitis).

–Diagnose idiopathic sudden sensorineural hearing loss when audiometry confirms a 30-dB hearing loss at 3 consecutive frequencies and no underlying condition can be identified.

–Evaluate patients with an MRI of the internal auditory canal, auditory brainstem responses, and an audiology exam.

–Treat with systemic or intratympanic steroids *within 14 d* of onset unless complete recovery occurs before treatment begins. Consider hyperbaric oxygen therapy only as an adjunct to steroids.

–Do not use antivirals, thrombolytics, vasodilators, or antioxidants for treatment or evaluate with CT scanning of the head or routine lab testing.

Practice Pearls

- Prompt diagnosis is important.
- Obtain audiometric testing as soon as possible, and *within 14 d*, to facilitate prompt treatment.
- Counsel patients with incomplete recovery of hearing about the benefits of hearing aids.

Source
  –https://www.entnet.org/quality-practice/quality-products/clinical-practice-guidelines/sudden-hearing-loss-update/

HOARSENESS

Management: Adults

Recommendations from

➤ AAO-HNS 2018
  –If hoarseness fails to resolve or improve spontaneously within 4 wk, refer for laryngoscopy.
  –Do not obtain neck imaging (CT or MRI) for chronic hoarseness prior to laryngoscopy.
  –Do not routinely use antibiotics or steroids to treat hoarseness.
  –Do not use antireflux medications, unless exhibiting signs or symptoms of gastroesophageal reflux disease.
  –Encourage or refer to voice therapy for all patients with continued hoarseness and a decreased voice-related quality of life.
  –Refer to surgeon for laryngeal cancer, benign laryngeal soft-tissue lesions, or glottis insufficiency.
  –Consider botulinum toxin injections for spasmodic dysphonia.

Practice Pearls

- Nearly one-third of Americans will have hoarseness at some point in their lives.
- Most, but not all, hoarseness is benign or self-limited; some of the most common causes are upper respiratory infection and vocal overuse.

Source
  –https://www.entnet.org//content/clinical-practice-guideline-hoarseness-dysphonia

LARYNGITIS, ACUTE

Management: Adults

Recommendations from

➤ Cochrane Database Systematic Reviews 2015
  –Insufficient evidence to support the use of antibiotics for acute laryngitis.
  –Erythromycin may provide some improvement in patient-reported symptoms, but cost and negative consequences of use outweigh benefit.

Source
  –http://www.cochrane.org/CD004783/ARI_antibiotics-to-treat-adults-with-acute-laryngitis

MENIERE DISEASE

Management: Adults

Recommendations from

> ### AAO-HNS 2020, AAFP 2020

Evaluation

–Consider diagnosis in patients presenting with all of the following:
- Vertigo: 2 or more episodes lasting 20 min to 12 h (definite) or up to 24 h (probable).
- Sensorineural hearing loss (persistent or fluctuating), tinnitus, or pressure in the affected ear.
- Symptoms not better accounted for by another disorder.

–Obtain audiogram when considering diagnosis of Meniere.

–Evaluate for vestibular migraine.

–Consider MRI of the internal auditory canal and posterior fossa in patients with asymmetric sensorineural hearing loss verified by audiometry.

–Do not routinely order vestibular function testing or electrocochleography.

Therapies

–Offer a limited course of vestibular suppressants (ie, promethazine, prochlorperazine, diazepam) to patients with Meniere disease to manage the vertigo during attacks.

–Consider diet restrictions: low sodium, minimal caffeine, minimal alcohol.

–Consider thiazide diuretics and/or betahistine for maintenance therapy to reduce symptoms or prevent Meniere disease attacks.

–Consider intratympanic steroids for patients with active Meniere disease not responsive to noninvasive treatment.

–Do not prescribe positive pressure therapy.

–Do not recommend physical therapy or vestibular therapy for acute vertigo attacks.

Practice Pearls

- Suspect Meniere in patients with spontaneous episodic dizziness and unilateral hearing loss, particularly in adults age 20–60.
- Additional symptoms can include nausea, vomiting, sudden falls, and headache.
- Additional coping mechanisms may include stress management skills: exercise, sleep, support groups, journaling, breathing exercises.

Source

–https://www.entnet.org/quality-practice/quality-products/clinical-practice-guidelines/menieres-disease/

ORAL CANCER

Screening: Adults

Recommendations from

> AAFP 2015, USPSTF 2013

–Insufficient evidence to recommend for or against routinely screening adults for oral asymptomatic cancer.

Practice Pearls

- Primary risk factors for oral cancer are tobacco and alcohol use.
- Additional risk factors include:
  - Male sex.
  - Older age.
  - Use of betel quid.
  - UV light exposure.
  - Infection with *Candida* or bacterial flora.
  - Compromised immune system.
- Recently, the human papillomavirus (HPV), which is transmitted sexually, has been recognized as an increasing risk factor for oropharyngeal cancer (another subset of head and neck cancer).

Sources
–http://www.aafp.org/online/en/home/clinical/exam.html
–http://www.ahrq.gov/clinic/uspstf/uspsoral.htm

Prevention: Adults and Children

Recommendations from

> National Cancer Institute 2018

–Avoid tobacco in any form, including smokeless.
–Reduce alcohol intake.
–Specifically, for lip cancer, avoid chronic sun exposure.

Practice Pearls

- Oropharyngeal squamous cell cancers (tonsil and base of tongue) are related to HPV infection (types 16 and 18) in 75% of patients. This correlates with sexual practices and number of partners and may be prevented by HPV vaccine. HPV (+), nonsmokers have improved cure rate by 35%–45%. (*N Engl J Med.* 2010;363:24, 82)
- There is inadequate evidence to suggest change in diet will reduce risk of oral cancer, though people who drink 3+ drinks a day have double the risk vs. nondrinkers. (*Cancer Causes Control.* 2011;22:1217)

Source
–https://www.cancer.gov/types/head-and-neck/hp/oral-prevention-pdq

OTITIS EXTERNA, ACUTE (AOE)

Management: Adults and Children Age ≥ 2 y

Recommendations from

➤ AAO-HNS 2014

–Use topical antibiotics for initial therapy of acute otitis externa.

–Do not prescribe systemic antimicrobials as initial therapy for diffuse, uncomplicated acute otitis externa.

–In the presence of a perforated tympanic membrane or tympanostomy tubes, prescribe a non-ototoxic topical antibiotic.

Practice Pearls

- Recommend reassessment of the diagnosis if the patient fails to respond within 72 h of topical antibiotics.
- If perforation is not suspected, acetic acid and neomycin/polymyxin B solutions are reasonable choices, but they should be avoided in setting of possible perforation because of ototoxicity.
- If perforation is suspected, quinolone solutions (ie, ofloxacin 0.3%, ciprofloxacin 0.3%/dexamethasone 0.1%) are often used to avoid risk of ototoxicity.
- Antibiotic corticosteroid combinations may be used, but evidence for their benefit is mixed.
- Reevaluate if there is no improvement in 24–72 h or no resolution by 2 wk.

Sources

–https://www.entnet.org/content/clinical-practice-guideline-acute-otitis-externa

–*Am Fam Physician.* 2023;107(2):145–151.

OTITIS MEDIA, ACUTE (AOM)

Prevention: Children and Adolescents

Recommendations from

➤ AAP 2013

–Do not use prophylactic antibiotics to reduce the frequency of episodes of AOM in children with recurrent AOM.

–Exclusive breastfeeding for at least the first 6 mo of life.

–Vaccinate all children to prevent bacterial AOM with pneumococcal and influenza vaccines.

–Avoid tobacco exposure.

Source

–*Pediatrics.* 2013;131(3):e964–e999.

Management: Children Age 3 mo to 18 y

Recommendations from

> AAP 2013

Evaluation
–Make diagnosis in children with an effusion and on one of the following findings:
  - Moderate or severe TM bulging.
  - Mild bulging and onset of ear pain in the past 24 h.
  - Erythema of the TM.
  - New onset of otorrhea not caused by otitis externa.

Therapies
–See Table 4–3 for treatment approaches based on age and findings.

–Educate caregivers about prevention of otitis media: encourage breast-feeding, feed child upright if bottle fed, avoid passive smoke exposure, limit exposure to groups of children, careful handwashing prior to handling child, avoid pacifier use >10 mo, ensure immunizations are up-to-date.

–Provide symptomatic relief with acetaminophen, ibuprofen, and warm compresses to the ear.

–Use amoxicillin as the first-line antibiotic for low-risk children.

–Use alternative medication if failure to respond to initial treatment within 72 h; penicillin allergy; presence of a resistant organism found on culture.

–Refer to an ear, nose, and throat (ENT) specialist for any complications of otitis media including mastoiditis, facial nerve palsy, lateral sinus thrombosis, meningitis, brain abscess, or labyrinthitis.

–Do not require routine rechecks at 10–14 d for children feeling well.

–Do not routinely prescribe antibiotics in children age 2–12 y with nonsevere AOM when observation is an option.

Practice Pearls

- Amoxicillin is first-line therapy for most children.
  - 80–90 mg/kg/d in 2 divided doses.
- Use amoxicillin-clavulanate if child has received antibiotics in prior 30 d.
- Alternative antibiotics:
  - Amoxicillin-clavulanate.
  - Azithromycin.
  - Cefdinir.
  - Cefixime.
  - Cefpodoxime.
  - Cefprozil.
  - Ceftriaxone.
  - Cefuroxime axetil.
  - Clarithromycin.
  - Erythromycin.
  - Loracarbef.

TABLE 4–3 ACUTE OTITIS MEDIA—APPROACHES TO TREATMENT		
Age	**Findings**	**Approach**
≥ 6 mo	Otorrhea, moderate-to-severe otalgia, otalgia > 48 h, or temperature > 102.2°F	Antibiotics × 10 d
6–23 mo	Bilateral AOM	Antibiotics × 10 d
6–23 mo	Unilateral AOM, no otorrhea, moderate-to-severe otalgia, otalgia > 48 h, or temperature > 102.2°F	Wait-and-see, or antibiotics × 10 d
≥ 24 mo	No otorrhea, moderate-to-severe otalgia, otalgia > 48 h, or temperature > 102.2°F	Wait-and-see, or antibiotics for 5–7 d

Sources
–*Pediatrics*. 2013;131:e964–e999.
–http://www.choosingwisely.org/societies/american-academy-of-family-physicians/
–*Am Fam Physician*. 2013;88(7):435–440.

OTITIS MEDIA WITH EFFUSION

Management: Children Age ≤ 12 y

Recommendations from

> NICE 2023

Evaluation
–Diagnose in children who have middle ear effusion without signs of acute inflammation or infection. Children may present with hearing difficulties, delayed speech and language development, ear discomfort, or tinnitus. These may lead to behavioral and attention issues, poor educational progress, and difficulties with balance.
–After initial diagnosis, reassess in 3 mo. Consider earlier intervention only if hearing loss is causing significant issues in daily living.

Therapies
–If no hearing loss, intervention is not indicated.
–If unilateral hearing loss persists at 3 mo, consider intervening or reassessing again in 3 mo.
–If bilateral hearing loss persists at 3 mo, intervene.
–Use interventions to restore hearing and promote normal development of speech, language, and behavior. Options include:
  • Hearing aids or bone conduction devices.
  • Auto-inflation.
  • Tympanostomy, with or without adenoidectomy.
–Do not use the following interventions:
  • Antibiotics.
  • Nasal corticosteroids.

- Oral corticosteroids.
- Antihistamines, PPI, anti-reflux medications, or decongestants.
- Homeopathy, cranial osteopathy, acupuncture, massage.

Source
–www.nice.org.uk/guidance/ng233

PHARYNGITIS, ACUTE

Management: Children and Adults with Acute Pharyngitis

Recommendations from
> IDSA 2012
>> –See Fig. 4–2.

RHINITIS, ALLERGIC

Management: Children and Adults

Recommendations from
> ICSI 2011, AAO-HSNF 2015

–Use intranasal steroids when symptoms affect quality of life.

–Use second-generation antihistamines if symptoms of itching or sneezing.

–Perform specific IgE serum or blood allergy testing if no response to treatment, uncertain diagnosis, or specific allergen identity is needed.

–Do not use leukotriene receptor antagonists as primary therapy.

Sources
–ICSI 2011; AAO-HNSF 2015.
–https://www.entnet.org//content/clinical-practice-guideline-allergic-rhinitis

SINUSITIS, PEDIATRICS

Management: Children

Recommendations from
> AAP 2013

–Presumptively diagnose acute sinusitis if child has acute URI and one of the following:
- Nasal discharge or persistent cough lasting more than 10 d.
- Worsening course.
- Severe onset with fever ≥ 102.2°F and purulent nasal discharge for at least 3 d.

–Do not obtain imaging studies for uncomplicated sinusitis.

–Obtain contrast-enhanced CT scan of sinuses for any suspicion of orbital or CNS involvement.

FIG. 4–2 APPROACH TO ACUTE PHARYNGITIS.

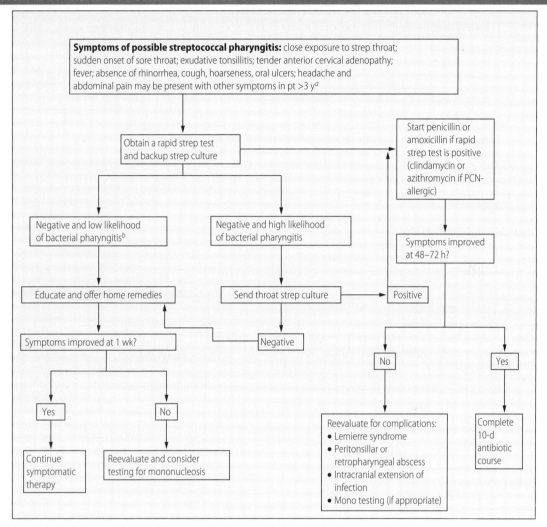

Symptoms of possible streptococcal pharyngitis: close exposure to strep throat; sudden onset of sore throat; exudative tonsillitis; tender anterior cervical adenopathy; fever; absence of rhinorrhea, cough, hoarseness, oral ulcers; headache and abdominal pain may be present with other symptoms in pt >3 y[a]

Obtain a rapid strep test and backup strep culture

Start penicillin or amoxicillin if rapid strep test is positive (clindamycin or azithromycin if PCN-allergic)

Negative and low likelihood of bacterial pharyngitis[b]

Negative and high likelihood of bacterial pharyngitis

Symptoms improved at 48–72 h?

Educate and offer home remedies

Send throat strep culture

Positive

Symptoms improved at 1 wk?

Negative

No

Yes

Yes

No

Reevaluate for complications:
- Lemierre syndrome
- Peritonsillar or retropharyngeal abscess
- Intracranial extension of infection
- Mono testing (if appropriate)

Complete 10-d antibiotic course

Continue symptomatic therapy

Reevaluate and consider testing for mononucleosis

[a]Diagnostic studies for GAS is not indicated for children <3 y because acute rheumatic fever is very rare in this age group.
[b]Low likelihood of GAS if rhinorrhea, cough, hoarseness, or oral ulcers.
Source: IDSA 2012 guidelines on group A Streptococcus (GAS) pharyngitis. https://doi.org/10.1093/cid/cis629

–Consider antibiotics for sinusitis with severe onset or worsening course:
- Amoxicillin $+/-$ clavulanate is first-line therapy.
- Persistent cough or rhinorrhea in the absence of severe symptoms may be managed with ongoing observation.

Practice Pearl
- Improvement of symptoms should occur within 72 h of antibiotic initiation.

Source
–https://guidelines.gov/summaries/summary/46939

SINUSITIS, ADULTS

Management: Adults

Recommendations from

> AAO-HNS 2015, AAAAI 2022
- –Classify sinusitis and manage according to Table 4–4.
- –Consider recommending analgesics, topical intranasal steroids, and/or nasal saline irrigation for symptomatic relief of sinusitis.
- –If the patient's condition worsens or fails to improve with the initial management option by 7 d after diagnosis or worsens during the initial management, reassess to confirm ABRS, exclude other causes of illness, and detect complications. If initially managed with antibiotic, change to a different agent.
- –If ABRS is confirmed in the patient initially managed with observation, begin antibiotic therapy.

Sources
–https://www.entnet.org//content/clinical-practice-guideline-adult-sinusitis
–https://www.jacionline.org/article/S0091-6749(22)01484-1/fulltext

TINNITUS

Management: Adults and Children

Recommendations from

> AAO-HNS 2014, American Speech-Language-Hearing Association 2018, NICE 2020
- –Obtain a thorough history and exam on patients with tinnitus. Elicit features such as unilateral or pulsatile tinnitus which may suggest more insidious etiology.
- –Refer for a comprehensive audiologic examination for unilateral or persistent tinnitus or any associated hearing impairment.
- –Only obtain imaging studies for unilateral tinnitus, pulsatile tinnitus, asymmetric hearing loss, or focal neurological abnormalities.

TABLE 4–4 TYPES OF SINUSITIS AND THEIR MANAGEMENT

Classification	Diagnostic Criteria	Management
Acute rhinosinusitis (ARS)	≤4 wk of purulent nasal drainage (anterior, posterior, or both) with nasal obstruction, facial pain/pressure/fullness, or both	Do not obtain radiographic imaging for patients who meet diagnostic criteria for ARS unless a complication or alternative diagnosis is suspected
Viral rhinosinusitis (VRS)	Symptoms or signs of ARS are present <10 d and the symptoms are not worsening	Analgesics, topical intranasal steroids, and/or nasal saline irrigation for symptomatic relief of VRS
Acute bacterial rhinosinusitis (ABRS)	Symptoms or signs of ARS fail to improve within 10 d or more beyond the onset of upper respiratory symptoms Symptoms or signs of ARS worsen within 10 d after an initial improvement (double worsening)	Offer watchful waiting (without antibiotics) or prescribe initial antibiotic therapy for adults with uncomplicated ABRS Offer watchful waiting only when there is assurance of follow-up such that antibiotic therapy is started if the patient's condition fails to improve by 7 d after ABRS diagnosis or if it worsens at any time When antibiotics are indicated, use amoxicillin with or without clavulanate for 5–10 d
Chronic rhinosinusitis (CRS)	Twelve weeks or longer of 2 or more of the following signs and symptoms: • Mucopurulent drainage (anterior, posterior, or both) • Nasal obstruction (congestion) • Facial pain/pressure/fullness • Decreased sense of smell AND inflammation is documented by one or more of the following findings: • Purulent (not clear) mucus or edema in the middle meatus or anterior ethmoid region • Polyps in nasal cavity or the middle meatus • Radiographic imaging showing inflammation of the paranasal sinuses Confirm a clinical diagnosis with objective documentation of sinonasal inflammation using anterior rhinoscopy, nasal endoscopy, or CT	Recommend saline nasal irrigation, topical intranasal corticosteroids, or both for symptom relief of CRS Do not prescribe topical or systemic antifungal therapy for patients with CRS

TABLE 4–4 TYPES OF SINUSITIS AND THEIR MANAGEMENT (*Continued*)		
Classification	**Diagnostic Criteria**	**Management**
CRS with nasal polyposis	Patients with CRS who have nasal polyps	Intranasal corticosteroids (stent, spray, and exhalation delivery systems) (low certainty evidence) Biologics (dupilumab, omalizumab, or mepolizumab) are typically reserved for patients with severe disease or failure of intranasal steroids (AAAAI 2022)

–Refer for a hearing aid for tinnitus with hearing loss.

–Consider cognitive behavioral therapy or sound therapy for persistent, bothersome tinnitus.

–Do not offer medical or herbal therapy, including betahistine, or transcranial magnetic stimulation for tinnitus (ASHA: "remain current" in the evidence or lack thereof for these approaches).

Practice Pearl

- Secondary etiologies of tinnitus include:
  - Infections: Lyme, syphilis, fungal, viral.
  - Metabolic: diabetes mellitus, hyperlipidemia, B_{12} deficiency.
  - Neurological: intracranial hypertension, idiopathic stapedial or tensor tympani muscle spasm, multiple sclerosis, palatal myoclonus, type I Chiari malformation, vestibular migraine.
  - Otologic: cerumen impaction, cholesteatoma, foreign body, Meniere disease, middle ear effusion, otitis, otosclerosis, patulous eustachian tube, tympanic membrane perforation, vestibular schwannoma.
  - Somatic: head/neck injury, temporomandibular joint dysfunction.
  - Traumatic: cerumen removal.
  - Vascular: arterial bruit, AVM, carotid artery pathology, Paget disease, vascular tumors, venous hum.
  - Medications: lidocaine/bupivacaine, carbamazepine, pregabalin, NSAIDs, aminoglycosides, macrolides, tetracyclines, vancomycin, several antineoplastics, loop diuretics, phosphodiesterase 5 inhibitors, atorvastatin, bupropion, varenicline, PPIs, HPV vaccine, Pneumovax, and several others.

Sources

–https://www.entnet.org//content/clinical-practice-guideline-tinnitus
–https://www.asha.org/Practice-Portal/Clinical-Topics/Tinnitus-and-Hyperacusis/
–https://www.nice.org.uk/guidance/ng155
–*Am Fam Physician.* 2021;103(11):663–671.

TONSILLECTOMY

Management: Children

Recommendations from

> AAO-HNS 2019

–Tonsillectomy is indicated for:
- Tonsillar hypertrophy with sleep-disordered breathing.
- Recurrent throat infections for ≥7 episodes of recurrent throat infection in last year; ≥5 episodes of recurrent throat infection per year in last 2 y; or at least 3 episodes per year for 3 y with documentation in the medical record for each episode of sore throat and ≥1 of the following: temperature > 38.3°C (101°F), cervical adenopathy, tonsillar exudate, or positive test for group A beta-hemolytic streptococcus.

–Do not routinely use perioperative antibiotics for tonsillectomy.

–Give post-tonsillectomy pain control, but do not use codeine in children less than age 12.

Source

–https://www.entnet.org/content/clinical-practice-guideline-tonsillectomy-children-update

TYMPANOSTOMY TUBES

Management: Children 6 mo to 12 y

Recommendations from

> AAO-HNS 2022

–Do not insert tympanostomy tubes for children with:
- A single episode of otitis media with effusion (OME) of <3 mo duration.
- Recurrent acute otitis media without effusion.

–Obtain a hearing test if OME persists for at least 3 mo or if tympanostomy tube insertion is being considered.

–Offer bilateral tympanostomy tube insertion to children with:
- Bilateral OME for at least 3 mo **AND** documented hearing impairment.
- Recurrent acute otitis media with effusions.
- Tympanostomy tube insertion is an option for chronic symptomatic OME associated with balance problems, poor school performance, behavioral problems, or ear discomfort thought to be due to OME.

–For children with chronic OME who are not surgical candidates, reevaluate every 3–6 mo until effusion resolves, significant hearing impairment develops, or abnormalities of tympanic membrane or middle ear are suspected.

–Only offer otic (not oral) antibiotics for children with uncomplicated acute otorrhea from tympanostomy tube. Do not offer antibiotics for prophylaxis of otorrhea.

Practice Pearl

- Prophylactic water precautions (avoidance of swimming or water sports or use of earplugs) are not necessary for children with tympanostomy tubes.

Sources

–http://www.guideline.gov/content.aspx?id=46909

–https://www.entnet.org/quality-practice/quality-products/clinical-practice-guidelines/tympanostomy-tubes-in-children/

VERTIGO, BENIGN PAROXYSMAL POSITIONAL (BPPV)

Management: Adults

Recommendations from

> AAO-HNS 2017

Evaluation

–Use the Dix–Hallpike maneuver to diagnose posterior semicircular canal BPPV.

–If the Dix–Hallpike test result is negative, use a supine roll test to diagnose lateral semicircular canal BPPV.

–Evaluate patients for an underlying peripheral vestibular or central nervous system disorder if they have an initial treatment failure.

–Do not routinely obtain radiologic imaging.

–Do not routinely order vestibular testing.

Therapies

–Consider observation as an acceptable initial management.

–Offer vestibular repositioning exercises such as the Epley maneuver for the initial treatment.

–Do not impose postprocedural postural restrictions for posterior canal BPPV.

–Do not routinely use antihistamines or benzodiazepines for patients with BPPV, as they can increase the risk of falls.

Practice Pearls

- BPPV is the most common vestibular disorder in adults, afflicting 2.4% of adults at some point during their lives.
- A positive Dix–Hallpike test is sufficient to diagnose BPPV, while a negative test is insufficient to rule it out if high pretest probability. (*Otolaryngol Clin North Am*. 2012;45(5):925–940)
- A demonstration of the Dix–Hallpike maneuver is available here: https://youtu.be/8RYB2QlO1N4
- A demonstration of the Epley maneuver is available here: https://youtu.be/jBzlD5nVQjk
- A demonstration of the Brandt–Daroff exercises is available here: https://youtu.be/voZXtTUdQ00

Source

–https://www.entnet.org//content/clinical-practice-guideline-benign-paroxysmal-positional-vertigo-bppv

GASTROINTESTINAL AND HEPATOBILIARY DISORDERS

ABNORMAL LIVER CHEMISTRIES

Management: Adults

Recommendations from

> ACG 2017, ACR 2023

–Elevations in liver function tests are encountered frequently in clinical practice and indicate hepatobiliary insult or obstruction.

–Albumin and prothrombin time serve as markers of hepatocellular synthetic function.

–Patterns of LFT elevation are characterized as "hepatocellular" and "cholestatic."

–See Figs. 5–1, 5–2, and 5–3 for a recommended approach to abnormal liver chemistries.

Sources
–*J Am Coll Radiol.* 2023;20(11S):S302–S314.
–*Am J Gastroenterol.* 2017;112(1):18–35.

ANAL FISSURES

Management: Adults

Recommendations from

> American Society of Colon and Rectal Surgeons (ASCRS) 2022

–Begin with nonoperative first-line treatments including:
- Sitz baths and fiber supplementation.
- Topical steroids or analgesics as needed for pain relief.
- Topical nitrates, with the understanding of increased risk for headaches.
- Topical calcium channel blockers.
- Botulinum toxin injections may be considered for chronic anal fissures.

–Consider operative treatment with lateral internal sphincterotomy unless the following contraindications are present:
- Women with prior obstetrical injuries.
- Patients with IBD.

FIG. 5–1 ALGORITHM FOR EVALUATION OF ASPARTATE AMINOTRANSFERASE (AST) AND/OR ALANINE AMINOTRANSFERASE (ALT) LEVEL.

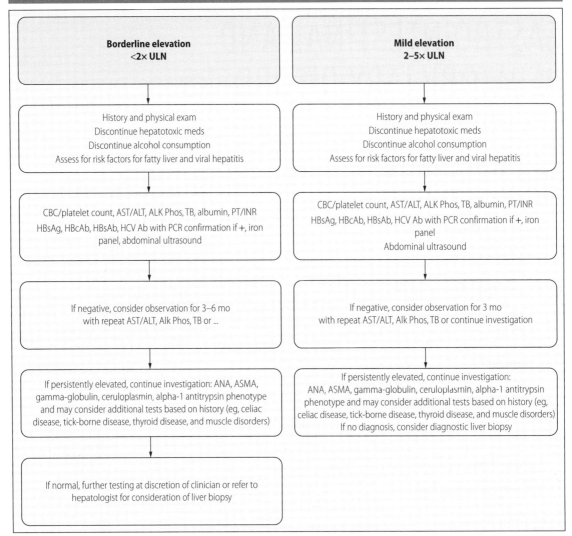

Source: Reproduced with permission from Kwo PY, Cohen SM, Lim JK. ACG clinical guideline: evaluation of abnormal liver chemistries. *Am J Gastroenterol.* 2017;112(1):18–35.

- History of anorectal operations.
- History of anal sphincter injury.

–Other operative treatment approaches are available for those with a high risk for fecal incontinence.

Source

–ASCRS. *Dis Colon Rectum.* 2022;66:190–199.

FIG. 5–2 ALGORITHM FOR EVALUATION OF ELEVATED SERUM ALKALINE PHOSPHATASE.

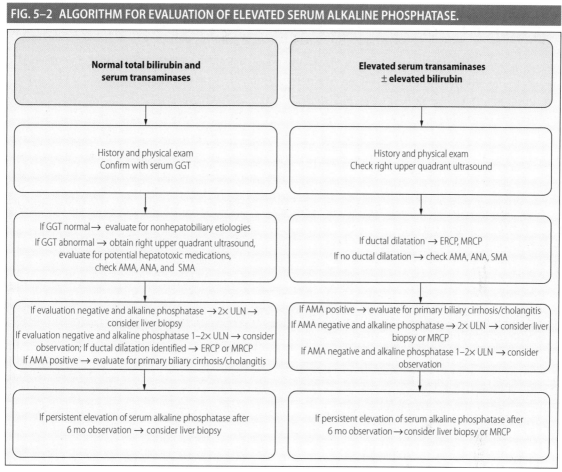

Normal total bilirubin and serum transaminases

History and physical exam
Confirm with serum GGT

If GGT normal → evaluate for nonhepatobiliary etiologies
If GGT abnormal → obtain right upper quadrant ultrasound, evaluate for potential hepatotoxic medications, check AMA, ANA, and SMA

If evaluation negative and alkaline phosphatase → 2× ULN → consider liver biopsy
If evaluation negative and alkaline phosphatase 1–2× ULN → consider observation; If ductal dilatation identified → ERCP or MRCP
If AMA positive → evaluate for primary biliary cirrhosis/cholangitis

If persistent elevation of serum alkaline phosphatase after 6 mo observation → consider liver biopsy

Elevated serum transaminases ± elevated bilirubin

History and physical exam
Check right upper quadrant ultrasound

If ductal dilatation → ERCP, MRCP
If no ductal dilatation → check AMA, ANA, SMA

If AMA positive → evaluate for primary biliary cirrhosis/cholangitis
If AMA negative and alkaline phosphatase → 2× ULN → consider liver biopsy or MRCP
If AMA negative and alkaline phosphatase 1–2× ULN → consider observation

If persistent elevation of serum alkaline phosphatase after 6 mo observation → consider liver biopsy or MRCP

Source: Reproduced with permission from Kwo PY, Cohen SM, Lim JK. ACG clinical guideline: evaluation of abnormal liver chemistries. *Am J Gastroenterol*. 2017;112(1):18–35.

BARRETT ESOPHAGUS (BE)

Screening: Adults

Recommendations from

> ASGE 2019

–Do not screen for BE in patients with gastroesophageal reflux disease (GERD) who are otherwise low risk.

–Screen moderate- to high-risk individuals using upper endoscopy (EGD) and biopsy.

• Moderate risk: GERD and ≥1 other risk factor: age > 50 y, male sex, White, obesity (BMI ≥ 30), central adiposity, tobacco use.

• High risk: family history of esophageal adenocarcinoma or BE.

FIG. 5–3 ALGORITHM FOR EVALUATION OF ELEVATED SERUM TOTAL BILIRUBIN.

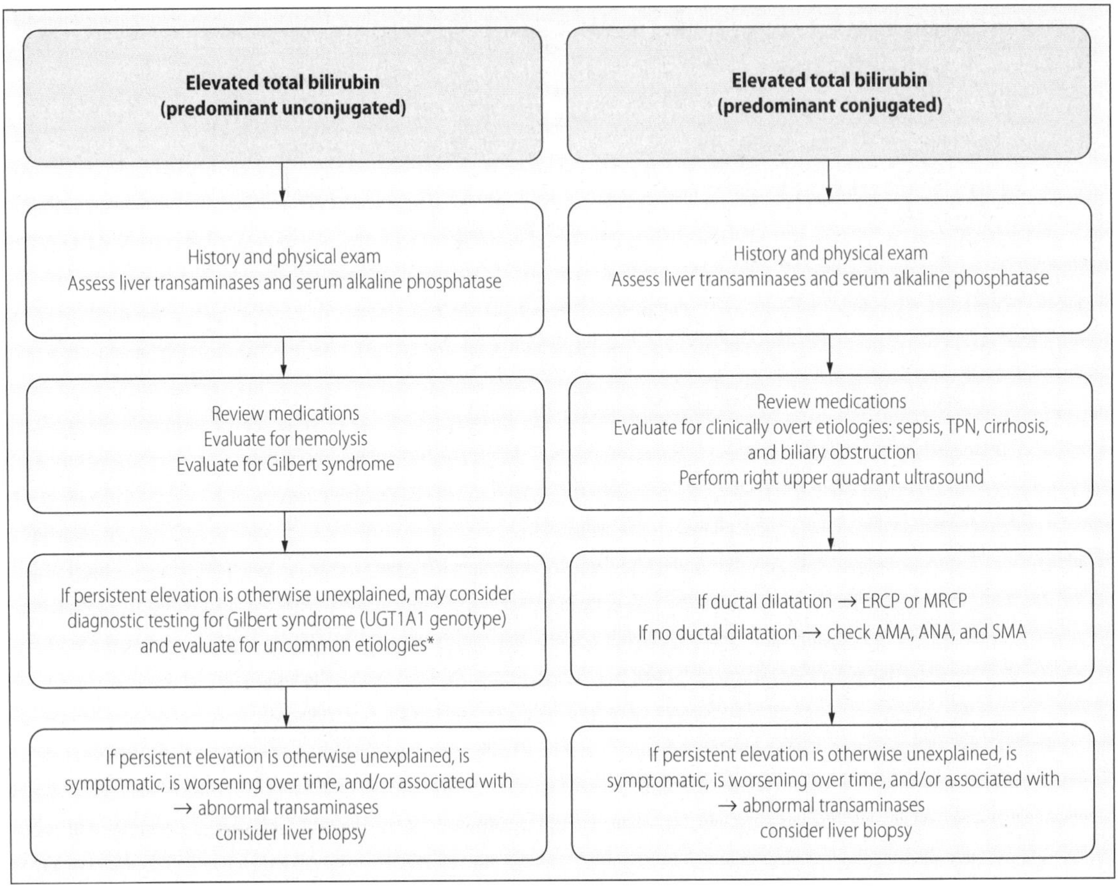

Elevated total bilirubin (predominant unconjugated)

↓

History and physical exam
Assess liver transaminases and serum alkaline phosphatase

↓

Review medications
Evaluate for hemolysis
Evaluate for Gilbert syndrome

↓

If persistent elevation is otherwise unexplained, may consider diagnostic testing for Gilbert syndrome (UGT1A1 genotype) and evaluate for uncommon etiologies*

↓

If persistent elevation is otherwise unexplained, is symptomatic, is worsening over time, and/or associated with → abnormal transaminases consider liver biopsy

Elevated total bilirubin (predominant conjugated)

↓

History and physical exam
Assess liver transaminases and serum alkaline phosphatase

↓

Review medications
Evaluate for clinically overt etiologies: sepsis, TPN, cirrhosis, and biliary obstruction
Perform right upper quadrant ultrasound

↓

If ductal dilatation → ERCP or MRCP
If no ductal dilatation → check AMA, ANA, and SMA

↓

If persistent elevation is otherwise unexplained, is symptomatic, is worsening over time, and/or associated with → abnormal transaminases consider liver biopsy

*Etiologies of elevated unconjugated bilirubin include Gilbert syndrome, Crigler-Najjar syndrome, hemolysis, ineffective erythropoiesis, resorption of large hematomas, neonatal jaundice, hyperthyroidism, medications, and post-blood transfusion. Etiologies of elevated conjugated bilirubin include bile duct obstruction, bile duct stricture, AIDS cholangiopathy, viral hepatitis, toxic hepatitis, drug-induced liver injury, acute alcohol-associated hepatitis, ischemic hepatitis, cirrhosis, primary biliary cirrhosis, primary sclerosing cholangitis, infiltrative liver disease (ie, sarcoid, tuberculosis, metastatic cancer), hepatocellular carcinoma, Wilson disease, autoimmune hepatitis, congestive hepatopathy, sepsis, TPN, intrahepatic cholestasis of pregnancy, benign postoperative jaundice, ICU or multifactorial jaundice, benign recurrent cholestasis, vanishing bile duct syndrome, and ductopenia. *Source:* Reproduced with permission from Kwo PY, Cohen SM, Lim JK. ACG clinical guideline: evaluation of abnormal liver chemistries. *Am J Gastroenterol.* 2017;112(1):18–35.

Practice Pearls

- Forty percent of persons with BE and esophageal cancer have no preceding GERD symptoms.
- Treat all persons with biopsy-proven BE with proton pump inhibitor (PPI) therapy, including asymptomatic individuals.

Sources

–*Gastrointest Endosc.* 2019;90(3):335–359.
–*Am J Gastroenterol.* 2016;111(1):30–50.
–*Barrett's Oesophagus and Stage 1 Oesophageal Adenocarcinoma: Monitoring and Management.* London: National Institute for Health and Care Excellence (NICE); 2023.

Management: Adults

Recommendations from

> AGA 2011, NICE 2023, ACG 2016

–Perform endoscopic surveillance (ES) in patients with Barrett esophagus (BE) at intervals determined by clinical assessment of a patient's cancer risk.

Guidelines Alert 5–1	
GUIDELINES DISCORDANT: FREQUENCY OF ENDOSCOPIC SURVEILLANCE	
Organization	**Frequency**
AGA	• If no dysplasia: endoscopic surveillance every 3–5 y • Low-grade dysplasia: endoscopic surveillance every 6–12 mo—consider radiofrequency ablation (RFA)—90% complete eradication of dysplasia • High-grade dysplasia: endoscopic surveillance every 3 mo if no eradication therapy
NICE	• Every 2–3 y for patients with long-segment (3 cm or longer) BE • Every 3–5 y for patients with short-segment (less than 3 cm) BE with intestinal metaplasia

Applying to Clinical Practice
• Without good data to determine the frequency of surveillance, the frequency will be determined in discussion between the gastroenterologist and the patient.

–Eradication therapy: radiofrequency ablation, photodynamic therapy, or endoscopic mucosal resection is preferred over endoscopic surveillance in high-grade dysplasia.
  • After complete eradication of intestinal metaplasia, arrange surveillance in 2 y, then every 3 y thereafter.
  • Patients who have not achieved complete eradication require surveillance every 6 mo for 1 y after the last endoscopy, then annually for 2 y, then every 3 y thereafter.

Guidelines Alert 5–2	
GUIDELINES DISCORDANT: LONG-TERM USE OF PPIs IN PATIENTS WITH BARRETT ESOPHAGUS	
AGA, AGC	Use PPIs long-term in patients with BE, even if asymptomatic
NICE	Insufficient evidence to recommend long-term use of PPIs to prevent the progression of esophageal dysplasia and cancer

Applying to Clinical Practice
• Routinely recommend the long-term use of PPIs in symptomatic patients with BE. Tailor the use of PPIs in asymptomatic patients based on individual risk profiles and patient preferences.

–Long-term use of PPIs.
  • Do not routinely recommend probiotics in patients with long-term PPI use to prevent infection.
  • Do not recommend that long-term PPI users routinely raise their calcium, vitamin B_{12}, or magnesium intake beyond the Recommended Dietary Allowance.

- Do not routinely screen or monitor long-term PPI users for bone mineral density, serum creatinine, magnesium, or vitamin B_{12}.
- Do not offer aspirin to prevent progression of esophageal dysplasia and cancer. (NICE)

Practice Pearls

- In patients with BE without dysplasia, esophageal cancer develops in 0.12% per year compared to 0.5% with low-grade dysplasia. Progression from high-grade dysplasia to cancer is 6% per year. (*N Engl J Med.* 2011;365:1375)
- Forty percent of patients with BE and esophageal cancer have no history of chronic GERD symptoms.
- The risk of developing cancer is higher among men, older patients (>65 y), and patients with long segments of Barrett mucosa or dysplasia. (*Am J Gastroenterol.* 2011;106:1231) (*Gut.* 2016;65:196)

Sources
   –https://www.gastrojournal.org/article/S0016-5085(11)00084-9/fulltext
   –https://www.gastrojournal.org/article/S0016-5085(16)35137-X/fulltext
   –https://www.gastrojournal.org/article/S0016-5085(17)30091-4/fulltext

CELIAC DISEASE

Screening: Adults

Recommendations from

➤ USPSTF 2017, AAFP 2017, ACG 2013
   –Do not routinely screen the general asymptomatic population for celiac disease.

Guidelines Alert 5–3 GUIDELINES DISCORDANT: POPULATION TO SCREEN FOR CELIAC DISEASE	
Organization	**Population**
USPSTF, AAFP	Insufficient evidence regarding screening of asymptomatic individuals
NICE	Do not screen the general population Screen first-degree relatives of individuals with celiac disease
ACG	Consider screening asymptomatic persons with type 1 diabetes mellitus every 1–2 y using serologic testing with IgA tissue transglutaminase antibody and total IgA level, as 3%–10% have concurrent celiac disease

Applying to Clinical Practice
- Most celiac testing is performed to evaluate symptoms.
- There is not good evidence to support asymptomatic screening.
- It may be reasonable to test those with type 1 diabetes or with strong family history.

Practice Pearls

- Serologic testing and biopsy must be performed while on gluten-containing diet.
- IgA tissue transglutaminase (TTG) antibody is the test of choice (>90% sensitivity and specificity), along with total IgA level. If equivocal tissue tTG, perform IgA endomysial antibody test.
- Symptoms of celiac disease include diarrhea, flatulence, and a range of extraintestinal manifestations, including anemia (malabsorption of iron and folic acid), dermatitis herpetiformis (IgA deposits), abnormal liver enzymes, peripheral neuropathy or ataxia, oral findings such as aphthous ulcers or enamel defects, and osteopenia/osteoporosis. While screening is generally discouraged by guidelines, testing for celiac disease is often indicated in the evaluation of these conditions.

Sources

–USPSTF. *JAMA*. 2017;317(12):1252.

–AAFP. *Clinical Recommendations: Screening for Celiac Disease*. 2017.

–*Am J Gastroenterol*. 2013;108(5):656–676.

–NICE. *Coeliac Disease: Recognition, Assessment and Management*. 2015.

–*Am Fam Physician*. 2014;89(2):99–105.

Management: Children and Adults

Recommendations from

> NICE 2017, ACG 2023

Evaluation

–Serologic testing for suspected celiac disease (CD):

- Test for total IgA and IgA tissue transglutaminase (tTG).
- Use IgA endomysial antibody test if IgA tTG is weakly positive.

–Refer individuals with positive serologic tests to a GI specialist for consideration of endoscopic duodenal biopsy to confirm the diagnosis.

–Children with high-level tTG IgA and positive endomysial antibody may not require biopsy for confirmation of diagnosis. (ACG)

–After diagnosis, monitor with antibody tests every 3–6 mo in the first year and once a year thereafter in stable patients responding to the gluten-free diet.

Therapies

–Gold standard treatment is adherence to gluten-free diet.

–Consider vaccinating against pneumococcal disease in those diagnosed with celiac disease. (ACG)

–For refractory celiac disease despite strict adherence to gluten-free diet:

- Review certainty of diagnosis.
- Consider coexisting conditions such as irritable bowel syndrome (IBS), lactose intolerance, microscopic colitis, or inflammatory bowel disease.

Practice Pearls

- The incidence has been increasing over the last 20 y.
- The highest incidence of celiac disease seroconversion is between 12 and 36 mo of age.
- Insufficient evidence to recommend for or against probiotics after diagnosis of celiac disease.

Sources
  –NICE. 2017. https://www.nice.org.uk/guidance/qs134
  –ACG. 2023. https://doi.org/10.14309/ajg.0000000000001874

CIRRHOSIS

Management: Adults with Cirrhosis and Ascites

Recommendations from

> AASLD 2013, EASL 2018, NICE 2023

Evaluation
  –Perform diagnostic paracentesis for all patients with new-onset ascites.
  - Do not routinely give platelets or fresh frozen plasma before performing paracentesis.
  - Ascitic fluid analysis: order cell count with differential, albumin, protein, and bedside inoculation of aerobic and anaerobic culture bottles.

Therapies
  –Alcohol cessation.
  –Low sodium diet.[1]
  –Control ascites with diuretics (see Guidelines Alert 5–4).
  –Restrict fluid intake if serum sodium is low (AASLD < 125 mmol/L; EASL < 130 mmol/L).
  –Consider liver transplantation for all patients with cirrhosis and ascites.
  –Avoid NSAIDs.
  –Use ACEI, ARB, and even beta-blockers cautiously. If used, monitor blood pressure carefully as an independent predictor of survival in patients with cirrhosis.
  –Avoid aminoglycosides. (EASL)
  –In patients with refractory ascites:
  - Avoid propranolol.
  - Avoid ACEI or ARB.
  - Consider oral midodrine, particularly if hypotensive.
  - Consider serial therapeutic paracentesis.
  - Consider transjugular intrahepatic portosystemic shunt (TIPS) in carefully selected patients.
  - Give albumin for large volume paracentesis (AASLD: give 6–8 g/L of ascitic fluid removed if >5 L; EASL: give 8 g/L ascitic fluid removed and consider even when <5 L).

---

[1] 2 g sodium/d is recommended by AASLD. EASL recommends 4.6–6.9 g/d which is equivalent to a no salt-added and no processed food diet.

–Offer prophylaxis for spontaneous bacterial peritonitis when indicated:
- Give prophylactic IV antibiotics to all patients with cirrhosis admitted for upper gastrointestinal bleeding (regardless of the presence of ascites).
- Give long-term oral trimethoprim-sulfamethoxazole or norfloxacin to any patient with a history of SBP. EASL: stop prophylaxis if long-term improvement with disappearance of ascites.
- Consider SBP prophylaxis if ascitic fluid protein < 1.5 g/dL in association with creatinine > 1.2 mg/dL or sodium < 130 mmol/L or bilirubin > 3 mg/dL.
- Consider liver transplant after first episode of SBP due to poor long-term survival. (EASL)
- Only use PPIs in those with clear indication due to possible increased risk for SBP. (EASL)

Guidelines Alert 5–4
GUIDELINES DISCORDANT: INITIATING DIURETICS TO CONTROL ASCITES

Organization	Diuretic Strategy
AASLD	Give furosemide and spironolactone in a 2:5 ratio
EASL	Start spironolactone at 100 mg/d Increase q3 d to max dose of 400 mg/d as tolerated If <2 kg/wk weight loss and patient reaches max dose or hyperkalemia develops in patient, add furosemide, starting at 40 mg/d Increase in 40 mg steps to maximum of 160 mg/d Consider substituting other loop diuretic if furosemide is not effective

Applying to Clinical Practice
- The EASL approach emphasizes spironolactone, as hyperaldosteronism may play a large role in fluid retention in cirrhosis.[a]
- Either approach is reasonable with close follow-up and lab monitoring of electrolytes and creatinine clearance.

[a]*Circ Heart Fail.* 2009;2:370–376.

Sources

–AASLD. 2013 https://www.aasld.org/sites/default/files/guideline_documents/ AASLDPracticeGuidelineAsciteDuetoCirrhosisUpdate2012Edition4_.pdf
–EASL. 2018. https://doi.org/10.1016/j.jhep.2018.03.024
–NICE. *Recommendations | Cirrhosis in Over 16s: Assessment and Management | Guidance | NICE.* 2023.

Management: Adults with Cirrhosis and Spontaneous Bacterial Peritonitis

Recommendations from

> **EASL 2018, AGA 2022, NICE 2023**

–Give cefotaxime 2 g IV q8 h for 5–7 d. Alternative is ofloxacin 400 mg PO BID.
–For locations with high bacterial resistance, use piperacillin/tazobactam or carbapenem. (EASL)

–Repeat paracentesis in 48 h to assess for reduction in leukocyte count of >25%. (EASL)

–Add albumin 1.5 g/kg/d on day 1 and 1 g/kg/d on day 3 if creatinine > 1 mg/dL, BUN > 30 mg/dL, or bilirubin > 4 mg/dL.

–Consider diagnosis of secondary bacterial peritonitis and obtain CT scan of abdomen and early surgery if high neutrophil count in ascitic fluid, multiple cultured organisms, or high ascitic protein count. (EASL)

Sources

–AASLD. 2013. https://www.aasld.org/sites/default/files/guideline_documents/AASLDPracticeGuidelineAsciteDuetoCirrhosisUpdate2012Edition4_.pdf

–EASL. 2018. https://doi.org/10.1016/j.jhep.2018.03.024

–NICE. *Recommendations | Cirrhosis in Over 16s: Assessment and Management | Guidance | NICE.* 2023.

Management: Adults with Cirrhosis and Portal Hypertensive Gastropathy (PHG) and Intestinopathy

Recommendations from

> **EASL 2018, AGA 2022. NICE 2023**

–Use nonselective beta-blockers, iron supplementation, and/or blood transfusion as first-line therapy for chronic hemorrhage from PHG.

–Consider TIPS for transfusion-dependent patients.

–Acute PHG bleeding can be treated similarly to variceal bleeding, but data are limited on efficacy of treatment.

Sources

–EASL. 2018. https://doi.org/10.1016/j.jhep.2018.03.024

–AGA. 2022. https://doi.org/10.1016/j.cgh.2022.08.033

–NICE. *Recommendations | Cirrhosis in Over 16s: Assessment and Management | Guidance | NICE.* 2023.

Management: Adults with Cirrhosis and Esophageal Varices

Recommendations from

> **NICE 2023**

–Screen for esophageal varices upon cirrhosis diagnosis with upper endoscopy unless already on propranolol or carvedilol.

–Screen every 3 y with upper endoscopy for patient's without known varices who are not taking propranolol or carvedilol.

–When using beta-blockers:
  • Use caution regarding blood pressure and heart rate lowering effect.
  • Start at low doses (carvedilol 3.125 mg BID, propranolol 40 mg BID).
  • Avoid propranolol and carvedilol in refractory ascites and severe hepatic impairment.

–If not able to tolerate propranolol or carvedilol, consider referring for endoscopic variceal ligation for medium/large esophageal varices.

Source

–NICE. *Recommendations | Cirrhosis in Over 16s: Assessment and Management | Guidance | NICE.* 2023.

Management: Adults with Cirrhosis and Renal Impairment/Hepatorenal Syndrome

Recommendations from

> EASL 2018, AGA 2022, NICE 2023

–Remove diuretics, nonselective beta-blockers, and nephrotoxic drugs immediately when impairment is suspected.

–Replace fluid losses as needed and rigorously search for infectious source.

–In patients with AKI and tense ascites, perform paracentesis and replace albumin regardless of the volume removed.

–For AKI where the serum creatinine doubles, give albumin at a dose of 1 g/kg/d for 2 d. Maximum dose of 100 g/d.

–When AKI is persistent despite attempts at correction, treatment for hepatorenal syndrome should be initiated with albumin at a dose of 1 g/kg on day 1, followed by 20–40 g daily after and one of the following:

- Terlipressin: has the best evidence but avoid when $SpO_2 < 90\%$ or Cr level > 5.
- Norepinephrine: slightly less efficacious compared to terlipressin.
- Midodrine + octreotide: inferior to the above therapies, but widely available.

–Treat to bring the serum creatinine to within 0.3 mg/dL of baseline. If hepatorenal syndrome recurs after treatment, repeat the course.

–The use of renal replacement therapy should be limited to AKI considered secondary to acute tubular necrosis, hepatorenal syndrome-AKI in potential candidates for liver transplantation, and AKI etiology unknown that is still being investigated.

Sources

–EASL. 2018. https://doi.org/10.1016/j.jhep.2018.03.024

–AGA. 2022. https://doi.org/10.1016/j.cgh.2022.08.033

–NICE. *Recommendations | Cirrhosis in Over 16s: Assessment and Management | Guidance | NICE.* 2023.

Management: Adults with Cirrhosis and Acute-on-Chronic Liver Failure

Recommendations from

> EASL 2018, AGA 2022, NICE 2023

–Acute-on-chronic liver failure has no particular therapy.

–Seek precipitating factors and treat.

–Expedite consideration for liver transplant.

–Suggest withdrawal of ongoing intensive care support if 4 or more organs are failing after 1 wk of adequate intensive treatment.

Sources
–EASL. 2018. https://doi.org/10.1016/j.jhep.2018.03.024
–AGA. 2022. https://doi.org/10.1016/j.cgh.2022.08.033
–NICE. *Recommendations | Cirrhosis in Over 16s: Assessment and Management | Guidance | NICE.* 2023.

Management: Adults with Cirrhosis and Coagulation Disorders

Recommendations from

➤ EASL 2018, AGA 2022, NICE 2023

–In patients with stable cirrhosis, extensive preprocedural testing with coagulation parameters such as INR or platelet count can likely be avoided.

–In patients with stable cirrhosis, there is a recommendation against the use of platelets, fresh frozen plasma, or thrombopoietin receptor agonists for bleeding prophylaxis.

–Standard in-hospital anticoagulation practices should be used for prevention of DVT/PE in hospitalized patients.

–Acute portal vein thrombosis as well as atrial fibrillation, when diagnosed, should be treated per standard anticoagulation recommendations in patients with stable cirrhosis.

Sources
–EASL. 2018. https://doi.org/10.1016/j.jhep.2018.03.024
–AGA. 2022. https://doi.org/10.1016/j.cgh.2022.08.033
–NICE. *Recommendations | Cirrhosis in Over 16s: Assessment and Management | Guidance | NICE.* 2023.

Management: Adults with Cirrhosis and Cardiopulmonary Complications

Recommendations from

➤ EASL 2018, AGA 2022, NICE 2023

–Assess systolic function with cardiac echo with dynamic stress testing (pharmacologic or exercise).

–Diastolic dysfunction may occur as an early sign of cardiomyopathy.

–Evaluate for prolonged QTc and discontinue medications as appropriate.

Sources
–EASL. 2018. https://doi.org/10.1016/j.jhep.2018.03.024
–AGA. 2022. https://doi.org/10.1016/j.cgh.2022.08.033
–NICE. *Recommendations | Cirrhosis in Over 16s: Assessment and Management | Guidance | NICE.* 2023.

Management: Adults with Cirrhosis and Hepatopulmonary Syndrome (HPS)

Recommendations from

➤ EASL 2018, AGA 2022, NICE 2023

–Assess for HPS in patients with tachypnea, digital clubbing, and/or cyanosis. Screen initially with pulse oximetry, and if $SpO_2 < 96\%$ obtain ABG and further workup as indicated.

–Characterize HPS with contrast (microbubble) echocardiography. Consider transesophageal study to exclude intracardiac shunts.

–Treat patients with HPS and severe hypoxemia with long-term oxygen therapy. It is unclear how this treatment affects survival.

–Liver transplant is the only proven effective treatment for HPS.

–Perform ABG every 6 mo to prioritize liver transplant recipients since severe hypoxemia (PaO_2 < 45–50 mmHg) predicts increased mortality post–liver transplant.

Sources
–EASL. 2018. https://doi.org/10.1016/j.jhep.2018.03.024
–AGA. 2022. https://doi.org/10.1016/j.cgh.2022.08.033
–NICE. *Recommendations | Cirrhosis in Over 16s: Assessment and Management | Guidance | NICE.* 2023.

Management: Adults with Cirrhosis and Portopulmonary Hypertension

Recommendations from

> ### EASL 2018, AGA 2022, NICE 2023

–Screen for portopulmonary hypertension with transthoracic echocardiogram and grade as mild, moderate, and severe based on mean pulmonary arterial pressure (mPAP).

–If there is evidence of portopulmonary hypertension, obtain a right heart catheterization.

–Stop beta-blockers and manage varices with endoscopic tools.

–Do not perform TIPS in patients with portopulmonary hypertension.

Sources
–EASL. 2018. https://doi.org/10.1016/j.jhep.2018.03.024
–AGA. 2022. https://doi.org/10.1016/j.cgh.2022.08.033
–NICE. *Recommendations | Cirrhosis in Over 16s: Assessment and Management | Guidance | NICE.* 2023.

Practice Pearls

- Confirm diagnosis of cirrhosis with ultrasound or MRI, which is preferred in obesity. (Bashir et al. *JACR.* 2020;17(5s))
- Preferred imaging modality to screen for hepatocellular carcinoma (HCC) is ultrasound or MRI with contrast. (Bashir et al. *JACR.* 2020;17(5s))

COLITIS, *CLOSTRIDIOIDES DIFFICILE*

Management: Adults

Recommendations from

> ### IDSA SHEA 2017

Evaluation
–In general, nucleic acid amplification test is preferred to enzyme immunoassay (EIA or toxin testing).

–If the institution uses only specimens from patients who are not taking laxatives and have at least 3 or more unformed stools in a 24-h period, then using the nucleic acid amplification test alone is satisfactory.

–Stool toxin test may be used in a multistep algorithm with glutamate dehydrogenase (GDH) to satisfy the recommendation.

–If the toxin test is negative, algorithm still recommends follow-up with the nucleic acid amplification test.

–Test for *C. difficile* or its toxins only on diarrheal stool (3 or more unformed stool in 24-h period).

–Avoid testing of stool on asymptomatic patients.

–Repeat testing (within 7 d) during the same episode of diarrhea is not recommended.

Therapies

–Discontinue inciting antibiotic agent as soon as possible.

–Avoid antiperistaltic agents.

–New guidelines recommend vancomycin and fidaxomicin, instead of metronidazole, as first-line treatments for *C. difficile*.

–Metronidazole can still be considered as first-line treatment in situations where accessibility to vancomycin and fidaxomicin is limited and in mild-to-moderate disease.

–Initial *C. difficile* infection: vancomycin 125 mg orally QID or fidaxomicin 200 mg BID for 10 d.

–Initial *C. difficile* infection, fulminant[1]: vancomycin 500 mg QID PO or by nasogastric tube. If ileus, consider adding rectal instillation of vancomycin. Intravenously administer metronidazole (500 mg q8 h) together with oral or rectal vancomycin, particularly if ileus is present.

–First recurrence, if metronidazole was used for the initial episode: vancomycin 125 mg given QID for 10 d.

–First recurrence, if standard regimen was used: a prolonged tapered and pulsed vancomycin regimen (eg, 125 mg QID for 10–14 d, BID for a week, QID for a week, and then q 2 or 3 d for 2–8 wk) or fidaxomicin 200 mg BID for 10 d.

–Second or subsequent recurrence: prolonged tapered and pulsed vancomycin regimen, or vancomycin 125 mg given QID for 10 d followed by rifaximin 400 mg TID for 20 d, or fidaxomicin 200 mg BID for 10 d, or fecal microbiota transplantation.

Practice Pearls

- Probiotics such as *Lactobacillus* and *Saccharomyces boulardii* have been associated with some reduction in *C. difficile* recurrence; however, significant results demonstrating efficacy in controlled clinical trials have yet to be seen. Thus, standard utilization of probiotics in the setting of *C. difficile* is not currently supported.

- Perform hand hygiene before and after contact with patient. Handwashing with soap and water is preferred if there is direct contact.

- Use disposable patient equipment when possible and ensure that reusable equipment is thoroughly cleaned and disinfected, preferentially with a sporicidal disinfectant.

---

[1] Fulminant *C. difficile* infection, previously referred to as severe, complicated CDI, is characterized by hypotension or shock, ileus, or megacolon.

- With regard to antibiotic stewardship in order to control increasing rates of *C. difficile*, the guidelines stress attempts to minimize the frequency and duration of high-risk antibiotic therapy and the number of antibiotic agents prescribed.

Source

–https://academic.oup.com/cid/article/66/7/e1/4855916

Management: Children

Recommendations from

> IDSA SHEA 2017

Evaluation

–Because of the high prevalence of asymptomatic carriage of toxigenic *C. difficile* in infants, do not routinely test for *C. difficile* infection in neonates or infants ≤12 mo of age with diarrhea.

–Colonization rates decrease with increasing age. By 2–3 y of age, approximately 1%–3% of children are asymptomatic carriers of *C. difficile* (a rate similar to that observed in healthy adults).

–In children ≥2 y of age, *C. difficile* testing is recommended for patients with prolonged or worsening diarrhea and risk factors (underlying inflammatory bowel disease, immunocompromising conditions, presence of a gastrostomy, or jejunostomy tube) or relevant exposures (contact with the health care system or recent antibiotics).

Therapies

–Discontinue inciting antibiotic agent as soon as possible.

–Avoid antiperistaltic agents.

–Either metronidazole or vancomycin is recommended for the treatment of children with an initial episode or first recurrence of nonsevere *C. difficile* infection.

–Initial *C. difficile* infection, nonsevere: metronidazole PO for 10 d (7.5 mg/kg/dose TID or QID) or vancomycin PO for 10 d (10 mg/kg/dose QID).

–Initial *C. difficile* infection, severe/fulminant: vancomycin PO/pr for 10 d (10 mg/kg/dose QID). Consider addition of IV metronidazole for 10 d (10 mg/kg/dose TID).

–First recurrence, nonsevere: metronidazole PO for 10 d (7.5 mg/kg/dose TID or QID) or vancomycin PO for 10 d (10 mg/kg/dose QID).

–Second or subsequent recurrence: prolonged tapered and pulsed vancomycin regimen,[1] or vancomycin for 10 d (10 mg/kg/dose QID) followed by rifaximin[2] for 20 d, or fecal microbiota transplantation.

Source

–https://academic.oup.com/cid/article/66/7/e1/4855916

---

[1] 10 mg/kg with max of 125 mg 4 times per day for 10–14 d, then 10 mg/kg with max of 125 mg 2 times per day for a week, then 10 mg/kg with max of 125 mg once per day for a week, and then 10 mg/kg with max of 125 mg every 2 or 3 d for 2–8 wk.

[2] No pediatric dosing for rifaximin is given, as it is not approved by the US Food and Drug Administration for use in children 12 and under.

COLORECTAL CANCER

Screening: Adults, Not High-Risk

Recommendations from

> ⯈ AAFP 2021, USPSTF 2021, ACS 2020, ACG 2021, US Multi-Society Task Force on Colorectal Cancer
> (USMSTF-CC) 2017, 2020, ACP 2023, Canadian Task Force (CTF) 2016, NCCN 2021, ASCO 2019
>> –Screen all adults, with age ranges, modalities, and frequencies varying by organization.
>> –Adults with elevated risk are outside the scope of these recommendations.[1]

Guidelines Alert 5–5 GUIDELINES DISCORDANT: POPULATION TO SCREEN FOR COLORECTAL CANCER		
Organization	**Ages and Frequencies**	**Modality**
AAFP	Age 50–75 y: screen all patients Age 76–85 y: individualize screening decision	No preference
ACS, USPSTF	Age 45–75 y: screen all patients Age 76–85 y: individualize screening decision Age > 85 y: do not screen	No preference
ACG, NCCN	Age 45–75 y: screen all patients Age > 75 y: individualize	ACG: prefer colonoscopy or fecal immunochemical test (FIT)

USMSTF-CC	Age 50–75 y: screen all patients (consider
	    starting at age 45 in Black persons)
	Age > 75 y: do not screen
	For patients with normal,[a] high-quality
	    colonoscopy, repeat colorectal cancer (CRC)
	    screening in 10 y[a]
		Prefer colonoscopy or FIT

ACP	Age 45–49 y: risk benefit discussion given
	    uncertainty of benefit vs. harms
	Age 50–75 y: screen all patients
	Age > 75 y or Life expectancy < 10 y: do not
	    screen
		No preference, do not use stool DNA,
		    computed tomography colonography,
		    capsule endoscopy, urine, or serum
		    screening tests for CRC

CTF	Age 50–74 y: screen all patients	Screen with stool-based test or flexible sigmoidoscopy, not colonoscopy
ASCO	Age 50–75 y: screen all patients	No preference

[1] Risk factors indicating need for earlier/more frequent screening: personal history of CRC or adenomatous polyps or hepatoblastoma, CRC or polyps in a first-degree relative age. (*Ann Intern Med.* 1998;128(1):900; *Am J Gastroenterol.* 2009;104:739; *N Engl J Med.* 1994;331(25):1669; 1995;332(13):861). Additional high-risk group: history of ≥30 Gy radiation to whole abdomen; all upper abdominal fields; pelvic, thoracic, lumbar, or sacral spine. Begin monitoring 10 y after radiation or at age 35 y, whichever occurs last (http://www.survivorshipguidelines.org). Screening colonoscopy in those age ≥ 80 y results in only 15% of the expected gain in life expectancy seen in younger patients. (*JAMA.* 2006;295:2357)

Applying to Clinical Practice

- Data suggests a rising incidence of colon cancer in the 45–49 y age group, moving many guidelines to lower their screening age from 50 to 45.
- AAFP opted against lowering its screening age until data is available to address these concerns:
  - Current studies were based on data modeling rather than prospective randomized trials and assumed 100% adherence, possibly enhancing the perceived benefit of screening.
  - It is not known whether tumors in younger adults benefit as much from early detection.
  - Lowering the screening age without ensuring robust systems for access may exacerbate health disparities.
  - Increasing access to screening in the 50–75 y age group would prevent more cancer at less cost.
- Colonoscopy or FIT test are the most recommended modalities but favor the study that the patient is most likely to be able to complete.

[a]Colonoscopy is considered normal where no adenoma, sessile serrated adenoma/polyp or sessile serrated polyp (SSP), hyperplastic polyp (HP) ≥ 10 mm, traditional serrated adenoma (TSA), or CRC was found. Individuals with only HPs < 10 mm are considered to have normal colonoscopy.

Practice Pearls

- Recommendations for follow-up testing after the initial colonoscopy are detailed in Table 5–1.
- Recommendations for screening in resource-limited settings are detailed in Table 5–2.
- USPSTF, ACG, ACS, and NCCN all recognize that evidence for initiating screening at age 45 is not as strong. USPSTF gives starting at age 45 a "B" recommendation, while starting at age 50 is an "A" recommendation. ACG "recommends" starting at age 50 and "suggests" starting at age 45. Incidence of colorectal adenocarcinoma in adults 40- to 49-y-old has increased by almost 15% from 2000–2002 to 2014–2016. (*Ann Intern Med.* 2021;174)
- Acceptable screening methods:[1, 2, 3]
  - Guaiac fecal occult blood test (gFOBT-guaiac based or FIT = fecal immunochemical test) annually.[4]
  - Flexible sigmoidoscopy every 5 y with reflex colonoscopy if abnormal.
  - FIT[5] annually plus flexible sigmoidoscopy every 10 y.
  - Colonoscopy every 10 y.
  - CT colonoscopy every 5 y.
- Follow-up/surveillance colonoscopy according to findings: refer to this chapter for updated USMSTF 2020 recommendations.
- FOBT alone decreased CRC mortality by 33% compared with those who were not screened. (*Gastroenterology.* 2004;126:1674)

---

[1] A positive result on an FOBT should be followed by colonoscopy. An alternative is flexible sigmoidoscopy and air-contrast barium enema.

[2] FOBT should be performed on 2 samples from 3 consecutive specimens obtained at home. A single stool guaiac during annual physical examination is not adequate.

[3] USPSTF did not find direct evidence that a screening colonoscopy is effective in reducing CRC mortality rates.

[4] Use the guaiac-based test with dietary restriction, or an immunochemical test without dietary restriction. Two samples from each of 3 consecutive stools should be examined without rehydration. Rehydration increases the false-positive rate.

[5] Population-based retrospective analysis: risk of developing CRC remains decreased for >10 y following negative colonoscopy findings. (*JAMA.* 2006;295:2366)

- Accuracy of colonoscopy is operator dependent—rapid withdrawal time, poor prep, and lack of experience will increase false-negatives. (*N Engl J Med*. 2006;355:2533) (*Ann Intern Med*. 2012;156:692) (*Gastroenterology*. 2015;110:72)
- Multitargeted DNA stool testing vs. iFOBT with more cancers detected (92.3% vs. 73.8%) but more false-positives with DNA test. (*N Engl J Med*. 2014;370:1287–1306)
- Percentage of US adults receiving some form of CRC screening increased from 44% in 1999 to 63% in 2008. The goal was 80% by 2018. (*CA Cancer J Clin*. 2015;65:30) (*Arch Intern Med*. 2011;171:647; 2012;172:575). However, the percentage increased from 58.7% in 2010 to 65.5% in 2018 (www.cdc.gov/mmwr/volumes/69/wr/mm6929a6.htm). In 2016, an estimated 134,000 new cases of CRC were diagnosed and 49,000 Americans died of CRC. Median age at diagnosis is 68. (*CA Cancer J Clin*. 2016;66:7)
- Colonoscopy vs. iFOBT testing in CRC with similar detection of cancer, but more adenomas identified in the colonoscopy group. (*N Engl J Med*. 2012;366:687,697)
- A normal screening colonoscopy may provide reassurance for up to 17 y. (*Ann Intern Med*. 2020;173(2):81–91)

Sources

–ACS. 2020. https://www.cancer.org/cancer/colon-rectal-cancer/detection-diagnosis-staging/acs-recommendations.html

–USPSTF. *JAMA*. 2016;315(23):2564–2575.

–AAFP. 2021. https://www.aafp.org/family-physician/patient-care/clinical-recommendations/all-clinical-recommendations/colorectal-cancer-adults.html

–ACG. *Am J Gastroenterol*. March 2021;116(3):458–479.

–ACP. *Ann Intern Med*. 2023;176(8):1092–1100.

TABLE 5–1 US MULTI-SOCIETY TASK FORCE RECOMMENDATIONS FOR FOLLOW-UP AFTER BASELINE SCREENING COLONOSCOPY IN AVERAGE-RISK ADULTS

	Baseline Colonoscopy	Size	Pathology	Recommended Surveillance Colonoscopy	Recommendation Strength
Normal	No adenoma, SSP, TSA, HP ≥ 10 mm, CRC; HP < 10 mm acceptable			10 y	High
Adenoma	1–2 adenomas	<10 mm	Tubular	7–10 y	Moderate
	3–4 adenomas	<10 mm	Tubular	3–5 y	Very low
	5–10 adenomas	<10 mm	Tubular	3 y	Moderate
	≥1 adenoma	≥10 mm		3 y	High
			Tubulovillous or villous histology	3 y	Moderate
			High-grade dysplasia	3 y	Moderate
	>10 adenomas			1 y	Very low
	Piecemeal resection	≥20 mm		6 mo	Moderate

TABLE 5–1 US MULTI-SOCIETY TASK FORCE RECOMMENDATIONS FOR FOLLOW-UP AFTER BASELINE SCREENING COLONOSCOPY IN AVERAGE-RISK ADULTS (*continued*)

	Baseline Colonoscopy	Size	Pathology	Recommended Surveillance Colonoscopy	Recommendation Strength
Polyp	≤20 HPs in rectum or sigmoid	<10 mm		10 y	Strong
	≤20 HPs proximal to sigmoid	<10 mm		10 y	Weak
	1–2 SSPs	<10 mm		5–10 y	Weak
	3–4 SSPs	<10 mm		3–5 y	Weak
	5–10 SSPs	<10 mm		3 y	Weak
	SSP	≥10 mm		3 y	Weak
	SSP		Dysplasia	3 y	Weak
	HP	≥10 mm		3–5 y	Weak
	TSA			3 y	Weak
	Piecemeal resection of SSP	≥20 mm		6 mo	Strong

Source: USMSTF. *Gastroenterol.* 2020;158:1131–1153.

TABLE 5–2 SCREENING IN HIGH-INCIDENCE SETTINGS STRATIFIED BY RESOURCE AVAILABILITY

Resource Setting[a]	Recommended CRC Screening Options
Basic	HSgFOBT annually (preferred) to every 2 y FIT annually (preferred) to every 2 y
Limited	HSgFOBT annually FIT annually FSIG every 5 y FSIG every 10 y *plus* FIT (preferred) or HSgFOBT annually
Enhanced	HSgFOBT annually FIT annually FSIG every 5 y FSIG every 10 y *plus* FIT (preferred) or HSgFOBT annually Colonoscopy every 10 y

TABLE 5–2 SCREENING IN HIGH-INCIDENCE SETTINGS STRATIFIED BY RESOURCE AVAILABILITY *(continued)*	
Resource Setting[a]	**Recommended CRC Screening Options**
Maximal	HSgFOBT annually
	FIT annually
	FSIG every 5 y
	FSIG every 10 y *plus* FIT (preferred) or HSgFOBT annually
	Colonoscopy every 10 y
	CT colonography
	FIT-DNA

[a]ASCO resource setting stratification:
Basic—Core, fundamental recourses/services essential for any public health/primary care system.
Limited—Second-tier resources/services intended to produce major improvements in outcomes/public health with limited financial means.
Enhanced—Third-tier resources/services that are optional but important.
Maximal—High-level/state-of-the-art resources/services associated with significantly higher cost and/or impracticality for broad use in resource-limited area.
Source: USPSTF 2021; American Society of Clinical Oncology (ASCO) Resource-Stratified Guideline for CRC screening in average-risk adults age 50–75 y in settings with high incidence of CRC. *J Global Oncol.* 2019;5:1–22.

–USMSTF. *Gastroenterol.* 2020;158:1131–1153.
–USMSTF. *Am J Gastroenterol.* 2017;112(7):1016–1030.
–CTF. *CMAJ.* 2016;188(5):340–348.
–NCCN. 2021. https://www.nccn.org/professionals/physician_gls/pdf/colorectal_screening.pdf
–ASCO. *J Global Oncol.* 2019;5:1–22.

Screening: Adults at High Risk of Colon Cancer

Recommendations from

⟫ **USMSTF on CRC 2017, NCCN 2021, ACG 2021**

–Screen adults with family history of early CRC[1] or advanced adenoma with colonoscopy every 5 y starting at age 40 y or 10 y prior to the earliest age of diagnosis of first-degree relative.

–Use Amsterdam I and II criteria to diagnose hereditary nonpolyposis CRC (HNPCC), with subsequent genetic screen for Lynch syndrome (LS).

- Amsterdam I criteria:
  ○ ≥3 relatives with histologically verified CRC, one of which is a first-degree relative of the other two. Diagnosis of familial adenomatous polyposis (FAP) excluded.
  ○ ≥2 generations with CRC.
  ○ ≥1 CRC diagnosis before age 50 y.
- Amsterdam II criteria:
  ○ ≥3 relatives with histologically verified HNPCC-associated cancer (colorectal, endometrial, small bowel, ureter, renal pelvis), one of which is a first-degree relative of the other two. Diagnosis of FAP excluded.
  ○ ≥2 generations with CRC.
  ○ ≥1 CRC diagnosis before age 50 y.

[1] First-degree relative diagnosed prior to age 60 or advanced adenoma in ≥ 2 first-degree relatives at any age.

–Lynch syndrome (LS): screening colonoscopy every 1–2 y for persons with LS or at-risk (first-degree relatives of those affected), starting at age 20–25 y, or 2–5 y before the youngest age of family CRC diagnosis if diagnosed before age 25 y.

–Family CRC Type X syndrome: screening colonoscopy every 3–5 y beginning 10 y before the age at diagnosis of the youngest affected relative.

Sources

–USMSTF. *Am J Gastroenterol.* 2017;112(7):1016–1030.
–NCCN. 2021. https://www.nccn.org/professionals/physician_gls/pdf/colorectal_screening.pdf
–ACG. *Am J Gastroenterol.* 2021;116(3):458–479.

Prevention: Adults

Recommendations from

> ### AAFP 2018, NCCN 2020

–Modifiable risk factors:
  - Diet:
    - Advise patients to increase consumption of fruits, nonstarchy vegetables, and whole grains. Preferentially optimize nutrition from natural food sources rather than dietary supplements.
    - Cholesterol: 2-fold increased risk of CRC with increased intake.
    - Fat: 25% increased risk of serrated polyps with increased fat intake.
    - Dairy: 15% reduced risk of CRC with >8 oz of cow's milk daily.
    - Fiber: no reduced risk of CRC or adenomatous polyps with increased fiber intake.
    - Red and processed meat: 22% increased risk of CRC with increased red and processed meat intake.
  - Lifestyle:
    - Alcohol: 8% increased risk of CRC and 24% increased risk of serrated polyps. Reducing alcohol intake does not clearly lower risk for CRC or polyps.
    - Cigarettes: 114% increased risk of high-risk adenomatous polyps and CRC in current smokers.
    - Obesity: bariatric surgery associated with 27% reduced risk of CRC in obese individuals. Increased BMI is associated with increased mortality from CRC.
    - Occupational physical activity: 25% decreased risk of colon cancer and 12% decreased risk of rectal cancer.
    - Recreational physical activity: 20% decreased risk of colon cancer and 13% decreased risk of rectal cancer.
  - Medications:
    - Statins: weak evidence that statin use ≥ 5 y is associated with a decreased risk of advanced adenomatous polyps.
    - Calcium: 26% reduced risk of adenomatous polyps; 22% reduced risk of CRC in individuals taking 1400 mg daily calcium compared to 600 mg.

–Polyp removal:
- Based on fair evidence, removal of adenomatous polyps reduces the risk of CRC, especially polyps >1 cm. (*Ann Intern Med.* 2011;154:22) (*Gastrointest Endosc.* 2014;80:471)
- Based on fair evidence, complications of polyp removal include perforation of the colon and bleeding estimated at 7–9 events per 1000 procedures.

–Interventions without benefit:
- Vitamin D.
- Folic acid.
- Antioxidants.

Sources
–*Am Fam Physician.* 2018;97(10):658–665.
–NCCN. *Colorectal Cancer Screening.* 2020:1–61.

CONSTIPATION

Management: Children

Recommendations from

➤ NICE 2010 (updated 2017)

–Assess all children for fecal impaction.
–If evidence of poor growth, test for celiac disease and hypothyroidism.
–Recommend polyethylene glycol (PEG) as first-line agent for oral disimpaction.
–Add a stimulant laxative if PEG therapy is ineffective after 2 wk.
–Use sodium citrate enemas for disimpaction only if all oral medications have failed.
–Use a maintenance regimen with PEG for several months after a regular bowel pattern has been established.
–Gradually taper maintenance dose over several months as bowel pattern allows.
–Recommend adequate fluid intake.

Practice Pearl

- Minimum fluid intake for age:
  - 1–3 y: 1300 mL.
  - 4–8 y: 1700 mL.
  - 9–13 y: 2200 mL.
  - 14–18 y: 2500 mL.

Source
–https://www.nice.org.uk/guidance/cg99

Management: Adults Not Using Opioids

Recommendations from

➤ AGA 2013, ACG 2023

–Perform digital examination to evaluate resting sphincter tone.

–Discontinue all medications that can cause constipation.

–Assess for hypercalcemia and hypothyroidism.

–Trial of laxatives and fiber:

- Bisacodyl.
- Milk of magnesia.
- PEG.
- Senna.

–Refractory constipation may require biofeedback or pelvic floor retraining. Severe cases of refractory slow transit constipation may require a total colectomy with ileorectal anastomosis.

Sources

–http://www.gastrojournal.org/article/S0016-5085%2812%2901545-4/fulltext

–American Gastroenterological Association–American College of… : Official Journal of the American College of Gastroenterology | ACG (lww.com).

Management: Adults with Opioid-Induced Constipation (OIC)

Recommendations from

➢ AGA 2019

–Use laxatives as first-line agents.

–For patients with laxative refractory OIC, use 1 of 3 peripherally acting mu-opioid receptor antagonists (PAMORAs). Avoid these agents in conditions that compromise blood-brain barrier, such as CNS infections, stroke, and traumatic brain injury, to avoid precipitating withdrawal or reversing analgesic effect. Available peripherally acting μ-opioid receptor antagonists:

- Naldemedine (high-quality evidence).
- Naloxegol (moderate-quality evidence).
- Methylnaltrexone (low-quality evidence).

–Not enough evidence to recommend for or against using lubiprostone (intestinal secretagogue) or prucalopride (selective 5-HT agonist).

Practice Pearls

- Traditional laxatives are divided into 4 categories: osmotic (eg, PEG/lactulose/magnesium citrate), stimulant (eg, bisacodyl/senna/sodium picosulfate), stool softener (eg, docusate), or lubricant (eg, mineral oil).
- There is limited evidence that routine use of stimulant laxatives for OIC is harmful to the colon despite previous concerns.
- Fiber has limited effect on OIC, except in patients with fiber-deficient diets.
- Enemas can sometimes be used as rescue therapy when OIC is refractory to oral treatments.

Source

–https://doi.org/10.1053/j.gastro.2018.07.016

DIARRHEA, ACUTE

Management: Adults

–Define acute diarrhea as ≥3 unformed stools in 24 h plus an enteric symptom (nausea, vomiting, abdominal pain/cramps, tenesmus, fecal urgency, moderate-to-severe flatulence).

–Give oral fluid therapy to all patients: fluid and salt intake, food including soups, broths, saltine crackers, broiled, and baked foods.

–Management of watery diarrhea:

- If mild, hydrate orally and consider loperamide 4 mg to control stool.
- If moderate-to-severe (ie, diarrhea is forcing a change to activity):
  - If travel-associated, give antibiotics.
  - If temperature < 100°F or febrile < 72 h, consider 48-h trial loperamide.
  - If febrile > 72 h, obtain stool cultures.

–Management of dysenteric diarrhea (grossly bloody stools):

- If severe illness (total disability) and febrile, treat empirically with azithromycin 1 g × 1 or 500 mg daily × 3 d.
- If nonsevere and afebrile, perform microbiologic assessment and tailor antimicrobials to results (see Table 5–3 for recommendations).

–Regardless of presentation, if diarrhea persists more than 14–30 d, evaluate with culture or other microbiologic assessment and target an antimicrobial to the results.

–Do not use probiotics or prebiotics for the treatment of acute diarrhea in adults.

TABLE 5–3 ACUTE DIARRHEA ANTIBIOTIC TREATMENT RECOMMENDATIONS		
Antibiotic[a]	**Dose**	**Treatment Duration**
Azithromycin[c, d]	1000 mg by mouth or	Single dose[b]
	500 mg by mouth	3-d course[d]
Ciprofloxacin	750 mg by mouth or	Single dose[b]
	500 mg by mouth	3-d course
Levofloxacin	500 mg by mouth	Single dose[b] or 3-d course
Ofloxacin	400 mg by mouth	Single dose[b] or 3-d course
Rifaximin[e]	200 mg by mouth 3 times daily	3-d course

ETEC, Enterotoxigenic *Escherichia coli*.

[a]Antibiotic regimens may be combined with loperamide, 4 mg first dose, and then 2 mg dose after each loose stool, not to exceed 16 mg in a 24-h period.

[b]If symptoms are not resolved after 24 h, complete a 3-d course of antibiotics.

[c]Use empirically as the first line in Southeast Asia and India to cover fluoroquinolone-resistant *Campylobacter* or in other geographical areas if *Campylobacter* or resistant ETEC are suspected.

[d]Preferred regimen for dysentery or febrile diarrhea.

[e]Do not use there is if clinical suspicion for *Campylobacter, Salmonella, Shigella,* or other causes of invasive diarrhea.

Source: Reproduced with permission from Riddle MS, DuPont HL, Connor BA. ACG clinical guideline: diagnosis, treatment, and prevention of acute diarrheal infections in adults. *Am J Gastroenterol.* 2016;111(5):602–622.

–Bismuth subsalicylates can be administered to control rates of passage of stool and may help travelers function better during bouts of mild-to-moderate illness.

–In patients receiving antibiotics for traveler's diarrhea, administer adjunctive loperamide therapy to decrease the duration of diarrhea and increase the chance for a cure.

–Discourage antibiotics for community-acquired diarrhea, as epidemiological studies suggest that most community-acquired diarrhea is viral in origin (norovirus, rotavirus, and adenovirus) and is not shortened by the use of antibiotics.

DIVERTICULITIS, ACUTE

Management: Adults

Recommendations from

> NICE 2020

–Offer oral antibiotics if patient is systemically unwell, immunocompromised, or has significant comorbidities.

–Offer IV antibiotics for complicated acute diverticulitis.

–Consider percutaneous drainage or surgery for abscesses >3 cm.

–Offer laparoscopic lavage or surgical resection for diverticular perforation with peritonitis.

–Consider elective resection in patients continuing to have symptoms, such as stricture or fistula, after recovering from acute complicated diverticulitis. There is no recommendation on the timing of surgery.

–Do not use 5-ASA or antibiotics to prevent recurrent acute diverticulitis.

Source

–https://www.nice.org.uk/guidance/ng147

DIVERTICULOSIS

Management: Adults

Recommendations from

> NICE 2020

–Recommend high-fiber diet and/or bulk-forming laxatives to reduce constipation.

–Avoid NSAIDs and opioid analgesia if possible.

–Consider antispasmodic if abdominal cramping.

Source

–https://www.nice.org.uk/guidance/ng147

Practice Pearl

• While commonly recommended, there is no evidence to support specific dietary restrictions (ie, seeds, nuts) to prevent diverticulitis in patients with diverticulosis.

DYSPEPSIA

Management: Adults

Recommendations from

> ### ACG/Canadian Association of Gastroenterology 2017

–Avoid routine motility studies for patients with functional dyspepsia unless there is a strong suspicion for gastroparesis in which case a motility study is indicated.

–See Fig. 5–4 for workup algorithm and Fig. 5–5 for management algorithm.

ESOPHAGEAL CANCER

Screening: Adults

Recommendations from

> ### ASGE 2017

–Follow-up intervals for biopsy-proven BE:
  • No dysplasia: follow-up EGD with biopsy every 3–5 y.

FIG. 5–4 WORKUP OF UNDIAGNOSED DYSPEPSIA.

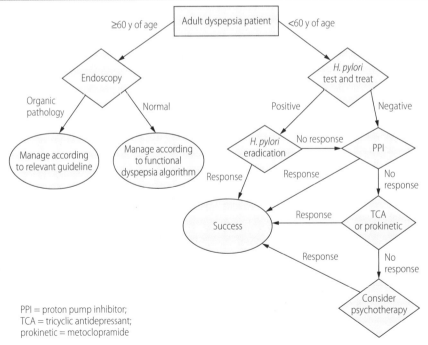

PPI = proton pump inhibitor;
TCA = tricyclic antidepressant;
prokinetic = metoclopramide

Source: Reproduced with permission from Moayyedi P, Lacy BE, Andrews CN, Enns RA, Howden CW, Vakil N. ACG and CAG clinical guideline: management of dyspepsia. *Am J Gastroenterol.* 2017;112(7):988–1013.

FIG. 5–5 MANAGEMENT OF FUNCTIONAL DYSPEPSIA.

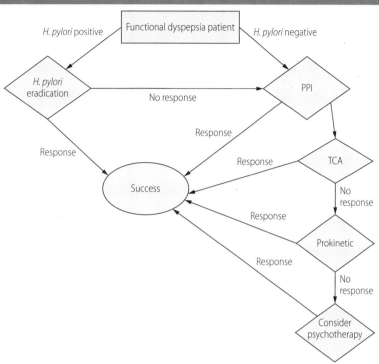

Source: Reproduced with permission from Moayyedi P, Lacy BE, Andrews CN, Enns RA, Howden CW, Vakil N. ACG and CAG clinical guideline: management of dyspepsia. *Am J Gastroenterol.* 2017;112(7):988–1013.

- Indeterminate dysplasia: repeat EGD with biopsy in 3–6 mo after optimizing PPI therapy.
- Low-grade dysplasia: endoscopic eradication therapy or ongoing annual endoscopic surveillance.
- High-grade dysplasia: endoscopic eradication therapy.

Practice Pearls

- In 2023, 21,560 new cases of esophageal cancer were diagnosed in the United States; 16,120 persons died from esophageal cancer.
- There is a 4-fold incidence of esophageal adenocarcinoma compared to squamous cell carcinoma.

Source

–*Gastrointest Endosc.* 2017;85(5):889–903.

Prevention: Adults

Recommendations from

⮞ **AAFP 2017**

–Minimize exposure to risk factors:

–Adenocarcinoma risk factors:

- Age 50–60 y.
- Male sex (8-fold risk).
- White race (5-fold risk).
- GERD (5- to 7-fold risk, depending on symptom frequency).
- Obesity (2.4-fold risk with BMI ≥ 30), particularly central adiposity.
- Smoking (2-fold risk).
- BE (premalignant).

–Squamous cell carcinoma risk factors:

- Age 60–70 y.
- Achalasia (10-fold risk).
- Smoking (9-fold risk).
- Alcohol use (3- to 5-fold risk with ≥3 drinks/d).
- Black race (3-fold risk).
- High-starch diet without fruits or vegetables.

Practice Pearls

- Longstanding GERD is associated with BE and increased risk of esophageal CA. (*PLOS*. 2014;9:e103508)
- Radiofrequency ablation of BE with moderate or severe dysplasia may reduce the risk of progression to malignancy. (*N Engl J Med*. 2009;360:2277–2288)
- Uncertain if elimination of GERD by surgical or medical therapy will reduce the risk of esophageal adenocarcinoma although a few trials show benefit. (*Gastroenterology*. 2010;138:1297)
- No trials in the United States have shown any benefit from the use of chemoprevention with vitamins and/or minerals to prevent esophageal cancer. (*Am J Gastroenterol*. 2014;109:1215) (*Gut*. 2016;65:548)

Source
–*Am Fam Physician*. 2017;95(1):22–28.

FECAL INCONTINENCE

Management: Adults

Recommendations from

⮞ **ASCRS 2023**

–Risk factors: older age, smoking, obesity, diabetes, vaginal delivery, pelvic surgery, anorectal surgery, Crohn disease, ulcerative colitis, IBS, celiac disease, constipation.

–Monitoring: use fecal incontinence severity scores (Wexner score, Vaizey score) and bowel diary to assess clinical intervention response.

–Conservative management: avoid triggers (caffeine, artificial sweeteners, lactose, gluten, supplements, prescription medications) and utilize fiber supplementation (thicken and optimize stool consistency).

–For patients with preexisting diarrhea consider loperamide or diphenoxylate-atropine.

–Supportive skin measures: protective barrier ointments (zinc oxide), gentle soaps, wipes, deodorants, and pads.

–Consider bowel training programs and biofeedback training/pelvic floor rehabilitation if there is no relief with conservative management.

–Consider colonoscopy to rule out colorectal pathology.

–Refer to a specialist for evaluation of anorectal physiology testing with manometry, sacral neuromodulation, and colostomy.

Source
–*Dis Colon Rectum.* 2023;66:647–661.

GALLSTONES

Management: Adults

Recommendations from

> **NICE 2014, EASL 2014**

Evaluation
–Obtain liver function tests and ultrasound.

–Suspect acute cholecystitis in a patient with fever, severe pain located in the right upper abdominal quadrant lasting for several hours, and right upper abdominal pain and tenderness on palpation.

–Consider magnetic resonance cholangiopancreatography (MRCP) if ultrasound has not detected common bile duct stones but the common bile duct is dilated, and liver function tests are abnormal.

Therapies
–Offer cholecystectomy for symptomatic gallstones or acute cholecystitis.

–Do not offer litholysis using bile acids alone or in combination with extracorporeal shock wave lithotripsy.

–Offer percutaneous cholecystostomy for acute cholecystitis or gallbladder empyema if surgery is contraindicated.

–Options for choledocholithiasis:
  • Cholecystectomy and intraoperative clearance of CBD stones.
  • ERCP prior to cholecystectomy.

Sources
–https://www.nice.org.uk/guidance/cg188

–http://www.easl.eu/medias/cpg/Prevention-diagnosis-and-treatment-of-gallstones/English-report.pdf

GASTRIC CANCER

Screening: Adults

Recommendations from

> ACG 2015

-Do not routinely screen average-risk adults given low incidence in the United States.

-Screen with EGD for specific high-risk subgroups.[1] For acute pancreatitis (AP) syndromes, start EGD screening for gastric and proximal small bowel tumors starting at age 25–30 y, with follow-up depending on the stage of duodenal polyposis.

Sources

-*Gastrointest Endosc.* 2016;84(1):18–28.

-*Am J Gastroenterol.* 2015;110(2):223–262.

Prevention: Adults

Recommendations from

> AAFP 2017

-Modifiable risk factors:

• *Helicobacter pylori*: classified as Group 1 (definite) carcinogen by the World Health Organization (WHO).

   ○ Screen for *H. pylori* in patients with peptic ulcer disease or gastric mucosa-associated lymphoid tissue lymphoma. (*Am J Gastroenterol.* 2007;102:1808–1825)

   ○ A study over 15 y showed a 40% reduction in risk of gastric cancer with *H. pylori* eradication. (*Ann Intern Med.* 2009;151:121) (*J Natl Cancer Inst.* 2012;104:488)

• Diet: increased risk with smoked foods (N-nitroso compounds), high salt diet. Decreased risk with fruit and nonstarch vegetable intake.

• Cigarette use: 60% increased risk in current male smokers and 20% increased risk in female smokers, compared to nonsmokers.

• Obesity: increased risk with BMI ≥ 30.

• Physical activity: 21% decreased risk.

• Male sex: 2-fold to 5-fold risk compared to women, though postmenopausal women have increased risk approaching that of men.

• First-degree relative with gastric cancer: 2.6-fold to 3.5-fold risk.

-Clinical consideration:

• Patients with hereditary susceptibility (HNPCC, e-cadherin mutation, Li–Fraumeni syndrome), pernicious anemia, atrophic gastritis, partial gastrectomy, or gastric polyps should be followed carefully for early cancer symptoms and for upper endoscopy at intervals according to risk.

---

[1] High-risk groups include those with gastric adenomas, pernicious anemia, gastric intestinal metaplasia, Lynch syndrome, familial adenomatous polyposis, and family history of gastric cancer.

Sources
    –*Am Fam Physician.* 2017;95(1):22–28.
    –*Gastrointest Endosc.* 2016;84(1):18–28.

GASTROESOPHAGEAL REFLUX DISEASE (GERD)

Management: Adults

Recommendations from

> NICE 2014, AGA 2023

–Recommend smoking cessation, avoiding recumbency until 3 h after eating, head of bed elevation, and weight reduction.

–Consider discontinuation of offending medications (calcium channel blockers, nitrates, theophylline, bisphosphonates, steroids, and NSAIDs).

–Consider testing for *H. pylori* after a 2-wk washout off PPIs.

–Empiric trial of PPI therapy.

–Consider laparoscopic fundoplication for patients who do not wish to continue with acid suppressive therapy long term.

–Consider specialist referral for:

- Dyspepsia refractory to meds.
- Consideration of surgery.
- Refractory *H. pylori* infection.
- BE.
- Extraesophageal symptoms (cough, asthma, laryngitis, dental erosions).

Practice Pearls

- Patients with heartburn and regurgitation are likely to have GERD; treat empirically for 4–8 wk with a PPI taken 30–60 min before a meal.
- If a once-daily PPI is ineffective, increase to twice-daily or switch to a different PPI.
- Alarm symptoms such as weight loss, dysphagia, and anemia should prompt endoscopy.
- For symptomatic GERD, start with a PPI rather than an H_2-antagonist.
- Consider screening for BE in men over 50 y who have had GERD symptoms for $\geq$5 y.
- Long-term PPI use may increase the risk of hypomagnesemia, hip fracture, *C. difficile* infection, vitamin B_{12} deficiency, and community-acquired pneumonia.

Sources
    –https://www.nice.org.uk/guidance/cg184
    –*Am Fam Physician.* 2015;91(10):692–697.
    –AGA. AGA clinical practice update on the diagnosis and management of extraesophageal gastroesophageal reflux disease: expert review. *Clin Gastroenterol Hepatol.* (cghjournal.org). 2023.

GASTROINTESTINAL BLEEDING, LOWER

Management: Adults

Recommendations from

> BSG 2019, ACG 2016

–Consider discharge home for urgent outpatient investigation only if a minor self-limited bleed and no other indication for hospitalization.

–Admit patients with major bleed for colonoscopy.

–Give 4–6 L PEG over 3–4 h.

–Perform colonoscopy within 24 h of presentation.

–For high-risk[1] or unstable patients:

- Resuscitate with IV fluids and blood transfusion as indicated.
- Exclude upper GI source with EGD emergently.
- Prep for colonoscopy unless UGI source is found. Consider nasogastric tube to facilitate prep.
- If remains unstable despite resuscitation or is intolerant to prep, pursue CT angiogram to localize bleed and coordinate radiologic intervention.

–In centers with 24/7 interventional radiology services, consider catheter angiography with the intent to embolize the site of bleeding prior to endoscopic investigation.

–Defer emergency laparotomy unless all effort has been made to localize the bleeding using radiologic and endoscopic modalities.

–If transfusion is required, use a restrictive transfusion threshold of 7 g/dL and target of 7–9 g/dL. If history of cardiovascular disease, the threshold is 8 g/dL with a target of 8–10 g/dL.

–Stop warfarin therapy at presentation. For low thrombotic risk patients, consider resuming in 7 d and for high-risk thrombotic patients (ie, prosthetic heart valve in mitral location, atrial fibrillation with prosthetic valve or mitral stenosis, <3 mo after venous thromboembolism) begin low-molecular-weight heparin after 48 h. If unstable from bleeding, reverse with prothrombin complex concentrate (PCC) and vitamin K.

–If patients with lower GI bleeds take aspirin for primary prophylaxis of cardiovascular events, discontinue it permanently. If on aspirin for secondary prevention of ASCVD, continue it.

–For patients with coronary stents in situ and on dual antiplatelet therapy, discuss with cardiology but do not stop routinely. For unstable hemorrhage patients, continue aspirin but stop P2Y12 receptor antagonist. Consider restarting P2Y12 receptor antagonist therapy in 5–7 d after bleeding is controlled.

–Stop oral anticoagulants at presentation. Consider treating with inhibitors (idarucizumab or andexanet) for life-threatening bleeding. Medication can be restarted in 7 d after hemorrhage.

–Consider platelet transfusion to maintain a platelet count of 50,000 in patients with severe bleeding and those requiring endoscopic hemostasis.

–Consider reversal of anticoagulation before endoscopy in patients with an INR > 2.5.

---

[1] Risk factors: persistent hemorrhage, SBP 100, INR > 1.2, altered mental status, syncope, antiplatelet or anticoagulant use, age >60, or creatinine > 1.5 mg/dL.

Practice Pearls

- A differential diagnosis for lower GI bleed includes angiodysplasias, malignancy, diverticular bleeding, hemorrhoids, infectious colitis, inflammatory bowel disease, ischemic colitis, and bleeding after polypectomy.
- In an outpatient setting, refer for urgent colonoscopy if painless bleeding and history of diverticular disease or polypectomy/biopsy in the past month, or if bleeding is associated with acute onset abdominal pain.
- Colonoscopy is also indicated to evaluate for inflammatory bowel disease or malignancy if intermittent pain, intermittent bleeding, weight loss, or bowel habit changes.
- In hemodynamically unstable patients, performing colonoscopy within the first 24 h does not improve outcomes.
- Patients with diverticular bleeding or angiodysplasia should avoid NSAIDs indefinitely.

Sources

–http://dx.doi.org/10.1136/gutjnl-2018-317807

–ACG clinical guideline: management of patients with acute lower gastrointestinal bleeding. *Am J Gastroenterol.* 2016;111:459–474.

–*Am Fam Physician.* 2020;101(4):206–212.

GASTROINTESTINAL BLEEDING, UPPER (UGIB)

Management: Adults

Recommendations from

> NICE 2016, EASL 2018

–Perform a formal risk assessment for patients with UGIB:
  - Blatchford score at first assessment.
  - Rockall score after endoscopy.

–Avoid platelet transfusions in patients who are not actively bleeding and are hemodynamically stable.

–For UGIB, give fresh frozen plasma if:
  - Fibrinogen < 100 mg/dL.
  - Partial thromboplastin time > 1.5× normal.

–Give PCC if patient with UGIB taking warfarin.

–Timing of endoscopy:
  - Immediately for unstable patients.
  - Within 24 h for stable patients.

–Management of nonvariceal bleeding:
  - Surgical clips.
  - Thermal coagulation.
  - Epinephrine injection.
  - Fibrin or thrombin glue.

- Recurrent bleeding can be assessed by repeat endoscopy or by interventional radiology angioembolization.
- PPIs.

–Management of variceal bleeding:
  - Esophageal variceal band ligation (EASL: within 12 h of admission).
  - Terlipressin or octreotide infusions.
  - Prophylactic third-generation cephalosporin.
  - Transjugular intrahepatic portosystemic shunt for recurrent esophageal variceal bleeding or gastric variceal bleeding.
  - Blood transfusion if necessary (EASL: use restrictive transfusion strategy with threshold of 7 g/dL and target of 7–9 g/dL).
  - Use balloon tamponade only as bridge therapy to definitive treatment and for a maximum of 24 h.
  - Stop beta-blockers and vasodilators and consider using lactulose as prophylaxis for hepatic encephalopathy.

–Prevention and treatment of variceal hemorrhage:
  - Primary prophylaxis for varices is indicated for high-risk varices—small varices with red signs, medium or large varices, or small varices in Child-Pugh C patients.
  - After banding and stabilization, initiate nonselective beta-blockers used to decrease risk.
  - Use propranolol or nadolol. Do not use carvedilol. Use caution in patients with ascites.
  - If intolerant to beta-blockers, consider patient for TIPS.

–Gastric varices:
  - Use nonselective beta-blockers as primary prevention.
  - Give medical therapy for acute gastric variceal hemorrhage as for esophageal variceal hemorrhage. During endoscopy, choose cyanoacrylate as sclerosing agent.
  - Consider TIPS or selective embolization through interventional radiology.

Practice Pearls

- Stop NSAIDs.
- Alcohol cessation if a factor.
- Low-dose aspirin can be resumed if needed for secondary prevention of vascular events once hemostasis has been achieved.
- Use of thienopyridine agents (eg, clopidogrel, ticagrelor, or prasugrel) ongoing only after discussion with appropriate specialist.

Sources
–NICE. 2012. https://www.nice.org.uk/Guidance/cg141
–EASL. 2018. https://doi.org/10.1016/j.jhep.2018.03.024

GASTROPARESIS

Management: Adults

Recommendations from

> ACG 2022

Evaluation

–Rule out other causes of symptoms (eg, iatrogenic gastric slowing from opiate use, mechanical obstruction).

–Diagnose using standard 3–4 h gastric emptying study after solid meal or via stable isotope breath testing (^{13}C-spirulina). Other diagnostics could include a wireless motility capsule.

–After diagnosis, treat all patients with small particle, nonfat, low nondigestible food content diet.

Therapies

–Ensure strict blood glucose control for all with diabetic gastroparesis.

–Consider pharmacologic management with the following medications:

- 5-HT$_4$ agonists.
- Domperidone.
- Metoclopramide.

–Consider the following therapies, which have been shown to improve symptoms but not affect gastric emptying.

- Antiemetics.
- Gastric electric stimulator.
- Acupuncture (specifically in the setting of diabetic gastroparesis).

–Avoid the following therapies:

- Central neuromodulators (haloperidol, nortriptyline).
- Ghrelin agonists.
- Herbal therapies such as Rikkunshito or STW5 (Iberogast).

–Consider pyloromyotomy in those with gastroparesis refractory to medical management.

Source

–ACG. 2022. https://doi.org/10.14309/ajg.0000000000001874

HELICOBACTER PYLORI INFECTION

Management: Adults

Recommendations from

> American College of Gastroenterology 2017

Evaluation

–Screen the following patients for *H. pylori* infection:

- Active peptic ulcer disease.

- A past history of peptic ulcer disease (unless previous cure of *H. pylori* infection has been documented).
- Low-grade gastric mucosa-associated lymphoid tissue lymphoma.
- Undiagnosed dyspepsia.
- Patients who are under the age of 60 y.
- Patients starting long-term treatment with an NSAID.
- Unexplained iron deficiency anemia.
- Idiopathic thrombocytopenic purpura.
- A history of endoscopic resection of early gastric cancer.

Therapies

–Treat all patients who test positive for *H. pylori*.

–Choice of therapy depends on prior antibiotic exposure and local resistance patterns.

–Consider clarithromycin triple therapy consisting of a PPI, clarithromycin, and amoxicillin or metronidazole for 14 d in regions where *H. pylori* resistance to clarithromycin is known to be <15% and in patients with no previous history of macrolide exposure for any reason.

–Consider bismuth quadruple therapy consisting of a PPI, bismuth, tetracycline, and a nitroimidazole for 10–14 d. Bismuth quadruple therapy is particularly useful in patients with any previous macrolide exposure or who are allergic to penicillin.

–Consider levofloxacin triple therapy consisting of a PPI, levofloxacin, and amoxicillin for 10–14 d.

–Consider concomitant therapy consisting of a PPI, clarithromycin, amoxicillin, and a nitroimidazole (eg, metronidazole) for 10–14 d.

–Whenever *H. pylori* infection is identified and treated, perform test of cure using a urea breath test, fecal antigen test, or biopsy-based testing at least 4 wk after the completion of antibiotic therapy and after PPI therapy has been withheld for 1–2 wk.

–Bismuth quadruple therapy or levofloxacin salvage regimens are the preferred treatment options if a patient received a first-line treatment containing clarithromycin.

Practice Pearls

- Given rising rates of clarithromycin resistance and the challenges of obtaining local resistance data, opt for bismuth quadruple therapy (bismuth/PPI/tetracycline/metronidazole) over triple therapy. Alternately, consider nonbismuth quadruple therapy using PPI/clarithromycin/amoxicillin/metronidazole.
- Testing options for *H. pylori*:
  - Urea breath test: highly sensitive/specific. Use for diagnosis and test of cure (4–6 wk after therapy). Stop PPI 2 wk prior to test. Requires fasting for 6 h.
  - Stool antigen tests: highly sensitive/specific. Cheaper than breath test. Stop PPI 2 wk prior to test (though PPI has less of an impact than for breath test).
  - Serum IgG test: cannot distinguish between active and past infection. Not affected by PPI or antibiotic use.
  - Endoscopic biopsy: can perform rapid urease testing if no PPI in prior 2 wk and no bismuth or antibiotic in prior 4 wk. Otherwise, can send to pathology for histologic evaluation.

Sources
  –ACG clinical guideline: treatment of *Helicobacter pylori* infection. *Am J Gastroenterol.*
   2017;112:212–238.
  –http://gi.org/guideline/treatment-of-helicobacter-pylori-infection/
  –*Am Fam Physician.* 2015;91(4):236–242.

HEPATITIS, ALCOHOLIC-ASSOCIATED (AH)

Management: Adults

Recommendations from

> EASL 2018, AASLD 2020, ACG 2024

Evaluation

–Suspect AH in patients with recent onset of jaundice and excessive alcohol consumption.
–Use prognostic scores, such as Maddrey Discriminant Function and MELD to identify severe
 AH (Maddrey Discriminant Function $\geq$ 32 or MELD > 20) who will likely benefit from
 corticosteroids.

Therapies

–If there are no contraindications to steroids (ie, uncontrolled infections or UGIB, AKI), give
 prednisolone 40 mg/d or methylprednisolone 32 mg/d for patients with severe AH to reduce
 short-term mortality. Medium- and long-term survivals do not change.
–Administer IV N-acetylcysteine in addition to prednisolone for patients with severe alcoholic
 hepatitis.
–Use the Lille model to assess response after 7 d of treatment. If the patient responds (Lille
 < 0.45), continue steroids for 28 d total. If no response (Lille $\geq$ 0.45), stop steroids and consider
 referral for liver transplant. Provide nutrition orally to maintain $\geq$35–40 kcal/kg body weight
 and 1.2–1.5 g/kg protein per day.
–There is insufficient evidence to support the use of universal administration of prophylactic
 antibiotics, granulocyte-colony stimulating factor, and pentoxifylline in AH.
–Consider early liver transplant evaluation in select patients at high risk of death who do not
 respond to medical management.

Sources
  –https://doi.org/10.1016/j.jhep.2018.03.018
  –https://doi:10.1002/hep.30866
  –*Am J Gastroenterol.* 2024;119:30–54

HEPATITIS B VIRUS (HBV) INFECTION

Screening: Adults

Recommendations from

> ## USPSTF 2020, CDC 2018, 2020, ASLD 2018

–Screen high-risk individuals using HBV surface antigen (HBsAg):

- Foreign-born persons from countries where HBV prevalence ≥2%.[1]
- US-born persons not vaccinated at birth whose parents were born in countries where HBV prevalence ≥8%.
- HIV-positive persons.
- Household contacts or sexual partners of persons with HBV infection.
- Men who have sex with men.
- Persons with injection drug use.
- Hemodialysis patients. (CDC)
- Persons needing immunosuppressive therapy, immunosuppression related to organ transplantation, and immunosuppression for rheumatologic or gastroenterological disorders. (CDC)
- Blood, organ, plasma, semen, or tissue donors. (CDC)
- People with elevated alanine aminotransferase levels (≥19 IU/L for women and ≥30 IU/L for men). (CDC)
- Infants born to HBV-infected mothers (HBsAg and antibody to hepatitis B surface antigen [anti-HBs] only are recommended). (CDC)

Sources

–USPSTF. *JAMA.* 2020;324(23):2415–2422.
–CDC. *MMWR Recomm Rep.* 12, 2018;67(1):1–31.
–CDC. 2020. www.cdc.gov/hepatitis/hbv/hbvfaq.htm
–https://www.aasld.org/sites/default/files/HBVGuidance_Terrault_et_al-2018-Hepatology.pdf

Management: Adults and Children

Recommendations from

> ## AASLD 2018

Evaluation

–Diagnostic criteria of chronic hepatitis B:

- HBsAg present for 6 mo.

---

[1] HBV prevalence ≥2% in Africa, Asia, South Pacific, Middle East (except Cyprus and Israel), Eastern Europe (except Hungary), Malta, Spain, indigenous populations of Greenland, Alaska natives, indigenous populations of Canada, Caribbean, Guatemala, Honduras, and South America. HBV prevalence ≥8% in Angola, Benin, Burkina Faso, Burundi, Cameroon, Central African Republic, Congo, Côte d'Ivoire, Djibouti, Equatorial Guinea, Gabon, Gambia, Ghana, Guinea, Liberia, Malawi, Mali, Mauritania, Mozambique, Namibia, Niger, Nigeria, Senegal, Sierra Leone, Somalia, South Sudan, Sudan, Swaziland, Togo, Uganda, Zimbabwe, Haiti, Kiribati, Nauru, Niue, Papua New Guinea, Solomon Islands, Tonga, Vanuatu, Kyrgyzstan, Laos, Vietnam, Mongolia, Yemen.

- Subdivided into HBsAg positive and negative. HBV-DNA levels are typically >20,000 IU/mL in HBsAg-positive CHB, and lower values (2000–20,000 IU/mL) are often seen in HBsAg-negative CHB.
- Normal or elevated ALT and/or AST levels.
- Liver biopsy results show chronic hepatitis with variable necroinflammation and/or fibrosis.

–Use quantitative HBV-DNA testing to guide treatment decisions.

–Obtain HBV genotyping in patients being considered for PEG-IFN therapy, otherwise not recommended.

–Do not test for viral resistance in treatment-naïve patients. Resistance testing can be useful in patients with past treatment experience, those with persistent viremia, or those who experience virologic breakthrough during treatment.

Therapies

–Recommend antiviral therapy for adults and alanine transaminase (ALT) > 2× normal, moderate-to-severe hepatitis on biopsy, compensated cirrhosis or advanced fibrosis, and HBV DNA > 20,000 IU/mL; or for reactivation of chronic HBV after chemotherapy or immunosuppression.

–Recommend antiviral therapy in children for ALT > 2× normal and HBV DNA > 20,000 IU/mL for at least 6 mo.

–If patients do not meet criteria for treatment, reassess regularly the need for future therapy.

- Test ALT in HBsAg-positive patients with persistently normal ALT every 3–6 mo.
- Test patients who are HBsAg positive with HBV DNA levels > 20,000 IU/mL and ALT levels less than 2 times the ULN to evaluate histologic disease severity with liver biopsy, elastography, or liver fibrosis biomarkers (FIB-4 or FibroTest).
- Screen all HBsAg-positive patients with cirrhosis with US examination with or without alfa fetoprotein (AFP) every 6 mo.

Source

–https://www.aasld.org/sites/default/files/HBVGuidance_Terrault_et_al-2018-Hepatology.pdf

HEPATITIS C VIRUS (HCV) INFECTION

Screening: Adults

Recommendations from

➤ AASLD 2020, AASLD-IDSA 2023, USPSTF 2020

–Offer one-time universal opt-out HCV screening, using anti-HCV antibody testing with reflex HCV RNA PCR, to all adults aged 18 y or older, regardless of risk factors.

–Screen all pregnant patients for HCV with each pregnancy.

–Individuals with increased risk[1] of HCV exposure:

- One-time HCV screening for age < 18 y.

[1] Risk factors for HCV infection: injection drug use, intranasal illicit drug use, men who have sex with men, long-term hemodialysis patients, percutaneous/parenteral exposures in an unregulated setting; health care providers and public safety workers after needlestick, sharps, or mucosal exposures to HCV-infected blood; children born to HCV-infected women, history of incarceration, prior recipients of blood transfusion(s) or organ transplant, HIV infection, sexually active persons about to start preexposure prophylaxis for HIV, unexplained chronic liver disease and/or chronic hepatitis, solid organ donors, and transplant recipients.

–Periodic repeat testing for all individuals as indicated.

–Annual screening for individuals who inject drugs and for men with HIV who have unprotected sex with men, including those with prior infections who were treated or cleared spontaneously.

Practice Pearls

- Anti-HCV antibodies typically develop 2–6 mo after exposure. HCV RNA is reliably detectable within 2–3 wk after exposure. In patients with negative anti-HCV antibody testing, perform HCV RNA testing for suspicion of acute HCV infection, or for unexplained liver disease in an immuno-compromised patient.
- In persons with acute hepatitis C, the infection resolves in 15%–25%; in the remaining persons in whom chronic infection develops, cirrhosis develops in 10%–20% within 20–30 y after infection and hepatocellular carcinoma develops in 1%–5%.
- Universal HCV screening is recommended because of the opioid epidemic, high efficacy of direct antiviral agent therapy, and long-term benefits of successful treatment.

Sources

–AASLD. *Hepatology*. 2020; 71(2):686–721.

–AASLD-IDSA. HCV guidance panel. Hepatitis C guidance 2023 update. *Clin Infect Dis*. 2023. https://doi.org/10.1093/cid/ciad319

–USPSTF. *JAMA*. 2020;323(10):970–975.

Management: Adults with Chronic HCV Infection

Recommendations from

➢ AASLD 2020, AASLD-IDSA 2023, AGA 2017, EASL 2020

Evaluation

–If antibody test positive, reflex to an HCV RNA or core antigen confirmation test.

–If in initial testing anti-HCV antibody is positive but RNA or core antigen is negative, test HCV RNA 12 to 24 wk later to confirm clearance. (EASL)

–Do not withhold treatment for patients with ongoing injection drug use.

–Initiate antiviral treatment for all adults with acute or chronic HCV infection, except those with a short life expectancy that will not improve with HCV therapy, liver transplant, or other therapies. Few contraindications exist otherwise.

–Consider urgent treatment for patients with significant cirrhosis, extrahepatic manifestations, recurrence after liver transplant, patients at risk for rapid progression because of comorbidities such as HIV or DM, and in individuals at high risk of transmitting HCV.

–Include the following in initial visits:

- History:
  - ○ HCV exposure risk factors and timing of exposure.
  - ○ Symptoms of advanced liver disease such as jaundice, ascites, variceal bleeding, fatigue, pruritus, and confusion.
  - ○ Extrahepatic manifestations.

- Prior HCV treatment.
- Other medical issues: diabetes, CVA, anemia, CKD, HIV, hepatitis B coinfection, depression, solid organ transplant recipient.
- Family history of cirrhosis, liver cancer, alcohol dependence.
- Social history of past and current alcohol use, current illicit drug use.
- Labs:
  - HCV RNA quantitative PCR.
  - HCV genotype (unless done previously). Resistance testing is not required prior to first-line treatment.
  - CBC.
  - Serum: creatinine, sodium, potassium, chloride, albumin, total protein, total bilirubin, ALT, AST, alkaline phosphatase, glucose, protime (INR).
  - Hepatitis A and B immune status.
  - Resistance-associated variant testing in patients with HCV genotype 1a who are using grazoprevir/elbasvir or prior treatment with a direct-acting antiviral agent.
  - Hepatic fibrosis severity testing, preferably noninvasively.
  - AFP.
  - Urine pregnancy test.
  - HIV antibody test.
  - Hepatic ultrasound.

Therapies

–Use a simple regimen with a single direct antiviral agent for treatment-naïve adults without cirrhosis or with compensated cirrhosis. Some regimens treat certain genotypes, and some are pangenotypic. Updated guidelines are available at www.HCVGuidelines.org.

–Conditions requiring a more complex treatment regimen include ESRD, HIV or HBsAg positive, pregnancy, known or suspected HCC, and history of liver transplant.

–Evaluate for drug-drug interactions (www.hep-druginteractions.org) prior to initiating therapy. Interactions exist between certain direct antiviral agents and HIV therapies, opiates, lipid-lowering drugs, antipsychotics, antiarrhythmics, antihypertensives, immunosuppressants, antiplatelet agents, anticoagulants, anticonvulsants, PPIs, and others.

–Interferon regimens are the only option for HCV infected or HIV/HCV infected with decompensated cirrhosis.

–There is very limited evidence for treating patients with mixed genotypes (ie, multiple genotypes of HCV infection concurrently). Consider using a pangenotypic regimen and if the optimal regimen or duration is unclear, consult a specialist.

–See Fig. 5–6 for treatment monitoring for 8, 12, and 16 wk regimens. (AGA)

–Vaccinate patients who lack antibodies for hepatitis A and B viruses. If cirrhotic, administer pneumococcal vaccine.

–Educate persons with current HCV infection on methods to reduce progression of liver disease (eg, alcohol abstinence) and avoid transmission to others.

–Insufficient evidence to recommend herbal therapy.

FIG. 5–6 Treatment Timeline for Direct Antiviral Hepatitis C Therapy

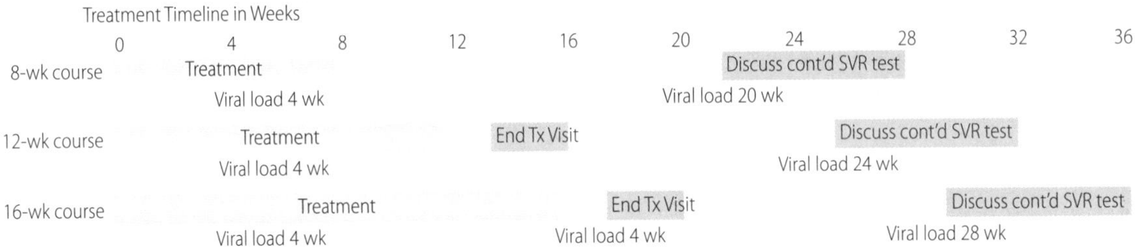

Treatment Timeline in Weeks

0	4	8	12	16	20	24	28	32	36

8-wk course — Treatment | Viral load 4 wk | Viral load 20 wk | Discuss cont'd SVR test

12-wk course — Treatment | Viral load 4 wk | End Tx Visit | Viral load 24 wk | Discuss cont'd SVR test

16-wk course — Treatment | Viral load 4 wk | End Tx Visit | Viral load 4 wk | Viral load 28 wk | Discuss cont'd SVR test

– Include the following in subsequent visits:
- For hepatic fibrosis stage 3 or 4:
  - EGD evaluation for esophageal varices.
  - Alfa fetoprotein fetoprotein.
  - Hepatic ultrasound (or, if images are inadequate, CT scan of abdomen with contrast).
  - Risk reduction/mitigation:
    - Hepatitis A and B vaccinations if not immune.
    - Age-appropriate vaccinations and cancer screening.
    - Counseling on alcohol abstinence.
    - Counseling on transmission/reinfection of HCV.
    - Management of comorbid conditions.
    - Counseling on adherence and consequences of treatment failure if being treated.

– Reassess labs within 12 wk of starting treatment which include CBC, INR, hepatic function panel (albumin, total and direct bilirubin, ALT/AST, alk phos), renal function (eGFR). (AGA)

– Refer patients with advanced cirrhosis, multiple treatment failures, coinfection with HIV or hepatitis B to hepatology clinic for proper management. (AGA)

– Declare sustained viral response if RNA or core antigen are undetectable 12–24 wk after the end of treatment.

– Long-term monitoring after successful treatment:
- Fibrosis score 0–2: no further monitoring; counsel on reinfection risk, HIV prevention.
- Fibrosis score 3–4: ongoing HCC monitoring q6 mo (hepatic ultrasound, AFP levels, LFTs, renal function, INR); yearly visits with hepatology.

Practice Pearl

- High-risk patients are defined as "history of injection drug use, transfusion or organ transplant before 1992, received clotting factors before 1987, history of long-term dialysis, HIV infection, persistently elevated liver enzymes, health care and public safety workers after needle sticks, sharps, or mucosal exposure to HCV-positive blood, and children born to HCV-positive women."

Sources
– https://doi.org/10.1002/hep.31060
– https://doi.org/10.1053/j.gastro.2017.03.039
– https://doi.org/10.1016/j.jhep.2020.08.018

–AASLD-IDSA. HCV guidance panel. Hepatitis C guidance 2023 update. *Clin Infect Dis.* 2023. https://doi.org/10.1093/cid/ciad319

Management: Adults with Acute HCV Infection

Recommendations from

➤ **AASLD 2020, EASL 2020**

–Initiate HCV treatment without awaiting spontaneous resolution. Use the same regimens recommended for chronic HCV infection.

–Assess sustained viral response at 12 and 24 wk as late relapses have been reported.

Sources
–https://doi.org/10.1002/hep.31060
–https://doi.org/10.1016/j.jhep.2020.08.018

Management: Children with HCV Infection

Recommendations from

➤ **AASLD 2020, EASL 2020**

–Treat patients >3-y-old if a direct antiviral agent regimen is available for their genotype and age range. Start treatment as soon as possible if the child has cryoglobulinemia, rashes, and glomerulonephritis or advanced fibrosis.

–Avoid interferon-based treatment regimens in children and adolescents.

–Surveil for HCC and varices in children with cirrhosis.

–Therapeutic dose of acetaminophen, steroids, chemotherapy, and organ and bone marrow transplant are not contraindicated in children with chronic hepatitis C.

–HCV is not transmitted through casual contact, so HCV-infected children do not pose a risk to other children. They can participate in school, sports, athletics, and regular childhood activities without restriction.

–Use universal precautions at school and in the home. Advise family members not to share toothbrushes, razors, or nail clippers. Advise family members to use gloves and dilute bleach to clean up blood.

Sources
–https://doi.org/10.1002/hep.31060
–https://doi.org/10.1016/j.jhep.2020.08.018

HEPATOCELLULAR CARCINOMA (HCC)

Screening: Adults

Recommendations from

➤ **AASLD 2018**

–For adults with cirrhosis (Child-Pugh class A and B), screen using ultrasound with or without AFP every 6 mo to improve overall survival.

–For Child class C cirrhosis, do not screen unless they are on a transplant waiting list, given the low anticipated survival associated with Child class C.

–For individuals with risk factors without cirrhosis, do not screen, given significantly lower risk of HCC.

Practice Pearls

- In 2023, there were an estimated 41,210 new diagnoses of HCC and 29,380 deaths due to this disease in the United States; 80% of HCC cases occur in persons with cirrhosis.
- Due to low-level evidence, HCC screening is considered controversial.
- Due to low sensitivity, AFP alone should not be used for screening unless ultrasound is not available.

Source
–AASLD. *Hepatology*. 2018;68(2):723–750.

Prevention: Adults

Recommendations from

➢ AASLD 2018, NCI 2019

–Modifiable risk factors: cirrhosis and associated risk factors:
- Chronic hepatitis B (HBV) infection.
- Hepatitis C (HCV) infection.
- Extensive alcohol use.
- Nonalcoholic steatohepatitis (NASH).
- Hereditary hemochromatosis.
- Primary biliary cholangitis.
- Wilson disease.
- Aflatoxin B1 (fungal toxin that contaminates corn, grains, and nuts that are not stored properly).

–**Prevention:**
- Vaccinate against hepatitis B.
- Treat hepatitis C infection.
- Achieve alcohol cessation.
- Treat underlying risk factors as applicable.

Sources
–AASLD. *Hepatology*. 2018;68(2):723–750.
–NCI. *Adult Primary Liver Cancer Treatment (PDQ)*. 2019.

HEREDITARY HEMOCHROMATOSIS (HH)

Screening: Adults

Recommendations from

➢ ACG 2019, AASLD 2011, AAFP 2013

–Screen family members, particularly first-degree relatives, of patients diagnosed with HH, using iron studies and serum *HFE* mutation analysis.

–If evidence of active liver disease, obtain iron studies (ferritin, transferrin saturation (TS)). If abnormal, evaluate for HH.

Practice Pearls

- HH is one of the most common genetic disorders among persons of northern European descent. There are 4 main HH categories based on which iron homeostasis proteins are affected. Screening indicated by positive family history should be tailored to a specific type of HH in the family. (ACG 2019)
- There is no established consensus regarding elevated ferritin or TS threshold levels that would warrant further evaluation for HH. Possible threshold values are serum ferritin > 200 mcg/L in women and > 300 mcg/L in men, and TS > 45%.
- There is fair evidence that clinically significant disease caused by hereditary hemochromatosis is uncommon in the general population. Male homozygotes for *C282Y* gene mutation have a 2-fold increase in the incidence of iron overload–related symptoms compared with women.
- There is poor evidence that early therapeutic phlebotomy improves morbidity and mortality in screening-detected vs. clinically detected individuals.
- Both men and women who have a heterozygote *C282Y* gene mutation rarely develop iron overload.
- For clinicians who choose to screen, one-time screening of non-Latino White men with serum ferritin level and TS has the highest yield.

Sources

–ACG. *Am J Gastroenterol.* 2019;114:1202–1218.
–AASLD. *Hepatology.* 2011;54(1):328–343.
–*Am Fam Physician.* 2013;87(3):183–190.

Management: Adults

Recommendations from

➢ AASLD 2011, EASL 2022

Evaluation

–Evaluate the following patients for hemochromatosis: asymptomatic patients with abnormal iron studies (increased ferritin and iron/TS), all patients with liver disease, patients with increased liver iron on liver biopsy or MRI, and first-degree relatives of patients with hemochromatosis.

–Combine TS and ferritin. If either is abnormal (TS > 45% or ferritin > upper limit of normal), obtain *HFE* mutation analysis.

–If TS is <45%, pursue a broader workup of hyperferritinemia.

–Test for the P.C282Y variant of *HFE* in individuals of European origin with iron overload and in adult first-degree relatives of patients with P.C282Y homozygous hemochromatosis.

–Use liver MRI to quantify hepatic iron concentrations and to assess extrahepatic organ involvement. Do not obtain a liver biopsy to assess hepatic iron overload.

–Obtain liver biopsy for diagnosis and prognosis in patients with phenotypic markers of iron overload who are not C282Y homozygotes or compound heterozygotes (C282Y, H63D), and for those who do not have an already known etiology for liver cirrhosis.

–Evaluate those diagnosed with hemochromatosis for presence and severity of liver cirrhosis and presence of extrahepatic manifestations.

–Screen for HCC every 6 mo.

Therapies

–Perform therapeutic phlebotomy weekly or biweekly until ferritin level 50 mcg/L during the induction phase to initially reduce ferritin stores.

–During the maintenance phase, continue phlebotomy, targeting ferritin levels of 50–100 mcg/L. It is typical to require 2–6 sessions per year.

–If C282Y homozygotes have elevated ferritin (but <1000 mcg/L), proceed to phlebotomy without liver biopsy.

–If end-organ damage is due to iron overload, undergo regular phlebotomy to keep ferritin between 50 and 100 mcg/L.

–Avoid vitamin C and iron supplements, limit red meats, and restrict alcohol intake.

–Monitor patients on a regular basis for reaccumulation of iron and undergo maintenance with targeted ferritin levels of 50–100 mcg/L.

–If phlebotomy is contraindicated, consider iron chelation therapy as a second line.

Practice Pearls

- Symptoms besides liver function abnormalities include skin pigmentation, pancreatic dysfunction with diabetes, arthralgias, erectile dysfunction, and cardiac involvement with ECG changes and heart failure (those with signs/symptoms of heart disease should be considered for cardiac MRI).

- Other rare mutations causing phenotypic hemochromatosis include transferrin receptor 2 mutation, ferroportin mutation, and H-ferritin mutation.

- The most devastating complication of hemochromatosis is a 20-fold increase in the risk of HCC. HCC develops in <1% of patients whose ferritin has never been >1000 mcg/L, while the risk rises considerably in patients with cirrhosis and ferritin level >1000 mcg/L. Screen these patients with hepatic ultrasound every 6 mo. Alfa fetoprotein is elevated in only 60% of patients with HCC and should not be used as a single screening test. (*Liver Cancer*. 2014;3:31)

- Patients with hemochromatosis are at increased risk for certain bacterial infections whose virulence is increased in the presence of iron overload. These include *Listeria monocytogenes* (most common in patients undergoing renal dialysis), *Yersinia enterocolitica*, and *Vibrio vulniticus* (uncooked seafood is a common source). Infections are made more virulent by iron overload of macrophages impairing their antibacterial activity.

- Secondary iron overload (most commonly secondary to a transfusion requirement due to blood or bone marrow disease) is best managed by iron chelation beginning when the ferritin rises above 1000 mcg/L. In contrast to HH, excess iron is deposited primarily in the reticuloendothelial system, although visceral iron overload does occur over time. (*Blood*. 2014;124:1212)

Sources
–Practice guidelines. *Hepatology*. 2011;54:328–343.
–EASL. 2022. https://doi.org/10.1016/j.jhep.2022.03.033

INFLAMMATORY BOWEL DISEASE, CROHN DISEASE

Management: Children, Young Adults, and Adults

Recommendations from
> ACR 2021, NICE 2019

Evaluation (ACR)
–For initial imaging of suspected Crohn, choose CT abdomen and pelvis with IV contrast, CT enterography, or MR enterography.
–For imaging in a Crohn flare, choose CT enterography, MR enterography, and/or CT abdomen and pelvis with IV contrast. Consider using more than one imaging modality to provide complementary information.

Therapies (NICE)
–Inducing remission in Crohn disease.
   - Glucocorticoids (prednisolone, methylprednisolone, or IV hydrocortisone) are recommended for first presentation or a single exacerbation in a 12-mo period.
   - Consider budesonide or 5-ASA, though less effective, if conventional glucocorticoids are contraindicated or intolerable and if disease is mild to moderate.
      ○ Add azathioprine or mercaptopurine to steroids if steroids cannot be tapered or ≥2 exacerbations in last 12 mo.
      ○ Assess thiopurine methyltransferase activity before offering azathioprine or mercaptopurine. Do not offer azathioprine or mercaptopurine if thiopurine methyltransferase activity is deficient. Consider low-dose thiopurines if thiopurine methyltransferase activity is below normal but not deficient.
   - Consider adding methotrexate in people who cannot tolerate azathioprine or mercaptopurine, or in whom thiopurine methyltransferase activity is deficient.
   - Monitor for neutropenia.
   - Infliximab or adalimumab is indicated with severe active Crohn disease refractory to conventional therapy.
      ○ Given for maximum of 12 mo at a time, or until treatment failure (ie, need for surgery), whichever is shorter.
–Maintaining remission.
   - Azathioprine or mercaptopurine as monotherapy in patients achieving remission with steroids.

- Methotrexate in patients who need methotrexate to induce remission or cannot tolerate thiopurines.
- Azathioprine and 3-mo postop metronidazole after complete macroscopic resection. Do not offer biologics or glucocorticosteroids. Do not offer a conventional glucocorticosteroid or budesonide to maintain remission.
- Offer colonoscopic surveillance.

–Surgery: consider when disease is limited to distal ileum and in patients whose disease is refractory to medical therapy or in children/young adults whose growth is impaired.

–Managing strictures: balloon dilation is an option for single stricture that is short, straight, and accessible by colonoscopy.

Surveillance

–Monitor for osteopenia or osteoporosis in children and young adults with risk factors, such as low BMI, pathologic fracture, or repeated glucocorticosteroid use. (NICE)

–For surveillance of stable Crohn, choose MR enterography or CT enterography. (ACR)

Practice Pearls

- Fecal calprotectin is a helpful diagnostic test to differentiate the presence of IBD from IBS.
- Avoid NSAIDs as they may exacerbate disease activity.
- Oral mesalamine has not consistently been demonstrated to be effective for induction of remission and achieving mucosal healing in patients with active Crohn disease.
- Consider using natalizumab for induction of symptomatic response and remission in patients with active Crohn disease, as it is more effective than placebo.
- Other treatments such as ustekinumab, novel anti-integrin therapy (with vedolizumab), and diet may be helpful.
- Surgery is required to treat enteric complications of Crohn disease; a resection of a segment of diseased intestine is the most common surgery.
- If a patient has risk factors, it may be helpful to take postoperative prophylaxis with anti-TNF agents.
- Avoid budesonide or 5-ASA for severe disease.
- Avoid azathioprine, mercaptopurine, or methotrexate as monotherapy.

Sources
–https://www.nice.org.uk/Guidance/cg152
–Kim et al. Crohn disease. *JACR*. 2020;17(5S).

INFLAMMATORY BOWEL DISEASE, ULCERATIVE COLITIS (UC)

Management: Adults

Recommendations from

➢ ACG 2019, AGA 2020

Guidelines Alert 5–6			
GUIDELINES DISCORDANT: INDUCTION OF REMISSION IN ULCERATIVE COLITIS			
Scenario	**ACG**	**AGA**	**NICE**
Mild proctitis	5-ASA suppositories or enema; rectal corticosteroids if refractory		
Mild, left-sided	Rectal plus oral 5-ASA	Rectal plus oral 5-ASA	Rectal 5-ASA Add oral 5-ASA after 4 wk if refractory
Mild-to-moderate, pancolonic	Oral 5-ASA (low-dose)	Oral 5-ASA (standard-dose, 2–3 g/d) Increase to high-dose (>3 g/d) and add rectal 5-ASA if refractory	Rectal plus high-dose oral 5-ASA Switch to high-dose oral 5-ASA plus oral corticosteroids after 4 wk if refractory
Moderate to severe	Anti-TNF monotherapy Consider oral budesonide MMX if anti-TNF is contraindicated Consider infliximab plus azathioprine as alternative to monotherapy Consider vedolizumab or tofacitinib for nonresponders	Use biologics, such as TNF-alpha inhibitors (eg, infliximab, adalimumab), integrin inhibitor (eg, vedolizumab), JAK inhibitors (eg, tofacitinib), or interleukin inhibitor (eg, ustekinumab). Start with infliximab or vedolizumab in patients naïve to biologics. Use tofacitinib or ustekinumab in nonresponders	
Acute severe	IV methylprednisolone 60 mg/d or hydrocortisone 100 mg 3–4×/d Consider infliximab or cyclosporine in patients not responding to corticosteroids in 3–5 d Test for *C. difficile* and give vancomycin if positive TPN for bowel rest	IV corticosteroids equivalent to 40–60 mg/d of methylprednisolone Use infliximab or cyclosporine in patients not responding to 3–5 d of IV corticosteroids	IV corticosteroids Consider IV cyclosporine after 72 h or if steroids contraindicated If cyclosporine contraindicated, consider infliximab

Recommendations

–Treat milder cases with salicylates. Treat more severe cases with biologics. Treat acute severe flares with short courses of high-dose corticosteroids.

–Maintain remission with salicylates, or with biologics if those were required to induce remission.

–Consider oral corticosteroids (eg, budesonide MMX, prednisone) in patients not responding to 5-ASA after 1 mo.

–CRC prevention:
  • Start colonoscopy screening and surveillance 8 y after diagnosis of UC.

- If UC and primary sclerosing cholangitis, obtain screening colonoscopy at the time of diagnosis and surveillance annually thereafter.
- Fecal DNA testing and CT colonography are not recommended due to insufficient evidence.
–Refractory UC: consider colectomy with moderate-to-severe UC who are refractory or intolerant to medical therapy.

Guidelines Alert 5–7		
GUIDELINES DISCORDANT: MAINTENANCE OF REMISSION IN ULCERATIVE COLITIS		
Scenario	ACG	NICE
Mild proctitis	Rectal 5-ASA	Rectal 5-ASA +/− oral 5-ASA
Mild, left-sided	Oral 5-ASA	Oral 5-ASA, low dose
Mild-to-moderate, pancolonic	Oral 5-ASA	Oral 5-ASA, low dose
Moderate-to-severe	Continue the biologic that induced remission If steroids were used, use thiopurines	
Acute severe	Continue infliximab if it was successful If cyclosporine was used, switch to thiopurine or vedolizumab	Consider oral azathioprine or mercaptopurine

Practice Pearls

- Addition of 5-ASA to anti-TNF therapy is not recommended if patient did not respond to 5-ASA prior to switching to biologics.
- Avoid corticosteroids to maintain remission.
- Patients with prominent arthritic symptoms may reasonably choose to use sulfasalazine 2–4 g/d if alternatives are cost-prohibitive.
- Patients who place a higher value on convenience and lower value on effectiveness may use oral rather than rectal administration.
- Patients who place a higher value on avoiding issues with the mesalamine enemas and do not mind lower effectiveness may use rectal corticosteroid foam preparations.
- For patients taking oral mesalamine, once daily dosing is recommended to increase adherence.
- There is no good evidence to support the use of probiotics for mild-to-moderate UC. There are limited data showing a benefit of curcumin as adjunctive therapy to 5-ASA in maintaining remission.
- Oral 5-ASA monotherapy can be considered in cases where topical monotherapy is indicated if patients decline topical treatment. However, inform patient that oral monotherapy may not be as effective.
- Consider oral azathioprine or oral mercaptopurine to maintain remission after two or more exacerbations in 12 mo that require treatment with systemic corticosteroids or if remission is not maintained by aminosalicylates.

- Monitor bone health, growth, and pubertal development in children and young adults with chronic active disease or who require frequent steroid therapy.
- Severity of UC is categorized by the Truelove and Witt's Severity Index in adults and by the Pediatric UC Activity Index in children.

Sources
  –https://doi.org/10.14309/ajg.0000000000000152
  –https://doi.org/10.1053/j.gastro.2018.12.009
  –https://doi.org/10.1053/j.gastro.2020.01.006
  –https://www.nice.org.uk/Guidance/cg166

IRRITABLE BOWEL SYNDROME (IBS)

Management: Adults

Recommendations from

> NICE 2015, AGA 2022

Evaluation
  –Consider IBS for any adult with any of these symptoms for at least 6 mo.
  - Abdominal pain.
  - Bloating.
  - Change in bowel habit.
  –Assess all patients with possible IBS for red flag indicators that argue against IBS.
  - Unintentional weight loss.
  - Rectal bleeding.
  - Anemia.
  - Abdominal mass.
  - Change in bowel habit to looser and more frequent stools if over 60 y.
  - Family history of IBD, colon cancer, or celiac disease.
  - Recent travel or immigration from high-risk areas.
  –Recommended for all patients with suspected IBS:
  - Complete blood count.
  - ESR.
  - C-reactive protein.
  - Antiendomysial antibody and antitissue transglutaminase antibody to rule out celiac disease.
  –For diarrhea-predominant IBS, consider these additional tests:
  - Fecal calprotectin/lactoferrin to rule out IBD.
  - Stool ova and parasites.
  - Giardia antigen or PCR.
  - 48-h stool bile acid to rule out bile acid malabsorption.

Therapies
  –Lifestyle recommendations for IBS:

- Eat regular meals.
- Drink at least 8 cups of noncaffeinated beverage daily.
- Limit intake of tea, coffee, and alcohol.
- Reduce intake of "resistant starch."
- Avoid sorbitol, an artificial sweetener, for diarrhea-predominant IBS.

–Pharmacologic therapy options for IBS-C:
  - Laxatives as needed, including PEG derivative laxatives.
  - Linaclotide, which aids in intestinal chloride and bicarbonate excretion.
  - Lubiprostone, which aids in the chloride influx into the GI lumen.
  - Plecanatide 3 mg daily, which stimulates enterocytes to secrete fluid/electrolytes.
  - Tenapanor 50 mg twice daily, which secretes water into the intestinal lumen.

–Pharmacologic therapy for IBS-D:
  - Alosetron, a 5-HT$_3$ antagonist (only in women with severe IBS not responsive to conventional therapy).
  - Eluxadoline, a mu and kappa opioid receptor agonist and delta opioid receptor antagonist, which has been found to be a particularly helpful analgesic (contraindicated if history of cholecystectomy or drink > 3 EtOH beverages/d).
  - Loperamide, peripheral opiate receptor that prolongs gut transit time.
  - Rifaximin, 14-d course, with re-treatment recommended for up to 2 times.

–Other pharmacologic therapy for IBS:
  - Avoid the use of SSRIs in those with IBS. (AGA)
  - Consider antispasmodic agents on an as-needed basis for pain.
  - Consider low-dose tricyclics (TCAs) as second-line treatment if antispasmodics or antimotility agents have not helped.
  - Consider cognitive behavioral therapy or hypnotherapy for refractory IBS.

Sources
–https://www.nice.org.uk/guidance/qs114
–https://doi.org/10.1053/j.gastro.2019.07.004
–https://doi.org/10.1053/j.gastro.2022.04.016

LIVER DISEASE, NONALCOHOLIC (NAFLD)

Management: Adults

Recommendations from

➤ AASLD 2017

Evaluation

–Exclude competing etiologies: significant alcohol consumption, hepatitis C, medications, parenteral nutrition, Wilson disease, autoimmune liver disease, and severe malnutrition.

–If incidental finding of hepatic steatosis on imaging:
- If LFTs are normal, assess metabolic risk factors (obesity, diabetes mellitus, dyslipidemia) and other causes of hepatic steatosis (significant alcohol consumption or medications).
- If signs/symptoms attributable to liver disease or abnormal LFTs, evaluate for NAFLD.

–Carry a high index of suspicion for NAFLD or NASH in patients with type 2 diabetes and metabolic syndrome. Consider a clinical decision tool such as the NFS or fibrosis-4 index to identify those at low or high risk for advanced fibrosis. Alternatives are using vibration-controlled transient elastography or MR elastography to assess fibrosis.

–Consider liver biopsy in patients:
- With high ferritin and high iron saturation liver to determine the extent of iron accumulation in the liver.
- At increased risk of steatohepatitis and/or advanced fibrosis.
- All patients with a competing etiology for hepatosteatosis which requires a liver biopsy to exclude.

Therapies

–Employ weight loss as first-line therapy. Weight loss of 3%–5% of body weight improves steatosis; weight loss of 7%–10% of body weight is needed to improve liver fibrosis. Consider bariatric surgery in select patients to help with weight loss.

–Use pharmacologic treatment only in those with biopsy-proven NASH and fibrosis.

–Do not use metformin or GLP-1 agonists to treat NASH.

–Consider pioglitazone only in patients who have biopsy-proven NASH after risks and benefits have been discussed.

–Vitamin E at 800 IU/d in nondiabetic biopsy-proven NASH patients improves liver histology. Do not use with diabetics, NAFLD without liver biopsy, NASH cirrhosis, or cryptogenic cirrhosis.

–Do not use ursodeoxycholic acid or omega-3 fatty acids to treat NAFLD or NASH.

–NAFLD patients are at high risk for cardiovascular disease and require aggressive lifestyle modifications and pharmacotherapy. NAFLD and NASH do not increase the risk of liver injury from statins.

–Screen patients with NASH cirrhosis for esophageal varices and HCC with the same frequency/modalities used for other types of cirrhosis. Noncirrhotic NASH patients do not require screening.

Source
–https://doi.org/10.1002/hep.29367

Management: Children

Recommendations from

> AASLD 2017

–Test children with fatty liver disease who are very young or not overweight for fatty acid oxidation defects, lysosomal storage diseases, and peroxisomal disorders in addition to the usual causes found in adults.

–Intensive lifestyle modifications are first-line treatment in children.

–Obtain a liver biopsy before starting pharmacotherapy in children.

–Do not use metformin.

–Vitamin E 800 IU/d in biopsy-proven NASH patients has been shown to improve liver histology. Discuss long-term use of vitamin E prior to starting treatment, as efficacy in children is unknown.

Source

–https://doi.org/10.1002/hep.29367

PANCREATIC CANCER

Screening: Adults

Recommendations from

> USPSTF 2019

–Do not screen asymptomatic adults.

–No established screening guidelines exist for individuals with inherited genetic cancer syndromes or familial pancreatic cancer.

Practice Pearls

- Cigarette smoking has consistently been associated with increased risk of pancreatic cancer. *BRCA2* mutation is associated with a 5% lifetime risk of pancreatic cancer; blood group O with lower risk, and diabetes with a 2-fold higher risk. (*J Natl Cancer Inst.* 2009;101:424) (*J Clin Oncol.* 2009;27:433)

- Patients with a strong family history (≥2 first-degree relatives with pancreatic cancer) should undergo genetic counseling and may benefit from interval screening with CA 19-9, CT scan, and magnetic resonance cholangiopancreatography. (*Nat Rev Gastroenterol Hepatol.* 2012;9:445–453)

Sources

–USPSTF. *JAMA.* 2019;322(5):438–444.

–*Gastroenterology.* 2019;156(7):2024–2040.

PANCREATITIS, ACUTE (AP)

Management: Adults

Recommendations from

> ACG 2013, AGA 2024, NICE 2020

Evaluation

–Diagnosis of AP requires the presence of 2 of the 3 following criteria:

- Abdominal pain consistent with the disease.

- Serum amylase and/or lipase greater than 3 times the upper limit of normal.
- Characteristic findings from abdominal imaging.

–Recommend a contrast-enhanced CT scan or MRI of the pancreas if the diagnosis is unclear or if symptoms are not improving within 72 h. Do not routinely image at initial presentation unless diagnosis is unclear.

–Obtain a biliary ultrasound in all patients with AP.

–Check serum triglyceride level in all patients without a history of alcohol abuse or gallstones.

–Consider ICU or intermediate-level monitoring for any organ dysfunction.

Guidelines Alert 5–8
GUIDELINES DISCORDANT: FLUIDS IN ACUTE PANCREATITIS

Organization	Fluid Strategy
ACG	Moderately aggressive initial fluid resuscitation (most patients need 3–4 L in the first 24 h). Prefer Lactated Ringer solution. Monitor for volume overload
AGA	Use judicious goal-directed therapy for fluid management for resuscitation

Applying to Clinical Practice
- While fluid losses due to third spacing are a risk in acute pancreatitis, it is possible to cause significant fluid overload with aggressive fluid infusions.
- A large 2022 study was halted early after showing no benefit and a higher incidence of fluid overload in patients with moderate-to-severe pancreatitis given 3 mL/kg/h of LR vs. those given 1.5 mL/kg/h.[a]

[a]N Engl J Med. 2022;387(11):989.

Therapies

–In mild AP, start oral feedings with clear liquids or low-fat diet immediately if there is no nausea and vomiting and the abdominal pain has resolved.

–In severe AP, use enteral nutrition to prevent infectious complications, starting within 72 h of presentation. Avoid parenteral nutrition unless the enteral route is not available, not tolerated, or not meeting caloric requirements.

–If gallstones present, perform a cholecystectomy before discharge to prevent a recurrence of AP.
- If cholangitis, perform ERCP within the first 24 h.
- If no cholangitis, defer ERCP for at least 72 h.

–Do not use prophylactic or empiric antibiotics, even for severe necrotizing AP.

–In patients with infected necrosis:
- Use antibiotics known to penetrate pancreatic necrosis, such as carbapenems, quinolones, and metronidazole, to delay or perhaps avoid intervention and decrease morbidity and mortality.
- Delay surgical, radiologic, and/or endoscopic drainage preferably for more than 4 wk to allow liquefaction of the contents and the development of a fibrous wall around the necrosis (walled-off necrosis), unless unstable.

Practice Pearls

- Nasogastric delivery and nasojejunal delivery of enteral feeding appear comparable in efficacy and safety.
- In addition to gallstones and alcohol, consider causes including metabolic (hypercalcemia, hyperlipidemia), prescription drugs, microlithiasis, hereditary causes, autoimmune pancreatitis, obstructing tumors, or anatomical anomalies.

Sources
–https://gi.org/guideline/acute-pancreatitis/
–www.nice.org.uk/guidance/ng104
–https://doi.org/10.1053/j.gastro.2018.01.032
–*Am J Gastroenterol.* 2024;119:419–437. https://doi.org/10.14309/ajg.0000000000002645

PANCREATITIS, CHRONIC (CP)

Management: Adults

Recommendations from

➢ ACG 2020

–Recommend alcohol and smoking cessation.

–Offer elective interventional procedures (eg, celiac plexus block) for pain palliation.

–Offer ERCP and/or EUS with pancreatic drainage for pain related to obstructive CP.

–Consider surgical approaches if endoscopic interventions are not effective.

–Consider antioxidants (eg, selenium, methionine, vitamins C, A, and D), which may reduce pain.

–Consider opiates only after all other therapies are exhausted.

–There are no data supporting the use of pancreatic enzyme supplements to reduce pain.

–Total pancreatectomy with islet autotransplantation is reserved for refractory pain despite all measures.

–For patients with exocrine pancreatic insufficiency:

- Recommend pancreatic enzyme replacement therapy to reduce complications of malnutrition.
- Measure zinc, magnesium, and fat-soluble vitamin levels, and bone density at baseline and periodically.

Source
–https://doi.org/10.14309/ajg.0000000000000535

PARACENTESIS

Management: Adults

Recommendations from

> AASLD 2012

 –Perform diagnostic abdominal paracentesis in inpatients and outpatients with clinically apparent new-onset ascites.
 –Include ascitic fluid cell count and differential, ascitic fluid total protein, and serum-ascites albumin gradient in initial lab assessment of ascites.
 –Do not routinely administer fresh frozen plasma prior to paracentesis.

Source
 –https://www.aasld.org/sites/default/files/guideline_documents/AASLDPracticeGuidelineAscite DuetoCirrhosisUpdate2012Edition4_.pdf

ULCERS, STRESS

Prevention: Adults

Recommendations from

> SHM 2013

 –Do not prescribe medications for stress ulcer prophylaxis to medical inpatients unless they are at high risk for GI complications.

Source
 –https://www.shmabstracts.com/abstract/evaluation-of-stress-ulcer-prophylaxis-for-patients-with-coagulopathy-secondary-to-chronic-liver-disease/

GENITOURINARY DISORDERS

BENIGN PROSTATIC HYPERPLASIA (BPH)

Management: Men Age > 45

Recommendations from

> AUA 2021, EUA 2022

Evaluation

–Evaluate patients with bothersome lower urinary tract symptoms (LUTS) with a medical history, physical examination, an International Prostate Symptom Score (IPSS), and urinalysis. (AUA)

–Do not routinely measure serum creatinine in men with BPH unless renal impairment is suspected. Assess renal function if hydronephrosis is present or if surgical treatment is being considered for LUTS.

–Do not recommend dietary supplements or phytotherapeutic agents for LUTS management.

–In patients with LUTS and no signs of bladder outlet obstruction by flow study, treat for detrusor overactivity.

- Alter fluid intake.
- Behavioral modification.
- Anticholinergic medications.

Therapies

–Treatment options for moderate-to-severe LUTS from BPH (International Prostate Symptom Score ≥ 8):

- Watchful waiting.
- Medical therapies:
    - Alpha-blockers.[1]
    - 5-Alpha-reductase inhibitors.[2]
    - Anticholinergic agents.
    - Combination therapy.

---

[1] Alpha-blockers: alfuzosin, doxazosin, silodosin, tamsulosin, and terazosin. All have equal clinical effectiveness.
[2] 5-Alpha-reductase inhibitors: dutasteride and finasteride.

- Transurethral needle ablation.
- Transurethral microwave thermotherapy.
- Transurethral laser ablation or enucleation of the prostate.
- Transurethral incision of the prostate.
- Transurethral vaporization of the prostate.
- Transurethral resection of the prostate.
- Laser resection of the prostate.
- Photoselective vaporization of the prostate.
- Prostatectomy.

–Reevaluate patients receiving medical therapy for symptoms within 4–12 wk with utilization of the International Prostate Symptom Score. Consider evaluating further symptoms with a post-void residual measurement and uroflowmetry.

–Refer for surgery when BPH causes renal insufficiency, refractory urinary retention secondary to BPH, recurrent urinary tract infections (UTIs), bladder stones, gross hematuria, refractory LUTS, and/or if unwilling to use other therapies.

Practice Pearls

- Combination therapy with alpha-blockers and 5-alpha-reductase inhibitors is effective for moderate-to-severe LUTS with significant prostate enlargement.
- Men with planned cataract surgery should be counseled of the associated risks of floppy iris syndrome with alpha-blockers and discuss with their ophthalmologists.
- 5-Alpha-reductase inhibitors should not be used for men with LUTS from BPH without prostate enlargement.
- Anticholinergic agents are appropriate for LUTS that are primarily irritative symptoms, and if patient does not have an elevated post-void residual (>250 mL).
- The choice of surgical method should be based on the patient's presentation, anatomy, surgeon's experience, and patient's preference.

Sources
–http://www.guidelines.gov/content.aspx?id=25635&search=aua+2010+bph
–https://www.auanet.org/guidelines/benign-prostatic-hyperplasia-(bph)-guideline

BLADDER CANCER (CA)

Screening: Adults

Recommendations from

➤ USPSTF 2021

–Current evidence is insufficient to assess the balance of benefits and harms of screening for bladder cancer in asymptomatic adults.

Practice Pearls

- There is inadequate evidence to determine whether screening for bladder CA has an impact on mortality. Based on fair evidence, screening for bladder CA would result in unnecessary diagnostic procedures and overdiagnosis (70% of bladder CA is in situ) with attendant morbidity. (NCI 2017)

- Urinary biomarkers (nuclear matrix protein 22, tumor-associated antigen p300, presence of DNA ploidy) do not have significant sensitivity or specificity to be utilized in clinical practice. Microscopic hematuria leads to a diagnosis of bladder CA in only 5% of patients.

- 81,180 cases of bladder CA were expected in 2022 in the United States, with the majority being noninvasive (70%), but still 17,100 Americans were expected to die of bladder CA in 2017. Bladder cancer is diagnosed almost twice as often in White individuals as in Black individuals of either sex. 550,000 new cases annually occur worldwide. Lifetime risk in the United States is 3.9% for men and 1.2% for women. (*World J Urol.* 2020 38:1895–1904) (*Ann Inter Med.* 2010;153:461) (*Eur Urol.* 2013;63:4) (American Cancer Society. *Cancer Facts & Figures 2022.* Atlanta: American Cancer Society; 2022)

- Maintain a high index of suspicion in anyone with a history of smoking (4- to 7-fold increased risk[1]), an exposure to industrial toxins (aromatic amines, benzene), arsenic exposure such as found in regions with high arsenic concentrations in drinking water, therapeutic pelvic radiation, cyclophosphamide chemotherapy, a history of *Schistosoma haematobium* cystitis, hereditary nonpolyposis colon CA (Lynch syndrome), and history of transitional cell carcinoma of ureter (50% risk of subsequent bladder CA). Large screening studies in these high-risk populations have not been performed.

- Voided urine cytology with sensitivity of 40% but only 10% positive predictive value, urinary biomarkers (nuclear matrix protein 22, telomerase) with suboptimal sensitivity and specificity. Screening for microscopic hematuria has <10% positive predictive value.

Sources
- https://www.aafp.org/pubs/afp/issues/2017/1015/p507.html
- http://www.cancer.gov
- https://www.uspreventiveservicestaskforce.org/uspstf/recommendation/bladder-cancer-in-adults-screening

ERECTILE DYSFUNCTION

Management: Men

Recommendations from
> EAU 2018, Endocrine Society 2018, AUA 2018

---

[1] Individuals who smoke are 4–7 times more likely to develop bladder CA than individuals who have never smoked. Additional environmental risk factors: exposure to aminobiphenyls; aromatic amines; azo dyes; combustion gases and soot from coal; chlorination by-products in heated water; aldehydes used in chemical dyes and in the rubber and textile industries; organic chemicals used in dry cleaning, paper manufacturing, rope and twine making, and apparel manufacturing; contaminated Chinese herbs; arsenic in well water. Additional risk factors: prolonged exposure to urinary *S. haematobium* bladder infections, cyclophosphamide, or pelvic radiation therapy for other malignancies.

Evaluation

–Perform a medical and psychosexual history on all patients.

–Perform a focused physical examination to assess CV status, neurologic status, prostate disease, penile abnormalities, and signs of hypogonadism.

–Check a fasting glucose, lipid profile, and morning fasting total testosterone levels.

–Do not routinely screen otherwise asymptomatic men for hypogonadism. (Endocrine Society)

Therapies

–Recommend exercise and decreased BMI.

–Refer for psychosexual therapy if psychogenic erectile dysfunction.

–Offer testosterone therapy for androgen deficiency (at least 2 morning testosterone levels that are below the normal limit) with associated signs and symptoms if no contraindications are present.[1]

–Selective phosphodiesterase 5 inhibitors (PDE5i) are first-line therapy for idiopathic erectile dysfunction.

–If PDE5i fails, consider intercavernosal injections or penile prosthesis.

Practice Pearls

- Selective PDE5i:
  - Avanafil (200 mg, half-life 6–17 h).
  - Sildenafil (100 mg, half-life 2–4 h).
  - Tadalafil (20 mg, half-life 18 h).
  - Vardenafil (20 mg, half-life 4 h).
- Avoid nitrates and use alpha-blockers with caution when prescribing a selective PDE5i.

Sources

–*J Clin Endocrinol Metab.* 2018;103(5):1–30.

–https://uroweb.org/guideline/male-sexual-dysfunction/

–https://www.auanet.org/guidelines/erectile-dysfunction-(ed)-guideline

HEMATURIA, MICROSCOPIC

Management: Adults

Recommendations from

➤ AUA 2020

–Define microscopic hematuria as >3 RBC per high-power field on microscopic examination of a properly collected specimen.

–Do not diagnose hematuria based on a positive dipstick alone.

–Use history and physical exam to determine risk factors for urothelial cancer and nonmalignant etiologies.

---

[1] Prostate CA, breast CA, signs of prostatism, men who intend fertility in the short term, PSA > 4 ng/mL or > 3 ng/mL and high-risk, or comorbidities that would be a contraindication.

TABLE 6–1   RISK-STRATIFIED EVALUATION OF MICROSCOPIC HEMATURIA

Risk Category	Definition of Risk Level	Initial Evaluation
Low risk	Meets all the following criteria: Women <50 y, Men <40 y <10 pack-year smoking 3–10 RBC/HPF No additional risk factors[a] No prior microhematuria episodes	Repeat urinalysis (UA) within 6 mo OR Cystoscopy and renal ultrasound, followed by computed tomography (CT) urogram if ultrasound negative and hematuria persists
Intermediate risk	Meets any of the following: Women 50–59 y; Men 40–59 y 10–30 pack-years smoking 11–25 RBC/HPF One or more risk factors[a] Previously low risk, no prior eval, and 3–25 RBC/HPF on repeat UA	Cystoscopy and renal ultrasound, followed by CT urogram if ultrasound negative and hematuria persists
High risk	Meets any of the following: Women and men age ≥ 60 y >30 pack-years smoking >25 RBC/HPF History of gross hematuria Previously low-risk, no prior eval and >25 RBC/HPF on repeat UA	Cystoscopy and CT urogram

[a]Higher risk factors for urothelial disease include smoking, prior pelvic radiation therapy, prior cyclophosphamide therapy, occupational exposures to benzene dyes or aromatic amines, family history of urothelial cancer or Lynch syndrome, or chronic indwelling foreign body in the urinary tract. *Source:* AUA 2020, p. 780.

–If a nonmalignant or gynecologic source is suspected, evaluate and treat.

–If an alternate source is not identified, or if hematuria persists despite treatment, perform risk stratification and evaluate according to Table 6–1.

–If initial evaluation is negative, consider repeat urinalysis in 12 mo. If that remains positive, consider further observation vs. repeating the evaluation.

–See Table 6–2 for specific imaging recommendations.

Source
–Barocas DA et al. Microhematuria: AUA/SUFU guideline. *J Urol.* 2020;204:778.

INFERTILITY, MALE

Management: Men

Recommendations from

> **EAU 2018**
–Assessment of male infertility includes semen analysis and scrotal ultrasound.

TABLE 6–2 AMERICAN COLLEGE OF RADIOLOGY (ACR) APPROPRIATENESS CRITERIA FOR HEMATURIA	
Clinical Situation	**Imaging Modality**
Microhematuria. No risk factors, or history of recent vigorous exercise, or presence of infection, or viral illness, or present or recent menstruation. Initial imaging	CT abd/pelvis without IV contrast (May be appropriate)
Microhematuria. Patients with risk factors, without any of the following: history of recent vigorous exercise, or presence of infection or viral illness, or present or recent menstruation, or renal parenchymal disease. Initial imaging	CT urogram with and without IV contrast (Usually appropriate) MR urogram with and without IV contrast CT abd/pelvis with and without IV contrast CT abd/pelvis with IV contrast US kidneys and bladder (May be appropriate)
Microhematuria. Pregnant patient. Initial imaging	US kidneys and bladder (Usually appropriate) MRU without IV contrast (May be appropriate)
Gross hematuria. Initial imaging	CT urogram with and without IV contrast MR urogram with and without IV contrast (Usually appropriate) CT abd/pelvis with and without IV contrast (or either alone) MRI abd/pelvis with and without IV contrast US kidneys and bladder (May be appropriate)

–If semen analysis is abnormal, check FSH, LH, and testosterone levels.

–If WBCs are present in semen analysis, consider empiric antibiotics for STIs, then repeat semen analysis after treatment.

–Refer patients with abnormal screens to a specialist in male infertility for potential treatments that may include clomiphene citrate, tamoxifen, human chorionic gonadotropin, dopamine agonists, or surgical treatments depending on the underlying etiology.

Practice Pearl

• Infertility is defined as the inability of a sexually active couple not using contraception to conceive in 1 y.

Source

–https://uroweb.org/guideline/male-infertility/#4

INTERSTITIAL CYSTITIS

Management: Adults

Recommendations from

➢ AUA 2022

–Diagnose based on symptoms and physical exam. Consider cystoscopy and/or urodynamics only if diagnosis is uncertain.

–Use multimodal pain management approaches including medications, stress management, and physical therapy. Avoid pelvic floor strengthening exercises.

–Reconsider diagnosis if there is no improvement with therapy.

–Consider pain management such as urinary analgesics, NSAIDs, and opioid and nonopioid analgesics.

–Consider medications including amitriptyline, cimetidine, hydroxyzine, and pentosan polysulfate. None has been established as superior to the others, as none have proven consistent long-term benefit and all have potential for adverse effect.

–Avoid long-term oral antibiotic therapy, hydrodistension, and long-term glucocorticoids.

Source

–Hanno PM et al. Diagnosis and treatment of interstitial cystitis/bladder pain syndrome. AUA. 2022.

OVERACTIVE BLADDER

Management: Adults

Recommendations from

➤ AUA 2024

Evaluation

–Evaluate patients with history, physical exam, and a urinalysis to exclude microhematuria and infection.

–Consider the following evaluation steps:

- Post-void residual to exclude urinary retention in patients with suggestive symptoms.
- Voiding diary and/or symptom questionnaire.

–Do not routinely perform urodynamics, cystoscopy, or urinary tract imaging in the initial evaluation.

Therapies

–Offer bladder training and behavioral therapies as first-line therapy: fluid management, caffeine reduction, physical activity/exercise, dietary modifications, and mindfulness.

–Consider noninvasive therapies: pelvic floor muscle therapy, transcutaneous tibial nerve stimulation, transvaginal electrical stimulation, and yoga.

–There is insufficient evidence for nutraceuticals, vitamins, supplements, or herbal remedies.

–Offer antimuscarinic agents or beta-3-agonists.

- Counsel on side-effect profiles.
- In older patients, counsel about the increased risk of developing cognitive impairment with antimuscarinic medications.
- Avoid antimuscarinics in patients with narrow-angle glaucoma, impaired gastric emptying, or a history of urinary retention.
- Reassess for side effects within 4–8 wk after initiating therapy.

–Use combination therapy if monotherapy is unsuccessful.

–If medication therapy unsuccessful, refer to urologist to consider minimally invasive therapies (eg, botulinum toxin injection, implantable tibial nerve stimulation, sacral neuromodulation), invasive therapies (eg, bladder augmentation cystoplasty, indwelling urinary catheters), or additional evaluation.

Practice Pearl

- One in 7 patients taking anticholinergics will have improvement in symptoms, while 1 in 6 will have dry mouth, 1 in 111 will have urinary retention, and 1 in 76 will stop the medication due to adverse effects. (*Am Fam Physician*. 2023;108(2):130–131)

Source
  –https://www.auajournals.org/doi/10.1097/JU.0000000000003985

PROSTATE CANCER

Screening: Men

Recommendations from

> USPSTF 2018, AUA 2018 and 2023, ACS 2016, EAU 2021, NCCN 2019

  –Discordant recommendations between organizations for prostate cancer screening.

Practice Pearls

- Prevalence: There were 1.4 million cases diagnosed in the world in 2020. It is estimated that 288,300 new cases and 34,700 deaths will occur in the United States in 2023. In the United States, the lifetime risk of being diagnosed with prostate cancer is approximately 11%, and the lifetime risk of dying of prostate cancer is 2.5%. Autopsy-detected prostate CA is about the same worldwide with a prevalence of 59% in men >79 y of age.
- Seventy-five percent of men with PSA > 3 ng/mL will have no cancer on subsequent biopsy. More than 10% of men screened will have a false-positive PSA elevation if tested annually for 4 y and >5% will undergo a negative biopsy. (AUA 2018)
- There is good evidence that PSA can detect early-stage prostate CA (2-fold increase in organcon-fined disease at presentation with PSA screening), but mixed and inconclusive evidence that early detection improves health outcomes or mortality.
  - Two long-awaited studies add to the confusion.
    - A US study of 76,000 men showed increased prostate CA in screened group, but no reduction in risk of death from prostate CA. Named the prostate, lung, colorectal, and ovarian cancer (PLCO) screening trial, it showed no evidence for overall survival benefit from PSA screening and postulated that many patients with low-grade cancers were treated aggressively, leading to morbidity and mortality. Subsequent evaluation found that approximately 90% of patients in the control arm had undergone PSA testing during the course of the trial. This fact makes the trial result uninterpretable.
    - A European study of 80,000 men showed a decreased rate of death from prostate CA by 20% but significant overdiagnosis (there was no difference in overall death rate). To prevent 1 death from prostate CA, 1410 men needed to be screened, and 48 cases of prostate CA were found. Patients older than age 70 y had an increased death rate in the screened group (*N Engl J Med*. 2009;360:1310, 1320) (*N Engl J Med*. 2012;366:981, 1047). It found that PSA screening did reduce prostate-specific mortality by 20%. In this trial, 781 men needed to be invited to screening to prevent 1 death.
  - What should be the response to this new data?
    - We can improve survival by recognizing low-risk patients to be followed by active surveillance and not exposed to treatment until evidence of disease progression.

- Recognized high-risk patients (Black men and men with first degree relatives with prostate cancer) should be screened early and frequently.
  - Average-risk men can be screened by PSA twice between the ages of 45 and 55 and if the PSA is 0.70 ng/mL, their risk of lethal prostate cancer is quite low.
- Guideline groups are presently working on new guidelines for PC screening to minimize over-treatment of this disease but at the same time screening a higher risk population for aggressive prostate cancer at a stage that can be treated with conservative intent. (*N Engl J Med.* 2017;376:1285) (*J Clin Oncol.* 2016;34:2705–2711, 3481–3491, 3499–3501)
- *Benefit:* Insufficient evidence to establish whether a decrease in mortality from prostate CA occurs with screening by DRE or serum PSA.
- *Harm:* Based on solid evidence, screening with PSA and/or DRE detects some prostate CAs that would never have caused important clinical problems. Based on solid evidence, current prostate CA treatments result in permanent side effects in many men, including erectile dysfunction and urinary incontinence. (NCI 2008)
- Men with localized, low-grade prostate CAs (Gleason score 2–4) have a minimal risk of dying from prostate CA during 20 y of follow-up (6 deaths per 1000 person-years) (*JAMA.* 2005;293:2095) (*N Engl J Med.* 2014;370:932)
- Many physicians continue to screen Black men and men with a strong FH of prostate cancer despite the guidelines (*J Urol.* 2002;168:483) (*J Natl Cancer Inst.* 2000;92:2009) (*JAMA.* 2014; 311:1143). Black men have a double risk of prostate cancer and a >2-fold risk of prostate cancer–specific death. These patients and those with first-degree relatives <65 y with prostate cancer are at high enough risk to justify PSA screening until a definitive study of this population is available. (*JAMA.* 2014;311:1143)
- Increase in prostate cancer distant metastases at diagnosis in the United States over the last 3 y. (*JAMA Oncol.* 2016;2:1657)
- Radical prostatectomy (vs. watchful waiting) reduces disease-specific and overall mortality in patients with early stage prostate CA (*N Engl J Med.* 2011;364:1708). This benefit was seen only in men age > 65 y. Active surveillance for low-risk patients is safe and increasingly used as an alternative to radical prostatectomy (*J Clin Oncol.* 2010;28:126) (*Ann Intern Med.* 2012;156:582). A gene signature profile reflecting virulence and treatment responsiveness in prostate CA is now available. (*J Clin Oncol.* 2008;26:3930) (*J Natl Compr Netw.* 2016;14:659)
- PSA velocity (>0.5–0.75 ng/y rise) is predictive for the presence of prostate CA, especially with a PSA of 4–10. (*Eur Urol.* 2009;56:573)
- Multiparametric MRI scanning is emerging as a tool for more accurate detection of early prostate cancer as well as distinguishing indolent from high-grade cancers. (*J Urol.* 2011;185:815) (*Nat Rev Clin Oncol.* 2014;11:346)
- PSA screening is confounded by the morbidity and mortality associated with the treatment of prostate cancer. Molecular profiling that can stratify patients into high-risk and low-risk groups is a critical need for individualized adaptive therapies, which could minimize toxicity and maximize benefit in many patients (oncotype, Decipher, and Polaris are now available to look at molecular profiling).
- Germline testing and genetic counseling is increasingly being used in the early detection of prostate CA. There are now several commercial screening panels to assess for prostate CA risk genes. It remains unclear when germline testing should be used and how this may impact localized and metastatic disease management.

Guidelines Alert 6–1
GUIDELINES DISCORDANT: APPROACH TO SCREENING FOR PROSTATE CANCER

Recommendation	Organization					
	AUA	USPSTF	ACS	EAU	NCCN	
Screening age, general population	Offer initial prostate-specific antigen (PSA) screen between age 45–50, then regular screening between ages 50–69, only if patient opts in after discussion of potential benefits and harms of screening: small potential benefit of reducing chance of dying from prostate cancer vs. overdiagnosis, overtreatment, and treatment complications	Ages 55–69 y, only if patient opts in after discussion of potential benefits and harms (small potential benefit of reducing chance of dying from prostate cancer vs. overdiagnosis, overtreatment, and treatment complications). No screening after age 70	Age 50+ if ≥10-y life expectancy; discuss risks and benefits	Data are lacking to determine appropriate screening age. Consider screening if patient prefers and has 10–15 y life expectancy	Age 45–75 after discussion of risks and benefits. Consider in age 75+ if healthy, especially if not screened prior	
Screening age, high-risk populations	Consider at age 40–45 if first-degree family history, BRCA1 and 2, or Black ancestry	Inadequate evidence to assess for mortality benefit from early screening in high-risk groups	Age 45 if first-degree relative dx before age 65 y or Black ancestry; age 40 if multiple first-degree relatives affected at early age	Age 45 if positive family history, if Black ancestry	Age 40–75 y if African ancestry, germline mutations that increase prostate cancer risk, or suspicious family history	
Preferred screening method, if elected	PSA alone, digital rectal exam (DRE) may be used to "ugment" PSA screening	PSA and DRE		Not defined	PSA; "strongly consider" DRE	

| Frequency of screening, if elected | Q2–4 y for ages 50–69 | PSA ≥ 2.5 ng/mL: annual PSA < 2.5 ng/mL: q2 y | Optimal interval unknown. Propose risk-adapted strategy based on initial PSA: q2 y if PSA > 1 ng/mL at age 40 or > 2 ng/mL at age 60. Otherwise delay at least 8 y | Optimal interval unknown. Risk-adapted strategy proposed PSA < 1 ng/mL at age 40, < 2 ng/mL at age 60: q8 y Initially at risk: PSA > 1 ng/mL at age 40, > 2 ng/mL at age 60: q2 y. Men with <15 y life expectancy unlikely to benefit from screening | |

Applying to Clinical Practice

- Prostate cancer is the most prevalent malignancy in men in high-income countries.
- PSA and DRE are imperfect screening tools as they capture many lesions that would not otherwise cause morbidity or mortality and can miss some highly aggressive cancers.
- Shared decision-making after a high-quality discussion of risks and benefits is ideal but often impractical.
- If screening is elected, start between age 45 and 55 y and stop by age 70 y.
- As "active surveillance" has gained favor over radiation or prostatectomy for many lower-risk prostate tumors, the harms of screening may be lower than represented in the modeling studies cited in guidelines.

Sources

–USPSTF. 2018. https://www.uspreventiveservicestaskforce.org/Page/Document/UpdateSummaryFinal/prostate-cancer-screening1

–*JAMA*. 2018;319(18):1901–1913.

–*Eur Urol*. 2017;71:618–629.

–https://www.auanet.org/guidelines/prostate-cancer-early-detection-guideline

–*NCCN Guidelines*. Version 1.2022. NCCN.org.

–http://www.cancer.org

–EUA-EANM-ESTRO-ESUR-ISUP-SIOG. *Guidelines on Prostate Cancer*. 2022.

Prevention Recommendation

–No evidence-based guidelines exist to guide recommendations for the prevention of prostate cancer.

Practice Pearls

- Diet: high dietary fat intake does not increase the risk for prostate CA but is associated with more aggressive cancers and shorter survivals.
- Medications:
  - Dutasteride: absolute risk reduction of 22.8%. No difference in prostate CA-specific or overall mortality. Concern raised by mild increase in more aggressive cancers in patients on dutasteride (Gleason score of 7–10). (*N Engl J Med*. 2010;302:1192; 2013;369:603)
  - Finasteride: decreased 7-y prostate CA incidence from 25% (placebo) to 18% (finasteride), but no change in mortality. Trial participants report reduced ejaculate volume (47%–60%); increased erectile dysfunction (62%–67%); increased loss of libido (60%–65%); increased gynecomastia (3%–4.5%).
- Vitamins and minerals:
  - Vitamin E/alfa-tocopherol—inadequate data—one study showed a 17% increase in prostate CA with vitamin E alone. (*JAMA*. 2011;306:1549)
  - Selenium—no study shows benefit in reducing risk of prostate CA.
  - Lycopene—largest trials to date show no benefit. (*Am J Epidemiol*. 2010;172:566)

Management: Men Who Have Survived Prostate Cancer

Recommendations from

➤ ASCO 2015

–Measure serum PSA (prostate-specific antigen) every 4–12 mo (depending on recurrence risk) for the first 5 y then recheck annually thereafter.

–Evaluate survivors with elevated or rising PSA levels as soon as possible by their primary treating specialist.

–Perform an annual digital rectal examination.

–Adhere to ASCO screening and early detection guidelines for 2nd cancers (increased risk of bladder and colon cancer after pelvic radiation).

–Assess for physical and psychosocial effects of PC and treatment:

- Anemia related to androgen deprivation therapy (ADT).
- Bowel dysfunction and symptoms especially rectal bleeding.
- Cardiovascular and metabolic effects for men receiving ADT—follow USPSTF guidelines for evaluation and screening for cardiovascular risk factors.
- Assess for distress and depression and refer to appropriate specialist.
- Osteoporosis and fracture risk in men on ADT—do baseline DEXA (dual energy X-ray absorptiometry) scan and support with calcium, vitamin D, and bisphosphonates as indicated.
- Sexual dysfunction—PDE5i may help—refer to appropriate specialist.
- Urinary dysfunction (incontinence and leakage)—refer to urology specialist.
- Vasomotor symptoms (hot flushes) in men receiving ADT—selective serotonin or noradrenergic reuptake inhibitors or gabapentin may be helpful. Low-dose progesterone may be helpful in refractory patients.

Practice Pearls

- General health promotion can be helpful:
  - Counsel patients to achieve and maintain a healthy weight by limiting consumption of high-caloric food and beverages.
  - Counsel survivors to engage in at least 150 min/wk of physical activity.
  - Improve dietary pattern with more fruits and vegetables and whole grains.
  - Encourage intake of at least 600 IU of vitamin D per day as well as sources of calcium not to exceed 1200 mg/d.
  - Counsel survivors to avoid or limit alcohol consumption to no more than 2 drinks/d.
  - Counsel survivors to avoid tobacco products.
- Rising PSA in patients with nonmetastatic PC:
  - A PSA ≥ 0.2 ng/mL on 2 consecutive tests is reflective of recurrent prostate cancer. These patients are treated with pelvic radiation with improvement in 10-y survival and freedom from recurrence. The earlier the radiation is started after a PSA rise, the better the outcome. Patients who have had previous radiation to the prostate occasionally undergo surgery but most are treated with ADT or cryoablation (*JCO.* 2009;27:4300–4305). A recent trial adding ADT to radiation in this setting increased disease-free progression. (*Eur Urol.* 2016;69:802)
  - Routine CT or bone scanning is not indicated but evaluate new symptoms even if PSA is not rising (transformation to small cell carcinoma in 5% of patients).
  - In newly relapsed patients with visceral metastasis and/or more than 4 separate bone lesions, a combination of concurrent androgen deprivation and taxotere chemotherapy is associated with a 15%–20% increased survival at 5 y vs. sequential therapy. (*N Engl J Med.* 2015;373:737) (*Lancet.* 2016;387:1163)

Source

–Prostate cancer survivorship care guidelines. *J Clin Oncol.* 2015;33:1078–1085.

TESTICULAR CANCER

Screening: Men

Recommendations from

➢ AAFP 2008, USPSTF 2011, AUA 2019 amended 2023

–Do not screen routinely.

–Treat a solid mass in the testis found on physical exam or imaging as malignant neoplasm until proven otherwise. The AUA considers this a "clinical principle."

–Evaluate suspected testicular mass using scrotal ultrasound with doppler. Do not use MRI for the initial evaluation.

–Reevaluate patients with normal serum human chorionic gonadotropin and AFP results and indeterminate findings on ultrasound in 6–8 wk with repeat imaging.

–Be aware of risk factors for testicular CA: previous testis CA (2%–3% risk of second cancer), cryptorchid testis, family history of testis CA, HIV (increased risk of seminoma), and Klinefelter syndrome.

Practice Pearls

• Inform patients with risk factors of their increased risk for developing testicular CA, and counsel about screening. Such patients may then elect to be screened or to perform testicular self-examination. Advise adolescent and young adult men to seek prompt medical attention if they notice a scrotal abnormality. (USPSTF 2011)

• *Benefits:* Based on fair evidence, screening would not result in appreciable decrease in mortality, in part because therapy at each stage is so effective.

• *Harms:* Based on fair evidence, screening would result in unnecessary diagnostic procedures and occasional removal of a noncancerous testis. (NCI 2011)

• In 2016, approximately 8850 men in the United States were diagnosed with testicular cancer, but only 400 men died of this disease. Worldwide, there are approximately 72,000 cases and 9000 deaths annually. (*CA Caner J Clin.* 2017;67:7)

• There is a 3- to 5-fold increase in testis cancer in White men vs. other ethnicities. (*N Engl J Med.* 2007;356:1835; 2014;371:2005)

Sources

–http://www.aafp.org/online/en/home/clinical/exam.html

–http://www.ahrq.gov/clinic/uspstf/uspstest.htm

URINARY INCONTINENCE, OVERACTIVE BLADDER

Management: Adults

Recommendations from

➢ AUA 2019

Evaluation

–Rule out urinary tract infection.

–Check a post-void residual to rule out overflow incontinence.

Therapies

–First-line treatments:
  - Bladder training.
  - Bladder control strategies.
  - Pelvic floor muscle training.

–Second-line treatments:
  - Antimuscarinic meds or beta-3-adrenoceptor agonists (ie, darifenacin, fesoterodine, oxybutynin, solifenacin, tolterodine, or trospium).
  - Contraindicated with narrow-angle glaucoma or gastroparesis.

–Third-line treatments:
  - Sacral neuromodulation.
  - Peripheral tibial nerve stimulation.
  - Intradetrusor botulinum toxin A.

–Avoid indwelling urinary catheters.

Source

–http://www.auanet.org/guidelines/overactive-bladder-(oab)-guideline

URINARY INCONTINENCE, STRESS

Management: Women

Recommendations from

➤ AUA 2017, ACP 2014

–Treat according to AUA algorithm (Fig. 6–1).

–Refer for pelvic floor muscle training and bladder training.

Source

–http://www.guideline.gov/content.aspx?id=48543

URINARY INCONTINENCE, MEN

Management: Men

Recommendations from

➤ EAU 2011

–Evaluate according to Fig. 6–2.

FIG. 6–1 AUA SUI ALGORITHM 2017.

Female Stress Urinary Incontinence: AUA/SUFU Evaluation and Treatment Algorithm

EVALUATION (INDICATIONS)

Initial evaluation

The initial evaluation of patients desiring to undergo surgical intervention should include the following components:

- History
- Physical exam
- Demonstration of SUI
- PVR assessment
- Urinalysis

Cystoscopy

Should not be performed unless there is a concern for lower urinary tract abnormalities

Urodynamics

May be omitted when SUI is clearly demonstrated

Additional evaluation

Additional evaluation **should** be performed in the following scenarios:

- Lack of definitive diagnosis
- Inability to demonstrate SUI
- Known/suspected NLUTD
- Abnormal urinalysis
- Urgency-predominant MUI
- Elevated PVR
- High-grade POP (if SUI not demonstrated with POP reduction)
- Evidence of significant voiding dysfunction

Additional evaluation **may** be performed in the following scenarios:

- Concomitant OAB symptoms
- Failure of prior anti-incontinence surgery
- Prior POP surgery

In patients who wish to undergo treatment, physicians should counsel regarding the availability of observation, pelvic floor muscle training, other nonsurgical options, and surgical interventions. Physicians should counsel patients on potential complications specific to the treatment options.

TREATMENT

Nonsurgical
- Continence pessary
- Vaginal inserts
- Pelvic floor muscle exercises

Surgical
- Bulking agents
- Midurethral sling (synthetic)
- Autologous fascia pubovaginal sling
- Burch colposuspension

If a midurethral sling surgery is selected, either the retropubic or transobturator midurethral sling may be offered. A single-incision sling may be offered to index patients if they are informed as to the immaturity of evidence regarding their efficacy and safety. Physicians must discuss the specific risks and benefits of mesh as well as alternatives to a mesh sling.

SPECIAL CASES

1. Fixed immobile urethra
- Pubovaginal sling
- Retropubic midurethral sling
- Urethral bulking agents

2. Concomitant surgery for POP repair and SUI
Any incontinence procedure

3. Concomitant NLUTD
Surgical treatment following appropriate evaluation and counseling

4. Child-bearing, diabetes, obesity, geriatric
Surgical treatment following appropriate evaluation and counseling

MUI, mixed urinary incontinence; NLUTD, neurogenic lower urinary tract dysfunction; OAB, overactive bladder; POP, pelvic organ prolapse; PVR, post-void residual; SUI, stress urinary incontinence.

Source: Reproduced with permission from Kobashi KC et al. Surgical treatment of female stress urinary incontinence: AUA/SUFU guideline. *J Urol.* 2017;198:875.

FIG. 6–2 INITIAL MANAGEMENT OF URINARY INCONTINENCE IN MEN: EAU 2011.

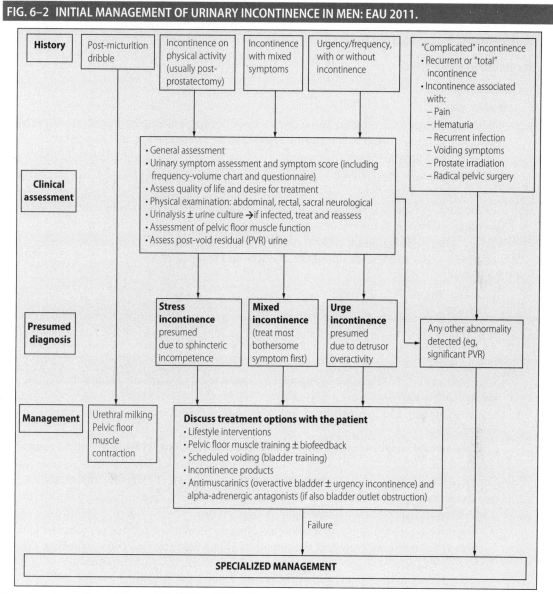

Source: Reproduced with permission from Thüroff JW et al. EAU guidelines on urinary incontinence. *Eur Urol.* 2011;59:387–400.

UROLITHIASIS

Management: Adults and Children

Recommendations from

> **EAU 2020, AUA 2016**

Evaluation

–Obtain noncontrast CT urogram using "low-dose protocols" if available for patients with acute flank pain. Consider contrast-enhanced CT scan if stone removal is planned and the renal anatomy needs to be assessed.

–Evaluate renal colic by obtaining:

- Urinalysis.
- Serum CBC, creatinine, uric acid, calcium, and albumin +/− intact parathyroid hormone.
- Stone analysis by X-ray crystallography or infrared spectroscopy.

–Obtain 24-h urine analysis for complicated calcium stone disease: calcium, oxalate, citrate, creatinine, urate, magnesium, phosphate, sodium, and potassium.

Therapies

–Analgesia options for renal colic:

- NSAIDs.
- Opiates.
- Alpha-blockers.

–Treat patients with hypercalciuria with a thiazide diuretic.

–Treat with an alkaline citrate for hypocitraturia, type 1 renal tubular acidosis, hypercalciuria, and hyperoxaluria.

–Advise adults with a history of urinary stones to drink sufficient water to maintain a urine output >2.5 L/d.

–Consider use of an alpha-receptor blocker to facilitate spontaneous passage of ureteral stones <10 mm.

–Consider active ureteral stone removal for persistent obstruction, failure of spontaneous passage, or the presence of severe, unremitting colic.

- Options include shockwave lithotripsy or ureteroscopy.
- Consider the stone composition before deciding on the method of removal, based on patient history, former stone analysis of the patient, or Hounsfield unit (HU) on unenhanced CT. Stones with density > 1000 HU (and with high homogeneity) on noncontrast-enhanced CT are less likely to be disintegrated by shockwave lithotripsy.

–For calcium stones and hypercalciuria:

- Limit sodium intake and consume 1–2 g/d of dietary calcium.
- Thiazide diuretic.

–For calcium oxalate stones:

- If high urinary oxalate, limit intake of oxalate-rich foods and maintain normal calcium consumption.
- If hyperuricosuria, treat with allopurinol.

–For uric acid stones and high urinary uric acid, limit intake of nondairy animal protein.

–For struvite stones refractory to surgical management, consider acetohydroxamic acid therapy.

–For uric acid or cystine stones, consider potassium citrate therapy to raise urinary pH to optimal level.

–Management of sepsis with obstructed kidney:

- • Urgent decompression with a ureteral stent or percutaneous nephrostomy tubes.
- • Start antibiotics immediately.

Practice Pearl

- • Patients at high risk for recurrent stone formation:
  - ≥3 stones in 3 y.
  - Infection stones.
  - Urate stones.
  - Children and adolescents with stones.
  - Cystinuria.
  - Primary hyperoxaluria.
  - Type 1 renal tubular acidosis.
  - Cystic fibrosis.
  - Hyperparathyroidism.
  - Crohn disease.
  - Malabsorption syndromes.
  - Nephrocalcinosis.
  - Family history of kidney stone disease.
  - High levels of vitamin D.

Sources

–https://uroweb.org/guideline/urolithiasis/

–http://www.auanet.org/guidelines/kidney-stones-surgical-management-guideline#x14007

HEMATOLOGIC DISORDERS

ANEMIA

Management: Adults and Children

Recommendations from

> **British Society of Gastroenterology 2011**
> –Evaluate with complete blood count, including Hb and mean corpuscular volume (MCV), reticulocyte count, ferritin level, total iron-binding capacity, and transferrin saturation. Calculate a reticulocyte index and Mentzer index.

Practice Pearl

- Iron deficiency anemia (IDA) and anemia of chronic disease (ACD), sometimes called anemia of inflammation, are the two most common causes of anemia. ACD is often underrecognized, with some hospital-based studies in the United States estimating the prevalence as high as 70%. See Table 7–1 for common causes of anemia.

TABLE 7–1 COMMON CAUSES OF ANEMIA						
Cause	MCV	Ferritin Level	RDW	Hb Electrophoresis	Iron/TIBC	Mentzer Index[a]
Iron deficiency anemia (IDA)	Low	<30	High	Normal	<10%	>13
Anemia of chronic disease (ACD)	Normal/ Decreased	High	Normal/ High	Normal	>15%	>13
IDA + ACD	Normal	<100	High	Normal	<20%	>13
Beta-thalassemia	Low	Normal	Normal	↑A_2, F hemoglobin	~20%	<13
Alpha-thalassemia	Low	Normal	Normal	Normal	~20%	<13
Hemoglobin E	Low	Normal	Normal	↑HgbE	~20%	<13
B_{12}/Folate deficiency	High	Normal	High	Normal	Normal	<13

[a]Mentzer index = MCV divided by red blood cell number (RBC) in millions.
RDW, red cell distribution of width; TIBC, total iron binding capacity.

ANEMIA, CHEMOTHERAPY ASSOCIATED

Management: Adults

Recommendations from

⪢ American Society of Hematology (ASH) 2019

–Offer erythrocyte-stimulating agents (ESAs) if Hb < 10 g/dL and curative intent. Consider RBC transfusion as alternative.

–Do not offer ESAs to cancer patients with anemia who are not on chemotherapy. Exception: patients with lower risk myelodysplastic syndromes and a serum erythropoietin < 500 IU/L.

–In patients with myeloma, non-Hodgkin lymphoma, or chronic lymphocytic leukemia, observe the response to treatment before considering an ESA.

–Counsel patients on the thromboembolic risks associated with ESAs.

–Epoetin beta and alfa, darbepoetin, and biosimilar epoetin alfa have equivalent safety and efficacy.

–Discontinue ESAs if there is no response within 6–8 wk.

–Consider iron replacement to improve Hb response and reduce RBC transfusions. See "Anemia of Chronic Disease" section for iron store assessment in inflammatory states.

Practice Pearl

- FDA-approved starting dose of epoetin is 150 U/kg 3 times/wk or 40,000 U weekly. For darbe-poetin, the dose is 2.25 μg/kg weekly or 500 μg every 3 wk subcutaneously.

Source
–*Blood Adv.* 2019;3(8):1197–1210.

ANEMIA, HEMOLYTIC (HA)

Management: Adults

Recommendations from

⪢ BSH 2016

Evaluation

–Diagnose when there is:
- Evidence of hemolysis (anemia, jaundice, elevated LDH, decreased haptoglobin, elevated reticulocyte index).
- A positive direct antiglobulin test.
- Alternative causes excluded.

–Categorize into primary autoimmune hemolytic anemia (AIHA), secondary AIHA, and drug-induced AIHA (DIIHA).

–Exclude cytomegalovirus (CMV) reactivation and parvovirus B19 infection if AIHA is associated with hematologic malignancy.

Therapy

–Give prednisolone 1 mg/kg/d for primary AIHA or secondary AIHA not responding to other treatments.

–In secondary AIHA, treating the associated condition often improves the AIHA.

–If DIIHA is suspected, stop the offending medication. Improvement usually occurs within 1–2 wk. The addition of steroids is of uncertain benefit though it is frequently used.

–If presenting with AIHA during remission of Hodgkin lymphoma, assess for recurrence. If remission is confirmed, treat for primary AIHA.

–Consider azathioprine, danazol, mycophenolate mofetil, and rituximab in AIHA due to systemic lupus erythematosus not responding to steroids.

–In metastatic malignancy, AIHA can respond to disease control or to corticosteroids.

–Use thromboprophylaxis, given the association between hemolysis and thrombosis.

–Transfuse for life-threatening anemia with ABO, Rh, and Kell-matched RBCs rather than waiting for full compatibility testing.

–Consider intravenous immunoglobulin (IVIG) as a rescue option in patients with AIHA.

Practice Pearls

- HA is caused by the patient's immune system acting against its own red cell antigens.
- Incidence is 1 per 100,000/y. Approximately half are secondary to an associated disorder. Of these, half are associated with malignancy, a third due to infection, and one-sixth due to collagen vascular disorders.
- Most cases of AIHA are warm agglutinins, but cold hemagglutinin diseases (CHAD) are also reported.
- Secondary causes of warm AIHA include neoplasms (chronic lymphocytic leukemia, lymphoma, solid organ tumors), infections (hepatitis C, HIV, CMV, VZV, pneumococcal infection, leishmaniosis, tuberculosis), and immune dysregulation (SLE, Sjögren, scleroderma, ulcerative colitis, primary biliary cirrhosis, sarcoidosis, posttransplantation).
- Secondary causes of cold AIHA include neoplasms (chronic lymphocytic leukemia, NHL, solid organ tumors), infections (mycoplasma, viral infections including infectious mononucleosis), autoimmune diseases, and postallogenic hematopoietic stem cell transplant.
- The most frequent benign associations to AIHA are ovarian teratoma and thymoma. Resection of the tumor consistently resolves the AIHA.
- Watch out for Evan syndrome: autoimmune thrombocytopenia plus AIHA, occurring either concurrently or consecutively. Neutropenia is also a common feature. Generally chronic, it affects both children and adults. Treatment is largely the same as for AIHA (first line: prednisone 1–2 mg/kg/d; second line: IVIG; third line: cyclosporine, MMF, azathioprine, danazol, rituximab, and splenectomy).

Source

–*Br J Hematol.* 2016;76(3):395–411.

ANEMIA, IRON DEFICIENCY (IDA)

Management: Adults

Recommendations from

> British Society of Gastroenterology 2021

Evaluation

–Assess dietary iron intake, malabsorption of iron, menstruation patterns, and blood donation.

–Confirm with iron studies (eg, serum ferritin, transferrin) before further investigation.

–Screen with upper and lower endoscopy for male and postmenopausal female patients unless history of recent significant non-GI blood loss. Consider CT colography if patient not suitable for endoscopy.

–Screen all patients with IDA for celiac disease (and *H. pylori*), but do not defer colonoscopy if the patient is >45 y, has marked anemia, or has a significant family history of colorectal cancer.

–Screen all patients for hematuria and workup accordingly.

–Avoid fecal occult blood testing and rectal exam.

–If the patient has undergone gastrectomy and has IDA, obtain upper and lower endoscopy if >40-y-old.

–If there is no response to iron replacement, perform an iron absorption test: check a baseline iron level and then a second iron level 2–4 h after ingesting a single 325-mg ferrous sulfate tablet with water. An increase in the iron level of at least 100 mcg/dL indicates adequate absorption.

–If upper and lower GI tracts are normal, obtain small bowel visualization with capsule endoscopy if the patient has symptoms of small bowel disease and/or continued anemia despite iron replacement. CT or MR enterography can be used if capsule is not available.

–Workup iron deficiency without significant anemia with GI evaluation in postmenopausal women and men >40-y-old.

Therapy

–Do not defer iron replacement while awaiting investigations into IDA unless colonoscopy is imminent.

–Dose ferrous sulfate, fumarate, or gluconate every other day dosing rather than BID dosing. Taking iron 15–30 min before a meal with orange juice or 500 mg of vitamin C may enhance absorption.

–Monitor for response to oral iron in the first 4 wk of treatment then continue for 3 mo.

–Monitor blood count every 6 mo after treatment to evaluate for recurrent IDA.

–If intolerant of iron, nonadherent, or not improving despite oral therapy, give intravenous iron sucrose (dose 200 mg once or twice a week until the calculated iron deficit is administered), ferric carboxymaltose (dose 1000 mg once weekly). Hemoglobin levels can take 8–10 wk to normalize. Reserve transfusion of RBC for cardiovascular instability or persistent symptomatic anemia despite IV iron therapy. See Tables 7–2 and 7–3 for potential complications of blood transfusion.

TABLE 7–2 NONINFECTIOUS COMPLICATIONS OF BLOOD TRANSFUSION

Complication	Incidence	Diagnosis	Rx and Outcome
Acute hemolytic transfusion reaction	1:40,000	Serum-free hemoglobin, Coombs	Fluids to keep urine output >1 mL/kg/h, pressors, treat disseminated intravascular coagulation, fatal in 1:1.8 × 10^6 RBC exposures
Delayed transfusion reaction (HTR)	1:3000–5000	Timing (10–14 d after tx)—(+) Coombs, ↑ LDH, indirect bilirubin, reticulocyte count—Ab often to Kidd or Rh	Identify responsible antigen, transfuse compatible blood if necessary
Febrile non-HTR	0.1%–1%	Exclude acute hemolytic transfusion reaction—↓ risk with leucocyte depletion—starts within 2 h of transfusion	Acetaminophen PO, support, and reassurance
Allergic (urticarial)	1%–3%	Urticaria, pruritus but no fever—caused by antibody to donor-plasma proteins	Hold tx—give antihistamines and complete tx when symptoms resolve
Anaphylactic	1:20,000–50,000	Hypotension, bronchospasm, urticaria, anxiety, rule out hemolysis	Epinephrine 1:1000—0.2–0.5 mL. SQ, steroids, antihistamine
Transfusion-related acute lung injury (TRALI)	1:10,000	HLA or neutrophil antibodies in donor blood hypoxia, bilateral lung infiltrates, and fever within 6 h of transfusion	Supportive care—steroids ineffective mortality—10%–20% (most common cause of transfusion-related fatality)

HTR: hemolytic transfusion reaction

TABLE 7–3 INFECTIOUS COMPLICATIONS OF TRANSFUSION

Transfusion-Transmitted Organism	Risk per Unit of Blood Transfused
HIV Hepatitis C Hepatitis B West Nile virus Cytomegalovirus (CMV)	1 in 1,467,000 1 in 1,149,000 1 in 282,000 Rare 70%–80% of donors are carriers, leukodepletion ↓ risk but in situation of significant immunosuppression gives CMV-negative blood
Bacterial infection	1 in 3000—5-fold more common in platelet vs. RBC transfusion
Parasitic infection (Babesiosis, malaria, Chagas disease)	Rare

Practice Pearls

- Symptoms of IDA: weakness, headache, irritability, fatigue, exercise intolerance, and restless leg syndrome. Symptoms may occur without anemia in patients with iron depletion (ferritin < 30 ng/mL). As many as 40% of patients with IDA will experience pica (appetite for clay, starch, and paper products) and/or pagophagia (craving for ice) which resolves rapidly with iron repletion.
- Rarely, in severe prolonged iron deficiency, dysphagia with esophageal webs (Plummer–Vinson syndrome), koilonychias (spoon nails), glossitis with decreased salivary flow, and alopecia can occur.
- Common causes of occult IDA: aspirin/NSAID use, colonic carcinoma, gastric carcinoma, benign gastric ulcerations, angiodysplasia, and celiac disease.
- Less common causes include *H. pylori* infection, gastrectomy, esophagitis, hematuria, gastric antral vascular ectasias, and small bowel tumors.
- Infrequent causes of IDA include *Ancylostoma duodenale* infection, epistaxis, intravascular hemolysis (especially paroxysmal nocturnal hemoglobinuria and microangiopathic hemolytic anemia), pulmonary hemosiderosis, autoimmune gastritis, and congenital IDA (germline mutation in the *TMPRSS6* gene which leads to reduction in iron absorption and mobilization). IDA is also associated with chronic kidney disease (CKD) and heart failure (HF) and can be multifactorial.
- Twenty percent to twenty-five percent of patients will have dose-dependent GI side effects from oral iron including abdominal pain, nausea, constipation, and diarrhea.
- In new IDA, a history of GI or bariatric surgery should not stop an investigation into other causes of IDA.
- A response of ≥ 10 g/L rise in Hgb after 2 wk of oral IRT is highly sensitive for a true IDA.
- IDA is common in young women, usually due to menstrual loss, pregnancy, or dietary insufficiency. Screen for celiac disease and limit other workup unless clinical suggestion for other etiology.
- IDA in older adults is common and multifactorial. Weigh risks and benefits of investigations based on comorbidities.

Sources
–https://gut.bmj.com/content/70/11/2030
–*Gut*. 2011;60(10):1309–1316.

ANEMIA OF CHRONIC DISEASE (ACD)

Management: Adults and Children

Recommendations from
➤ ASH 2019, BJH 2011

Evaluation
–Anemia is defined as Hb < 12 g/dL in women and Hb < 13 g/dL in men, usually, normochromic and normocytic pattern.

–Test for concomitant iron deficiency and determine potential responsiveness to iron therapy and long-term iron requirements every 3 mo (every 1–3 mo for people receiving hemodialysis):
  - Percentage of hypochromic cells > 6%, reticulocyte hemoglobin content < 29 pg, or transferrin saturation < 20%, and serum ferritin < 100 mg/L are consistent with iron deficiency.
  - The ratio of the serum transferrin receptor to the log of the serum ferritin can also be used to establish the presence of IDA. A ratio < 1 makes ACD likely, whereas a ratio > 2 suggests that iron stores are deficient, with or without ACD.

–Do not order transferrin saturation or serum ferritin alone to assess iron deficiency in people with ACD or CKD.

–Test as appropriate for kidney and liver function, thyroid function, folic acid, cobalamin (B_{12}), or vitamin D (negative regulator of hepcidin expression).

Therapy

–Treat the underlying inflammatory or malignant process.

–In people with anemia of CKD, treat clinically relevant hyperparathyroidism to improve the management of the anemia.

–In people treated with iron, serum ferritin levels should not rise above 800 mcg/L.

–Treat with transfusion only if patient is clinically unstable or rapid correction of Hb is needed, eg, before surgery.

–Do not initiate ESA therapy in the presence of absolute iron deficiency without also managing the iron deficiency (oral or parenteral).

–Offer treatment with ESAs to patients with ACD/anemia of CKD who are likely to benefit in terms of quality of life and physical function. ESA should not be used if hemoglobin > 10 g/dL. The main benefit of ESA is to reduce transfusion need.

–ESA is not to be used in patients with curable malignancies or in patients with cancer not on chemotherapy. Side effects of thrombosis and potentially increased cancer growth should be discussed with the patient.

–Goal Hb is typically 10–12 g/dL for adults, young people, and children 2 y and older, and between 9.5 and 11.5 g/dL for children younger than 2 y of age. Rate of rise goal is typically 1–2 g/dL/mo.

–Avoid blood transfusions in people with anemia of CKD in whom kidney transplant is a treatment option due to antibody formation.

–For patients with anemia of CKD who are iron deficient and not on ESA therapy, consider a trial of oral iron before offering intravenous iron therapy. If intolerant of oral iron or target Hb levels are not reached within 3 mo, offer IV iron therapy. If the patients are receiving hemodialysis, offer IV iron.

–For patients who are iron deficient, receiving ESA therapy, and receiving hemodialysis, offer IV iron.

Practice Pearls

- Frequent causes of ACD include infections (viral, bacterial, parasitic, fungal), malignancies, auto-immune diseases (rheumatoid arthritis, systemic lupus erythematosus, vasculitis, sarcoidosis, inflammatory bowel disease), CKD, and HF.

- IDA frequently occurs concomitantly with ACD.
- Classically, ACD has a mild-to-moderate anemia, normochromic and normocytic, with a low reticulocyte index. Inflammation is typically evident through inflammatory markers such as the white blood cell count, platelet count, C-reactive protein, or erythrocyte sedimentation rate.
- Routine measurement of erythropoietin is not recommended.
- Epoetin and darbepoetin are equal in efficacy. FDA-approved starting dose of epoetin is 150 U/kg 3 times/wk or 40,000 U weekly. For darbepoetin, the dose is 2.25 mcg/kg weekly or 500 mcg every 3 wk subcutaneously.
- When patients stop chemotherapy for any reason, stop ESAs and substitute transfusion therapy according to FDA guidelines.

Source
–*Br J Hematol.* 2011;154(3):289–300.

ARTERIAL THROMBOSIS AND THROMBOEMBOLISM

Management: Adults with COVID-19

Recommendations from
> CHEST 2023

Therapy
–Hospitalized patients with COVID-19:
- History of acute coronary syndrome (ACS):
  - Continue antiplatelet therapy. Consider change ticagrelor or clopidogrel to prasugrel if concern for drug-drug interaction with COVID-19 medications.
  - Continue dual antiplatelet therapy (DAPT).
  - In patients with COVID-19 and myocardial injury without acute coronary syndrome, do not initiate DAPT.
  - In patients on DAPT and therapeutic parenteral anticoagulation, individualize therapy based on bleeding risk with DAPT.
- History of stroke:
  - If on antiplatelet therapy, do not change oral or subcutaneous anticoagulation.
  - Continue antiplatelet therapy and deep vein thrombosis (DVT) prophylaxis.
- Acute stroke:
  - Treat with recanalization therapy with either medical or endovascular treatment as indicated.
  - Treat with antiplatelet therapy for stroke or TIA as indicated for non-COVID-19 patient.
- Atrial fibrillation:
  - If needing to discontinue oral anticoagulation, switch to therapeutic parenteral anticoagulation, either LMWH or UFH.
  - New onset: outpatient, start anticoagulation based on CHA_2DS_2-VASc.

- Peripheral arterial disease:
  - Stable disease: continue antiplatelet therapy with DVT prophylaxis with DVT prophylaxis. Individualize treatment if therapeutic anticoagulation is needed when choosing to continue antiplatelet therapy.
  - Unstable disease: consult vascular surgery early for consideration for intervention.

Source
–*CHEST.* 2023;164(6):1531–1550.

CANCER

Prevention: Adults

Recommendations from
➤ ACS 2020
  –Achieve and maintain a healthy body weight throughout life.
  –Be physically active:
  - Adults should get 150–300 min of moderate-intensity physical activity/wk, or 75–150 min of vigorous-intensity physical activity/wk. Exceeding the upper limit of 300 min is optimal.
  - Children and adolescents should get at least 1 h of moderate- or vigorous-intensity activity each day.
  - Limit sedentary behavior.
  –Follow a healthy eating pattern at all ages:
  - A healthy eating pattern includes foods high in nutrients, a variety of vegetables and fruits, and whole grains.
  - A healthy eating pattern limits or does not include red and processed meats, sugar-sweetened beverages, highly processed foods, and refined grain products.
  –Avoid alcohol. People who choose to drink should limit consumption to no more than 1 drink/d for women and 2 drinks/d for men.

CANCER CACHEXIA

Management: Adults

Recommendations from
➤ ASCO 2020
  –In adults with cachexia from advanced cancer, especially lung and GI malignancies, give low-dose olanzapine 2.5 to 5 mg oral daily to improve weight gain and appetite.
  –In those who cannot tolerate olanzapine, trial progesterone analogs (megestrol) or corticosteroid.

Source
–ASCO rapid recommendations. *J Clin Oncol.* 2023;41(25):4178–4179.

COBALAMIN (B$_{12}$) AND FOLATE (B$_9$) DEFICIENCY

Management: Adults

Recommendations from

> BJH 2014

Evaluation

–There is no gold standard test for the diagnosis of cobalamin deficiency. Serum cobalamin lacks sensitivity and specificity (a cutoff of 200 ng/L results in a sensitivity of 95% but a specificity of 50%).

–Consider cobalamin or folate deficiency when CBC shows oval macrocytes or hypersegmented neutrophils in the presence of an elevated MCV.

–Cobalamin and folate assays should be assessed concurrently.

–Consider plasma total homocysteine (tHcy) and/or plasma methylmalonic acid (MMA) as supplementary tests if there is clinical suspicion of cobalamin deficiency but intermediate cobalamin level. Both are elevated in cobalamin deficiency. Total homocysteine is a sensitive marker, but methylmalonic acid is more specific. Holotranscobalamin, the active fraction of plasma cobalamin, may be a suitable assay for assessment of cobalamin status in the future.

–Test all patients with anemia, neuropathy, or glossitis, suspected of having pernicious anemia for anti-intrinsic factor antibodies regardless of cobalamin levels. Do not test for antigastric parietal cell antibodies.

–Test for anti-intrinsic factor antibodies in patients with low-serum cobalamin levels in the absence of anemia and who do not have other causes of deficiency. Patients found to have a positive test should have lifelong cobalamin therapy.

Therapy

–Treat promptly, as neurologic symptoms may be irreversible if treatment is delayed.

–For patients with neurologic symptoms, give parenteral cobalamin 1000 mcg IM daily or every other day for 2 wk. Then give 1000 mcg IM q3 mo or 1000–2000 mcg PO daily. Oral crystalline cyanocobalamin is as effective as parenteral unless anti-intrinsic factor antibodies.

–Retest serum cobalamin levels after 2–4 mo to ensure normalization.

–A serum folate level < 7 nmol/L (3 mcg/L) is indicative of folate deficiency. Routine RBC folate testing is not necessary.

–In the presence of strong clinical suspicion of folate deficiency, despite a normal level, an RBC folate assay may be undertaken, having ruled out B$_{12}$ deficiency.

–The dose of folic acid necessary for treatment depends on the cause of the deficiency. Folic acid 0.8 mg PO daily is typically sufficient; however, 5 mg daily is necessary in hemolytic states and patients on hemodialysis.

Practice Pearls

• The interpretation of cobalamin testing should be considered in relation to the clinical circumstances. Falsely low-serum cobalamin levels may be seen in the presence of folate deficiency. Moreover, neurologic symptoms due to cobalamin deficiency can occur in the presence of a normal MCV.

- The most frequently cited causes of cobalamin deficiency include *H. pylori*, *Giardia lamblia*, fish tapeworm, pernicious anemia, gastric resection, celiac disease, tropical sprue, Crohn disease, low dietary intake (ie, vegan diet), metformin use, and achlorhydria due to atrophic gastritis or proton pump inhibitors.
- The incidence of B_{12} deficiency in the older adults (>70-y-old) is 5%–10%.
- Pernicious anemia (the most common cause of B_{12} deficiency) is an autoimmune illness with antibodies to gastric parietal cells and intrinsic factor resulting in gastric atrophy and malabsorption of food-derived B_{12}. It is associated with Hashimoto disease, type 1 diabetes, vitiligo, and hypoadrenalism.
- Independent of the etiology of B_{12} deficiency, oral B_{12} (1000–2000 mg) daily will correct lower B_{12} levels due to intrinsic-factor independent absorption.
- Causes of low folic acid levels include poor diet (lack of legumes and green leafy vegetables), goat's milk (as opposed to cow's milk in children), alcohol use disorder, pregnancy, increased RBC turnover (thalassemia, hemolytic anemias, sickle cell anemia), and hemodialysis.
- Patients with elevated MCV who are folate deficient must have B_{12} deficiency ruled out since treatment with folate in patients with B_{12} deficiency will accelerate peripheral neuropathy.
- Drugs that can cause folate deficiency and B_{12} deficiency include trimethoprim, pyrimethamine, methotrexate, and phenytoin.
- When treating B_{12} and folate deficiency, the MCV may decrease due to acquired iron deficiency as iron is incorporated into red cell precursors in response to B_{12} and/or folate therapy.

Source
–*Br J Haematol.* 2014;166(4):496–513.

PERIOPERATIVE MANAGEMENT OF ANTITHROMBOTIC THERAPY

Management: Adults on Anticoagulants or Antiplatelet Agents Undergoing Procedures

Recommendations from

➢ ACCP 2022
   – Direct Oral Anticoagulants (DOACs):
   - In patients undergoing elective surgery or procedures, stop the agent 1–2 d prior. Generally, 1 d for low-to-moderate bleed risk surgeries[1] and 2 d for high bleed risk surgeries.[2] If on dabigatran and CrCl < 50 mL/min, stop 4 d prior for high bleed risk.
   - Do not bridge perioperatively with heparin.
   - Do not routinely test for DOAC coagulation function perioperatively.
   - Resume DOAC > 24 h after the procedure.

---

[1] Low-to-moderate surgeries include arthroscopy, cutaneous or lymph node biopsies, foot/hand surgeries, coronary angiography, GI endoscopy or colonoscopy (+/– biopsy), abdominal hysterectomy, laparoscopic cholecystectomy, abdominal hernia repair, hemorrhoidal surgery, and bronchoscopy +/– biopsy.
[2] High bleed risk surgeries include major surgery with extensive tissue injury, cancer, major orthopedic, reconstructive plastics, major thoracic, urologic or GI, TURP, nephrectomy, resection of colon polyp, bowel resection, percutaneous endoscopic gastrostomy placement, ERCP, surgery involving kidneys/liver/spleen, cardiac, intracranial, or spinal surgery, any surgery >45 min, neuraxial anesthesia, and epidural injections.

–Antiplatelets:
  • Continue aspirin in patients with an indication for aspirin who are undergoing elective noncardiac surgery.
  • If interruption is required, stop aspirin ≤7 d prior.
  • Stop clopidogrel 5 d prior to elective noncardiac surgery (ticagrelor: 3–5 d, prasugrel: 7 d).
  • Do not use preoperative platelet function testing.
  • Resume antiplatelet agents ≤24 h after.
  • Minor procedures (dental, dermatologic, ophthalmologic): if on single agent, do not interrupt. If on both, stop P2Y$_{12}$ inhibitor but continue ASA.
  • Antiplatelets for coronary stents:
    ○ If on ASA and P2Y$_{12}$ inhibitor due to stents placed prior 6–12 wk, continue both or stop one agent within 7–10 d of surgery.
    ○ If on ASA and P2Y$_{12}$ inhibitor due to stents placed prior to 3–12 mo, stop the P2Y$_{12}$ and continue ASA.
    ○ If antiplatelet drugs must be interrupted, do not bridge.
    ○ If dual antiplatelets are required, delay elective surgeries.
–VKA therapy (eg, warfarin):
  • Stop warfarin ≥5 d prior to the procedure.
  • Resume <24 h after at their usual dose.
  • Do not routinely give preoperative vitamin K.
  • Minor procedures (dental, dermatologic, ophthalmologic): do not stop warfarin unless there is unusually high bleeding risk. Consider hemostatic agent such as tranexamic mouthwash for dental procedures.
  • Generally, avoid heparin bridging when patients with the following conditions require interruption for an elective surgery/procedure:
    ○ Atrial fibrillation. Consider bridge for high-risk patients (conditional recommendation, very low certainty): those with stroke/TIA in past 3 mo, prior perioperative stroke, or CHA2DS2-VASC score ≥ 7.
    ○ VTE. Consider bridge for those with VTE in past 3 mo, severe thrombophilia, or active cancer.
    ○ Mechanical heart valve, low VTE risk. Bridge higher risk patients: those with older-generation mechanical valve, mechanical mitral valve with stroke risk factors, thrombotic event in past 3 mo, or history of perioperative stroke.
    ○ Colonoscopy with polypectomy.
–Bridging strategy.
  • If bridging with low-molecular-weight heparin, give the last dose approximately 24 h prior to the procedure, and resume at least 24 h after.
  • In patients undergoing high bleed-risk surgery, consider giving half the total daily dose the day prior to surgery rather than the full dose.

Source
–*CHEST.* 2022;162(5):e207–e243.

HEPARIN-INDUCED THROMBOCYTOPENIA (HIT)

Management: Adults

Recommendations from

> American Society of Hematology 2018

Evaluation

–If platelets drop 30%–50%, suspect HIT and use the 4T scoring model (see Table 7–4) to assess likelihood of HIT.

- If intermediate-to-high probability, treat for HIT and send immunologic (enzyme-linked immunosorbent assay [ELISA]) and functional testing (platelet serotonin release assay).
- Do not test for or empirically treat for HIT in patients with a low-probability 4T score.

TABLE 7–4 DIAGNOSTIC TOOL FOR DIAGNOSIS OF HIT			
4 Ts	**2 Points**	**1 Point**	**0 Point**
Thrombocytopenia	• Fall in platelet count > 50% and nadir of ≥20,000 **AND** • No surgery in preceding 3 d	• >50% fall in platelets but with surgery in preceding 3 d • 30%–50% platelet fall with nadir 10–19,000	• <30% fall in platelets • Any platelet fall with nadir < 10,000
Timing of platelet fall	• 5–10 d after start of heparin • Platelet fall < 5 d with heparin exposure within past 30 d	• Platelet fall after day 10 • Platelet fall < 5 d with heparin exposure in past 100 d	• Platelet fall ≤ day 4 without exposure to heparin in last 100 d
Thrombosis or other sequelae	• Confirmed new venous or arterial thrombosis • Skin necrosis at heparin injection sites • Anaphylactoid reaction to IV heparin	• Progressive or recurrent thrombosis while on heparin • Erythematous skin reaction at heparin injection sites	• Thrombosis suspected
Other causes of thrombocytopenia	• No alternative cause of platelet drop evident	• At least 1 other possible cause of drop in platelet count	• Definite or highly likely cause present • Sepsis • Chemotherapy within 20 d • Disseminated intravascular coagulation • Drug-induced ITP • Posttransfusion purposes
High probability: 6–8 pts; intermediate probability: 4–5 pts; low probability: ≤3 pts.			

Therapy

–If elevated 4T score, stop heparin and start nonheparin anticoagulation (argatroban, bivalirudin, danaparoid, fondaparinux, or a DOAC) until HIT immunoassay returns negative or platelets are >150,000/mcL.

–Avoid platelet transfusion unless life-threatening bleeding.

–Screen for bilateral lower extremity DVT with ultrasound. Consider screening for upper extremity DVT if upper extremity central venous catheter.

Practice Pearls

- The median platelet count in HIT is 60,000 and seldom falls below 20,000.
- The development of HIT is not related to the degree of exposure to heparin. A single flush of an IV line or 1 dose of prophylactic heparin can trigger the HIT syndrome. If HIT is not recognized, further administration of heparin will lead to a significant increased risk of clot, morbidity, and mortality. (*N Engl J Med.* 2006;355:809–817) (*JAMA.* 2004;164:361–369)
- The 4T scoring system is most accurate in the low-risk subset, with a negative predictive value of 0.998. (*Blood.* 2012;120:4160–4167)

Source

–*Blood Adv.* 2018;2(22):3360–3392.

IMMUNE THROMBOCYTOPENIA (ITP)

Management: Adults

Recommendations from

➤ ASH 2019

Evaluation

–Diagnosis of exclusion. There is no reliable diagnostic test (including antiplatelet antibody studies). Test for hepatitis C and HIV, and other underlying illnesses suggested by exam.

–Assess for risk factors:

- Drug induced (trimethoprim-sulfamethoxazole, rifampin, carbamazepine, vancomycin, quinine derivatives, and many more).
- Systemic lupus erythematosus/Sjögren syndrome, and other rheumatologic diseases.
- Infections—hepatitis C, HIV, CMV, *H. pylori*, Epstein–Barr virus (EBV), varicella.
- Indolent lymphomas and breast and colon cancer.
- Vaccinations—mostly in children.
- Common variable immunodeficiency—almost exclusively in children.

Therapy

–Observe if platelet count > 30,000 and asymptomatic; do not give steroids except when comorbidities exist, procedures are anticipated, or age > 60-y-old.

–Treat if platelet count < 30,000 with or without bleeding.

- Use corticosteroids (prednisone 0.5–2 mg/kg daily with taper) (preferred over observation, even if no bleeding).

- Consider IVIG with corticosteroids when a more rapid rise in platelet count is needed (ie, prior to surgery).
- Second-line therapy: rituximab.
- If corticosteroids are contraindicated: IVIG or anti-D immune globulin (in patients who are Rh(+) and spleen in place).
- IVIG dose: 1 g/kg as a 1-time dose that may be repeated as necessary. (*Lancet Haematol.* 2016;3:e489) (*Blood.* 2016;127:296) (See Table 7–5.)

–If unresponsive or relapsed, consider splenectomy and/or thrombopoietin receptor agonists.

–Treatment of specific forms of secondary ITP (see Table 7–6).

- HCV-associated: consider antiviral therapy in absence of contraindications. Use IVIG as initial therapy.

TABLE 7–5 FIRST-LINE THERAPY FOR ITP		
Corticosteroids	**RR**	**% With Sustained Response**
Prednisone 0.5–2 mg/kg/d for 2 wk followed by taper	70%–80%	10-y disease-free—13%–15%
Dexamethasone 40 mg daily for 4 d every 2–4 wk for 1–4 cycles	90%	As high as 50% (2–5 y follow-up)
IV anti-D immune globulin 50–75 mcg/kg—warning regarding brisk hemolysis and rare disseminated intravascular coagulation	80%	Usually lasts 3–4 wk, but may persist for months in some patients
IVIG 0.4 g/kg/d × 5 d or 1 g/kg/d for 1–2 d	80%	Transient benefit lasting 2–4 wk

TABLE 7–6 SELECTED SECOND-LINE THERAPY OPTIONS IN ADULT ITP	
TPO Receptor Agonist	**RR**
Eltrombopag 25–75 mg PO daily	70%–80%
Romiplostim 1–10 mcg/kg SQ weekly	80%–90%
Immunosuppression	
Azathioprine 1–2 mg/kg	40%
Cyclosporine 5 mg/kg/d for 6 d then 2.5–3 m/kg/d to titrate blood levels of 100–200 mg/mL	50%–60%
Cytoxan 1–2 mg/kg PO or IV (0.3–1 g/m²) for 113 doses every 2–4 wk	30%–60%
Rituximab 375 mg/m² weekly × 4	50%–60% respond—sustained >3–5 y in 10%–15%
Uncertain Mechanism	
Danazol 200 mg 2–4× daily (orally)	~50%
Vinca alkaloid 1–2 mg IV weekly to max of 6 mg	~30% variable

- HIV-associated: start ART first unless patient has significant bleeding complications. If ITP therapy is required, use corticosteroids, IVIG, anti-D immune globulin, and romiplostim or eltrombopag. Refractory patients should have a splenectomy.
- *H. pylori*–associated: eradication therapy of newly diagnosed active *H. pylori* infection (stool antigen, urea breath test, endoscopic biopsy) will result in resolution of ITP in 25%–35% of patients.

Practice Pearl

- TTP (thrombotic thrombocytopenic purpura) should always be excluded. Symptoms: ill appearing, low-grade fever, myalgia, chest pain, and altered mental status. Labs: thrombocytopenia and a hemolytic anemia with red cell fragmentation, elevated reticulocyte count, and significant elevation of lactate dehydrogenase. This is a *medical emergency* and should be treated urgently with plasma exchange. See next section for more details.

Sources
- *Blood Adv.* 2019;3(23):3829–3866.
- *Blood.* 2016;128:1547.
- *Blood.* 2011;117:4190–4207.
- *Blood.* 2010;115:168–186.

Management: Children

Recommendations from

> ### American Society of Hematology (ASH) 2011

- Do not obtain bone marrow (BM) examination in children and adolescents with typical features of ITP (isolated thrombocytopenia, large, morphologically normal platelets, asymptomatic except for bleeding).
- Initially, observe regardless of platelet count unless moderate-to-severe bleeding.
- If moderate-to-severe bleeding, admit for a single dose of IVIG (0.8–1 g/kg) or short-course corticosteroid is the first line.
- Consider splenectomy for pediatric patients with chronic or persistent ITP who have significant or persistent bleeding and lack of responsiveness or intolerance to other standard therapies.
- Children with a history of ITP who are unimmunized should receive their scheduled first MMR vaccine. Check titers subsequently and only give further vaccines if immunity is insufficient.

Practice Pearls

- Treatment focuses on severity of bleeding, not platelet cell count. In a study of 505 children with platelets < 20,000 and skin bleeding, only 3 patients developed severe bleeding and none had intracranial hemorrhage.
- Response rate to splenectomy is 70%–80%, but unless a child has severe unresponsive disease, delay the splenectomy for at least 12 mo since 20%–30% will have spontaneous remission.

Sources
   –*Pediatr Blood Cancer.* 2009;53:652–654.
   –*Blood.* 2010;115:168–186.
   –*Blood.* 2013;121:4457–4462.
   –*Blood.* 2014;124:3295.

HEMOPHILIA A AND B

Management: Adults and Children

Recommendations from

> NHF 2018

   –Hemophilia A is a loss of factor VIII (FVIII) activity. Hemophilia B is a loss of factor IX (FIX) activity. Usually congenital, though can develop acquired hemophilia due to cancer, SLE, or other autoimmune diseases.
   –Treat with the corresponding recombinant (r) or plasma-derived (pd) factor concentrates.
   –Do not use cryoprecipitate unless there is a risk of loss of life or limb and no FVIII concentrate is available.
   –Consider desmopressin (DDAVP, intranasal or parenteral) for patients with mild hemophilia A who have been documented by a DDAVP trial to have a significant rise in FVIII.
   –For patients with hemophilia A or B with high titer inhibitors, immune tolerance induction is the best option for inhibitor eradication.
   –Treatment for patients with hemophilia with inhibitor antibodies include:
   • FEIBA (activation prothrombin complex concentration) contains activation factors IIa, VIIa, and Xa and is used to bypass an inhibitor to FVIII or FIX. It is plasma derived.
   • NovoSeven RT (recombinant-activated factor VII concentrate) contains activated FVIIa and is used to bypass inhibitors to FVIII or FIX.
   • Hemlibra (emicizumab-kxwh) is a bispecific FIXa- and FX-directed monoclonal antibody that bridges FIXa and FX, bypassing the FVIII inhibitor to prevent or treat bleeding in patients with hemophilia A and inhibitors.
   • There is a significant risk of thrombosis with the use of these agents. Do not exceed recommended doses.
   –Treat patients with acquired hemophilia A with NovoSeven RT or Obizur, a recombinant porcine factor VIII (rpFVIII). Often the human FVIII inhibitor does not cross-react with the porcine FVIII, allowing for cessation of bleeding with Obizur treatment.
   –Confirm hepatitis A and B immunity for all patients with hemophilia. Immunize seronegative patients.

Source
   –https://www.hemophilia.org/Researchers-Healthcare-Providers/Medical-and-Scientific-Advisory-Council-MASAC/MASAC-Recommendations/Guidelines-for-Emergency-Department-Management-of-Individuals-with-Hemophilia-and-Other-Bleeding-Disorders

NEUTROPENIA WITHOUT FEVER

Management: Adults

Recommendations from

> IDSA/ASCO 2018, NIH 2012, ASH 2012

Evaluation

–Neutropenia is defined as an ANC < 1500 cells/mcL.

- Mild: 1500–1000 cells/mcL.
- Moderate: 1000–500 cells/mcL.
- Severe: <500 cells/mcL.

–Most commonly due to chemotherapy but consider other etiologies including solid malignancies with BM invasion, lymphoproliferative malignancies (eg, natural killer cell lymphomas, hairy cell leukemia, and chronic lymphocytic leukemia), radiation therapy, autoimmune etiologies (eg, SLE, rheumatoid arthritis), viral (eg, CMV, EBV, HIV), parasitic (eg, malaria), medications (eg, quinidine, aminopyrine, cephalosporin, hydralazine, penicillins, heavy metals, phenothiazine), and genetic (eg, aplastic anemia, paroxysmal nocturnal hemoglobinuria, May-Hegglin anomaly).

–Consider BM biopsy if etiology is not evident.

Therapy

–Manage chemotherapy-associated neutropenia by dose modification, dose interval delays, and/or prophylaxis with G-CSFs.

–Use antibiotic (fluoroquinolone) and antifungal (oral triazole or parenteral echinocandin) prophylaxis for patients at high risk for febrile neutropenia or profound, protracted neutropenia (defined as ANC < 100 for >7 d, eg, most patients with AML/MDS or hematopoietic stem cell transplant treated with myeloablative conditioning regimens).

–If HSV is seropositive and undergoing hematopoietic stem cell transplant or leukemia induction therapy, use HSV prophylaxis (eg, acyclovir, valacyclovir).

–Use *Pneumocystis jirovecii* prophylaxis (eg, TMP-SMX, dapsone, aerosolized pentamidine, atovaquone) for patients receiving chemotherapy regimens with >20 mg prednisone equivalents daily for >1 mo or purine analog usage.

–If high risk of hepatitis B virus reactivation, treat with a nucleoside reverse transcription inhibitor (eg, entecavir or tenofovir).

–Offer yearly influenza vaccination with inactivated vaccine to all patients receiving chemotherapy and all family and household contacts and health care providers.

–Administer COVID-19 vaccination in 3 doses (not booster dose for third vaccine) and continue precautions due to impaired immune response.

–Use standard precautions (hand hygiene and respiratory hygiene/cough etiquette) to avoid transmission to reduce transmission of pathogens in the health care setting.

–Avoid prolonged contact with environmental airborne fungal spores, ie, demolition sites, prolonged gardening/digging, and home renovation.

Practice Pearls

- Risk factors for neutropenia include older age, comorbidities, and a history of multiple cytotoxic chemotherapy regimens.
- Bone marrow transplantation and chemotherapy for hematologic malignancies are associated with a higher incidence of neutropenia than chemotherapy for solid tumor malignancies.

Sources

–www.ncbi.nlm.nih.gov/books/NBK507702/

–https://www.idsociety.org/covid-19-real-time-learning-network/vaccines/vaccines-information-faq/#

–*J Clin Oncol.* 2018.36:3043–3054.

–*J Clin Oncol.* 2018.36:1443–1453.

–*Clin Adv Hematol Oncol.* 2012;10(12):825–826.

–*Hematol Am Soc Hematol Educ Program.* 2012(1):174–182.

MULTIPLE MYELOMA/MONOCLONAL GAMMOPATHY OF UNDETERMINED SIGNIFICANCE

Management: Adults

Recommendations from

> NICE 2016, EMN 2014, EMN 2018, ASCO 2019

–Classic findings of multiple myeloma are "CRAB": hypercalcemia, renal failure, anemia, and bony lesions/pain, in addition to clonal BM plasma cells.

–Use serum protein electrophoresis and serum-free light-chain assays to confirm the presence of a paraprotein-indicating possible myeloma (MM) or monoclonal gammopathy of undetermined significance (MGUS).

–If serum protein electrophoresis is abnormal, order immunofixation to confirm the presence of a paraprotein-indicating possible myeloma or MGUS.

–Do not use serum protein electrophoresis, immunofixation, serum-free light-chain assay, or urine electrophoresis alone to exclude a diagnosis of myeloma.

–Order whole-body MRI as first-line imaging for all people with a plasma cell disorder suspected to be myeloma.

- Consider whole-body low-dose CT if whole-body MRI is unsuitable or the patient declines.
- Only consider skeletal survey if whole-body MRI and low-dose CT are unsuitable or the person declines them.
- Do not use isotope bone scans to identify myeloma-related bone disease.

–Confirm diagnosis using BM aspirate and trephine biopsy based on plasma cell percentage and flow cytometry morphology.

–Diagnostic criteria for MM are:

- Involved/uninvolved serum-free light-chain ratio ≥ 100 and the involved serum-free light-chain level > 100 mg/dL.
- Clonal BM plasma cells $\geq 60\%$.
- Two or more focal lesions on MRI.

–MGUS is differentiated from MM by the absence of end-organ damage (ie, hypercalcemia, renal insufficiency, anemia, and bone lesions), decreased amount of serum monoclonal protein (<30 g/L in MGUS), and decreased amount of BM plasma cells (<10% in MGUS).

- MGUS carries 1% annual risk of progression to other lymphoproliferative disorder.
- Typically, IgG or IgA MGUS progresses to MM while IgG MGUS progresses to Waldenstrom macroglobulinemia.
- Waldenstrom macroglobulinemia is defined by the presence of an IgM monoclonal gammopathy and ≥10% clonal plasma cells in the BM, as opposed to <10% in IgM MGUS.

–Test for hepatitis B, hepatitis C, and HIV before starting myeloma treatment.
–Monitor smoldering myeloma every 3 mo for the first 5 y with CBC, CMP, bone profile, serum protein electrophoresis, serum-free light-chain assay.

- Do not routinely offer skeletal surveys.

–Image any new bone symptoms promptly (MRI, CT FDG PET-CT).

Practice Pearls

- Myeloma is still an incurable disease, although the spectrum of disease is highly variable.
- MGUS is present in approximately 3.5% of the population over age 50 y.

Sources
–www.nice.org.uk/guidance/ng35
–*Leukemia.* 2018;32(8):1697–1712.
–*Haematologica.* 2015;100(10):1254–1266.
–https://www.asco.org/practice-patients/guidelines/hematologic-malignancies

SICKLE CELL DISEASE

Management: Adults and Children

Recommendations from

> NHLBI 2014, ASH 2021

Evaluation
–Evaluate patients with symptoms of dyspnea on exertion for possible pulmonary hypertension.
–If a partner of a patient with SCA has unknown sickle cell disease or thalassemia status, refer the partner for hemoglobinopathy screening.
–Test women with SCD who have been transfused and are anticipating pregnancy for red cell alloantibodies. If she has red cell alloantibodies, test her partner for the corresponding red cell antigens.
–Screen via brain scan to assess for silent stroke.

Therapy
–Give oral penicillin prophylaxis to children <5-y-old and older who have had splenectomy or invasive pneumococcal infection. Dose (125 mg for age < 3 y and 250 mg for age > 3 y) twice daily. Consider withholding from children with HbSC diseases and HbS-beta thalassemia who have not had splenectomy.

–Assure that people of all ages with SCD have been vaccinated against *Streptococcus pneumoniae*. All infants with SCD should receive the complete series of the 13-valent conjugate pneumococcal vaccine series beginning shortly after birth and the 23-valent pneumococcal polysaccharide vaccine at 2 y, with a second dose at age 5 y. Give all other vaccines according to ACIP harmonized vaccine schedule.

–Ensure every patient with SCD has a reproductive plan. Provide contraceptive counseling to prevent unintended pregnancy and preconception counseling if pregnancy is desired. Progestin-only contraceptives, levonorgestrel IUDs, and barrier methods have no restrictions for use in women with SCD. If the benefits are considered to outweigh the risk, combined hormonal contraceptives (pills, patches, rings) may be used in women with SCD.

–Use an individualized prescribing and monitoring protocol to promote rapid, effective, and safe analgesic management and resolution of vasoocclusive crises. Use NSAIDs as an adjuvant analgesic in the absence of contraindications as well as adjunctive nonpharmacologic approaches to treat pain such as local heat application and distraction.

- In adults and children with SCD and a vasoocclusive crisis, do not administer a blood transfusion unless there are other indications for transfusion.
- In adults and children with SCD and a vasoocclusive crisis and an oxygen saturation < 95% on room air, administer oxygen.
    ○ Reassess pain every 30–60 min.

–Chronic pain: tailor treatment plan and consider nonopioid medications with careful consideration for opioid therapy.

–Advise that patients seek immediate medical attention for temperatures greater than 101.3°F (38.5°C) due to the risk of severe bacterial infections. Evaluate fevers immediately with a history and physical exam, CBCD, reticulocyte count, blood culture, and urine culture when UTI is suspected.

–In children with SCD and a temperature > 101.3°F (38.5°C), promptly administer ongoing empiric parenteral antibiotics that provide coverage against *S. pneumoniae* and gram-negative enteric organisms. Subsequent outpatient management using an oral antibiotic is feasible in people who do not appear ill.

–In adults with SCD who have pain that interferes with daily activities and quality of life, treat with hydroxyurea.

–In infants 9 mo of age and older, children, and adolescents with SCD, offer treatment with hydroxyurea regardless of clinical severity to reduce SCD-related complications.

–Discontinue hydroxyurea in persons who are pregnant or breastfeeding.

–In people with HbS-beta thalassemia or HbSC who have recurrent sickle cell–associated pain that interferes with daily activities, consult a sickle cell expert for consideration of hydroxyurea therapy.

–Transfuse RBCs to bring the Hb level to 1 g/dL prior to undergoing a surgical procedure involving general anesthesia. Blood transfusion is not indicated for uncomplicated painful crisis, priapism, asymptomatic anemia, recurrent splenic sequestration, and acute kidney injury unless there is multisystem organ failure. Test RBC with extensive profiling.

–Consider immune suppression therapy in patients with high risk for immune response to transfusion.

–Chronic transfusion therapy is recommended for a child with TCD > 200 cm/s and adults and children with previous clinically overt stroke.

Surveillance

–Screen annually for proteinuria beginning at age 10. If positive, perform a first morning void urine albumin-creatinine ratio, and if abnormal, consult a renal specialist.

–Refer all patients to an ophthalmologist for annual dilated eye exam beginning at age 10.

–Screen children with SCD annually with transcranial Doppler beginning at age 2 and continuing until at least age 16. Refer children with conditional (170–199 cm/s) or elevated (>200 cm/s) transcranial Doppler results. Do not screen patients with genotypes other than SCD.

–Monitor for iron overload in chronic transfusion therapy with liver function tests, serum ferritin levels, liver biopsy, and MRIs. Administer iron chelation therapy, in consultation with a hematologist, to patients with SCD with documented transfusion-acquired iron overload.

–Consider hematopoietic stem cell transplant in the setting of stroke or high stroke risk or recurrent acute chest syndrome ideally from sibling donor.

Practice Pearls

- More than 2 million US residents are estimated to be either heterozygous or homozygous for the sickle cell mutation.
- Black persons are affected most commonly, but Latino/Latina persons as well as persons of southern European, Middle Eastern, or Indian descent may also be affected.
- Clinical improvement with hydroxyurea may take 3–6 mo. Watch for thrombocytopenia and neutropenia with hydroxyurea treatment.
- RBC units that are to be transfused to individuals with SCD should include matching for C, E, and K antigens.

Sources

–ASH clinical practice guidelines on sickle cell disease. *Blood Adv.* 2020;4(2):327–355.

–NHLBI. *Evidence-Based Management of Sickle Cell Disease.* 2014. http://www.nih.gov/guidelines

THROMBOTIC THROMBOCYTOPENIA PURPURA (TTP)

Management: Adults and Children

Recommendations from

➤ ASH 2017, BJH 2023

Evaluation

–Classic pentad (present in only 10% of cases) is microangiopathic hemolytic anemia (jaundice, anemia, schistocytes, low haptoglobin, elevated LDH, increased reticulocyte count), thrombocytopenia (epistaxis, bruising, retinal hemorrhage, hemoptysis), renal impairment (proteinuria, microscopic hematuria), fever (>37.5°C), and neurologic signs (confusion, encephalopathy, coma, headache, paresis, aphasia, dysarthria, visual problems), often with insidious onset.

- Revised diagnostic criteria state that TTP must be suspected even with only thrombocytopenia and microangiopathic hemolytic anemia.
- Up to 35% of patients do not have neurologic symptoms. Renal failure requiring hemodialysis on presentation is more indicative of HUS than in TTP. Median platelet count is 10,000–30,000/mcL at presentation.
  - Diagnosis based on clinical history, exam, and lab testing.
- If TTP is suspected, order ADAMTS-13 activity and anti-ADAMST-13 activity prior to starting treatment.
  - Treat empirically. Do not wait for confirmatory tests.
- Lab tests: ADAMTS-13 assay (activity/antigen and inhibitor/antibody), CBCD, reticulocyte count, peripheral blood smear, haptoglobin, coagulation studies, CMP, cardiac troponins, LDH, urinalysis, Coombs, blood type and antibody screen, TSH, HIV, hepatitis A/B/C viruses, and autoantibodies (ANA/RF/LA/ACLA), stool culture (for pathogenic *E. coli*).
- Consider CT chest/abdomen pelvis (to look for possible underlying malignancy).
- Check a pregnancy test in women of childbearing age.
- Consider ECG or echocardiogram and brain imaging (CT or MRI).

Therapy

- TTP is a medical emergency requiring transfer to hospital: 3 units of fresh-frozen plasma should be given while a large-bore catheter is placed for plasma exchange, which should begin within 4–8 h of presentation.
- Start plasma exchange (TPE) with 40 mL/kg body weight plasma volume exchanges. The volume of exchange can be reduced to 30 mL/kg body weight as clinical conditions and lab studies improve.
- Avoid platelet transfusion.
- Give caplacizumab 10 mg pre-TPE and monitor for bleeding events and delay administration if planned procedures, but do not discontinue once started.
- Continue daily TPE for a minimum of 2 d after platelet count > 150,000 and then stopped.
- Consider steroids (eg, IV methylprednisolone 10 mg/kg/d or 1 g/d × 3 d, then 2.5 mg/kg/d), although benefits are uncertain.
- In patients with neurologic and/or cardiac pathology (associated with increased mortality), use rituximab at a dose of 375 mg/m² weekly for 4 doses.
- Start anti-CD20 within 3 d of acute admission with rituximab. Obinutuzumab can be offered to those with anaphylaxis or acute serum sickness to rituximab.
- Consider other immunomodulation in refractory or relapsing TTP.
- Start DVT prophylaxis when platelet count is ≥50,000.

Surveillance

- Monitor ADAMTS-13 lifelong.
- Offer support for anxiety/depression.
- Offer pre-emptive anti-CD20 therapy when ADAMTS-13 activity < 20 IU/dL or higher with symptoms.

Practice Pearls

- Mortality rate of 10%–20% even with appropriate management.
- TTP results from congenital or autoimmune loss of ADAMTS-13 activity. Loss of ADAMTS-13 prevents cleavage of large high-molecular-weight vWF. vWF binds to platelet receptor GPIB and the resulting complex obstructs the microvasculature leading to red cell fragmentation, thrombocytopenia, and organ ischemia.
- Differential diagnosis primarily of thrombocytopenia and microangiopathic hemolytic anemia includes autoimmune hemolysis/Evans syndrome, DIC, pregnancy-associated conditions (eg, HELLP, eclampsia, hemolytic uremic syndrome [HUS]), drugs (quinine, simvastatin, interferon, calcineurin inhibitors), malignant hypertension, infections (CMV, adenovirus, herpes simplex virus, meningococcus, pneumococcus, fungal), autoimmune diseases (lupus nephritis, acute scleroderma), vasculitis, malignancy, catastrophic antiphospholipid syndrome.
- Plasma exchange is not a curative therapy but does protect the patient until antibody levels decline either spontaneously or with the use of corticosteroids and rituximab.
- Precipitating factors: drugs (quinine, ticlopidine, clopidogrel, simvastatin, trimethoprim, interferon, and combined oral contraceptive pills), HIV infection, and pregnancy (usually in the second trimester).
- HUS clinically resembles TTP, but has a different pathophysiology, and total plasma exchange is of minimal benefit. This illness is commonly caused by bacterial toxins (*Shiga*-like toxin from *E. coli*) or drugs (quinine, gemcitabine, mitomycin C). It is also associated with malignancy and autoimmune disease. In HUS, there is disruption of the endothelium and release of high-molecular-weight vWF that overwhelms the cleaving capacity of ADAMTS-13. An antibody to ADAMTS-13 is not involved. Renal failure dominates the clinical picture, and 15%–20% die of the disease. (*Br J Haematol.* 2010;148:37) (*N Engl J Med.* 2014;371:654)

Sources

–*Br J Haematol.* 2023;203(4):546–563.

–*Blood.* 2017;129(21):2836–2846.

THROMBOPHILIAS

Management: Adults

Recommendations from

> NICE 2016, ACOG 2018, Anticoagulation Forum 2016, BSH 2012

Evaluation

–The most common thrombophilias include factor V Leiden (FVL), protein C deficiency, protein S deficiency, antithrombin deficiency, prothrombin gene *20210 A/G* mutation (PGM), and antiphospholipid syndrome (APS).

–Do not perform thrombophilia testing at the time of VTE diagnosis or during the first 3 mo of anticoagulation.

- Genotype-based tests (FVL, PGM) and antibody titers (cardiolipin and beta-2 glycoprotein I) can be performed at any point.

- The remaining thrombophilia tests need to be performed 2–4 wk after discontinuation of anticoagulants.
- Only test for thrombophilias when the results will be used to improve or modify management.
    - Do not offer thrombophilia testing to patients who are continuing anticoagulation treatment.
    - Do not offer thrombophilia testing to patients who have had provoked VTE.
    - Consider testing for hereditary thrombophilias or antiphospholipid antibodies in patients who have had unprovoked DVT or pulmonary embolism (PE) if it is planned to stop anticoagulation.
- Do not routinely offer thrombophilia testing to first-degree relatives of people with a history of DVT or PE and thrombophilia.
    - This includes patients contemplating estrogen use. Even with a negative thrombophilia screen, they still have an elevated risk of VTE. Only do so if the test will change your management.
    - An exception would be patients who are pregnant or planning to become pregnant as it could change treatment plans.
- Do not rely solely on a positive thrombophilia evaluation to recommend extended anticoagulation following an episode of provoked VTE where the other provoking factor has resolved.
- Testing for APS requires a dual screening testing (eg, DRVVT and aPTT). If either of these is positive, a confirmatory test is performed (eg, high phospholipid concentration, platelet-neutralizing reagent, or LA-insensitive reagent).
    - Diagnosis is based on the presence of either vascular thrombosis or pregnancy morbidity plus the presence of lupus anticoagulant, anticardiolipin IgG and/or IgM, or anti-beta-2 glycoprotein-I.
- Patients < 50-y-old with ischemic stroke should be screened for APS.
    - Do not routinely offer APS screening in patients > age 50.
    - Antiplatelet therapy is as effective as warfarin for ischemic stroke associated with a single positive APS test result.
- Order a baseline PT when starting warfarin therapy for APS with thrombosis. If this is prolonged, an alternative PT reagent for which the baseline is normal (ie, not affected by lupus anticoagulant) should be used.
- Screen women with recurrent pregnancy loss (≥3 losses) before 10-wk gestation with normal fetal anatomy/genomics for APS.

Therapy

- Do not start primary thromboprophylaxis for incidentally discovered APS.
- Always emphasize improvement in modifiable VTE risk factors: obesity, tobacco use, exogenous estrogen use.

Practice Pearls

- Testing for thrombophilias in a patient with unprovoked VTE: the 2-step method. After 3 mo of anticoagulation, FVL, PGM, cardiolipin, and beta-2 glycoprotein-I antibodies are ordered. If negative, anticoagulation is stopped and 2–4 wk later a D-dimer, lupus anticoagulant, protein C deficiency, protein S deficiency, and antithrombin deficiency are ordered. A final decision on anticoagulation can then be made on the basis of results.

- FVL is the most common inherited thrombophilia, with estimated carrier frequency in the United States in White persons 5%, Latino/Latina persons 2%, Black persons 1%, Asian persons 0.5%, and American Indian persons 1%.
- PGM in the United States is present in approximately 4% of White persons, 4% in Latino/Latina persons, 1% of Black persons, and 0.3% in American Indian persons.
- The prevalence of protein C deficiency heterozygosity depends on the cutoff used, but may be as high as 1.5%.

VENOUS THROMBOEMBOLISM (VTE)

Prevention: Hospitalized Adults, Not Requiring Surgery

Recommendations from

> NICE 2023, ASH 2018, ACCP 2016, ACP 2011

–In acutely ill patients (hospitalized, not in ICU/CCU), determine risk for VTE using Padua Prediction Score or IMPROVE score (Table 7–7). (ASH)

–Note that many scoring tools are not validated in the setting of active COVID-19 infection.

–Consider determining risk of bleeding using IMPROVE bleeding score or risk factors (Tables 7–8 and 7–9). (ASH)

TABLE 7–7 RISK FACTORS FOR VTE IN HOSPITALIZED MEDICAL PATIENTS	
Risk Factor	**Points**
Padua Predictive Scale	
Active cancer[a]	3
Previous VTE	3
Reduced mobility[b]	3
Underlying thrombophilic disorder[c]	3
Recent (<1 mo) trauma or surgery	2
Age (≥70 y)	1
Congestive HF or respiratory failure	1
Acute MI or stroke	1
Acute infection or inflammatory disorder	1
Obesity (BMI ≥ 30)	1
Thrombophilic drugs (hormones, tamoxifen, erythroid-stimulating agents, lenalidomide, bevacizumab)	1

TABLE 7–7   RISK FACTORS FOR VTE IN HOSPITALIZED MEDICAL PATIENTS (continued)

Risk Factor	Points
High risk: ≥4 points—11% risk of VTE without prophylaxis	
Low risk: <3 points—0.3% risk of VTE without prophylaxis	
IMPROVE VTE Risk Scale	
Previous VTE	3
Known thrombophilia	2
Lower limb paralysis	2
Active cancer	2
Immobilization ≥ 7 d	1
ICU/CCU stay	1
Age ≥ 60 y	1
Score	Risk of VTE
0–1	0.5%
2–3	1.5%
≥4	5.7%

[a]Local or distant metastases and/or chemotherapy or radiation in prior 6 mo.
[b]Bedrest with bathroom privileges for at least 3 d.
[c]Antithrombin, protein C/S, factor V Leiden, prothrombin, or antiphospholipid defects.

TABLE 7–8   RISK FACTORS FOR BLEEDING (CHEST. 2011;139:69–79)

Risk Factor[a, b]	N = % of Patients	Overall Risk
Active gastroduodenal ulcer	2.2	4.15
GI bleed < 3 mo previous	2.2	3.64
Platelet count < 50,000	1.7	3.37
Age ≥ 85 y (vs. 40 y)	10	2.96
Hepatic failure (INR[c] ≥ 1.5)	2	2.18
Renal failure (GFR[d] < 30 mL/min/1.73 m²)	11	2.14
ICU admission	8.5	2.10
Current cancer	10.7	1.78
Male sex	49.4	1.48

[a]Although not studied in medical patients, antiplatelet therapy would be expected to increase risk of bleeding.
[b]Go to www.outcomes-umassmed.org/IMPROVE/risk_score/vte/index.html to calculate the risk of bleeding for individual patients.
[c]International normalized ratio.
[d]Glomerular filtration rate.

TABLE 7–9 IMPROVE BLEEDING RISK SCALE	
Risk Factor	Points
Renal failure (GFR 30–59 mL/min/1.73 m^2)	1
Male vs. female	1
Age 40–80 y	1.5
Current cancer	2
Rheumatic disease	2
Central venous catheter	2
ICU/CCU stay	2.5
Renal failure (GFR < 30 mL/min/1.73 m^2)	2.5
Hepatic failure (INR > 1.5)	2.5
Age ≥ 85 y	3.5
Platelets < 50,000	4
Bleeding in last 3 mo	4
Active gastroduodenal ulcer	4.5
Score	Bleeding risk (major/any)
<7	0.4%/1.5%
≥7	4.1%/7.9%

–Do not use pharmacologic prophylaxis or mechanical prophylaxis in low-risk patients.

–Use VTE prophylaxis for all hospitalized patients with COVID-19.

–Use thromboprophylaxis with LMWH in acutely ill hospitalized patients at elevated risk: equivalent of enoxaparin 40 mg SQ daily; fondaparinux 2.5 mg SQ daily. Only use low-dose unfractionated heparin (UFH) 5000 units BID or TID in patients with significant renal disease. UFH has a 10-fold increased risk of heparin-induced thrombocytopenia (HIT). Women are 2.5 times likely to develop HIT compared to men. Continue for duration of hospital stay.

–If not using pharmacologic prophylaxis because of bleeding risk, use mechanical (use intermittent pneumatic compression [IPC] or graduated compression stockings [GCS]).

–If unable to use pharmacologic or mechanical prophylaxis, consider aspirin.

–Do not use both pharmacologic and mechanical prophylaxis together.

–Do not use DOACs for prophylaxis unless on DOAC for some other reason.

–Do not use VTE prophylaxis in chronically ill (including nursing home), outpatients with minor risk factors, or low-risk long-distance travelers (≥4 h).

–For high-risk long-distance travelers (Table 7–10): use GCS or LMWH.

TABLE 7–10 HEREDITARY THROMBOPHILIC DISORDERS

Disorder	% of US Population	Increase in Lifetime of Risk of Clot
Resistance to activated protein C (factor V Leiden mutation)	5–6	3×
Prothrombin gene mutation	2–3	2.5×
Elevated factor VIII (≥175% activity)	6–8	2–3×
Elevated homocysteine	10–15	1.5–2×
Protein C deficiency	0.37	10×
Protein S deficiency	0.5	10×
Antithrombin deficiency	0.1	25×
Homozygous factor V Leiden	0.3	60×

Practice Pearls

- Routine ultrasound screening for DVT is not recommended in any group.
- 150,000–200,000 deaths from VTE in the United States per year. Hospitalized patients have a VTE risk that is 130-fold greater than that of community residents. (*Mayo Clin Proc.* 2001;76:1102)
- Neither heparin nor warfarin is recommended prophylactically for patients with central venous catheters.
- In higher risk long-distance travelers, frequent ambulation, calf muscle exercises, aisle seat, and below-the-knee GCS are recommended over aspirin or anticoagulants.
- Treat hospitalized inpatients with solid tumors without additional risk factors for VTE (history of DVT, thrombophilic drugs, immobilization) with prophylactic dose LMWH.
- Be cautious in patients with CrCl < 20–30 mL/min—UFH or dalteparin (half-dose) preferred.
- Consider adjusted LMWH dose in patients < 50 kg or ≥ 110 kg in weight. Monitor with heparin anti-10a activity testing.
- Inferior vena cava (IVC) filter indicated in patients with diagnosed DVT with or without PE who cannot be anticoagulated because of bleeding. There are no other situations where a filter has been proven to be beneficial. Do not use IVC filter prophylactically.
- Although several studies have shown survival benefits for VTE prophylaxis in surgical patients, this has not been proven in medical patients. (*N Engl J Med.* 2007;356:1438; 2011;365:2463)

Sources

−*Blood Adv.* 2018;2:3198–3225.
−American Society of Hematology. *Guidelines for Management of Venous Thromboembolism: Prophylaxis for Hospitalized and Nonhospitalized Medical Patients.* 2018.
−*JAMA.* 2012;307:306.
−*Ann Intern Med.* 2011;155:625–632.
−*CHEST.* 2016;149:315–352.
−http://www.uwhealth.org/files/uwheath/docs/anticoagulation/VTE

Prevention: Adults Undergoing Surgery

Recommendations from

➤ ACCP 2016

–Stratify surgical risk:

- Low risk: <40 y, minor surgery,[1] no risk factors,[2] Caprini score < 2 (Table 7–11).
- Intermediate risk: minor surgery plus risk factors, age 40–60 y, major surgery with no risk factors, Caprini score 3–4.
- High risk: major surgery plus risk factors, high-risk medical patient, major trauma, spinal cord injury, craniotomy, total hip or knee arthroplasty (THA, TKA), thoracic, abdominal, pelvic cancer surgery.

–Employ preventive measures:

- Early ambulation: consider mechanical prophylaxis and IPC or GCS.
- UFH 5000 U SQ q8–12 h should ONLY be used in patients with renal disease with a CrCl < 20–30 mL/min.
- LMWH equivalent to enoxaparin 40 mg SQ 2 h before surgery then daily or 30 mg q12 h SQ starting 8–12 h postop.

TABLE 7–11 CAPRINI RISK STRATIFICATION MODEL FOR PERIOPERATIVE VTE			
1 Point	**2 Points**	**3 Points**	**5 Points**
• Age 41–60 y • Minor surgery • BMI ≥ 25 • Swollen legs • Varicose veins • Pregnancy or postpartum • History of recurrent spontaneous abortion • Sepsis (<1 mo) • Lung disease • History of acute MI • Congestive HF (<1 mo) • History of inflammatory bowel disease • Medical patient at bed rest	• Age 61–74 y • Arthroscopic surgery • Major open surgery ≥ 45 min • Laparoscopic surgery • Malignancy • Confined to bed • Immobilizing cast • Central venous catheter	• Age ≥ 75 y • History VTE • Family history of VTE • Factor V Leiden • Prothrombin gene mutation • Lupus anticoagulant • Elevated homocysteine • Other congenital or acquired thrombophilia	• Stroke (<1 mo) • Elective arthroplasty; hip, pelvis, or leg fracture • Acute spinal cord injury (<1 mo)
		Caprini score < 3: low risk Caprini score 3–4: intermediate risk Caprini score ≥ 5: high risk	

[1] Eye, ear, laparoscopy, cystoscopy, and arthroscopic operations.
[2] Prior VTE, cancer, stroke, obesity, congestive HF pregnancy, thrombophilic medications (tamoxifen, raloxifene, lenalidomide, thalidomide, erythroid-stimulating agents).

- Fondaparinux 2.5 mg SQ daily starting 8–12 h postop.
- LMWH: equivalent to enoxaparin 40 mg SQ 2 h preoperative then daily or 30 mg SQ q12 h starting 8–12 h postop and also use mechanical prophylaxis with IPC or GCS.
- Extend prophylaxis for as long as 28–35 d in high-risk patients. In THA, TKA ortho patients, acceptable VTE prophylaxis also includes rivaroxaban 10 mg/d, dabigatran 225 mg/d, adjusted dose warfarin, and aspirin, although LMWH is preferred. DOACs are likely to play a larger role in the future as trials continue to show superiority over warfarin. (*Ann Intern Med.* 2013;159:275) (*Thromb Haemot.* 2011;105:444)
- If high risk of bleeding, use IPC alone. (*Ann Intern Med.* 2012;156:710, 720) (*JAMA.* 2012;307:294)
- Do not use UFH for prophylaxis if CrCl is ≥20 mL/min. There is a 10-fold increased risk of HIT compared to LMWH.

Practice Pearls

- Seventy-five percent to ninety percent of surgical bleeding is structural. VTE prophylaxis adds minimally to risk of bleeding.
- With creatinine clearance < 20 to 30 mL/min UFH with partial thromboplastin time monitoring is preferred (decrease dose if partial thromboplastin time is prolonged). In all other situations, LMWH or DOACs are preferred to reduce the risk of HIT.
- Patients with liver disease and prolonged international normalized ratio (INR) are still at risk for clot. Individualize risk-to-benefit ratio of VTE prophylaxis.
- Epidural anesthesia: before placing catheter wait 18 h after daily prophylactic dose of LMWH and 24 h after prophylactic dose of fondaparinux. For patients on twice daily therapeutic LMWH anticoagulation or once daily LMWH, wait more than 24 h before placing epidural catheter. Patients on DOACs should hold their anticoagulation for 3–5 d. After placing or removing an epidural catheter hold on starting anticoagulation for 6–8 h.
- Do not place prophylactic IVC filter for high-risk surgery.
- For cranial and spinal surgery patients at low risk for VTE use mechanical prophylaxis: high-risk patients should have pharmacologic prophylaxis added to mechanical prophylaxis once hemostasis is established and bleeding risk decreased.
- Patients at high risk for bleeding[1] with major surgery should have mechanical prophylaxis (IPC, GCS): initiate anticoagulant prophylaxis if risk is lowered.
- Surgical patients receive indicated prophylaxis 60% of the time compared to 40% in medical patients.

Sources

–*CHEST.* 2016;149:315.

–http://www.fda.gov/Drugs/ResourcesForYou/Consumers/ucm390574.htm

---

[1] Selected factors in the rising risk of major bleeding complications:

General risk factors: active bleeding, previous major bleed, known untreated bleeding disorder, renal or liver failure, thrombocytopenia, acute stroke, uncontrolled high BP, concomitant use of anticoagulants, or antiplatelet therapy.

Procedure-specific risk factors: major abdominal surgery—extensive cancer surgery, pancreatic-duodenectomy, hepatic resection, cardiac surgery, thoracic surgery (pneumonectomy or extended resection). Procedures where bleeding complications have especially severe consequences: craniotomy, spinal surgery, spinal trauma.

Management: Adults with Deep Vein Thrombosis (DVT) and/or Pulmonary Embolism

Recommendations from

➢ ESC 2019, ACCP 2021, ACP 2015, ASH 2018

  –Use a validated tool to diagnose PE that considers clinical probability.
- For suspected initial DVT, use Wells score for DVT (Table 7–12) to determine pretest probability and therefore diagnostic algorithm (Figs. 7–1 to 7–3).

  –Pulmonary embolism rule-out criteria (PERC rule) is not validated in those with COVID-19.
- If D-dimer or US cannot be obtained within 4 h, consider interim therapeutic anticoagulation while awaiting results.

  –Collect baseline blood tests before starting anticoagulation (CBC, renal and hepatic function, PT, APPT), but do not delay starting anticoagulation while awaiting results.
- For suspected recurrent lower extremity DVT, use the diagnostic algorithm in Fig. 7–4.
- For suspected pulmonary embolism, use Wells score for PE (Table 7–13) or Revised Geneva Score for PE, creatinine clearance, and age-adjusted D-dimer to guide diagnostic strategy.

  –Start anticoagulation while initiating workup if PE is suspected.

  –Use D-dimer in outpatient settings, or where the probability of PE is low, to reduce unnecessary imaging.

  –Use pretest probability to determine further testing (ASH) (Fig. 7–5):
- If low or intermediate PTP of PE (≤5% up to 20%), order D-dimer in an attempt to exclude the diagnosis. If D-dimer positive, order VQ scan or CT pulmonary angiography.
- If high PTP of PE (≥50%), order CT pulmonary angiography as the initial test, or VQ scan if not feasible.

TABLE 7–12 WELLS SCORE FOR DVT	
Symptoms	**Points**
Malignancy, treatment, or palliation within 6 mo	+1
Bedridden recently > 3 d or major surgery within 4 wk	+1
Calf swelling > 3 cm compared to the other leg	+1
Collateral superficial veins present	+1
Entire leg swollen	+1
Localized tenderness along the deep venous system	+1
Pitting edema, confined to symptomatic leg	+1
Paralysis, paresis, or recent plaster immobilization of the lower extremity	+1
Previously documented DVT	+1
Alternative diagnosis to DVT as likely or more likely	−2
Low—0 (3% risk of DVT), Moderate—1 or 2 (20% risk of DVT), High—3 or greater (75% risk of DVT). *Source:* Goldhaber SZ, Bounameaux H. Pulmonary embolism and deep vein thrombosis. *Lancet.* 2012;379:1835.	

FIG. 7–1 DIAGNOSTIC ALGORITHM FOR SUSPECTED LOW PRETEST PROBABILITY INITIAL LOWER EXTREMITY DEEP VEIN THROMBOSIS (DVT).

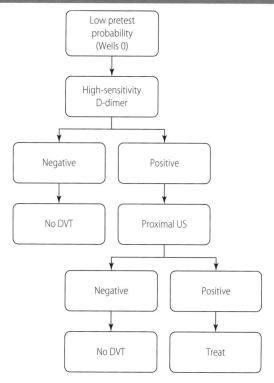

- If low PTP of DVT (≤10%), order D-dimer in an attempt to exclude the diagnosis. If D-dimer is positive, order ultrasound.
- If intermediate or high PTP of PE (25% up to ≥50%), order ultrasound of the legs. If initial ultrasound is negative in high-risk patient, follow up with serial ultrasounds.

–If pulmonary embolism rule-out criteria score is negative, consider foregoing additional testing for PE. (ASH)

–CT pulmonary angiogram (CTPA) is the definitive diagnostic study for PE.

–VQ scan can rule out PE if normal and can confirm PE if "high probability."

–In patients with isolated distal DVT consider repeat US once weekly ×2 wk over anticoagulation if no severe symptoms or risk for extension. If the thrombus does not extend, do not start anticoagulation. If found to have extension to distal veins, consider anticoagulation; if extension to proximal veins, recommend anticoagulation.

–In patients with subsegmental PE without proximal DVT of lower extremity, recommend clinical surveillance over anticoagulation if low risk for recurrent VTE. If at high risk for recurrent VTE, initiate anticoagulation over clinical surveillance.

FIG. 7–2 DIAGNOSTIC ALGORITHM FOR SUSPECTED MODERATE PRETEST PROBABILITY INITIAL LOWER EXTREMITY DEEP VEIN THROMBOSIS (DVT).

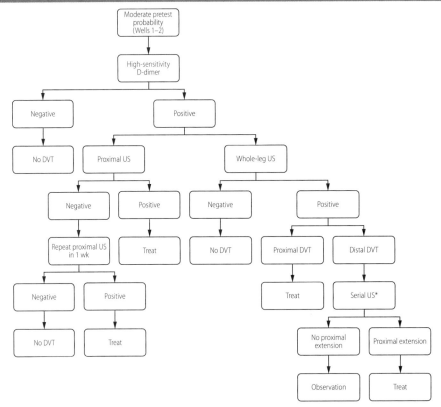

*Treat distal DVT only if patient is at high risk for proximal extension or severely symptomatic.

–In patients with cerebral vein/venous sinus thrombosis, recommend anticoagulation for at least 3 mo.

–In patients with low-risk PE, recommend outpatient treatment over hospitalization.

–In acute DVT, anticoagulation is recommended over interventional techniques. (In high-risk PE, admit for unfractionated heparin and consider catheter-directed thrombolysis or embolectomy; Fig. 7–6.)

–If low-risk PE (age < 80, no cancer, no COPD, HR < 110, SBP > 100, O_2 saturation ≥ 90%, no RV dysfunction, adequate social support, and access to medical care), may discharge home from ER on oral anticoagulation (Table 7–14).

–Offer apixaban or rivaroxaban as first line if there are no contraindications; if not an option, offer LMWH ×5 d followed by dabigatran or edoxaban or LMWH with VKA ×5 d or until INR is at least 2 × 2 readings then VKA alone.

FIG. 7–3 DIAGNOSTIC ALGORITHM FOR SUSPECTED HIGH PRETEST PROBABILITY INITIAL LOWER EXTREMITY DEEP VEIN THROMBOSIS (DVT).

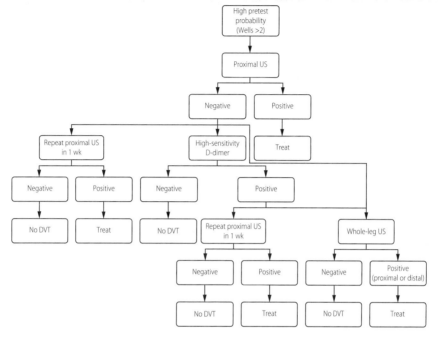

In patients with extensive unexplained leg swelling, if there is no DVT on proximal CUS or whole-leg US and D-dimer testing has not been performed or is positive, the iliac veins should be imaged to exclude isolated iliac DVT.

–Consider regular monitoring for therapeutic levels in patients <50 kg or >120 kg to ensure effectiveness.

–If oral therapy, use DOAC rather than VKA if able (ie, no severe renal impairment, CrCl > 15 mL/min), pregnancy/breastfeeding, antiphospholipid syndrome, etc. If VKA is necessary, bridge with parenteral anticoagulant until INR is 2–3 (Table 7–15).

–Consider IVC filter only if absolute contraindication to anticoagulation or if recurrent PE despite anticoagulation.

–Remove IVC filter when anticoagulants are no longer contraindicated and have been established.

–ESC: duration of therapy: ≥3 mo (see Table 7–16).

  • If major reversible/transient risk factor, stop anticoagulation after 3 mo.
  • If recurrent VTE without major reversible/transient risk factor, continue indefinitely.
  • If first VTE and minor or persistent risk factor, consider extending anticoagulation indefinitely.
  • If first VTE without identifiable risk factor, consider extending beyond 3 mo vs. discontinuing at 3 mo.

–If extending therapy (in the absence of cancer), consider reducing DOAC dose after 6 mo (apixaban 2.5 mg BID or rivaroxaban 10 mg daily). (ESC 2019)

FIG. 7–4 EVALUATION OF SUSPECTED RECURRENT DVT.

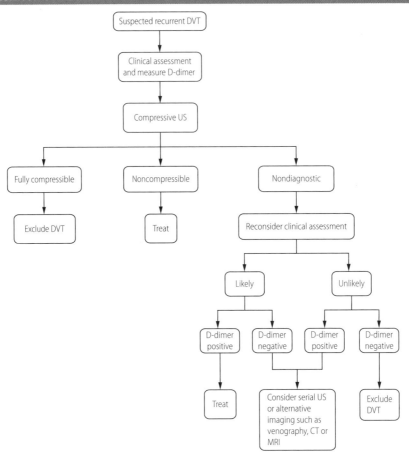

TABLE 7–13 WELLS SCORE FOR PE

Symptoms	Points
Clinical signs and symptoms of DVT	+3
PE is #1 diagnosis OR equally likely	+3
Heart rate > 100	+1.5
Immobilization at least 3 d OR surgery in the previous 4 wk	+1.5
Previous, objectively diagnosed PE or DVT	+1.5
Hemoptysis	+1
Malignancy, treatment, or palliation within 6 mo	+1

Low—less than 2 (2%–3% risk of PE), Moderate—2–6 (20%–30% risk of PE), High—6 or greater (>70% risk of PE).
Source: Goldhaber SZ, Bounameaux H. Pulmonary embolism and deep vein thrombosis. *Lancet.* 2012;379:1835.

–If extended therapy is indicated but oral anticoagulants are not tolerated or declined, use aspirin or sulodexide instead. (ESC 2019)

–Aspirin 75 mg or 150 mg daily is recommended.

–ACCP: duration based on location (Fig. 7–5).

–If pregnant, use LMWH at weight-based dose using weight from early pregnancy. Do not use DOACs.

FIG. 7–5 DIAGNOSTIC ALGORITHM FOR SUSPECTED PULMONARY EMBOLISM.

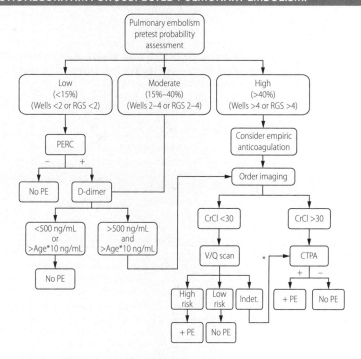

*Consider empiric treatment for PE after risk/benefit analysis.

FIG. 7–6 TREATMENT ALGORITHM FOR CONFIRMED PULMONARY EMBOLISM.

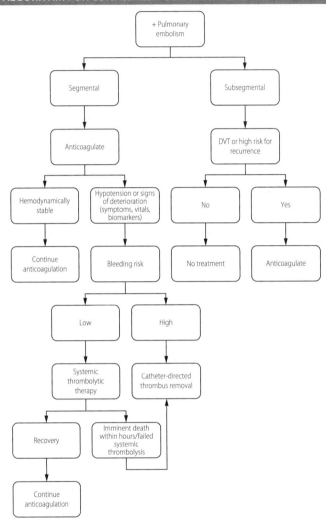

TABLE 7–14 RECOMMENDED ANTICOAGULANT SELECTION AND DURATION OF ANTICOAGULATION BASED ON RISK FACTORS AND LOCATION OF DVT

Limb	Prox vs. Dist	Provoked	Cancer	Bleeding Risk	Anticoagulants	Duration
Upper	Prox	Yes	Yes		No specific recommendations	Indefinite
			No		No specific recommendations	3 mo
		No	No	High	No specific recommendations	3 mo
				Low	No specific recommendations	Indefinite
	Dist[a]	Yes	Yes		No specific recommendations	Indefinite
			No		No specific recommendations	3 mo
		No	No	High	No specific recommendations	3 mo
				Low	No specific recommendations	Indefinite
Lower	Prox	Yes	Yes		LMWH over VKA, direct thrombin, or Xa inhibitors	Indefinite
			No		Dabigatran, rivaroxaban, apixaban, or edoxaban over VKA	3 mo
		No	No	High	Dabigatran, rivaroxaban, apixaban, or edoxaban over VKA	3 mo
				Low	Dabigatran, rivaroxaban, apixaban, or edoxaban over VKA	Indefinite
	Dist[a]	Yes	Yes		LMWH over VKA, direct thrombin, or Xa inhibitors	Indefinite
			No		Dabigatran, rivaroxaban, apixaban, or edoxaban over VKA	3 mo
		No	No	High	Dabigatran, rivaroxaban, apixaban, or edoxaban over VKA	3 mo
				Low	Dabigatran, rivaroxaban, apixaban, or edoxaban over VKA	Indefinite

VKA, vitamin K antagonist.

[a] In general, treatment of isolated distal upper or lower extremity DVT is not recommended unless there are severe symptoms or a high risk for or evidence of proximal extension on ultrasound.

TABLE 7–15 RECOMMENDED ANTICOAGULANT SELECTION AND DURATION OF ANTICOAGULATION FOR PULMONARY EMBOLISM BASED ON RISK FACTORS AND LOCATION OF PULMONARY EMBOLISM

Location	Provoked	Cancer	Bleeding Risk	Anticoagulants	Duration
Segmental	Yes	Yes		LMWH over VKA, direct thrombin, or Xa inhibitors	Indefinite
		No		Dabigatran, rivaroxaban, apixaban, or edoxaban over VKA	3 mo
	No	No	High	Dabigatran, rivaroxaban, apixaban, or edoxaban over VKA	3 mo
			Low	Dabigatran, rivaroxaban, apixaban, or edoxaban over VKA therapy	Indefinite
Subsegmental[a]	Yes	Yes		LMWH over VKA, direct thrombin, or Xa inhibitors	Indefinite
		No		Dabigatran, rivaroxaban, apixaban, or edoxaban over VKA	3 mo
	No	No	High	Dabigatran, rivaroxaban, apixaban, or edoxaban over VKA	3 mo
			Low	Dabigatran, rivaroxaban, apixaban, or edoxaban over VKA	Indefinite

VKA, vitamin K antagonist.
[a]In general, treatment of a subsegmental PE is not recommended unless there is a concomitant DVT or high risk for recurrence.

TABLE 7–16 NEW ORAL ANTICOAGULANTS[a] AND WARFARIN

Agent	Target	Dosing	Monitoring	Half-life	Time to Peak Plasma Concentration	Specific Reversible Agent
Warfarin	Vitamin K epoxide	Once daily	INR–adjusted	40 h	72–96 h	Vitamin K[b]
						PCC
Dabigatran	Thrombin	Fixed—once or twice daily	None	14–17 h	2 h	Idarucizumab[c]
Rivaroxaban	Factor Xa	Fixed—once or twice daily	None	5–9 h (50-y-old)	2.5–4 h	Andexxa[c]
				9–13 h (older adults)		
Apixaban	Factor Xa	Fixed twice daily	None	8–15 h	3 h	None[c]
Edoxaban	Factor Xa	Give once daily	None	10–14 h	1–2 h	None[c]

[a]Do not use new oral anticoagulants in patients with mechanical valves. Warfarin is superior.
[b]If significant bleed on warfarin, give vitamin K, and 4-factor prothrombin complex concentrate (PCC/K–centra) or recombinant FVIIa if not controlled.
[c]If significant bleed, aggressively treat source of bleed; consider 4-factor PCC, recombinant FVIIa or Andexxa.

Practice Pearls

- Iodinated contrast agents for CTPA are safe at least to a creatinine clearance of 30, if not lower. (*Ann Emerg Med.* 2018;71(1):44–53)

- Knee-high GCS (GCS s) with 30–40 mmHg pressure at ankles for 2 y will reduce postthrombotic syndrome risk by 50%.

- In patients with acute lower extremity DVT, suggest against using compression stockings to prevent PTS (*CHEST.* 2021;160(6):e545–e608). Can consider use for management of leg symptoms after DVT. (*NICE.* 2020;NG158:1–47)

- Risk factors for warfarin bleeding—age > 65 y, history of stroke, history of GI bleed, and recent comorbidity (MI, Hct < 30, creatinine > 1.5, diabetes). If all 4 factors are present, there is 40% risk of significant bleed in 12 mo; 0.4% of patients taking warfarin die of bleeding yearly. (*CHEST.* 2016;149:315) (*Am J Med.* 2011;124:111)

- Calf and iliofemoral thrombosis have increased incidence of false-negative compression ultrasound—recommend CT or MR venogram or venography for suspected iliofemoral thrombosis, and for calf thrombosis, follow-up compression ultrasound (CUS) in 5–7 d is acceptable.

- Consider high thrombophilic risk in patients with recurrent VTE or patients with first unprovoked VTE who have the following characteristics:
  - Age < 50-y-old.
  - Family history of VTE.
  - Unusual site of thrombosis.
  - Massive venous thrombosis.

- In unprovoked VTE, 3% of patients are found to have associated malignancy, with another 10% diagnosed with cancer over the next 2 y. (*N Engl J Med.* 1998;338:1169) (*Ann Intern Med.* 2008;149:323) (*N Engl J Med.* 2015;373:697)

- In patients with the antiphospholipid antibody syndrome and a new venous thrombosis, transition to warfarin is superior to using the new oral anticoagulants with adjusted target INR of 2.5. (*Am J Hematol.* 2014;89:1017) (*CHEST.* 2021;160(6):e545–e608).

- The presence of a permanent IVC filter does not mandate continuous anticoagulation unless documented recurrent clot problems.

- Asymptomatic PE (found incidentally on chest CT) should be treated with same protocol as symptomatic PE.

- In patients with superficial thrombosis of lower extremity with risk of progression, consider anticoagulation with fondaparinux 2.5 mg daily (or rivaroxaban 10 mg daily as alternative) for 45 d.

- If anticoagulation treatment fails, increase the dose of change to anticoagulant with different mechanisms of action (after evaluating for adherence and other sources of hypercoagulability).

- Consider catheter-directed thrombolytic therapy for symptomatic iliofemoral DVT with symptoms < 14 d, good functional status, life expectancy ≥ 1 y, and low bleeding risk.

- In patients with confirmed antiphospholipid syndrome, suggest adjusted dose VKA (target INR 2.5) over DOAC during the treatment phase.

Sources

    –*NICE.* 2023;NG158:2–55.

    –*CHEST.* 2021;160(6):e545–e608.

    –*J Thromb Hemost.* 2018:16(9);1891–1894. https://doi.org/10.1111/jth.14219

    –*Blood Adv.* 2018;2(22):3226.

    –*Blood Adv.* 2018;2(22):3257.

    –*CHEST.* 2016;149(2):315–352.

    –*Blood.* 2016;127;696–702.

Management: Adults with Cancer and Venous Thromboembolism

Recommendations from

> NICE 2020, ACCP 2021, ESC 2019, International Society on Thrombosis and Hemostasis 2018

Guidelines Alert 7–1	
GUIDELINES DISCORDANT: MANAGEMENT OF VTE IN PATIENTS WITH ACTIVE CANCER	
Recommendations from:	**Guidance**
NICE	If active cancer, treat for 3–6 mo, consider stopping if provoked or HAS-BLED $\geq$ 4 and can't be modified vs. continuing indefinitely if unprovoked and low bleeding risk
ACCP	If active cancer, use oral Xa inhibitor (apixaban, edoxaban, or rivaroxaban) over LMWH (apixaban or LMWH may be a preferred option in luminal GI malignancies)
ESC	If active cancer, use LMWH, but consider edoxaban or rivaroxaban as alternatives if cancer is not GI. Treat for at least 6 mo, but consider extending indefinitely or until cure
International Society on Thrombosis and Hemostasis	Employ shared decision-making, as overall data are lacking. Consider edoxaban or rivaroxaban as first-line therapy for patients with acute VTE, low bleeding risk, and no drug-drug interactions. Otherwise, use LMWHs to treat acute VTE in cancer

Applying to Clinical Practice
- Factor Xa inhibitors (rivaroxaban, edoxaban) are as effective as LMWH and are better tolerated.
- GI cancers may be the exception, as the bleeding risk with factor Xa inhibitors is much higher.
- Duration should generally be at least 6 mo and determined in consultation with the treating oncologist.

Sources

    –*CHEST.* 2021;160(6):e545–e608.

    –*NICE.* 2020;NG158:1–47.

    –https://doi.org/10.1111/jth.14219

    –*Eur Heart J.* 2020:41;543–603.

VON WILLEBRAND DISEASE

Management: Adults and Children

Recommendations from

> ASH 2021, NHF 2018, NHLBI 2007

Evaluation

–Suspect in patients with mucous membrane bleeding, excessive bruising, or bleeding (eg, excessive menstrual bleeding, history of postpartum hemorrhage, excessive bleeding after dental work or a surgical procedure).

–Diagnose based on history and physical examination, CBC, partial thromboplastin time, PT/INR, fibrinogen, PFA-100 (if available), and VWD assays (VWF:Ag, VWF:RCo, and FVIII).

Therapy

–Treat significant bleeding related to type 1, 2A, 2M, 2N VWD with DDAVP.[1] If hemostasis is not achieved with DDAVP, use FVIII or recombinant VWF concentrate.

–Treat significant bleeding related to type 2B and 3 VWD with FVIII concentrate or recombinant VFW concentrate.

–Manage minor bleeding (eg, epistaxis, simple dental extraction, menorrhagia) with DDAVP without laboratory monitoring.

–For patients with cardiovascular disease, give necessary antiplatelet agents or anticoagulation. Desmopressin is generally contraindicated.

–For patients having mucosal procedures, give tranexamic acid alone in patients with mild-to-moderate VWD (VWF activity level ≥ 0.50 IU/mL).

–For patients having minor surgery with mild-to-moderate VWD, antifibrinolytics combined with DDAVP and tranexamic acid are generally effective.

–Refer all major surgeries and bleeding events to hospitals with 24-h laboratory capability, a hematologist, and a surgeon skilled in the management of bleeding disorders. Target FVIII and VWF activity levels ≥ 0.50 IU/mL for >3 d after surgery.

–In women who do not desire pregnancy, offer combined oral contraceptives or the levonorgestrel intrauterine device for menorrhagia in VWD.

–Women with VWD who desire pregnancy should speak with a genetic counselor and a pediatric hematologist.

–Women who desire pregnancy can be treated preferentially with tranexamic acid over DDAVP, antifibrinolytics, or VWF concentrate.

–Women with VWD who are pregnant should achieve VWF/RCo and FVIII levels of at least 50 IU/dL before delivery and maintain that level for at least 3–5 d afterward.

–Women who desire neuraxial anesthesia during labor, target VWF activity level to 0.50–1.5 IU/mL.

–Use tranexamic acid (IV or PO 25 mg/kg TID for 10–14 d, or longer if blood loss remains heavy) in the postpartum period.

–Do not use cryoprecipitate except in an emergency situation when none of the above-mentioned products are available.

[1] IV DDAVP dosing is 0.3 mcg/kg IV over 30 min. Intranasal dosing of Stimate (1.5 mg/mL DDAVP solution, 0.1-mL puff) is 150 mcg (1 puff) for persons who weigh <50 kg and 300 mcg (2 puffs) for persons weighing 50 kg or more.

Sources

–*Blood Adv.* 2021;5(1):280–300.
–*Blood Adv.* 2021;5(1):301–325.

Practice Pearls

- The prevalence of protein S deficiency is unknown, but in 1 case-control study it accounted for 1% of VTEs. Pregnancy, female sex, and estrogen use reduce the levels of protein S. Use of sex-specific reference intervals and testing prior to pregnancy or while not receiving estrogen preparations is preferred.
- Antithrombin deficiency heterozygosity prevalence is approximately 1 per 2500 people or 0.04%.
- The presence of hereditary thrombophilia does not affect survival in patients with a history of VTE or the risk of postthrombotic syndrome.
- Patients with an unprovoked DVT and negative thrombophilia evaluation have the same recurrence rate for VTE as patients with an unprovoked DVT and positive thrombophilia evaluation.
- Heterozygosity for FVL or PGM does not increase the predicted risk of recurrence to a clinically significant degree after an unprovoked VTE.
- Family history of thrombosis alone carries an increased risk of thrombosis, even with a negative thrombophilia evaluation.
- Degree of postthrombotic symptoms, D-dimer levels after a minimum of 3 mo of anticoagulation, and residual vein thrombosis do modify the risk of recurrence in unprovoked VTE.

Sources

–https://www.acog.org/clinical/clinical-guidance/practice-bulletin/articles/2018/07/inherited-thrombophilias-in-pregnancy
–*J Thromb Thrombol.* 2016;41(1):154–164.
–*Br J Hematol.* 2012;159(10):28–38.

INFECTIOUS DISEASES

BACTERIURIA, ASYMPTOMATIC

Management: Adults

Recommendations from

> IDSA 2019

–Do not treat asymptomatic bacteriuria with antibiotics.
–Only screen pregnant persons and patients undergoing urologic procedures.
–Treat asymptomatic bacteriuria in pregnant patients for 4–7 d.

Practice Pearl

- Delirium in older patients is often caused by urinary tract infections (UTIs). However, in the absence of overt urinary symptoms or signs of systemic infection, empiric treatment of bacteriuria does not improve patient-oriented outcomes. (*JAMA Intern Med.* 2019;179(11):1519–1527)

Source
–https://doi.org/10.1093/cid/ciy1121

COLITIS, *CLOSTRIDIOIDES DIFFICILE*

Prevention: Adults

Recommendations from

> ACG 2013, CID 2018

–Develop antibiotic stewardship programs to minimize the frequency and duration of high-risk antibiotic therapy.
–Place patients with suspected *C. difficile* infection (CDI) preemptively on contact precautions pending the *C. difficile* test results.
–Maintain contact precautions for at least 48 h after diarrhea has resolved.
–Perform hand hygiene before and after contact of a patient with CDI and after removing gloves with either soap or water.

–Use gloves and gowns on entry to the room of a patient with known or suspected CDI and remove gowns and gloves before leaving the patient's room.

–Prevent transmission by using single-use disposable equipment. Thoroughly clean and disinfect reusable medical equipment, preferentially with a sporicidal disinfectant. Dedicated nondisposable equipment should be kept in the patient's room.

–Disinfect environmental surfaces using an Environmental Protective Agency (EPA)–registered disinfectant with *C. difficile* sporicidal label claim or minimum chlorine concentration of 5000 ppm.

–Although there is an epidemiological association between proton pump inhibitor (PPI) use and CDI, there is insufficient evidence for discontinuation of proton pump inhibitors as a measure for preventing CDI.

–Although there is moderate evidence that probiotics containing *Lactobacillus rhamnosus* GG and *Saccharomyces boulardii* decrease the incidence of antibiotic-associated diarrhea, there is insufficient data to recommend administration of probiotics for primary prevention of CDI. Still, short-term use of probiotics appears to be safe and effective when used along with antibiotics in patients who are not immunocompromised or severely ill.

Sources
–*Am J Gastroenterol.* 2013;108(4):478.
–*Clin Infect Dis.* 2018;66(7):e1–e48.
–*Cochrane Database Syst Rev.* 2017;12:CD006095.

COMMON COLD

Management: Adults

Recommendations from

> Annals of Internal Medicine 2016

–Do not prescribe antibiotics for the common cold to adults without chronic lung disease or immunocompromising conditions.

Practice Pearls

- Harm from antibiotics outweighs benefits, as all causes of the common cold are viral.
- Evidence-based therapies for cold symptoms include the following:
  - Ipratropium (4 puffs QID) for cough.
  - NSAIDs for headache, earache, muscle, and joint pains.
  - Acetaminophen for rhinorrhea.
  - Decongestants, with or without antihistamines, for congestion.
  - Zinc (80–92 mg/d within 3 d of symptom onset) to reduce duration.
  - Honey, in children.
- Nasal saline, oral fluid intake, nasal oxymetazoline, and many herbal therapies lack quality evidence of efficacy.

- Therapies proven to be no more effective than placebo include antibiotics, antivirals, antihistamines, cough suppressants and expectorants, nasal steroids, steam, vitamins D and E, and echinacea.

Sources

–http://annals.org/aim/fullarticle/2481815/appropriate-antibiotic-use-acute-respiratory-tract-infection-adults-advice-high

–*Am Fam Physician.* 2019 Sep 1;100(5):281–289.

CORONAVIRUS DISEASE 2019 (COVID-19)

The CDC maintains updated guidelines at https://www.covid19treatmentguidelines.nih.gov/.

Management: Adults in the Community

Recommendations from

> NIH 2024, IDSA 2024, ACP 2024

–Provide symptomatic care: antipyretics, analgesics, and antitussives.

–Encourage adequate nutrition and rehydration.

–Reduce the risk of SARS-CoV-2 transmission.

–Consider pharmacologic therapy for patients who are at high risk of progressing to severe COVID-19 (please see Tables 8–1 and 8–2 for risk factors and treatment prioritization).

–Preferred pharmacologic therapies for those at high risk of progression to severe COVID-19, listed in order of preference (NIH):

- Ritonavir-boosted nirmatrelvir (Paxlovid): start as soon as possible and within 5 d of symptoms onset (300-mg nirmatrelvir/100-mg ritonavir BID × 5 d, GFR 30–60 mL/min/1.73 m² 150 mg/100 mg BID ×5 d, GFR < 30 mL/min/1.73 m² not recommended).
- Remdesivir: start as soon as possible and within 7 d of symptoms onset (200 mg day 1 followed by 100 mg on days 2 and 3, pediatric dosing 5 mg/kg on day 1 and 2.5 mg/kg on days 2 and 3).
- Molnupiravir: start as soon as possible within 5 d of symptoms onset (800 mg daily × 5 d only in nonpregnant patients ≥ 18 y).

–Consider FDA-qualified high-titer COVID-19 convalescent plasma within 8 d of symptom onset only for ambulatory patients with mild-to-moderate COVID-19 at high risk for progression to severe disease who have no other treatment options.

–Refer for in-person evaluation when patients have persistent or progressive dyspnea, especially those with O_2 saturation of 94% or less on room air or have symptoms that suggest high acuity (eg, chest pain or tightness, dizziness, confusion, or other mental status changes).

Sources

–https://www.cdc.gov/coronavirus/2019-ncov/hcp/

–www.idsociety.org/COVID19guidelines.

–https://www.covid19treatmentguidelines.nih.gov

–*BMJ.* 2020;370:m3379.

TABLE 8–1 CDC LIST OF MEDICAL CONDITIONS THAT INCREASE RISK OF PROGRESSION TO SEVERE COVID-19
Conclusive Higher-Risk

Condition
Asthma
Cancer
  • Hematologic malignancies
Cerebrovascular disease
Chronic kidney disease: people receiving dialysis
Chronic lung diseases limited to:
  • Bronchiectasis
  • COPD (chronic obstructive pulmonary disease)
  • Interstitial lung disease
  • Pulmonary embolism
  • Pulmonary hypertension
Chronic liver diseases limited to:
  • Cirrhosis
  • Metabolic dysfunction-associated steatotic liver disease
  • Alcohol-associated liver disease
  • Autoimmune hepatitis
Cystic fibrosis
Diabetes mellitus, type 1
Diabetes mellitus, type 2
Disabilities, including Down syndrome
Heart conditions (such as heart failure, coronary artery disease, or cardiomyopathies)
HIV (human immunodeficiency virus)
Mental health conditions limited to:
  • Mood disorders, including depression
  • Schizophrenia spectrum disorders
Neurologic conditions limited to dementia
Obesity (BMI > 30 or >95th percentile in children)
Physical inactivity
Pregnancy and recent pregnancy
Primary immunodeficiencies
Smoking, current and former
Solid organ or blood stem cell transplantation
Tuberculosis (TB)
Use of corticosteroids or other immunosuppressive medications

Conditions Suggestive of Higher Risk
Children with certain underlying conditions Overweight (BMI > 25 but <30) Sickle cell disease Substance use disorders
Source: https://www.cdc.gov/coronavirus/2019-ncov/hcp/clinical-care/underlyingconditions.html

TABLE 8–2 NIH PATIENT RISK GROUPS FOR PRIORITIZING COVID-19 THERAPY

Tier	Risk Groups
1	• Immunocompromised individuals who are not expected to mount an adequate immune response to COVID-19 vaccination or SARS-CoV-2 infection due to their underlying conditions, regardless of their vaccine status • Unvaccinated individuals who are at the highest risk for severe disease (anyone aged ≥75 y or anyone aged ≥65 y with additional risk factors)
2	• Unvaccinated individuals who are at risk for severe disease and who are not included in Tier 1 (anyone aged ≥65 y or anyone aged <65 y with clinical risk factors)
3	• Vaccinated individuals who are at high risk for severe disease (anyone aged ≥75 y or anyone aged ≥65 y with clinical risk factors) • Vaccinated individuals who have not received a COVID-19 vaccine booster dose are likely to be at higher risk for severe disease; patients who have not received a booster dose and who are within this tier should be prioritized for treatment
4	• Vaccinated individuals who are at risk for severe disease (anyone aged ≥65 y or anyone aged <65 with clinical risk factors) • Vaccinated individuals who have not received a COVID-19 vaccine booster dose are likely to be at higher risk for severe disease; patients who have not received a booster dose and who are within this tier should be prioritized for treatment

Source: https://www.covid19treatmentguidelines.nih.gov/. Updated February 29, 2024.

Management: Hospitalized Adults

Recommendations from

> ### NIH 2024, IDSA 2024, ACP 2024, NICE 2024

–Awake-prone positioning of severely ill patients hospitalized with COVID-19 requiring supplemental oxygen (includes high-flow nasal oxygen) or noninvasive ventilation. (NICE)

–For severe and critical COVID-19 disease, use corticosteroids, interleukin-6 receptor blockers (tocilizumab or sarilumab), and baricitinib (Janus kinase inhibitor). All three may be combined.

–Corticosteroids:
  • Do not use for patients not requiring hospitalization or supplemental oxygen.
  • If discharged from hospital without supplemental oxygen, stop steroids.
  • If discharged from hospital with supplemental oxygen, insufficient evidence exists to guide decision.

–Consider home pulse oximetry monitoring for patients safe for discharge home with risk factors for progression to severe disease.

–Do not use fluvoxamine outside of clinical trials given currently limited data.

–Do not use inhaled corticosteroids for ambulatory patients with mild-to-moderate COVID-19 in absence of other indications.

–Do not use chloroquine, hydroxychloroquine, HIV protease inhibitors, famotidine, colchicine, nitazoxanide, ciclesonide, or antibiotic therapy in the absence of other indications.

–Do not use anticoagulants or antiplatelet therapy in outpatients in the absence of other indications.

–Do not stop ACE inhibitors, statin therapy, NSAIDs, or corticosteroids being used for comorbid conditions.

–See Table 8–3 for guidance on other unproven therapies.

Practice Pearls

- Convalescent plasma showed a reduction in hospitalizations and medical visits, however, unclear evidence given limited events, may be more effective if containing high titers of neutralizing antibodies and used earlier in presentation.
- Remdesivir reduced hospitalizations and medical visits up to day 28.
- Nirmatrelvir/ritonavir resulted in reduced all-cause mortality and fewer COVID-19-related hospitalizations, but contraindication with drugs highly dependent on CYP3A clearance or potent CYP3A inducers and should check all drug interactions before initiation (no studies in children).
- Molnupiravir showed a reduction in COVID-19-related mortality and COVID-19-related hospitalizations (not recommended in children due to possible effects on bone and cartilage growth).
- There are insufficient data on whether a longer course of ritonavir-booster nirmatrelvir or molnupiravir will prevent viral rebound or symptom recurrence. There are also insufficient data on the efficacy of administering a second course of antiviral therapy to treat viral rebound or symptom recurrence.
- When deciding between outpatient treatment options, consider age, symptom duration, renal function, drug interactions, and product availability. No data exist for combining these treatment options.
- In the United States, neutralizing antibody treatments were found to be largely inactive against the most common variants and are no longer recommended for pre- or postexposure prophylaxis (PrEP) or for treatment.
- Bacterial coinfection was found to be uncommon, and procalcitonin was not an effective tool for discontinuing antibiotics compared to clinical judgment. WBC and CRP were shown to decrease in patients with bacterial infections compared to COVID-19 and may be a useful guide for antibiotic discontinuation.
- Limited studies exist on outcomes for children, but remdesivir and corticosteroids are commonly used given low risk of adverse events, and recent studies support the use of remdesivir down to patients weighing 3.5 kg.

Sources

–https://www.cdc.gov/coronavirus/2019-ncov/hcp/

–www.idsociety.org/COVID19guidelines

–https://www.covid19treatmentguidelines.nih.gov

–*BMJ.* 2020;370:m3379.

–www.nice.org.uk/guidance/ng191

TABLE 8–3 COMPARISON OF RECOMMENDATIONS FOR VARIOUS THERAPIES IN NONSEVERE DISEASE, IN THE NONHOSPITAL SETTING

	CDC	WHO
Ivermectin	Do not use	Do not use
Convalescent plasma	Insufficient evidence in nonhospitalized patients or in patients with impaired immunity. Do not use in hospitalized patients	Do not use
Supplements (vitamin C, vitamin D, zinc)	Insufficient evidence	Not assessed in guideline
JAK inhibitors (baricitinib, ruxolitinib, tofacitinib)	Do not use	Do not use

CORONAVIRUS DISEASE 2019 (COVID-19), LONG

Management: Adults

Recommendations from

> NICE 2021

–Long COVID-19 includes both ongoing symptomatic COVID-19 (from 4 to 12 wk) and post-COVID-19 syndrome (after 12 wk).

–Aggressively evaluate for life-threatening causes of concerning symptoms including hypoxia, exertional hypoxia, signs of severe lung disease, or cardiac chest pain.

–Consider labs including CBC, CMP, CRP, ferritin, BNP, A1c, and TSH as directed by symptoms.

–Consider an exercise tolerance test such as the 1-min sit to stand test. If postural symptoms, assess with a 3-min or 10-min active stand test.

–Consider a chest X-ray 12 wk after COVID-19 diagnosis if there are ongoing respiratory symptoms.

–Provide sources of advice and support, including information about common symptoms.

–Insufficient evidence to recommend vitamins and supplements.

–Advise a gradual, phased return to work or school.

–Develop a personalized rehabilitation plan attending to physical, psychologic, and psychiatric symptoms.

Source

–https://www.nice.org.uk/guidance/ng188/

COCCIDIOIDOMYCOSIS (VALLEY FEVER)

Management: Adults

Recommendations from

> IDSA 2016

–Test for coccidioidomycosis in patients presenting with pneumonia in endemic regions (southwest United States).

–Do not start treatment for a mild infection.

–Do not treat asymptomatic chronic cavitary coccidioidal pneumonia.

–Use fluconazole as the first-line therapy, 400–1200 mg PO daily, including during pregnancy. Check renal function prior to initiating therapy.

–Refer to infection disease specialist for extrapulmonary, disseminated coccidioidomycosis.

Source

–https://academic.oup.com/cid/article/63/6/e112/2389093

DIABETIC FOOT INFECTIONS

Management: Adults

Recommendations from

> IDF 2023, IWGDF 2023, NICE 2019

Evaluation

–Assess glycemic control.

–Assess arterial perfusion and need for revascularization.

–Debride callus if necrotic tissue; to fully visualize wound, measure depth and extent.

–Check C-reactive protein (CRP), erythrocyte sedimentation rate, procalcitonin when the clinical exam is equivocal.

–Obtain X-ray of all new diabetic foot infections.

–Obtain cultures: tissue or bone specimen preferred; deep swab only after debriding wound.

–If considering osteomyelitis:

  • Obtain inflammatory markers.

  • Obtain MRI if the diagnosis of osteomyelitis remains in doubt after inflammatory markers and X-rays.

  • Consider PET scan as an alternative to MRI.

  • Bone biopsy is preferred to tissue biopsy.

Therapies

–Consider hospitalization for a severe infection or moderate infection with clinically significant comorbidities.

–Offload diabetic foot ulcers.

–Request surgical consultation for deep abscesses, compartment syndrome, and necrotizing soft tissue infection.

–Request vascular consultation in those with PAD and foot ulcer with infection.

–Choose an antibiotic based on the suspected pathogen and severity.

–Treat clinically infected wounds with antibiotics:

- 1–2 wk for mild-to-moderate infections, with empiric antibiotics that cover gram-positive organisms.
- 3–4 wk for more serious skin and soft tissue infections, with empiric antibiotics that cover gram-positive, gram-negative, and anaerobic bacteria.
- 6 wk for osteomyelitis (or up to 3 wk with surgically resected osteomyelitis with positive margins).

Practice Pearls

- Antibiotic choice should be guided by severity and local resistance patterns. Common choices include:
  - Mild infection, suspect MSSA or strep: dicloxacillin, cephalexin, clindamycin, or amoxicillin-clavulanate.
  - Mild infection, suspect MRSA: trimethoprim-sulfamethoxazole (TMP-SMX), minocycline, or doxycycline.
  - Moderate-to-severe infections, suspect MSSA, strep, or Enterobacter: IV therapy with levo-floxacin, cefoxitin, ceftriaxone, ampicillin/sulbactam, moxifloxacin, ertapenem, tigecycline, or imipenem/cilastatin.
  - Moderate-to-severe infections, suspect MRSA: IV therapy with linezolid, daptomycin, vanco-mycin, or ceftaroline.
  - Moderate-to-severe infections, suspect pseudomonas: piperacillin/tazobactam or carbapenems.
- A deep space infection may have deceptively few superficial signs.
- The diabetic foot care team should include:
  - Diabetologist.
  - Surgeon with expertise managing DM foot problems.
  - DM nurse specialist.
  - Podiatrist.
  - Tissue viability nurse.
  - Biomechanic and orthotic specialist.
- Do not treat diabetic foot ulcers with:
  - Electrical stimulation therapy, topical antiseptics, silver preparations, autologous platelet-rich plasma gel, regenerative wound matrices, growth factors, or hyperbaric oxygen therapy.

Sources

–https://www.idf.org/e-library/guidelines/119-idf-clinical-practice-recommendations-on-diabetic-foot-2017.html

–https://onlinelibrary.wiley.com/doi/full/10.1002/dmrr.3280

–https://www.nice.org.uk/guidance/ng19

–https://www.idsociety.org/practice-guideline/diabetic-foot-infections/

ENDOCARDITIS, INFECTIOUS

Prevention: Adults

Recommendations from

> AHA 2007, AHA/ACC 2014, AHA/ACC 2017, AAPD 2014

–Maintain optimal oral health and hygiene. This is more important in reducing the risk of infective endocarditis (IE) than prophylactic antibiotics for dental procedures.

–There is insufficient evidence to support the use of topical antiseptics for IE prevention.

–Prevent rheumatic fever by promptly recognizing and treating streptococcal pharyngitis.

–The effectiveness of antibiotic prophylaxis in preventing IE in patients undergoing dental procedures is unknown.

–Do not use antibiotic prophylaxis for mitral valve prolapse, rheumatic heart disease, or most cases of congenital heart disease.[1]

–Offer IE prophylaxis[2] only for patients with underlying cardiac conditions (patients with prosthetic valves,[3] previous history of IE, certain cardiac transplant recipients,[4] and selected patients with congenital heart disease and residual defects) who will undergo selected dental, respiratory, GI, GU, skin, and soft tissue procedures.

  • Dental procedures: consider antibiotic prophylaxis for qualifying patients undergoing dental procedures that involve the gingival tissues or periapical region of a tooth and for those procedures that perforate the oral mucosa.

  • Respiratory procedures: consider antibiotic prophylaxis for qualifying patients undergoing invasive respiratory tract procedures that involve incision or biopsy of the respiratory mucosa.

  • GI/GU procedures: do not use antibiotic prophylaxis solely to prevent IE for GU or GI tract procedures, unless there is ongoing enterococcal infection in qualifying patients. Treat patients with an enterococcal UTI or whose urine is colonized with *Enterococcus* with an antibiotic to eradicate enterococci from the urine prior to an elective cystoscopy or other urinary tract manipulation. If the urinary tract procedure is not elective, treat concurrently with antibiotics that are active against enterococci.

---

[1] Exceptions: (1) Unrepaired cyanotic congenital heart disease, including palliative shunts and conduits; (2) completely repaired congenital heart defect with prosthetic material or device, whether placed by surgery or by catheter intervention, during first 6 mo after the procedure; (3) repaired congenital heart disease with residual defects (eg, shunts or valvular regurgitation) at the site of or adjacent to the site of a prosthetic patch or prosthetic device.

[2] Standard prophylaxis regimen: amoxicillin (adults 2 g; children 50 mg/kg orally 1 h before procedure). If unable to take oral medications, give ampicillin (adults 2.0 g IM or IV; children 50 mg/kg IM or IV within 30 min of procedure). If penicillin-allergic, give clindamycin (adults 600 mg; children 20 mg/kg orally 1 h before procedure) or azithromycin or clarithromycin (adults 500 mg; children 15 mg/kg orally 1 h before procedure). If penicillin-allergic and unable to take oral medications, give clindamycin (adults 600 mg; children 20 mg/kg IV within 30 min before procedure). If allergy to penicillin is not anaphylaxis, angioedema, or urticaria, options for nonoral treatment also include cefazolin (1 g IM or IV for adults; 50 mg/kg IM or IV for children); and for penicillin-allergic, oral therapy includes cephalexin 2 g PO for adults or 50 mg/kg PO for children (IM, intramuscular; IV, intravenous; PO, by mouth, orally).

[3] Prosthetic cardiac valves, including transcatheter-implanted prostheses and homografts, or prosthetic material used for cardiac valve repair (annuloplasty rings, chords).

[4] Only those who develop cardiac valvulopathy.

- Skin/soft tissue procedures: consider antibiotic prophylaxis for qualifying patients undergoing surgical procedures involving infected skin, skin structure, or musculoskeletal tissue using an agent that is active against staphylococci and beta-hemolytic streptococci. Advise against body piercing.
- Arrange perioperative prophylactic antibiotics with staphylococcal coverage for patients undergoing surgery for placement of prosthetic intravascular or intracardiac materials (eg, prosthetic valves).
- Give long-term antistreptococcal prophylaxis for secondary prevention of rheumatic fever in patients with RHD, specifically mitral stenosis.
- Continue IE prophylaxis indefinitely in postcardiac transplant patients with a structurally abnormal valve.
- Do not use antibiotic prophylaxis for the following procedures and events:
  - Routine anesthetic injections through noninfected tissue.
  - Taking dental radiographs.
  - Placement of removable prosthodontic or orthodontic appliances.
  - Adjustment of orthodontic appliances or placement of orthodontic brackets.
  - Shedding of deciduous teeth.
  - Bleeding from trauma to the lips or oral mucosa.
  - Bronchoscopy without incision of the respiratory tract mucosa.
  - Diagnostic esophagogastroduodenoscopy or colonoscopy.
  - Vaginal or cesarean delivery.
  - Hysterectomy.
  - Tattooing.
  - Coronary artery bypass graft surgery.

Practice Pearls

- IE is much more likely to result from frequent exposure to random bacteremia associated with daily activities (eg, chewing food, tooth brushing, flossing, use of toothpicks, use of water irrigation devices) and dental disease than from bacteremia caused by a dental, GI, or GU procedure.
- Antibiotic prophylaxis may reduce the incidence and duration of bacteremia but does not eliminate bacteremia.
- Only an extremely small number of cases of IE might be prevented by antibiotic prophylaxis even if it were 100% effective.

Sources
- *Circulation.* 2007;116:1736–1754.
- *J Am Coll Cardiol.* 2014;63(22):e57.
- *J Am Coll Cardiol.* 2017;70(2):252–289.
- *Am Acad Pediatr Dent.* 2014;40(6):386–391.

GONORRHEA AND CHLAMYDIA

Screening: Women < 25 y

Recommendations from

> **CDC 2015, AAP 2014, USPSTF 2021**
>   –Screen all women < 25 y who are sexually active and ≥25 y if at increased risk.[1]
>   –There is insufficient evidence for or against screening nonpregnant persons > 25 y without risk factors.

Guidelines Alert 8–1	
GUIDELINES DISCORDANT: RECOMMENDED SCREENING INTERVAL FOR GONORRHEA AND CHLAMYDIA	
Organization	**Interval**
CDC, AAP	Screen annually
USPSTF	Screen when sexual history reveals new or persistent risk factors since last negative test. Insufficient data to determine universal screening interval

Applying to Clinical Practice
- The AAP and CDC prefer the simplicity and regularity of an annual screen.
- The USPSTF notes that the optimal interval between screening tests has not been studied.
- Screening rates remain low despite the universal recommendation, so clinicians and health systems should prioritize a screening program that effectively increases rates in their population.

Practice Pearls

- In addition to the public health benefit of identifying and treating a communicable disease, infections in women are often asymptomatic but may lead to pelvic inflammatory disease which can lead to chronic pelvic pain, ectopic pregnancy, and infertility.
- Women aged <25 y are at highest risk for gonorrhea infection. Other risk factors that place women at increased risk include a previous gonorrhea infection, the presence of other sexually transmitted infections (STIs), new or multiple sex partners, sex partner with concurrent partners, sex partner who has an STI, inconsistent condom use, commercial sex work, history of incarceration and drug use.

Sources
  –CDC. *Sexually Transmitted Diseases Guidelines*. 2015.
  –*Pediatrics*. 2014;134(1):e302.
  –USPSTF. *Chlamydia and Gonorrhea: Screening*. 2021.

---

[1] Women aged <25 y are at highest risk for gonorrhea infection. Other risk factors that place women at increased risk include a previous gonorrhea infection, the presence of other STIs, new or multiple sex partners, inconsistent condom use, commercial sex work, and drug use.

Screening: Men

Recommendations from

> CDC 2015, USPSTF 2014

–Test annually in men who have sex with men, regardless of condom use. Increase frequency to q3–6 mo if high risk activity.

–There is insufficient evidence for or against routine screening in other men.

–Consider screening in high prevalence clinical settings.

Practice Pearls

- Chlamydia and gonorrhea are reportable infections to the Public Health Department in every state.
- Men are more likely than women to have symptomatic infection and are at lower risk of permanent sequelae such as infertility, making the rationale for asymptomatic screening less evident.
- Urine nucleic amplification acid test (NAAT) for chlamydia and/or gonorrhea for men who have had insertive intercourse and women with vaginal/penile intercourse.
- NAAT of rectal swab for persons who have had receptive anal intercourse.
- NAAT of oropharyngeal swab for persons engaged in oral sexual intercourse.

Sources

–USPSTF. *Chlamydia and Gonorrhea: Screening.* 2014.

–CDC. *Sexually Transmitted Diseases Guidelines.* 2015.

GONORRHEA, OPHTHALMIA NEONATORUM

Prevention: Newborns

Recommendations from

> USPSTF 2019

–Give all newborns prophylactic ocular topical medication against gonococcal ophthalmia neonatorum.

Practice Pearls

- Erythromycin 0.5% ointment is the only agent available in the United States for this application.
- Canadian Paediatric Society recommends against universal prophylaxis, given incomplete efficacy of erythromycin, rarity of the condition, and disruption in maternal-infant bonding. Instead, they recommend screening mothers for gonorrhea and chlamydia infection and, if infected with gonorrhea at the time of delivery, treating the infant with ceftriaxone. (*Paediatr Child Health.* 2015;20:93–96)

Source

–USPSTF. *Ocular Prophylaxis for Gonococcal Ophthalmia Neonatorum.* 2019.

HERPES SIMPLEX VIRUS (HSV), GENITAL

Screening: Adults

Recommendations from

➢ CDC 2015, USPSTF 2023

–Do not screen routinely for HSV with serologies.

Practice Pearl

- In women with a history of genital herpes, routine serial cultures for HSV are not indicated in the absence of active lesions.

Sources

–https://www.uspreventiveservicestaskforce.org/uspstf/recommendation/genital-herpes-serologic-screening
–CDC. *Sexually Transmitted Diseases Treatment Guidelines*. 2015.

HUMAN IMMUNODEFICIENCY VIRUS (HIV)

Screening: Adults

Recommendations from

➢ AAFP 2019, USPSTF 2019, CDC 2015, ACP 2009

–Screen everyone in recommended age groups.
–Consider screening high-risk individuals[1] of other ages.

Guidelines Alert 8–2
GUIDELINES DISCORDANT: POPULATION TO SCREEN FOR HIV

Organization	Age Range
USPSTF, AAFP	15–65 y
CDC	13–64 y
ACP	13–75 y

Applying to Clinical Practice
- AAFP and USPSTF declined to lower screening age to 13, given relatively low prevalence and possibility of false-positives.
- ACP extended screening to age 75 based on a VA study of rising HIV prevalence in 65–75 y age group.

---

[1] Risk factors for HIV: men who have had sex with men after 1975; multiple sexual partners; history of injection drug use; prostitution; history of sex with an HIV-infected person; history of STI; history of blood transfusion between 1978 and 1985; or persons requesting an HIV test.

Practice Pearls

- Optimal screening interval is not defined, but consider testing annually with patients at higher risk, as many HIV diagnoses are made within 2 y of a negative test.[1]
- Educate and counsel all high-risk patients regarding HIV testing, transmission, risk-reduction behaviors, and implications of infection.
- If acute HIV is suspected, use plasma RNA test also.
- False-positive results with electroimmunoassay: nonspecific reactions in persons with immunologic disturbances (eg, systemic lupus erythematosus or rheumatoid arthritis), multiple transfusions, recent influenza, or rabies vaccination.
- Confirmatory testing is necessary using Western blot or indirect immunofluorescence assay.
- Awareness of HIV positively reduces secondary HIV transmission risk and high-risk behavior and viral load if on antiretroviral therapy (ART). (CDC, 2006)

Sources

–AAFP. *Clinical Recommendations: HIV Infection, Adolescents and Adults.* 2013.
–CDC. *Sexually Transmitted Diseases Treatment Guidelines.* 2015.
–USPSTF. *Screening for HIV Infection.* 2019.
–ACP. *Ann Intern Med.* 2009;150(2):125–131.

Prevention: Adults at High Risk of Acquiring HIV

Recommendations from

> **CDC 2021, USPSTF 2019, BHIVA/BASHH 2018**

–Offer PrEP with effective ART to adolescents and adults who are at high risk for HIV acquisition. (See Fig. 8–1 for high risk characteristics.)
–Before beginning PrEP, ensure documented negative HIV Ag/Ab test within 1 wk of initial prescription, no signs/symptoms of acute HIV infection, CrCl ≥ 30 mL/min, and no contraindicated medications. If high-risk exposure in the preceding 4 wk, obtain HIV viral load.
–Obtain baseline hepatitis B and C, syphilis, and gonorrhea and chlamydia testing at all sites of intercourse.
–Prescribe once daily emtricitabine/tenofovir disoproxil fumarate (F/TDF), up to a 90-d supply.
–For men and transgender women, consider emtricitabine/tenofovir alafenamide (F/TAF) as an alternative. (CDC)
–Consider the 2-1-1 alternate dosing schedule, only for adult men who have sex with men who prefer it to daily use:
  - Take F/TDF 2 pills 2 to 24 h before sex (closer to 24 h is preferred).
  - Take F/TDF 1 pill 24 h after the initial 2-pill dose.
  - Take F/TDF 1 pill 48 h after the initial 2-pill dose.
  - If sex on consecutive days, take 1 pill daily until 48 h after the last sexual event.
  - If there is a gap of <7 d between the last pill and the next sexual event, resume 1 pill daily.
  - If there is a gap of ≥7 d between the last pill and the next sexual event, start again with 2 pills.
  - Prescribe no more than 30 pills without follow-up.

[1] *MMWR Morb Mortal Wkly Rep.* 2012;61(24):441.

FIG. 8–1 HIGH-RISK CHARACTERISTICS FOR PrEP ELIGIBILITY

Sexually active adults and adolescents weighing at least 35 kg who have engaged in anal or vaginal sex in the last 6 mo and have:
- A sexual partner with HIV, especially with an unknown or detectable viral load.
- Syphilis, chlamydia, or gonorrhea infection in the last 6 mo for transgender women and men who have sex with men.
- Syphilis or gonorrhea infection in the last 6 mo for heterosexual adults.
- History of inconsistent or no condom use with sexual partners whose HIV status is unknown.
- Persons who inject drugs and have a drug injecting partner who has HIV.
- Persons who engage in transactional sex.

–Follow up 4 wk after initiation to assess tolerance.

–Assess for HIV infection at least every 3 mo, as PrEP regimens are inadequate therapy for HIV.

–Screen for STIs and hepatitis C every 3–6 mo.

–Obtain renal panel every 6 mo, or every 12 mo if eGFR is >90 mL/min/1.73 m^2.

–Test for pregnancy as indicated.

–If on F/TAF, assess weight and cholesterol levels annually.

Practice Pearls

- PrEP is highly effective and widely underutilized.
- Clinicians should look for opportunities to offer PrEP to anyone at increased risk of acquiring HIV.
- Consider PrEP on a case-by-case basis. Although guidelines describe particular "at-risk groups," evaluate each patient as an individual and offer PrEP if risk is elevated.
- Suggested eGFR for individuals starting TDF-FTC is >60 mL/min/1.73 m^2.
- Start individuals with eGFR < 60 mL/min/1.73 m^2 on a case-by-case basis.
- Start hepatitis B vaccination in persons who are nonimmune.
- Hold PrEP if patient has symptoms suggestive of HIV and high risk of seroconversion.
- Positive HIV test is an absolute contraindication to starting PrEP.
- PrEP can be continued during pregnancy and breastfeeding.
- Report information regarding the use of PrEP during pregnancy to the Antiretroviral Pregnancy Registry.
- Women using depot medroxyprogesterone, PrEP is likely to counteract and increase in HIV acquisition. An alternative form of contraception, if available, should be offered.
- There are no known interactions between TDF-FTC and feminizing or masculinizing hormones.
- A discussion about side effects including impact upon bone density should be held at PrEP initiation and maintenance visits.
- In those at risk for reduced bone density, FRAX tool can guide need for DEXA scan and potential treatment.
- Robust adherence support is required at PrEP initiation and maintenance.
- PrEP provision should include condom provision and behavioral support.
- TDF alone can be offered to heterosexual men and women where FTC is contraindicated.

Sources

–USPSTF. *Preexposure Prophylaxis for the Prevention of HIV Infection US Preventive Services Task Force Recommendation Statement*. 2023.

–*JAMA*. 2019;321(22):2203–2213.

–*BHIVA/BASHH Guidelines on the Use of HIV Pre-exposure Prophylaxis (PrEP)*. 2018.

–BASHH. *2021 UK Guideline for the Use of Post-Exposure Prophylaxis (PEP)*. 2021.

–Centers for Disease Control and Prevention: US Public Health Service. Preexposure prophylaxis for the prevention of HIV infection in the United States—2021 Update: a clinical practice guideline. https://www.cdc.gov/hiv/pdf/risk/prep/cdc-hiv-prep-guidelines-2021.pdf. Published December 2021.

Prevention: Adults Who Have Recently Been Exposed to HIV

Recommendations from

> ### CDC 2021, USPSTF 2019, BHIVA/BASHH 2018

–Offer PEP to reduce the risk of HIV transmission in the following scenarios:

- After receptive anal intercourse with an index partner of unknown HIV status or known to be HIV-positive with an unknown or detectable HIV viral load.
- After receptive vaginal sex with an index partner known to be HIV-positive with an unknown or detectable HIV viral load.
- After an occupational exposure (sharps or mucosal splash) from an index case known to be HIV-positive with an unknown or detectable HIV viral load.
- For people who inject drugs after sharing needles/equipment if their index injecting partner is known to be HIV-positive with an unknown or detectable HIV viral load.

–PEP first-line regimen is TDF 245 mg/emtricitabine (FTC) 200 mg fixed dose combination plus raltegravir 1200 mg once daily for 28 d.

–Initiate PEP as soon as possible after exposure, preferably within 24 h. Do not initiate PEP beyond 72 h after exposure.

–Test for the following after all exposures:

- Creatinine and eGFR.
- Alanine transaminase.
- HIV-1 antigen (Ag)/antibody (Ab).
- If not known to be vaccinated with documented hepatitis B surface antigen (HBsAg) > 10 IU: hepatitis B serology (HBsAg, HBsAb, and hepatitis B core antibody [HBcAB]).
- If sexual exposure: obtain additional studies including chlamydia, gonorrhea, and syphilis testing, HCV screening in men who have sex with men and others at risk for hepatitis C.
- If occupational exposure: obtain additional testing including hepatitis C screening in all.
- Obtain a pregnancy test for all women of childbearing age considering PEP.

–Consider PEP in the following circumstances:

- Insertive vaginal intercourse with an index partner known to be HIV-positive with an unknown or detectable HIV viral load.
- Insertive anal intercourse with an index partner of unknown HIV status.

–Do not use PEP for the following scenarios:
- Sharps and splash injuries, sharing of injecting equipment, receptive or insertive vaginal intercourse when the index case is from a high-risk group but the HIV status is unknown.
- Human bite if the index case is HIV-positive with an unknown or detectable HIV viral load. Consider, however, for patients who fulfill ALL of the following criteria: (a) the biter's saliva was visibly contaminated with blood, (b) the biter is known or suspected to have a plasma HIV viral load > 3.0 log copies/mL, and (c) the bite resulted in severe and/or deep tissue injuries.

–PEP special populations: pregnant and breastfeeding mothers.
- Pregnancy and breastfeeding should not alter the decision to start PEP.
- For women who are pregnant, raltegravir 400 mg twice daily is preferred as a third agent.
- For women at risk for pregnancy or known to be within the first 6 wk of pregnancy who cannot use first-line PEP for any reason, avoid the use of dolutegravir as an alternative third agent, though acceptable after 6 wk of pregnancy.

Sources

–USPSTF. *Preexposure Prophylaxis for the Prevention of HIV Infection US Preventive Services Task Force Recommendation Statement.* 2019.

–*JAMA.* 2019;321(22):2203–2213.

–*BHIVA/BASHH Guidelines on the Use of HIV Pre-exposure Prophylaxis (PrEP).* 2018.

–BASHH. *2021 UK Guideline for the Use of Post-Exposure Prophylaxis (PEP).* 2021.

–Centers for Disease Control and Prevention: US Public Health Service. Preexposure prophylaxis for the prevention of HIV infection in the United States—2021 Update: a clinical practice guideline. https://www.cdc.gov/hiv/pdf/risk/prep/cdc-hiv-prep-guidelines-2021.pdf. Published December 2021.

Management: Adults

Recommendations from

> IDSA 2018, USPSTF 2023, HHS 2022

Evaluation

–Obtain a comprehensive present and past medical history, physical examination, medication/social/family history, and review of systems, including HIV-related information upon initiation of care.

–Assess for the presence of depression, substance abuse, or domestic violence.

–Baseline labs upon initiation of care: HIV serostatus; CD4 count; quantitative HIV RNA by PCR (viral load); HIV genotyping and genotypic resistance testing; CBCD, chemistry panel, G6PD testing; fasting lipid profile; random or fasting glucose; hepatitis A/B/C serology; HLA B5701 test (if abacavir will be used); tropism testing (if the use of a CCR5 antagonist is being considered); urinalysis; pregnancy test; Pap smear in women.[1]

–Screening labs: *M. tuberculosis* testing (PPD or interferon-gamma release assay); toxoplasma antibodies; hepatitis B panel, HCV antibodies; Venereal Disease Research Laboratory (VDRL);

---

[1] CBCD, complete blood count with differential; G6PD, glucose-6-phosphate dehydrogenase; NAAT, nucleic acid amplification test; PCR, polymerase chain reaction; PPD, purified protein derivative; VDRL, Venereal Disease Research Laboratory.

urine NAAT for gonorrhea; and urine NAAT for chlamydia (except in men aged <25 y); anti-CMV IgG in lower risk groups (populations other than men who have sex with men or injection drug users), trichomoniasis in all women, *Chlamydia trachomatis* in all women ≤ 25 y of age.

–Monitoring labs:
  • HIV viral load 4–8 wk after initiation or modification or ART and q4–6 wk until undetectable then every 3–6 mo.
  • CD4 every 3 mo if <300, CD4 every 6 mo if ≥300 for first 2 y, after 2 y with consistently suppressed viral load, every 12 mo for 300–500 and optional if >500. Monitor CBCD yearly when no longer monitoring CD4.
  • Chemistries every 6 mo.
  • STI screening and TB screening tests should be repeated periodically depending on symptoms and signs, behavioral risk, and possible exposures.
  • Lipid panel 1–3 mo after initiation or modification.
–Ask all women of childbearing age living with HIV about their plans and desires regarding pregnancy upon initiation of care and routinely thereafter.
–Pap smear with HPV or reflex to HPV based on age in women every 6 mo and annually thereafter if results are normal. For ASC-US Pap result, if reflex HPV testing is negative, a repeat Pap test in 6–12 mo or repeat co-testing in 12 mo is recommended. For any result ≥ ASC-US on repeat cytology, referral to colposcopy is recommended.
–Perform individualized assessment of risk for breast cancer and inform them of the potential benefits and risks of screening mammography for women ages 40–49 y. Perform a mammogram annually for age > 50 y.

Therapies
–Educate patients on high-risk behaviors to minimize the risk of HIV transmission.
–Start ART as soon as feasibly possible.
–Start ART within the first 2 wk after the initiation of treatment for most opportunistic infections:
  • Within 4–6 wk after starting antifungals for cryptococcal meningitis.
  • Within 2–8 wk after starting TB treatment in patients with CD4 >50.
  • Start immediately in patients with HIV and cancer with special attention to drug interactions.
–Use one of these antiretroviral regimens for most patients with HIV:
  • Bictegravir/TAF/emtricitabine.
  • Dolutegravir + emtricitabine or lamivudine + TAF or TDF.
  • Dolutegravir/lamivudine (except if HIV RNA > 500,000 copies/mL, CD4 < 200, on active treatment for opportunistic infection, HBV coinfection and not without HIV genotyping so not to be started on the day of diagnosis).
  • Raltegravir + emtricitabine or lamivudine + TAF or TDF.
–For patients with history of CAB-LA (long-acting injectable cabotegravir) use for PrEP, recommend INSTI genotypic resistance testing before initiation and treating with darunavir/cobicistat or darunavir/ritonavir + TAF or TDF + emtricitabine or lamivudine pending results.

- For pregnant persons/women of childbearing age, recommend: dolutegravir, raltegravir, atazanavir/ritonavir, darunavir/ritonavir (dosed twice daily), or efavirenz, PLUS either TDF/emtricitabine or TDF/lamivudine.
- Pregnant persons taking ART should be switched to a recommended regimen after review of genotype testing and ART therapy. Selection of a regimen should be individualized.
- Efavirenz is teratogenic.
- Tenofovir should be used cautiously with renal insufficiency.
- Ritonavir-boosted atazanavir and rilpivirine should not be used with high-dose proton pump inhibitors.
- Regimens that include INSTIs have higher rates of weight gain, greater in dolutegravir, bictegravir.
- Patients on rifamycin-based TB treatment should be on ART with 2 nRTIs plus efavirenz (600 mg/d), raltegravir (800 mg BID), or dolutegravir (50 mg BID).
- Cabotegravir (CAB) + rilpivirine RPV is not recommended as initial ART, patients desiring long-acting injectable regimen should first attain viral suppression on one of the above regimens then transition to a month of oral CAB/RPV with proof of maintenance of suppression before transitioning to injectable.

–How and when to switch between ART therapies:
- To simplify the regimen in patients with viral suppression, switch from 3-drug to 2-drug regimens to reduce AEs and adherence. Recommended regimens include dolutegravir/rilpivirine, boosted PPT/lamivudine, dolutegravir/lamivudine, and long-acting injectable cabotegravir/rilpivirine q4 wk.
- Virologic failure (HIV RNA > 200 copies/mL on 2 consecutive measurements): NNRTI failure → dolutegravir + 2 nRTIs, INSTI failure → boosted PI + 2 nRTIs, raltegravir or elvitegravir failure → dolutegravir BID + 1 fully active other agent, multiclass (>3) resistance → construct new regimen from new classes of drugs.
- Development of concomitant disease including kidney, liver, cardiovascular, or bone disease, weight gain, cancer, autoimmune disease, or solid organ transplant may require switching regimens.

–Screen for HLA-B*5701 before starting abacavir.

–Interruption of ART is recommended for drug toxicity, intercurrent illness, or operations that preclude oral intake.

–Management of a patient with prior antiretroviral exposure is complex and should be managed by an HIV specialist if changing regimens.

–Vaccinate for pneumococcal infection, influenza, varicella, hepatitis A, HPV, and HBV according to standard immunization charts.

Surveillance

–Laboratory testing:
- Screen non-HIV-infected high-risk patients every 3 mo as long as risk persists and offer PrEP (TDF/emtricitabine daily, double dose on the first day for MSM).
- While on PrEP, screen quarterly with combined HIV Ab/Ag, genital and nongenital GC/Ch, syphilis, and pregnancy, and screen annually for estimated CrCl and hepatitis C Ab.

- If high-risk exposure within 72 h, screen with rapid HIV antibody test; if negative, offer PEP (3-drug ART regimen within first 24–72 h and continued × 28 d) and obtain testing for Cr, hepatitis B sAg, STIs, and HIV Ab/Ag or HIV RNA.
- If positive for HIV, obtain HIV RNA, CD4, reverse transcriptase-prodrug resistance genotype testing, kidney and liver function, lipid levels, CBC, glucose, pregnancy, viral hepatitis A/B/C, TB, and STI testing, but do not delay initiation of ART while awaiting results (add serum cryptococcal Ag if CD4 < 100).
- Within 6 wk of starting ART, repeat HIV RNA; if levels have not declined considerably in adherent patient, then perform genotypic resistance testing.
- If viral suppression is considered stable, monitor HIV RNA levels every 3 mo until 1 y of suppression, then monitor every 6 mo.
- If previously achieved suppression and HIV RNA > 50, quickly repeat HIV RNA and assess adherence and tolerability.
- Measure CD4 counts every 6 mo until >250 × 1 y then only repeat if ART failure or immunosuppressive condition.

–Recommend coreceptor tropism assay whenever a CCR5 coreceptor antagonist is considered.

Practice Pearls

- This guideline focuses on antiretroviral management in HIV-1-infected individuals.
- The following regimens can be considered for HIV-2-infected individuals: ibalizumab, lenacapavir, boosted darunavir, or dolutegravir.
- Alternative regimens for specific clinical scenarios or patient characteristics are beyond the scope of this book.
- Baseline evaluation should include:
  - Patient's readiness for ART.
  - Psychosocial assessment.
  - Substance abuse screening.
  - Mental illness screening.
  - HIV risk behavior screening.
  - Health insurance and coverage status.
  - Discussion of risk reduction and disclosure to sexual and/or needle-sharing partners.
- Initial labs:
  - CD4 T-cell count.
  - HIV-1 antibody testing.
  - HIV RNA viral load.
  - Genotypic drug-resistance testing.
  - CBCD, chemistry panel, LFTs, urinalysis.
  - Serologies for hepatitis B and C.
  - Fasting glucose or A1c and lipid panel.
  - Pregnancy test.
  - STI screening.
- Specific ART recommendations are updated regularly at the CDC's website: https://clinicalinfo. hiv.gov/en/guidelines.

- Screen for anogenital HPV with anal Pap testing for men who have sex with men, women with abnormal cervical Pap smear results, and persons with a history of genital warts.
- Test for serum testosterone level in men complaining of fatigue, ED, or decreased libido.
- Chest X-ray should be obtained in persons with pulmonary symptoms or who have a positive PPD test result.
- Screen for STI via mode of intercourse, ie, anal, vaginal, or oral swab for gonorrhea and chlamydia.
- Patient should be informed that maintaining HIV RNA < 200 with ART prevents sexual transmission to partners.
- Patients starting ART should use another form of protection (condoms, PrEP, abstinence) for the first 6 mo of treatment and until viral load <200.
- Do not have to wait for results of all tests to be back to initiate ART (except those to confirm HIV diagnosis), but should obtain all labs above before starting ART and follow up to adjust therapy as appropriate.

Sources

–http://aidsinfo.nih.gov/guidelines/html/1/adult-and-adolescent-arv-guidelines/0
–*JAMA*. 2020;324(16):1651–1669. doi:10.1001/jama.2020.17025
–*Clin Infect Dis*. 2014;58(1):e1–e34, http://academic.oup.com/cid/article/58/1/e1/374007#74163693
–https://www.idsociety.org/globalassets/idsa/practice-guidelines/guidelines-for-prevention-and-treatment-of-opportunistic-infections-in-hiv-infected-adults-and-adolescents.pdf
–https://www.cdc.gov/std/gonorrhea/stdfact-gonorrhea.htm

Management: Children

Recommendations from

⟩ HHS 2018, IDSA 2019, HHS 2022

Evaluation

–Obtain a comprehensive present and past medical history, physical examination, medication/social/family history, and review of systems, including HIV-related information upon initiation of care.

–Assess for the presence of depression, substance abuse, or domestic violence.

–Baseline labs upon initiation of care: HIV serostatus; CD4 count; quantitative HIV RNA by PCR (viral load); HIV genotyping and genotypic resistance testing; CBCD, chemistry panel, G6PD testing; fasting lipid profile; random or fasting glucose; hepatitis A/B/C serology; HLA B5701 test (if abacavir will be used); tropism testing (if the use of a CCR5 antagonist is being considered); urinalysis; pregnancy test.[1]

–Screening labs: *M. tuberculosis* testing (PPD or interferon-γ release assay); toxoplasma antibodies; hepatitis B panel, HCV antibodies; VDRL.

Therapies

–Specific ART recommendations are updated regularly at the CDC's website: https://clinicalinfo.hiv.gov/en/guidelines.

---

[1] CBCD, complete blood count with differential; G6PD, glucose-6-phosphate dehydrogenase; NAAT, nucleic acid amplification test; PCR, polymerase chain reaction; PPD, purified protein derivative; VDRL, Venereal Disease Research Laboratory.

Surveillance

–Monitoring labs:

- HIV viral load 4–8 wk after initiation or modification or ART and q4–6 wk until undetectable, then every 3–6 mo.
- CD4 every 3 mo if <300, CD4 every 6 mo if ≥300 for first 2 y, after 2 y with consistently suppressed viral load, every 12 mo for 300–500 and optional if >500 monitor CBCD yearly when no longer monitoring CD4.
- Chemistries every 6 mo.
- STI screening and TB screening tests should be repeated periodically depending on symptoms and signs, behavioral risk, and possible exposures.
- Lipid panel 1–3 mo after initiation or modification.

–ART is recommended for all children, regardless of symptoms or CD4 count.

–HIV genotypic resistance testing is recommended:

- At the time of diagnosis.
- Prior to initiation of therapy.
- For all treatment-naïve children.

–Evaluate for possible side effects and evaluate response to therapy in all children 1–2 wk after initiation of ART or changing ART regimen.

–Recommend laboratory testing for toxicity and viral load response at 2–4 wk after treatment initiation.

–Check absolute CD4 T lymphocyte (CD4) cell count and plasma HIV RNA (viral load) and evaluate therapy adherence, effectiveness, and toxicities every 3–4 mo. CD4 count can be monitored every 6–12 mo in children who are adherent to therapy and have had CD4 counts well above the threshold for opportunistic infections, sustained viral suppression, and stable clinical status for 2–3 y.

Sources

–Panel on Antiretroviral Therapy and Medical Management of Children Living with HIV. *Guidelines for the Use of Antiretroviral Agents in Pediatric HIV Infection.*

–http://aidsinfo.nih.gov/contentfiles/lvguidelines/pediatricguidelines.pdf

HUMAN IMMUNODEFICIENCY VIRUS (HIV), OPPORTUNISTIC INFECTIONS

Prevention: Adults with HIV

Recommendations from

> CDC 2014, WHO 2018, NIH 2013

–See Table 8–4.

–ART to avoid advanced immune deficiency constitutes primary prophylaxis against candidiasis, coccidioidomycosis, cryptococcosis, cryptosporidiosis, cystoisosporiasis, and giardiasis in children.

TABLE 8–4 PROPHYLAXIS TO PREVENT FIRST EPISODE OF OPPORTUNISTIC DISEASE AMONG HIV-INFECTED ADULTS

Opportunistic Infection	Indication	First Choice Therapy	Alternative Regimens
Pneumocystis jirovecii pneumonia (PCP)	CD4+ count < 200 cells/mcL or oropharyngeal candidiasis CD4+ < 14% or history of AIDS-defining illness CD4+ count ≥ 200 but < 250 cells/mcL if monitoring CD4+ count every 3 mo is not possible and ART initiation delayed Note: Additional PCP prophylaxis is not needed if already receiving pyrimethamine/sulfadiazine for treatment/suppression of toxoplasmosis	TMP-SMX, 1 DS PO daily or 1 SS daily	TMP-SMX 1 DS PO, TIW, or Dapsone 100 mg PO daily or 50 mg PO BID, or Dapsone 50 mg PO daily + pyrimethamine 50 mg PO weekly + leucovorin 25 mg PO weekly, or [Dapsone 200 mg + pyrimethamine 75 mg + leucovorin 25 mg] PO weekly, or Aerosolized pentamidine 300 mg via Respirgard II nebulized every month, or Atovaquone 1500 mg PO daily, or [Atovaquone 1500 mg + pyrimethamine 25 mg + leucovorin 10 mg] PO daily
Toxoplasma gondii encephalitis	*Toxoplasma* IgG-positive patients with CD4+ count <100 cells/mcL Seronegative patients receiving PCP prophylaxis not active against toxoplasmosis should have toxoplasma serology retested if CD4+ count declines to <100 cells/mcL; prophylaxis should be initiated if seroconversion occurred Note: Patients receiving primary prophylaxis for *T. gondii* are also covered for PCP prophylaxis	TMP-SMX 1 DS PO daily	TMP-SMX 1 DS PO TIW, or TMP-SMX 1 SS PO daily, or Dapsone 50 mg PO daily + pyrimethamine 50 mg PO weekly + leucovorin 25 mg PO weekly, or [Dapsone 200 mg + pyrimethamine 75 mg + leucovorin 25 mg] PO weekly, or Atovaquone 1500 mg PO daily, or [Atovaquone 1500 mg + pyrimethamine 25 mg + leucovorin 10 mg] PO daily Note: (1) Screen for G6PD prior to administration with dapsone or primaquine (2) Screen for latent TB prior to initiating treatment with pyrimethamine

TABLE 8–4 PROPHYLAXIS TO PREVENT FIRST EPISODE OF OPPORTUNISTIC DISEASE AMONG HIV-INFECTED ADULTS (continued)			
Opportunistic Infection	Indication	First Choice Therapy	Alternative Regimens
Mycobacterium tuberculosis infection (TB) (treatment of latent TB infection [LTBI])	(+) Screening test for LTBI, no evidence of active TB, and no prior treatment for active or latent TB (+) Diagnostic test for LTBI and no evidence of active TB, but close contact with a person with infectious pulmonary TB A history of untreated or inadequately treated healed TB (ie, old fibrotic lesions) regardless of diagnostic tests for LTBI and no evidence of active TB (AII)	(Rifapentine [see dose below] plus isoniazid (INH) 900 mg plus pyridoxine 50 mg) PO once weekly for 12 wk Note: Rifapentine is recommended only for persons receiving efavirenz, raltegravir, or once daily dolutegravir-based ART regimen Weight-based rifapentine dose: *Weighing 32.1–49.9 kg:* 750 mg PO once weekly *Weighing* > 50 kg: 900 mg PO once weekly *or* (INH 300 mg plus rifampin [RIF] 600 mg plus pyridoxine 25–50 mg) PO daily for 3 mo For persons exposed to drug-resistant TB, selection of drugs after consultation with public health authorities	(INH 300 mg plus pyridoxine 25–50 mg) PO daily for 9 mo, *or* RIF 600 mg PO daily for 4 mo, *or* (Rifapentine [see dose below] plus INH 300 mg plus pyridoxine 25–50 mg) PO once daily for 4 wk Weight-based rifapentine dose: *Weighing* < 35 kg: 300 mg PO once daily *Weighing* 35–45 kg: 450 mg PO once daily *Weighing* > 45 kg: 600 mg PO once daily
Mycobacterium avium complex (MAC) disease	CD4+ count < 50 cells/mcL in those who are not on fully suppressive ART—after ruling out active disseminated MAC infection. Not recommended for those who immediately initiate ART	Azithromycin 1200 mg PO once weekly; or clarithromycin 500 mg PO BID; or azithromycin 600 mg PO twice weekly	Rifabutin (dosage adjustment based on drug-drug interactions with ART); rule out active TB before starting RFB

TABLE 8–4 PROPHYLAXIS TO PREVENT FIRST EPISODE OF OPPORTUNISTIC DISEASE AMONG HIV-INFECTED ADULTS *(continued)*

Opportunistic Infection	Indication	First Choice Therapy	Alternative Regimens
Streptococcus pneumoniae infection	History of prior pneumococcal vaccination or unknown vaccine history	Administer either 15-valent pneumococcal conjugate vaccine (PCV15) or 20-valent pneumococcal conjugate vaccine (PCV20) If PCV15 is used, a dose of 23-valent pneumococcal polysaccharide vaccine (PPSV23) should be administered at least 8 wk later. No additional pneumococcal vaccine doses are recommended For people with HIV who previously started or completed a pneumococcal vaccination series, there is no need to restart the series People with HIV who previously received only the 13-valent pneumococcal conjugate vaccine (PCV13) should receive PPSV23 at least 8 wk later People with HIV who have received PCV13 and PPSV23 should receive a booster PPSV23 at least 5 y after the first dose. If they were <65 at the time of the second dose, they should receive a third and final dose at or after age 65, at least 5 y after the second PPSV23 dose People with HIV who have only received PPSV23 may receive a PCV (either PCV20 or PCV15) ≥1 y after their last PPSV23 dose. When PCV15 is used in those with history of PPSV23 receipt, it need not be followed by another dose of PPSV23	

TABLE 8–4 PROPHYLAXIS TO PREVENT FIRST EPISODE OF OPPORTUNISTIC DISEASE AMONG HIV-INFECTED ADULTS (continued)

Opportunistic Infection	Indication	First Choice Therapy	Alternative Regimens
Influenza A and B virus infection	All HIV-infected patients	Inactivated or recombinant influenza vaccine annually Do not use live-attenuated influenza vaccine	
Syphilis	For patients with exposure to a partner diagnosed with syphilis < 90 d prior or for partners diagnosed >90 d prior with unknown serologic tests or uncertain follow-up	Benzathine penicillin (PCN) G 2.4 million units IM × 1	For PCN allergy: Doxycycline 100 mg PO BID × 14 d, or Ceftriaxone 1 g IM/IV daily × 8–10 d, or Azithromycin 2 g PO × 1 (BII) (not recommended for MSM or pregnant persons)
Histoplasma capsulatum infection	CD4+ count < 150 cells/mcL and at high risk because of occupational exposure or live in a community with a hyperendemic rate of histoplasmosis (>10 cases/100 patient y)	Itraconazole 200 mg PO daily	
Coccidioidomycosis	New positive IgM or IgG serologic test in a patient from a disease-endemic area, and CD4+ count < 250 cells/mcL	Fluconazole 400 mg PO daily	

TABLE 8–4 PROPHYLAXIS TO PREVENT FIRST EPISODE OF OPPORTUNISTIC DISEASE AMONG HIV-INFECTED ADULTS (continued)

Opportunistic Infection	Indication	First Choice Therapy	Alternative Regimens
Varicella-zoster virus (VZV) infection	*Preexposure prevention:* Patient with CD4+ count > 200 cells/mcL who have not been vaccinated, have no history of varicella or herpes zoster, or who are seronegative for VZV Note: Routine VZV serologic testing in HIV-infected adults/adolescents is not recommended *Postexposure prevention:* Close contact in susceptible persons (not vaccinated, no history of chickenpox or shingles, or VZV seronegative) with a person who has active varicella or herpes zoster	*Preexposure prevention:* Primary varicella vaccination (Varivax), 2 doses (0.5 mL SQ) administered 3 mo apart If vaccination results in disease because of vaccine virus, treat with acyclovir *Postexposure prevention:* Varicella-zoster immune globulin (VZIG) 125 IU/10 kg (maximum of 625 IU) IM, administered as soon as possible within 10 d after exposure Note: Varicella-zoster immune globulin can be obtained only under a treatment IND (1-800-843-7477, FFF Enterprises) No need to redose if patient receives monthly IVIG > 400 mg/kg with last dose within previous 3 wk	*Preexposure prevention:* VZV-susceptible household contacts of susceptible HIV-infected persons should be vaccinated to prevent potential transmission of VZV to their HIV-infected contacts *Alternative postexposure prevention* (not studied in the HIV population): Preemptive acyclovir 800 mg PO 5 ×/d for 5–7 d Valacyclovir 1 g PO TID × 5–7 d Varicella vaccines should be delayed >72 h after administration of antivirals These two alternatives have not been studied in the HIV population
HPV infection	Patients aged 13–26 y and shared decision-making for those 27–45 y	HPV recombinant vaccine 9 valent (types 6, 11, 16, 18, 31, 33, 45, 52, 58) 0.5 mL IM at 0, 1–2, and 6 mo	Consider additional vaccination with recombinant 9-valent vaccine for patients who completed vaccination with recombinant bivalent or quadrivalent series (unclear who benefits or how cost-effective this is)
Hepatitis A virus (HAV) infection	HAV-susceptible patients with chronic liver disease, or who are injection-drug users, or men who have sex with men	Hepatitis A vaccine 1 mL IM × 2 doses—at 0 and 6–12 mo Reassess IgG antibody response 1 mo after vaccination; revaccinate nonresponders when CD4 count > 200 cells/mcL	If susceptible to both HAV and HBV, combined vaccine (Twinrix) 1 mL IM as a 3-dose series (0, 1, and 6 mo) or 4-dose series (day 0, day 7, days 21–30, and 12 mo)

TABLE 8–4 PROPHYLAXIS TO PREVENT FIRST EPISODE OF OPPORTUNISTIC DISEASE AMONG HIV-INFECTED ADULTS *(continued)*

Opportunistic Infection	Indication	First Choice Therapy	Alternative Regimens
Hepatitis B virus (HBV) infection	No evidence of prior exposure to HBV (anti-HBs < 10 IU/mL) should be vaccinated with HBV vaccine, including patients with CD4+ count <200 cells/mcL Vaccinate early before CD4 falls <350 cells/mcL Patients with CD4 <200 cells/mcL may not respond to vaccination; consider delayed revaccination Vaccine nonresponders (anti-HBs <10 IU/mL 1–2 mo after vaccine series)	HBV vaccine IM (Engerix-B 20 mcg/mL or Recombivax HB 10 mcg/mL) at 0, 1, and 6 mo or 0, 1, 2, and 6 mo *or* Vaccine conjugated to CpG (Heplisav-B) IM at 0 and 1 mo (2-dose series can only be used if both doses are Heplisav-B) *or* Combined HAV and HBV vaccine (Twinrix) 1 mL IM as a 3-dose (0, 1, and 6 mo) or 4-dose series (days 0, 7, 21–30, and 12 mo) If anti-HBs ≤ 10 IU/mL after 1–2 mo from receipt of the vaccine, revaccinate with additional 4-dose series; consider delayed revaccination until sustained increase in CD4 count on ART *Patients with isolated anti-HBc:* Vaccinate × 1 standard dose of HBV. If anti-HBs <100 IU in 1–2 mo, vaccinate with full series and retest anti-HBs	Some experts recommend double dose of either HBV vaccine
Hepatitis B virus (HBV) infection in vaccine nonresponders	Defined as anti-HBs < 10 IU/mL 1 mo after a vaccination series For patients with low CD4+ count at the time of first vaccination series, certain specialists might delay revaccination until after a sustained increase in CD4+ count with ART (CIII)	Revaccinate with a second vaccine series (BIII)	Consider double doses of either HBV vaccine (BI)

TABLE 8–4 PROPHYLAXIS TO PREVENT FIRST EPISODE OF OPPORTUNISTIC DISEASE AMONG HIV-INFECTED ADULTS *(continued)*

Opportunistic Infection	Indication	First Choice Therapy	Alternative Regimens
Malaria	Travel to disease-endemic area	Recommendations are the same for HIV-infected and noninfected patients. One of the following 3 drugs is usually recommended, depending on location: atovaquone/proguanil, doxycycline, or mefloquine. Refer to the following website for the most recent recommendations based on region and drug susceptibility: http://www.cdc.gov/malaria/	
Talaromyces (Penicillium) marneffei infection	Patients with CD4 < 100 cells/mcL who have extended exposure to rural areas of Thailand, Vietnam, or Southern China	Itraconazole 200 mg PO daily	Fluconazole 400 mg PO once weekly

BID, twice daily; BIW, two times weekly; DS, double strength; IM, intramuscular; PO, by mouth; SS, single strength; SQ, subcutaneous; TIW, three times weekly.
Source: From the clinical practice guidelines at *CDC MMWR.* 2009;58(RR04):1–198.

Sources

–Centers for Disease Control and Prevention. Revised Surveillance Case Definition for HIV Infection—United States, 2014. *MMWR Recomm Rep.* 2014;63(RR-03):1–10.

–NIH. *Guidelines for the Prevention and Treatment of Opportunistic Infections in Adult and Adolescents with HIV.* 2023.

IMMUNIZATIONS

Management: All

Recommendations from

➢ **Advisory Committee on Immunization Practices (ACIP) 2024**

–Simultaneously administering all vaccines for which a person is eligible at the time of a visit increases the probability that a child, adolescent, or adult will be vaccinated fully by the appropriate age.

–Routine physical examinations and procedures (eg, measuring temperatures) are not prerequisites for vaccinating persons who appear to be healthy.

–The National Childhood Vaccine Injury Act of 1986 requires health care personnel and vaccine manufacturers to report to Vaccine Adverse Event Reporting System specific adverse events that occur after vaccination.

–See Table 8–5 for changes to the 2024 immunization schedule.

TABLE 8–5   ACIP CHANGES IN THE 2024 IMMUNIZATION SCHEDULE
See Appendix for Full Immunization Schedule for Children and Adults
ACIP CHANGES IN THE 2024 PEDIATRIC IMMUNIZATION SCHEDULE *RSV: give nirsevimab during RSV season for all infants ages less than 8 mo and children 8 to 19 mo who are at increased risk for severe RSV disease. *COVID-19: starting at 6 mo, one or more doses of updated (2023–2024 formula) *Tdap: dose recommended at age 11–12 y is the adolescent Tdap booster dose. *Source:* Wodi, et al. ACIP schedule for children and adolescents ages 18 years or younger US, 2024. *MMWR.* 2024; 73(1):6–10.
ACIP CHANGES IN THE 2024 ADULT IMMUNIZATION SCHEDULE *RSV: shared clinical decision-making for adults aged >= 60 y and seasonal administration during pregnancy (use of Abrysvo during 32–36 wk gestation starting September through January) *Influenza: persons with a history of egg allergy can be vaccinated with any influenza vaccine indicated for the recipient's age and health status *COVID-19: all adults are recommended to receive at least 1 dose of an updated (2023–2024 formula) *Inactivated poliovirus: adults who are known or suspected to be unvaccinated or incompletely vaccinated to complete the 3-dose inactivated poliovirus primary vaccination series. One time, lifetime inactivated poliovirus booster dose to adults who have completed the primary series and who are at increased risk for exposure to poliovirus *Hepatitis B: shared clinical decision-making for persons >= 60 y with diabetes *Source:* Murthy, et al. ACIP schedule for adults 19 years and older US, 2024. *Morbidity and Mortality Weekly Report (MMWR).* 2024; 73(1); 11–15.

Source
  –CDC. *Pinkbook Course Book: Epidemiology of Vaccine Preventable Diseases*. www.cdc.gov/
  vaccines/pubs/pinkbook/index.html

INFLUENZA

Prevention: Adults and Children

Recommendations from

> CDC 2022, AAP 2022

  –Vaccinate for influenza yearly in all persons aged >6 mo.
  –All children aged 6 mo to 8 y should receive 2 doses of the vaccine (>4 wk apart) during their first season of vaccination.
  –Use any licensed influenza vaccine product appropriate for age and health status. One product is not recommended over another (eg, inactivated vs. live attenuated).
  –For children that require 2 doses, offer vaccines as soon as they become available, with the recommended dose(s) ideally received by the end of October.
  –For most adults, particularly 65 y and older, the goal is to immunize after August due to concern of waning immunity.
  –Continue vaccinations as long as influenza virus circulates and vaccine is available.
  –Adults 65 y and older should preferentially receive any one of the following higher dose or adjuvanted influenza vaccines: quadrivalent high-dose inactivated influenza vaccine, quadrivalent recombinant influenza vaccine, or quadrivalent adjuvanted inactivated influenza vaccine. If none of these are available, then any other age-appropriate influenza vaccine should be used.
  –Influenza vaccine is contraindicated only if history of severe allergic reaction is found. Egg allergy is not a contraindication, though persons with history of severe reaction should be monitored after receiving the vaccine.
  –Individuals who have experienced Guillain-Barre syndrome within 6 wk of a previous influenza vaccine are not contraindicated to receiving the flu vaccine but should have a detailed discussion on the risk and benefits of future influenza vaccinations.
  –Contraindications for use of live-attenuated flu vaccine:
  • Less than 2 y of age or greater than 49-y-old.
  • History of severe allergic reaction (eg, anaphylaxis) to any component of the vaccine (other than egg) or to a previous dose of any influenza vaccine.
  • Concomitant aspirin or salicylate-containing therapy in children and adolescents.
  • Children aged 2 through 4 y who have received a diagnosis of asthma or with history of wheezing during the preceding 12 mo.
  • Children and adults who are immunocompromised due to any cause, including but not limited to medications, congenital or acquired immunodeficiency states, HIV infection, congenital, or functional asplenia.
  • Close contacts and caregivers or severely immunosuppressed persons who require a protective environment.

- Pregnancy.
- Cerebrospinal fluid leak.
- Cochlear implants.
- Receipt of influenza antiviral medication within the previous 48 h for oseltamivir and zanamivir, 5 d for peramivir, and 17 d for baloxavir.

–Precautions for use of live-attenuated influenza vaccine:

- Moderate or severe acute illness with or without fever.
- Nasal congestion that may interfere with administration should result in deferral or switch to another type of influenza vaccine.
- History of Guillain-Barre syndrome within 6 wk of receipt of influenza vaccine.
- Asthma in persons aged 5 y and greater.
- Other underlying medical conditions that might predispose to complications from influenza (eg, chronic pulmonary, cardiovascular, renal, hepatic, neurologic, hematologic, or metabolic disorders).

Practice Pearl

- Highest-risk groups for influenza complications are:
  - Children aged 6 mo to 5 y.
  - Adults aged ≥50 y.
  - Persons with chronic medical conditions or who are immunocompromised.[1]
  - Pregnant individuals or people who will be pregnant during the influenza season or breastfeeding.
  - Residents of extended-care facilities.
  - Morbidly obese (BMI > 40) persons.
  - Health care personnel.
  - Household contacts of persons with high-risk medical conditions or caregivers of children aged <5 y or adults aged >50 y.
  - Children and adolescents receiving long-term aspirin therapy.
  - American Indians or Alaska Natives.
  - People with a history of influenza-associated encephalopathy.

Sources

–*Pediatrics.* 2022;150(4):e2022059274.

–*MMWR Prevention and Control of Seasonal Influenza with Vaccines: Recommendations of the Advisory Committee on Immunization Practices* (ACIP). US 2022-23:2022;71 (No. RR-1).

Prevention: Children and Adults Exposed to Influenza

Recommendations from

> CDC 2021, AAP 2021

The following situations warrant chemoprophylaxis:

–Children at high risk for complications who cannot receive vaccine, or within 2 wk of receiving vaccine.

---

[1] Chronic heart, lung, renal, liver, hematologic, cancer, metabolic, neuromuscular or neurodevelopmental, or seizure disorders, severe cognitive dysfunction, diabetes, HIV infection, or immunosuppression.

–Family members or health care providers who are unimmunized and likely to have ongoing exposure to high-risk or unimmunized children younger than 24 mo of age.

–Unimmunized staff and children in an institutional setting during an outbreak.

–PrEP for close contacts of infected person who are at high risk of complications if less than 48 h since exposure.

–Consider as supplement to vaccine if immune compromised.

Practice Pearls

- Influenza vaccination is the best way to prevent influenza.
- Antiviral chemoprophylaxis is not a substitute for influenza vaccination.
- Agents for chemoprophylaxis of influenza A (H1N1) and B: zanamivir or oseltamivir.
- Children at high risk for complications include those with chronic diseases such as asthma, diabetes, cardiac disease, immune suppression, and neurodevelopmental disorders.
- If child < 3 mo of age, use of oseltamivir for chemoprophylaxis is not recommended unless situation is judged critical due to limited data in this age group.

Sources

–Recommendations for Prevention and Control of Influenza in Children, 2021–2022. *Pediatrics*. 2021;148(4):e2021053744.

–CDC. https://www.cdc.gov/flu/professionals/antivirals/summary-clinicians.htm

Management: Adults

Recommendations from

➤ CDC 2020

–Test for concomitant SARS-CoV-2 (COVID-19).

–Prioritize treatment: start antiviral treatment as soon as possible for any patient with suspected or confirmed influenza if hospitalized; severe, complicated, or progressive illness; or higher risk for influenza complications, while awaiting lab confirmation.

- Lab-confirmed cases of influenza within 48 h of symptom onset.
- Strongly suspected influenza within 48 h of symptom onset.
- Hospitalized patients with severe, complicated, or progressive lab-confirmed influenza or influenza-like illness with high likelihood of complications even if >48 h from symptom onset.
  - Children aged younger than 2 y or adults aged 65 y and older.
  - Persons with chronic pulmonary (including asthma), cardiovascular (except hypertension alone), renal, hepatic, hematologic (including sickle cell disease), metabolic (including diabetes mellitus), or neurologic disorders (including disorders of the brain, spinal cord, peripheral nerve, and muscle, such as cerebral palsy, epilepsy [seizure disorders], stroke, intellectual disability, moderate-to-severe developmental delay, muscular dystrophy, or spinal cord injury).
  - Persons with immunosuppression, including that caused by medications or by HIV infection.

- Women who are pregnant or postpartum (within 2 wk after delivery).
- Persons aged younger than 19 y who are receiving long-term aspirin therapy.
- American Indians/Alaska Natives.
- Persons who are extremely obese (ie, BMI equal to or greater than 40).
- Residents of nursing homes and other long-term care facilities.

–Antiviral chemoprophylaxis after exposure to a person with influenza is recommended for:
- Prevention of influenza in persons at high risk for influenza complications during the first 2 wk following vaccination.
- Patients at high risk for complications from influenza who have contraindications to the influenza vaccine.
- Patients with severe immune deficiencies or others who might not respond to influenza vaccination, such as persons receiving immunosuppressive medications.
- Do not give if more than 48 h have elapsed since first exposure to a person with influenza.

–Antiviral treatment options include oseltamivir, zanamivir, and peramivir.
- Oseltamivir (oral) for influenza A or B:
  - Treatment dose: 75 mg PO BID × 5 d.
  - Chemoprophylaxis dose: 75 mg PO QD × 7 d following last known exposure.
  - Will need to be renally dosed for patients with decreased GFR.
- Zanamivir (inhaled) for influenza A or B:
  - Treatment dose: 10 mg (two 5-mg inhalations) BID × 5 d.
  - Chemoprophylaxis dose: 10 mg (two 5-mg inhalations) QD × 7 d after last known exposure.
  - Avoid in patients with underlying respiratory disease (eg, asthma, COPD).
- Peramivir (IV) for influenza A or B:
  - Treatment dose: 600 mg IV once for creatinine clearance ≥ 50 mL/min × 1 dose.
  - 200 mg IV once for creatinine clearance 30–49 mL/min.
  - 100 mg IV once for creatinine clearance 10–29 mL/min.
  - ESRD patients on dialysis should receive a dose after dialysis at a dose adjusted based on creatinine clearance.
  - Not recommended for chemoprophylaxis.
  - Baloxavir (oral):
    - Treatment dose: 40 to <80 kg = 40 mg × 1; ≥80 kg = 80 mg.
  - Do not use as chemoprophylaxis.

Sources

–http://www.cdc.gov/mmwr/preview/mmwrhtml/rr6001a1.htm
–https://www.cdc.gov/flu/professionals/antivirals/summary-clinicians.htm#:~:text=The%20 recommended%20treatment%20course%20for,oral%20baloxavir%20for%201%20day

Management: Children

Recommendations from

➢ ACIP 2011, CDC 2020

–Prioritize treatment: start antiviral treatment as soon as possible for any patient with suspected or confirmed influenza if hospitalized; severe, complicated, or progressive illness; or higher risk for influenza complications, while awaiting lab confirmation.

–Treatment indicated if symptom onset within 48 h and:

• Any child hospitalized with presumed influenza or with severe, complicated, or progressive illness attributable to influenza, regardless of influenza immunization status.

• Influenza infection of any severity in children at high risk for complications of influenza infection.

• Children aged <2 y.

–Chemoprophylaxis indicated as above for adults.

–Antiviral treatment options include oseltamivir and zanamivir.

• Oseltamivir for influenza A or B treatment dose (5 d):

  ○ If <1-y-old: 3 mg/kg/dose BID.

  ○ If 1 y or older, dose varies by child's weight:

   ○ 15 kg or less, the dose is 30 mg BID.

   ○ >15 to 23 kg, the dose is 45 mg BID.

   ○ >23 to 40 kg, the dose is 60 mg BID.

   ○ >40 kg, the dose is 75 mg BID.

• Oseltamivir chemoprophylaxis dose (7 d):

  ○ Not recommended for <3 mo of age.

  ○ If child is 3 mo or older and younger than 1 y: 3 mg/kg/dose QD.

  ○ If 1 y or older, dose varies by child's weight:

   ○ 15 kg or less, the dose is 30 mg QD.

   ○ >15 to 23 kg, the dose is 45 mg QD.

   ○ >23 to 40 kg, the dose is 60 mg QD.

   ○ >40 kg, the dose is 75 mg QD.

• Zanamivir for influenza A or B:

  ○ Treatment dose (7 y or older): 10 mg (two 5-mg inhalations) BID × 5 d.

  ○ Chemoprophylaxis dose (5 y or older): 10 mg (two 5-mg inhalations) QD × 7 d.

  ○ Avoid in patients with underlying respiratory disease (eg, asthma, COPD).

• Peramivir (IV) for influenza A or B: (2–12 y of age).

  ○ Treatment dose: 12 mg/kg/dose infusion over 15 min (max 600 mg).

  ○ Not recommended for chemoprophylaxis.

• Baloxavir (oral) ≥12 y:

  ○ Treatment dose: >40 to <80 kg = 40 mg × 1; ≥80 kg = 80 mg.

  ○ Do not use for chemoprophylaxis.

Practice Pearls

- Consider an influenza nasal swab for diagnosis during influenza season in:
  - Persons with acute onset of fever and respiratory illness.
  - Persons with fever and acute exacerbation of chronic lung disease.
  - Infants and children with fever of unclear etiology.
  - Severely ill persons with fever or hypothermia.
- Rapid influenza antigen tests have 70%–90% sensitivity in children and 40%–60% sensitivity in adults.
- Direct or indirect fluorescent antibody staining is useful in screening tests.
- Influenza PCR may be used as a confirmatory test.

Source
–http://www.cdc.gov/mmwr/preview/mmwrhtml/rr6001a1.htm

LYME DISEASE

Management: Adults and Children

Recommendations from

> AAN 2020, IDSA 2006

Evaluation
–Diagnose clinically if 1 or more lesions are consistent with erythema migrans.
–If lesions are suggestive but low risk, perform antibody testing on an acute phase sample followed by antibody testing on convalescent phase serum sample if initial testing negative.
–Use serum antibody testing over cerebrospinal fluid PCR or culture sample testing for Lyme neuroborreliosis.
–Tick can be submitted for speciation at most labs or health department. Do not test the tick for *B. burgdorferi* as it does not predict clinical infection.
–Do not routinely test for Lyme disease in workup of psychiatric illness, but can be considered in the evaluation of some neurologic disorders.

Therapies
–Promptly remove attached tick and mouthparts by mechanical means (ie, tweezer). Do not burn or apply noxious chemicals or petroleum products to coax detachment.
–Prophylaxis dose: if *I. scapularis* tick is attached for ≥36 h, prophylaxis can be started within 72 h of removal, bite was from identified *Ixodes* spp. vector in an area where Lyme is endemic.
  - Treat adults with a single dose of doxycycline 200 mg.
  - Treat children ≥ 8 y with doxycycline 4.4 mg/kg to max 200 mg.
–Early illness:
  - Adults: doxycycline 100 mg PO BID × 10 d (amoxicillin or cefuroxime × 14 d, if doxycycline contraindication). Azithromycin as second-line therapy × 7 d.
  - Children (≥8 y): amoxicillin, cefuroxime axetil.
–Treat pregnant patients similar to other adults, but do not use doxycycline.

–Early neurologic Lyme:
- Adults: ceftriaxone 2 g IV × 14–21 d.
- Children: ceftriaxone 50–75 mg/kg/d IV × 14 d.
- Alternative agents: cefotaxime, IV PCN, or oral doxycycline.

–Lyme carditis: perform ECG only if suggestive symptoms:
- Adults: ceftriaxone 2 g IV × 14–21 d, transition to PO doxycycline when appropriate to complete course.

–Late Lyme arthritis:
- Adults: doxycycline 100 mg PO BID × 28 d.
- Consider ceftriaxone IV for 2–4 wk if no or minimal response to initial oral antibiotic course.
- Children: amoxicillin 50 mg/kg/d divided TID (max 500 mg/dose) × 28 d.

Source
–https://www.idsociety.org/practice-guideline/lyme-disease/

MOLLUSCUM CONTAGIOSUM

Management: Adults and Children

Recommendations from

⮞ BASHH 2021

–Diagnose clinically.

–Avoid autoinoculation via shaving, electrolysis, and waxing. Do not squeeze lesions full of infectious virus.

–Avoid transmission, which occurs via sex, close contact, or fomite spread: do not share linens. Cover lesions with waterproof bandages prior to swimming. Condoms may reduce transmission. Do not share sex toys.

–Treatment options:
- Observation, as lesions usually resolve spontaneously in 12–18 mo.
- Liquid nitrogen.
- Podophyllotoxin 0.5%.
- Emollients and mild topical steroids.
- If HIV positive: treat lesions with above agents, start ART.
- Alternative regimens: cautery and curettage if few lesions. Light-emitting and pulsed dye laser, imiquimod 5%.

Source
–https://www.bashhguidelines.org/media/1309/mc-2021.pdf

OTITIS MEDIA, ACUTE

Management: Children

Recommendations from

> NICE 2022, AAP 2019, CDC 2017

Evaluation

–See Fig. 8–2 for diagnostic and treatment pathway.

–Diagnose when bulging tympanic membrane with effusion or otorrhea (not due to otitis externa).

Therapies

–When appropriate, use nonantibiotic treatments (as most cases resolve without antibiotic treatment):

- Prescribe acetaminophen or ibuprofen; ensure correct dosing.
- Offer eardrops with anesthetic or analgesic to improve pain.
- Do not prescribe decongestants, antihistamines, or oral steroids.

–Antibiotic strategy:

- Consider watchful waiting with backup antibiotic prescription if there is no improvement at 48 h with pain control for mild unilateral cases in children 6–23 mo or >24 mo with unilateral or bilateral illness.

FIG. 8–2 DIAGNOSIS AND TREATMENT OF AOM IN CHILDREN.

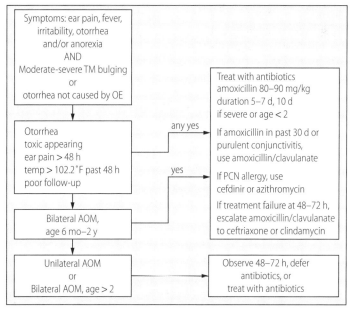

Source: Adapted from Am Fam Physician. 2019;100(6):350–356.

- Antibiotic selection: use amoxicillin first-line 125–500 mg TID (based on age). Amoxicillin-clavulanate has more side effects.
- Clarithromycin (NICE) or cefdinir (AAP) are alternatives in allergy or intolerance.
- Use amoxicillin-clavulanate if not improved in 2–3 d on amoxicillin or had taken amoxicillin within the past 30 d (0.25 mL/kg of 125/31 mg suspension based on weight and age).
- Duration of antibiotic: 5–7 d, consider 10 d if <2 or severe.
- Do not use prophylaxic antibiotics not recommended.

Practice Pearls

- Usually self-limited, caused by viruses and bacteria (commonly: *Streptococcus pneumoniae, Haemophilus influenzae, Moraxella catarrhalis,* and *Streptococcus pyogenes*).
- Complications: temporary hearing loss and tympanic membrane perforation (antibiotics do not affect rates of these complications).
- Antibiotics do not reduce pain at 24 h. There is a small benefit to pain at 23 d. They do reduce tympanic membrane perforations, but the effect is small.
- Antibiotic benefits are greatest for children ≤ 2 y and children with otorrhea suggesting perforation.
- Risk factors include age < 5 y, craniofacial anomalies, family history, birth weight < 2.5 kg, male sex, birth < 37 wk EGA, prior ear infections, recent viral URI, and White ethnicity.
- Potentially modifiable risk factors include exposure to tobacco smoke and air pollution, crowded living conditions, GERD, lack of breast feeding, pacifier use after 6 mo, and supine bottle feeding.

Sources
–https://www.nice.org.uk/guidance/ng91
–https://www.cdc.gov/antibiotic-use/clinicians/pediatric-treatment-rec.html
–*Pediatrics.* 2013;131(3):e964–e999.
–*Am Fam Physician.* 2019;100(6):350–356.

RESPIRATORY TRACT INFECTIONS, LOWER (COMMUNITY-ACQUIRED PNEUMONIA)

Management: Adults

Recommendations from

➢ ATS 2019, ESCMID 2011, IDSA 2007, NICE 2023, ACP 2023

Evaluation
–Use severity-of-illness score to determine if inpatient treatment is appropriate:
- CURB-65: confusion, uremia, respiratory rate, low blood pressure, age ≥ 65.
- Pneumonia severity index.
- Severe community-acquired pneumonia: 1 major or 3 minor (IDA):
  ○ Minor:
    ○ Respiratory rate ≥ 30 breath/min.

- - PaO$_2$/FiO$_2$ ratio ≤ 250.
    - Multilobar infiltrates.
    - Confusion/disorientation.
    - Uremia (BUN ≥ 20 mg/dL).
    - Leukopenia (WBC ≤ 4000 cells/mcL).
    - Thrombocytopenia (platelet count ≤ 100,000/mcL).
    - Hypothermia (temp ≤ 36°C).
    - Hypotension requiring "aggressive fluid resuscitation."
  - Major:
    - Septic shock.
    - Respiratory failure requiring mechanical ventilation.
- Obtain chest radiograph; if suspected or confirmed sepsis with a nonspecific chest radiograph, CT chest with or without IV contrast is usually appropriate.
- Sputum evaluation and blood cultures are not recommended for outpatients (only for moderate-to-high severity).
- Routine testing for antigens is not recommended, ie, pneumococcal or *Legionella*, unless severe illness (former) or community outbreak (latter) (only for moderate-to-high severity).
- CRP (point of care): if <2: do not prescribe antibiotics; delay antibiotic if >2, but <10 and reassess in 48 h; prescribe antibiotics if >10.
- Test for influenza during endemic time; rapid test preferred.
- Do not use procalcitonin to guide antibiotic initiation.
- Consider inflammatory markers, notably CRP, at baseline and to trend 48–72 h after hospital admission if improvement is uncertain.
- Do not routinely order follow-up chest imaging if symptoms are improving.

Therapies
- Empiric therapy based on local antibiotic resistance patterns:
  - Previously healthy, no risk for drug-resistant *Streptococcus pneumoniae*:
    - Amoxicillin 1 g PO TID.
    - Doxycycline 100 mg PO BID.
    - Macrolide (azithromycin, clarithromycin, or erythromycin) only in areas where resistance < 25%.
  - Comorbidities (chronic heart, lung, liver, or renal disease; diabetes; alcohol use disorder; malignancy; asplenia; immune suppression; antimicrobials in past 3 mo):
    - Combination therapy:
      - Amoxicillin/clavulanate 500 mg/125 mg PO TID or 875 mg/125 mg PO BID or 2000 mg/125 mg PO BID.
      - Cephalosporin (cefpodoxime 200 mg PO BID or cefuroxime 500 mg PO BID).
      - Macrolide (azithromycin 500 mg PO first day, then 250 mg PO daily or clarithromycin 500 BID) or doxycycline 100 mg PO BID.
  - Monotherapy:
    - Respiratory fluoroquinolone (moxifloxacin 400 mg PO daily, gemifloxacin 320 mg PO daily, or levofloxacin 750 mg PO daily).

o Beta-lactam + macrolide.

o If high rate of *S. pneumoniae* macrolide-resistance (MIC ≥ 16 mcg/mL), then consider alternative agent to a macrolide.

–Duration of antibiotics: 5 d; consider longer duration if delayed improvement of symptoms.

Practice Pearls

- Consider aspiration pneumonia in patients with pneumonia and dysphagia. Do not add anaerobic coverage unless lung abscess or empyema is suspected.
- Steroids are not routinely recommended solely for pneumonia.
- For *S. pneumoniae*:
  - Erythromycin MIC > 0.5 mg/L predicts clinical failure.
  - PCN MIC ≤ 8 mg/L predicts IV PCN susceptibility.
- Influenza in patients being treated for community-acquired pneumonia: treat with anti-influenza treatment independent of duration of symptoms prior to diagnosis, but not the converse.
- A CRP < 2 mg/dL at presentation with symptoms > 24 h makes pneumonia highly unlikely; a CRP > 10 mg/dL makes pneumonia likely.
- Indications for antibiotics in lower respiratory tract infections:
  - Suspected pneumonia.
  - Acute exacerbation of COPD with increased dyspnea, sputum volume, and sputum purulence for 5 d of antibiotic therapy.

Sources

–https://academic.oup.com/cid/article/44/Supplement_2/S27/372079

–http://www.escmid.org/fileadmin/src/media/PDFs/4ESCMID_Library/2Medical _Guidelines/ ESCMID_Guidelines/Woodhead_et_al_CMI_Sep_2011_LRTI_GL_fulltext.pdf

–https://www.acr.org/Clinical-Resources/ACR-Appropriateness-Criteria

–https://www.atsjournals.org/doi/full/10.1164/rccm.201908-1581ST

–https://www.nice.org.uk/guidance/cg191

–https://pubmed.ncbi.nlm.nih.gov/33819054/

Management: Infants and Children

Recommendations from

➢ IDSA 2011

Evaluation

–Use rapid viral detection tests. Avoid urinary antigen tests and blood cultures in children being treated as outpatients.

–Avoid chest X-ray unless ill enough to be hospitalized or failed initial antibiotic therapy. Avoid routine follow-up imaging to document improvement.

Therapies

–Hospitalize children with respiratory distress or hypoxia (<90%), or if <6 mo old.

–As viral etiologies cause the majority of pneumonia-like illness in preschool-aged children, do not routinely prescribe antibiotics.

–If there is evidence of bacterial origin, use amoxicillin, as *S. pneumoniae* is the most common etiology.

–If there is evidence of atypical pathogens, use macrolides. Test for *M. pneumoniae* if results can be available quickly enough to guide therapy.

–If influenza virus is prevalent in the community, start anti-influenza therapy immediately while awaiting diagnostic test results.

–Consider 10-d duration of antibiotics, though shorter durations may be acceptable for milder illness.

–After initiating therapy, follow up in 48–72 h to ensure improvement.

Practice Pearl

- For outpatients, a duration of 5 d of amoxicillin 75–100 mg/kg/d is equivalent to a duration of 10 d. (*JAMA Pediatr.* 2021;175(5):475–482)

Source
–*Clin Infect Dis.* 2011:53(7):e25–e76.

RESPIRATORY TRACT INFECTIONS, UPPER

See above section on Common Cold.

SEXUALLY TRANSMITTED INFECTIONS

Prevention: Adults and Adolescents

Recommendations from

➤ USPSTF 2020

–Counsel all sexually active adolescents and adults at increased risk for STIs.

–Population at risk: patients diagnosed with an STI within the past year, not consistently using condoms, having multiple sex partners or having a partner(s) at high risk for STIs, belonging to a population that has a high STI prevalence (such as persons seeking STI testing or attending an STI clinic, sexual and gender minorities, persons living with HIV, persons with injection drug use, persons who exchange sex for money or drugs, persons who have recently been in a correctional facility, and some racial/ethnic minority groups).

–Provide behavioral counseling to sexually active adolescents and to adults at increased risk:

- Deliver counseling in person, refer patients to outside counseling services, or inform patients about media-based interventions.
- Interventions that include group counseling, involve more than 120 min of counseling, and are delivered over several sessions have the strongest effect in preventing STIs.
  - Counseling interventions shorter than 30 min delivered in a single session may also be effective.
- Provide information on common STIs and STI transmission; aim to increase motivation or commitment to safer sex practices; and provide training in condom use, communication about safer sex, problem solving, and other pertinent skills.

Source
    –*JAMA*. 2020;324(7):674–681.

Management: Adults and Adolescents

Recommendations from

➢ CDC

    –See Table 8–6 for recommended treatment regimens for various STIs.

SINUSITIS

Management: Adults and Children

Recommendations from

➢ EPOS 2020, CDC 2017, NICE 2017, IDSA 2012

Evaluation

–Do not obtain sinus radiographs.

Therapies

–Advise patients that etiology is usually viral, course self-limited lasting for 2–3 wk.

–Treat with decongestants, nasal irrigation, and zinc > 75 mg/d within 24 h of symptom onset.

–Consider nasal steroid and systemic steroid, as they have small beneficial effect.

–Avoid vitamin C and homeopathy, herbal medication (BNO1016 and *Pelargonium sidoides* drops) as there is limited evidence, and antihistamines which offer no benefit.

–Avoid antibiotics early in illness.

–If persistent symptoms (>10 d) or if severe (>3–4 d + fever or purulent discharge) or change in symptoms (eg, "double sickening"), consider no antibiotic or backup antibiotic and/or nasal corticosteroid (off-label). (NICE 2017)

–If systemic symptoms or high-risk comorbidity or signs of more serious illness, offer antibiotics.

–Antibiotics: (CDC)

- Adult > 18-y-old:
    ○ Amoxicillin or amoxicillin-clavulanate × 10 d.
    ○ Macrolides not recommended due to resistance.
    ○ PCN allergy: doxycycline or respiratory fluoroquinolone (levofloxacin or moxifloxacin).
- Children ≤ 18-y-old:
    ○ Amoxicillin or amoxicillin-clavulanate × 10 d.
    ○ Intractable vomiting: ceftriaxone IM × 1, then oral antibiotics.

Sources
    –https://epos2020.com/Documents/supplement_29.pdf
    –https://academic.oup.com/cid/article/54/8/1041/364141
    –https://www.cdc.gov/antibiotic-use/community/for-hcp/outpatient-hcp/adult-treatment-rec.html
    –https://www.nice.org.uk/guidance/ng79

TABLE 8–6 SEXUALLY TRANSMITTED DISEASES TREATMENT GUIDELINES

Infection	Recommended Treatment	Alternative Treatment
Chancroid	• Azithromycin 1 g PO × 1 • Ceftriaxone 250 mg IM × 1	• Ciprofloxacin 500 mg PO BID for 3 d • Erythromycin base 500 mg PO TID for 7 d
Genital HSV, first episode	• Acyclovir 400 mg PO TID × 7–10 d[a] • Famciclovir 250 mg PO TID × 7–10 d[a] • Valacyclovir 1 g PO BID × 7–10 d[a]	• Acyclovir 200 mg PO 5 times a day for 7–10 d[a]
Genital HSV, suppressive therapy	• Acyclovir 400 mg PO BID • Valacyclovir 500 mg or 1 g PO daily • Famciclovir 250 mg PO BID	
Genital HSV, episodic therapy for recurrent disease	• Acyclovir 800 mg PO TID × 2 d • Acyclovir 800 mg PO BID × 5 d • Valacyclovir 500 mg PO BID × 3 d • Valacyclovir 1 g PO daily × 5 d • Famciclovir 125 mg PO BID × 5 d • Famciclovir 1000 mg PO BID × 1 d • Famciclovir 500 mg PO × 1 then 250 mg BID × 2 d	
Genital HSV, suppressive therapy for HIV-positive patients	• Acyclovir 400–800 mg PO BID–TID • Famciclovir 500 mg PO BID • Valacyclovir 500 mg PO BID	
Genital HSV, episodic therapy for recurrent genital HSV in HIV-positive patients	• Acyclovir 400 mg PO TID × 5–10 d • Famciclovir 500 mg PO BID × 5–10 d • Valacyclovir 1 g PO BID × 5–10 d	
Granuloma inguinale (donovanosis)	• Azithromycin 1 g PO once per week or 500 mg daily for at least 3 wk and until all lesions have completely healed	• Doxycycline 100 mg PO BID × ≥3 wk • Erythromycin 500 PO QID × 3 wk • TMP-SMX 160/800 mg PO BID × 3 wk • Continue all regimens until lesions are completely healed
		• Erythromycin base 500 mg PO QID × ≥3 wk • TMP-SMX 1 double-strength (160/800 mg) tablet PO BID × ≥3 wk • Continue all of these treatments until all lesions have completely healed

TABLE 8-6 SEXUALLY TRANSMITTED DISEASES TREATMENT GUIDELINES *(continued)*

Infection	Recommended Treatment	Alternative Treatment
Lymphogranuloma venereum	• Doxycycline 100 mg PO BID for × 21 d	• Azithromycin 1 g PO weekly × 3 wk • Erythromycin base 500 mg PO QID × 21 d
Primary and secondary syphilis in adults	• Benzathine PCN G 2.4 million units IM × 1	• Doxycycline 100 mg PO BID × 14 d • Tetracycline 500 mg PO QID × 14 d • Amoxicillin 3 g + probenecid 500 mg, both PO BID × 14 d
Primary and secondary syphilis in infants and children	• Benzathine PCN G 50,000 units/kg IM, up to the adult dose of 2.4 million units × 1	
Early latent syphilis in adults	• Benzathine PCN G 2.4 million units IM × 1	
Early latent syphilis in children	• Benzathine PCN G 50,000 units/kg IM, up to the adult dose of 2.4 million units × 1	
Late latent syphilis or latent syphilis of unknown duration in adults	• Benzathine PCN G 2.4 million units IM weekly × 3 doses	• Doxycycline 100 mg PO BID × 4 wk
Late latent syphilis or latent syphilis of unknown duration in children	• Benzathine PCN G 50,000 units/kg, up to the adult dose of 2.4 million units, IM weekly × 3 doses	
Tertiary syphilis	• Benzathine PCN G 2.4 million units IM weekly × 3 doses	• Doxycycline 100 mg PO BID × 4 wk
Neurosyphilis	• Aqueous crystalline PCN G 3–4 million units IV q4 h × 10–14 d	• Procaine PCN 2.4 million units IM daily × 10–14 d PLUS • Probenecid 500 mg PO QID × 10–14 d
Syphilis, pregnant persons	• Pregnant persons should be treated with the PCN regimen appropriate for their stage of infection	• No good alternatives. Recommend PCN allergy test and desensitization if patient has reported PCN allergy
Congenital syphilis	• Aqueous crystalline PCN G 50,000 units/kg/dose IV q12 h × 7 d; then q8 h × 3 more days	• Procaine PCN G 50,000 units/kg/dose IM daily × 10 d • Benzathine PCN G 50,000 units/kg/dose IM × 1

TABLE 8–6   SEXUALLY TRANSMITTED DISEASES TREATMENT GUIDELINES (continued)

Infection	Recommended Treatment	Alternative Treatment
Older children with syphilis	• Aqueous crystalline PCN G 50,000 units/kg IV q4–6 h × 10 d	
Nongonococcal urethritis	• Doxycycline 100 mg PO BID × 7 d	• Azithromycin 1 g PO × 1 • Azithromycin 500 mg PO × 1, then 250 mg PO × 4 d
Recurrent or persistent urethritis	• Metronidazole 2 g PO × 1 • Tinidazole 2 g PO × 1 • Azithromycin 1 g PO × 1	
Cervicitis[b]	• Doxycycline 100 mg PO BID × 7 d	• Azithromycin 1 g PO × 1
Chlamydia infections in adolescents, adults[b]	• Doxycycline 100 mg PO BID × 7 d	• Azithromycin 1 g PO × 1 • Levofloxacin 500 mg PO daily × 7 d
Chlamydia infections in pregnancy[b]	• Azithromycin 1 g PO × 1	• Amoxicillin 500 mg PO TID × 7 d • Erythromycin base 500 mg PO QID × 7 d • Erythromycin ethylsuccinate 800 mg PO QID × 7 d
Ophthalmia neonatorum from *C. trachomatis*	• Erythromycin base or ethylsuccinate 50 mg/kg/d PO QID × 14 d	
Ophthalmia neonatorum prophylaxis	• Erythromycin (0.5%) ophthalmic ointment in each eye × 1	
Ophthalmia neonatorum caused by gonococcus	• Ceftriaxone 25–50 mg/kg, not to exceed 250 mg, IV/IM × 1	
C. trachomatis pneumonia in infants	• Erythromycin base or ethylsuccinate 50 mg/kg/d PO QID × 14 d	
Chlamydia infections in children ≥ 45 kg	• Erythromycin base or ethylsuccinate 50 mg/kg/d PO QID × 14 d	
Chlamydia infections in children ≥ 45 kg and age ≥ 8 y	• Azithromycin 1 g PO × 1	

TABLE 8–6   SEXUALLY TRANSMITTED DISEASES TREATMENT GUIDELINES *(continued)*

Infection	Recommended Treatment	Alternative Treatment
Chlamydia infections in children age ≥ 8 y	• Azithromycin 1 g PO × 1 • Doxycycline 100 mg PO BID × 7 d	
Uncomplicated gonococcal infections of the cervix, urethra, pharynx, or rectum in adults or children ≥ 45 kg	• Ceftriaxone 500 mg IM × 1 if <150 kg. If >150 kg, ceftriaxone 1 g IM × 1 • Empirically treat for chlamydia if not ruled out with testing with doxycycline 100 mg BID × 7 d	• If cephalosporin allergy: • Gentamicin 240 mg IM × 1 + azithromycin 2 g PO × 1 • If ceftriaxone not available: cefixime 800 mg PO × 1 • Empirically treat for chlamydia if not ruled out with testing with doxycycline 100 mg BID × 7 d
Gonococcal conjunctivitis in adults or children ≥ 45 kg	• Ceftriaxone 1 g IM × 1	
Gonococcal meningitis or endocarditis in adults or children ≥ 45 kg	• Ceftriaxone 1 g IV q12 h • Empirically treat for chlamydia if not ruled out with testing with doxycycline 100 mg BID × 7 d	
Disseminated gonococcal infection in adults or children ≥ 45 kg	• Ceftriaxone 1 g IV/IM daily • Empirically treat for chlamydia if not ruled out with testing with doxycycline 100 mg BID × 7 d	• Cefotaxime 1 g IV q8 h • Ceftizoxime 1 g IV q8 h
Prophylactic treatment of infants born to mothers with gonococcal infection	• Ceftriaxone 25–50 mg/kg, not to exceed 250 mg, IV/IM × 1	
Uncomplicated gonococcal infections of the cervix, urethra, pharynx, or rectum in children ≥ 45 kg	• Ceftriaxone 125 mg IM × 1 if <150 kg	
Gonococcal infections with bacteremia or arthritis in children or adults	• Ceftriaxone 50 mg/kg (maximum dose 1 g) IM/IV daily × 7 d	

TABLE 8–6   SEXUALLY TRANSMITTED DISEASES TREATMENT GUIDELINES *(continued)*

Infection	Recommended Treatment	Alternative Treatment
Bacterial vaginosis	• Metronidazole 500 mg PO BID × 7 d[c] • Metronidazole gel 0.75%, 1 applicator (5 g) IVag daily × 5 d • Clindamycin cream 2%, 1 applicator (5 g) IVag qhs × 7 d[d]	• Tinidazole 2 g PO daily × 3 d • Clindamycin 300 mg PO BID × 7 d • Clindamycin ovules 100 mg IVag qhs × 3 d
Bacterial vaginosis in pregnancy	• Metronidazole 500 mg PO BID × 7 d • Metronidazole 250 mg PO TID × 7 d • Clindamycin 300 mg PO BID × 7 d	
Trichomoniasis	• Women: metronidazole 400 to 500 mg PO BID × 7 d[c] • Men: metronidazole 2 g PO × 1 d[c]	• Tinidazole 2 g PO × 1 (women and men)
Candida vaginitis	• Butoconazole 2% cream 5 g IVag × 3 d • Clotrimazole 1% cream 5 g IVag × 7–14 d • Clotrimazole 2% cream 5 g IVag × 3 d • Nystatin 100,000-unit vaginal tablet, 1 tablet IVag × 14 d • Miconazole 2% cream 5 g IVag × 7 d • Miconazole 4% cream 5 g IVag × 3 d • Miconazole 100-mg vaginal suppository, 1 suppository IVag × 7 d • Miconazole 200-mg vaginal suppository, 1 suppository IVag × 3 d • Miconazole 1200-mg vaginal suppository, 1 suppository IVag × 1 • Tioconazole 6.5% ointment 5 g IVag × 1 • Terconazole 0.4% cream 5 g IVag × 7 d • Terconazole 0.8% cream 5 g IVag × 3 d • Terconazole 80-mg vaginal suppository, 1 suppository IVag × 3 d	• Fluconazole 150-mg PO × 1

TABLE 8–6　SEXUALLY TRANSMITTED DISEASES TREATMENT GUIDELINES *(continued)*

Infection	Recommended Treatment	Alternative Treatment
Severe pelvic inflammatory disease	• Cefotetan 2 g IV q12 h PLUS • Doxycycline 100 mg PO/IV q12 h OR • Cefoxitin 2 g IV q6 h	• Ampicillin/sulbactam 3 g IV q6 h PLUS • Doxycycline 100 mg PO/IV BID OR • Clindamycin 900 mg IV q8 h PLUS • Gentamicin loading dose IV or IM (2 mg/kg of body weight), followed by a maintenance dose (1.5 mg/kg) q8 h. Single daily dosing (3–5 mg/kg) can be substituted

Mild-to-moderate pelvic inflammatory disease	• Ceftriaxone 500 mg IM × 1 PLUS
	• Doxycycline 100 mg PO BID × 1 d PLUS
	  metronidazole 500 mg PO BID × 14 d[c] OR
	• Cefoxitin 2 g IM × 1 and probenecid 1 g PO × 1 PLUS
	• Doxycycline 100 mg PO BID × 14 d ±
	  metronidazole 500 mg PO BID × 14 d[c]	

Epididymitis	• Ceftriaxone 500 mg IM × 1, if <150 kg; if >150 kg, ceftriaxone 1 g IM × 1 PLUS • Doxycycline 100 mg PO BID × 10 d For men who practice insertive anal sex: • Ceftriaxone 500 mg IM × 1 PLUS • Levofloxacin 500 mg PO daily × 10 d OR • Ofloxacin 300 mg PO BID × 10 d	• Fluoroquinolone monotherapy can be considered if enteric organism and gonorrhea ruled out • Levofloxacin 500 mg PO daily × 10 d • Ofloxacin 300 mg PO BID × 10 d
External genital warts	Provider-administered: • Cryotherapy liquid nitrogen or cryoprobe • TCA or BCA 80%–90% • Surgical removal by tangential scissor excision, tangential shave excision, curettage, or electrosurgery	Patient-applied: • Podofilox 0.5% solution or gel • Imiquimod 5% cream • Sinecatechins 15% ointment

TABLE 8–6   SEXUALLY TRANSMITTED DISEASES TREATMENT GUIDELINES (*continued*)

Infection	Recommended Treatment	Alternative Treatment
Cervical warts	• Cryotherapy with liquid nitrogen • Surgical removal by tangential scissor excision, tangential shave excision, curettage, or electrosurgery • TCA or BCA 80%–90% applied only to warts • Recommend consulting with specialist in management • Biopsy to exclude high-grade SIL must be performed before treatment is initiated	
Vaginal warts	• Cryotherapy with liquid nitrogen • Surgical removal by tangential scissor excision, tangential shave excision, curettage, or electrosurgery • TCA or BCA 80%–90% applied only to warts	
Urethral meatal warts	• Cryotherapy with liquid nitrogen • Surgical removal by tangential scissor excision, tangential shave excision, curettage, or electrosurgery	
Anal warts	• Cryotherapy with liquid nitrogen • Surgical removal by tangential scissor excision, tangential shave excision, curettage, or electrosurgery • TCA or BCA 80%–90% applied only to warts	• Surgical removal by tangential scissor excision, tangential shave excision, curettage, or electrosurgery
Proctitis	• Ceftriaxone 500 mg IM × 1, if <150 kg; if >150 kg, ceftriaxone 1 g IM × 1 PLUS • Doxycycline 100 mg PO BID × 7 d (extend to 21 d if bloody discharge, ulceration, or positive for rectal chlamydia)	

TABLE 8–6 SEXUALLY TRANSMITTED DISEASES TREATMENT GUIDELINES (continued)

Infection	Recommended Treatment	Alternative Treatment
Pediculosis pubis	• Permethrin 1% cream rinse applied to affected areas and washed off after 10 min • Pyrethrins with piperonyl butoxide applied to the affected area and washed off after 10 min	• Malathion 0.5% lotion applied for 8–12 h and then washed off • Ivermectin 250 mcg/kg PO, repeated in 2 wk
Scabies	• Permethrin cream (5%) applied to all areas of the body from the neck down and washed off after 8–14 h • Ivermectin 200 mcg/kg PO, repeat in 2 wk	• Lindane (1%) 1 oz of lotion (or 30 g of cream) applied in a thin layer to all areas of the body from the neck down and thoroughly washed off after 8 h • Crotamiton 10% apply thin layer

BCA, bichloroacetic acid; BID, twice a day; h, hour(s); HSV, herpes simplex virus; IM, intramuscular; IV, intravenous; IVag, intravaginally; PO, by mouth; q, every; qhs, at bedtime; QID, 4 times a day; SIL, squamous intraepithelial lesion; TCA, trichloroacetic acid; TID, 3 times a day; TMP-SMX, trimethoprim-sulfamethoxazole.

[a]Treatment can be extended if healing is incomplete after 10 d of therapy.

[b]Consider concomitant treatment of gonorrhea.

[c]Avoid alcohol during treatment and for 24 h after treatment is completed. Consider high-dose metronidazole for treatment failure: 2 g daily for 5–7 d or 800 mg TID × 7 d.

[d]Clindamycin cream may weaken latex condoms and diaphragms during treatment and for 5 d thereafter.

Sources: Adapted from *CDC Guidelines: Sexually Transmitted Infection Guidelines.* 2021. https://www.cdc.gov/std/treatment-guidelines/default.htm. *MMWR Recomm Rep.* 2021;70(4): 1–187.

British Association for Sexual Health and HIV National Guideline on the Management of *Trichomonas vaginalis.* 2021. https://pubmed.ncbi.nlm.nih.gov/35701863/

–https://www.cdc.gov/mrsa/pdf/flowchart_pstr.pdf

–https://www.sanfordguide.com/products/digital-subscriptions/sanford-guide-to-antimicrobial-therapy-mobile/

SKIN AND SOFT TISSUE INFECTIONS

Management: Adults and Children

Recommendations from

> **IDSA 2014, ACP 2021**

Therapies

–Impetigo and ecthyma:
  - Gram stain pus or exudate.
  - Treat with topical mupirocin or retapamulin BID × 5 d.
  - Oral therapy: start with dicloxacillin or cephalexin. If MRSA is present, doxycycline, clindamycin, or trimethoprim-sulfamethoxazole (TMP-SMX) for 5–6 d.

–Purulent infections:
  - Gram stain recommended.
  - Perform incision and drainage.
  - Use antibiotics if signs of systemic infection to cover for MRSA.

–MSSA antibiotics:
  - Dicloxacillin 500 mg PO TID.
  - Cephalexin 500 mg PO QID.

–MRSA antibiotics:
  - TMP-SMX 160/800 PO BID; if BMI > 40, 2 tab PO BID (lacks coverage for Group A streptococcus, not recommended in the third trimester of pregnancy, age < 2 y).
  - Clindamycin 300–450 mg PO BID; if BMI > 40, use higher dose.
  - Doxycycline or minocycline 100 mg PO BID; not for use in pregnancy, age < 8 y, less effective for *Streptococcus* spp.
  - RIF; many drug interactions.
  - Linezolid; consult infectious disease specialist; many severe side effects, may be used in renal dysfunction.

–Recurrent abscesses:
  - Rule out pilonidal cyst, hidradenitis suppurativa, or foreign body.
  - Drain and culture drainage.
  - Treat with antibiotics for 5–10 d directed by culture result.
  - Consider 5-d decolonization: intranasal mupirocin BID, daily chlorhexidine bath, and daily decontamination of personal items.
  - Evaluate for neutrophil disorders.

–Erysipelas and cellulitis:
  - Routine cultures are not recommended.

- Culture blood and local aspirate if history of malignancy on chemotherapy, neutropenia, cell-mediated immunodeficiency, immersion injury, or animal bite.
- Treat with antibiotics to cover streptococci for 5 d.
- Treat underlying conditions, ie, edema.
- If systemic illness, deep infection, severely immunocompromised, or delirium, then treat with intravenous antibiotics.

–Animal bites (dog or cat):
- Treat with amoxicillin-clavulanate for 3–5 d, if immunocompromised, asplenic, advanced liver disease, antecedent edema, moderate-to-severe injury, involve the hands or face, or involve periosteum or joint.
- Evaluate for rabies prophylaxis.
- Evaluate tetanus status. If >10 y from vaccination, give Tdap.
- Do not perform primary closure, except face following copious irrigation and debridement.

Sources

–https://www.idsociety.org/practice-guideline/skin-and-soft-tissue-infections/

–https://www.cdc.gov/mrsa/pdf/flowchart_pstr.pdf

–https://www.sanfordguide.com/products/digital-subscriptions/sanford-guide-to-antimicrobial-therapy-mobile/

–https://pubmed.ncbi.nlm.nih.gov/33819054/

SYPHILIS

Screening: Adults and Adolescents

Recommendations from

> USPSTF 2022, AAFP 2016, CDC 2015

–Screen all high-risk[1] persons.

Practice Pearls

- Screen and confirm method:
  - Option one (traditional screening method): nontreponemal test (VDRL test or rapid plasma reagent test) should be used for initial screening. If positive, confirm with a treponemal antibody detection test (eg, fluorescent treponemal antibody absorption test).
  - Option two (reverse sequence method): automated treponemal test (eg, enzyme-linked or chemiluminescence immunoassay). If positive, confirm with a nontreponemal test.
- There is limited evidence on screening interval for the general population; however, men who have sex with men or persons with HIV infection may benefit from screening at least annually.
- Syphilis is a reportable disease in every state.

[1] High risk includes men who have sex with men; persons with HIV infection or other sexually transmitted infections; those who use illicit drugs; and persons with a history of sex work, military service, or incarceration.

Sources
    –*JAMA*. 2022;328(12):1243–1249.
    –AAFP. *Clinical Recommendations: Syphilis*. 2016.
    –CDC. *Sexually Transmitted Diseases Treatment Guidelines*. 2015.

Management: Adults, Children, and Infants

Recommendations from

➤ IDSA 2011, CDC 2021

Evaluation

–Diagnosis: test all persons who have syphilis for HIV, offer PrEP, and retest for HIV in 3 mo if primary test is negative.

–Cerebrospinal fluid analysis is indicated if:

- Early syphilis infection and neurologic symptoms.
- Late latent syphilis.

–Obtain cerebrospinal fluid examination, for patients with early syphilis who do not achieve a >4-fold decline in rapid plasma reagent titers within 12 mo.

Therapies

–See treatment section in Table 8–6.

–Use PCN G 2.4 million units IM for early syphilis.

–Doxycycline is a second-line therapy for early syphilis in PCN-allergic patients.

–Ceftriaxone is a second-line therapy for neurosyphilis in PCN-allergic patients.

–Evaluate and treat sexual partners within preceding 90 d.

–If re-treatment is necessary, use PCN G 2.4 million units IM × 3 wk, unless neurologic involvement.

Practice Pearls

- PCN G is the only treatment in pregnancy. If PCN allergy, pursue desensitization therapy.
- Avoid doxycycline in pregnancy.
- Infants and children: benzathine PCN G 50,000 U/kg IM up to adult dose 2.4 million units. If secondary syphilis is suspected, consult infectious disease specialist.
- Treat HIV-positive patients with primary or secondary syphilis as HIV-negative persons.

Sources
    –http://cid.oxfordjournals.org/content/53/suppl_3/S110.abstract
    –https://www.cdc.gov/std/treatment-guidelines/p-and-s-syphilis.htm

SURGICAL SITE INFECTIONS

Prevention: Adults

Recommendations from

> NICE 2020

–Offer patients and caregivers:
- Clear, consistent information and advice throughout all stages of their care including risks of surgical site infections, what is being done to reduce them, and how they are managed.
- Information and advice on how to care for their wound after discharge.
- Information and advice about how to recognize a surgical site infection and who to contact if they are concerned.
- Always inform patients after their operation if they have been given antibiotics.

–Preoperative phase:
- Advise patients to shower or have a bath using soap, either the day before, or on the day of, surgery.
- Consider nasal mupirocin in combination with a chlorhexidine body wash before procedures in which *Staphylococcus aureus* is a likely cause of a surgical site infection. (This should be locally determined and taken into account: type of procedure, individual patient risk factors, increased risk of side effects in preterm infants, and potential impact of infection.)
- Do not use mechanical bowel preparation routinely to reduce the risk of surgical site infection.

–Antibiotic prophylaxis:
- Give antibiotic prophylaxis to patients before clean surgery involving the placement of a prosthesis or implant, clean-contaminated surgery, or contaminated surgery.
- Do not use antibiotic prophylaxis routinely for clean nonprosthetic uncomplicated surgery.
- Use the local antibiotic formulary and always take into account the potential adverse effects when choosing specific antibiotics for prophylaxis.
- Give antibiotic treatment (in addition to prophylaxis) to patients having surgery on a dirty or infected wound.
- Inform patients before the operation, whenever possible, if they will need antibiotic prophylaxis, and afterward if they have been given antibiotics during their operation.

–Postoperative phase:
- Use an aseptic nontouch technique for changing or removing surgical wound dressings.
- Use sterile saline for wound cleansing up to 48 h after surgery.
- Advise patients that they may shower safely 48 h after surgery.
- Use tap water for wound cleansing after 48 h if the surgical wound has separated or has been surgically opened to drain pus.
- Use topical antimicrobial agents for wound healing by primary intention.

- Do not use topical antimicrobial agents for surgical wounds that are healing by primary intention to reduce the risk of surgical site infection. Dressings for wound healing by secondary intention.
- Do not use Eusol and gauze, or moist cotton gauze or mercuric antiseptic solutions to manage surgical wounds that are healing by secondary intention.
- Use an appropriate interactive dressing to manage surgical wounds that are healing by secondary intention.
- Ask a tissue viability nurse (or another health care professional with tissue viability expertise) for advice on appropriate dressings for the management of surgical wounds that are healing by secondary intention.
- When surgical site infection is suspected by the presence of cellulitis, either by a new infection, or an infection caused by treatment failure, give the patient an antibiotic that covers the likely causative organisms. Consider local resistance patterns and the results of microbiological tests in choosing an antibiotic.

Source
  –www.nice.org.uk/guidance/ng125

TRICHOMONAS

Screening: Women

Recommendations from

> CDC 2015

  –Consider screening women in high-prevalence settings (STI clinics, correctional facilities) and at increased risk (multiple sex partners, commercial sex, illicit drug use, history of STI).

Source
  –CDC. *Sexually Transmitted Diseases Treatment Guidelines*. 2015. https://www.cdc.gov/std/tg2015/trichomoniasis.htm

TUBERCULOSIS (TB), ACTIVE PULMONARY

Management: Adults and Children

Recommendations from

> IDSA 2017, NICE 2016, ATS 2019

  Evaluation
  –Do not routinely test for TB. Screen those who spend time with TB patients, are from an endemic country, who live/work in high-risk setting, or are health care workers.
  –Screening: perform interferon-gamma release assay if >5 y with suspected infection, risk for disease progression, concern for latent MTB (LTBI), or history of BCG vaccination.
  –Tuberculin skin test is an alternative if interferon-gamma release assay is not available, costly, or burdensome.

–Suspected active MTB:

  • Perform a chest X-ray in all patients with symptoms.

–Obtain 3 early-morning sputum samples for AFB smear and culture.

–Tuberculin skin test preferred in patients <5 y.

–Mandatory screening due to law: interferon-gamma release assay preferred to tuberculin skin test. Perform second test if initial test is positive in asymptomatic individuals. Diagnose infection if tests are positive twice.

Therapies

–Report suspect to local public health office for case management and contact screening.

–Isolate patients in negative pressure rooms within the hospital.

–Test for RIF resistance, especially if at risk for drug resistance.

–Decision to initiate therapy depends on multiple factors. Refer to a clinician with expertise in TB management.

–If initiating treatment, start patients on RIPE therapy: RIF, INH, pyrazinamide, and ethambutol. All regimens include an intensive initial phase with four drugs followed by a continuation phase with INH and RIF alone.

–Preferred regimen: RIPE 5 or 7 d/wk × 8 wk then INH + RIF 5 or 7 d/wk × 18 wk. This has greater efficacy and lower risk of resistance than the alternate regimens below.

–Alternate regimen, if direct observed therapy is challenging: RIPE 5 or 7 d/wk × 8 wk then INH + RIF 3 d/wk × 18 wk.

–Alternate regimen, to simplify direct observed therapy further: RIPE 3 d/wk × 8 wk then INH + RIF 3 d/wk × 18 wk. Use with caution in HIV or cavitary disease, as missed doses can lead to failure/relapse/resistance.

–Simplest acceptable regimen, not for use in HIV, smear positive or cavitary lung disease, or if missed doses are likely: RIPE 7 d/wk × 2 wk, then RIPE 2 d/wk × 6 wk, then INH + RIF 2 d/wk × 18 wk.

–Cavitation on initial chest X-ray with positive cultures at 2 mo of therapy may require extending continuation phase to 31 wk.

–When using INH, give pyridoxine 25–50 mg/d if any risk of neuropathy (pregnancy, breastfeeding, HIV, diabetes, alcohol use disorder, malnutrition, chronic kidney disease, advanced age).

Practice Pearls

• Consider sputum for nucleic acid amplification for mycobacterium TB complex if the person has HIV disease, or there is a need for large contact tracing or rapid diagnosis.

• TB treatment regimens are modified based on TB sensitivities.

• Consider de-escalation of hospital isolation after 2 wk of therapy if:
  - Resolution of cough.
  - Afebrile for a week.
  - Immunocompetent patient.
  - No extensive disease by X-ray.
  - Initial smear grade was 2+ or less.

• If sputum cultures remain positive after 3 mo of treatment, repeat drug sensitivity testing and assess adherence with regimen.

Sources

–https://www.atsjournals.org/doi/10.1164/rccm.201909-1874ST

–Nahid P et al. Official American Thoracic Society/Centers for Disease Control and Prevention/ Infectious Diseases Society of America clinical practice guidelines: treatment of drug-susceptible tuberculosis. *Clin Infect Dis.* 2016;63(7):e147–e195. doi:10.1093/cid/ciw376. Translated and reproduced by permission of Oxford University Press on behalf of the Infectious Diseases Society of America.

–https://academic.oup.com/cid/article/64/2/111/2811357

–https://guidelines.gov/summaries/summary/49964

Management: Adults with Suspected or Proven Drug-Resistant TB

Recommendations from

⟩ ATS 2019, WHO 2011

–Perform rapid drug susceptibility testing of INH and RIF at the time of TB diagnosis. If INH resistance is detected, check for fluoroquinolone resistance.

–Use at least 5 drugs during the intensive phase (5–7 mo), followed by 4 drugs during the continuation phase (additional 15–21 mo after culture conversion to negative).

–Use sputum smear microscopy and culture to monitor patients with MDR-TB.

–Repeat drug sensitivity testing if cultures remain positive at 3 mo of adherent treatment.

–Add a later-generation fluoroquinolone, bedaquiline, linezolid, clofazimine, and cycloserine. Add ethambutol only if there are no better options for the 5-drug regimen.

Sources

–https://www.atsjournals.org/doi/10.1164/rccm.201909-1874ST

–http://whqlibdoc.who.int/publications/2011/9789241501583_eng.pdf

TUBERCULOSIS (TB), LATENT

Screening: Adults

Recommendations from

⟩ USPSTF 2023

–Screen for latent TB infections (LTBI) in those with increased risk (see practice pearl below for a list of those typically considered high risk).

–Screen using either the tuberculin skin test or the interferon-gamma release assay.

Management: Adults and Children

Recommendations from

⟩ NICE 2016, CDC 2020

–Offer high-risk individuals younger than 35 y with latent TB:

 • 3 mo of rifapentine and INH (with pyridoxine) (adults and children ≥ 2 y).

–4 mo of daily RIF (HIV-negative, adults and children of all ages).

–3 mo of INH and RIF (HIV-negative, adults and children of all ages).

   • 6 or 9 mo of INH (with pyridoxine) (alternative regimen).

–Offer adults HIV, HBV, and HCV testing before starting treatment for latent TB.

–Offer high-risk individuals between 35 and 65 y latent TB therapy if hepatotoxicity is not a concern.

Practice Pearl

- High-risk patients with latent TB:
  - Persons born outside of the United States.
  - Persons who have lived, or are living, in congregate settings.
  - HIV-positive.
  - Younger than 5 y.
  - Excessive alcohol intake.
  - Injection drug users.
  - Solid organ transplant recipients.
  - Hematologic malignancies.
  - Undergoing chemotherapy.
  - Prior jejunoileal bypass.
  - Diabetes.
  - Chronic kidney disease.
  - Prior gastrectomy.
  - Receiving treatment with antitumor necrosis factor medication or other biologic agents.
  - Consider those who have contact with persons with active TB.

Sources

–https://guidelines.gov/summaries/summary/49964

–https://www.cdc.gov/mmwr/volumes/69/rr/rr6901a1.htm

–https://www.uspreventiveservicestaskforce.org/uspstf/recommendation/latent-tuberculosis-infection-screening

URINARY TRACT INFECTIONS (UTI)

Management: Adults

Recommendations from

> ACOG 2008, EAU 2023, IDSA 2011, NICE 2018, AUA 2019

Evaluation

–Perform a urinalysis or dipstick testing for symptoms of a UTI: dysuria, urinary frequency, suprapubic pain, or hematuria.

–Send urine culture in men, pregnant persons, children, those with a history of resistant bacteria, suspect pyelonephritis, symptoms do not resolve, or atypical symptoms.

Therapies

–Use acetaminophen rather than NSAIDs for pain control.

–There is no evidence for cranberry products or urine alkalization for treatment.

–Duration of antibiotics (consider any previous culture results and sensitivities):
- Uncomplicated cystitis: 3–7 d (nitrofurantoin requires 5–7 d).
- Uncomplicated pyelonephritis: 7–10 d.
- Complicated pyelonephritis or UTI: 3–5 d after control/elimination of complicating factors and defervescence.

–Empiric antibiotics for uncomplicated cystitis[1]:
- TMP-SMX 800 mg/160 mg BID × 3 d (not recommended if local resistance rate > 20%).
- Nitrofurantoin monohydrate 100 mg BID × 5 d.
- Fosfomycin 3 g PO × 1 (second line).
- Beta-lactam antibiotics are alternative agents.[2]

–Empiric antibiotics for complicated UTI or uncomplicated pyelonephritis:
- Ceftriaxone or cefuroxime.
- Aminoglycosides.

–Fluoroquinolones: only use if there are not alternative antimicrobials.

–Empiric antibiotics for complicated pyelonephritis:
- Fluoroquinolones: only use if there are not alternative antimicrobials.
- Piperacillin-tazobactam.
- Carbapenem.
- Aminoglycosides.

–Consider a fluoroquinolone for symptoms of pyelonephritis or for refractory UTI, but only use if there are not alternative antimicrobials.

–Special circumstances: (NICE 2018)
- Pregnant persons: cephalexin 500 mg BID or TID × 7–10 d.
- Men: nitrofurantoin, TMP-SMX, ciprofloxacin, or levofloxacin.

Practice Pearls

- EAU recommends 7 d of antibiotics for men with otherwise uncomplicated cystitis.
- EAU suggests the following options for antimicrobial prophylaxis of recurrent uncomplicated UTIs in nonpregnant persons:
  - Nitrofurantoin 50 mg PO daily.
  - TMP-SMX 40/200 mg daily.
- EAU suggests the following options for antimicrobial prophylaxis of recurrent uncomplicated UTIs in pregnant persons:
  - Cephalexin 125 mg PO daily.
- Once urine culture and sensitivity results are known, antibiotics can be adjusted to the narrowest spectrum antibiotic.

Sources
–http://www.guidelines.gov/content.aspx?id=12628
–http://www.uroweb.org/gls/pdf/Urological%20Infections%202010.pdf

---

[1] TMP-SMX only if regional *Escherichia coli* resistance is low.
[2] Amoxicillin-clavulanate, cefdinir, cefaclor, or cefpodoxime-proxetil. Cephalexin may be appropriate in certain settings.

–http://www.guidelines.gov/content.aspx?id=25652

–http://guidelines.gov/content.aspx?id=12628

–http://cid.oxfordjournals.org/content/52/5/e103.full.pdf+html

–http://nice.org.uk/guidance/ng111

–http://nice.org.uk/guidance/ng109

–https://www.sanfordguide.com/products/digital-subscriptions/sanford-guide-to-antimicrobial-therapy-mobile/

–https://www.auanet.org/guidelines/recurrent-uti

Management: Children 2–24 mo

Recommendations from

> AAP 2016, NICE 2022, AAP 2021

–Diagnose a UTI if patient has pyuria, abnormal urinalysis, and ≥50,000 colonies/mL single uropathogenic organism.

–Obtain midstream sample for urine dipstick and culture prior to antibiotics. Bagged specimens can be used for urinalysis, but not for culture. Collect catheterized specimen or suprapubic aspiration for culture only if urinalysis suggests infection.

–Obtain blood cultures if toxic appears.

–Obtain a renal and bladder ultrasound in all infants 2–24 mo with a febrile UTI.

–Treat febrile UTIs with 7–14 d of antibiotics and tailor antibiotics to culture result.

–Assume upper UTI with bacteriuria and fever (and flank pain).

–Antibiotic prophylaxis is not indicated for a history of febrile UTI.

–A voiding cystourethrogram is indicated if ultrasound reveals hydronephrosis, renal scarring, or other findings of high-grade vesicoureteral reflux, and for recurrent febrile UTIs.

Practice Pearls

- Urine obtained through catheterization has a 95% sensitivity and 99% specificity for UTI.
- Bag urine cultures have a specificity of approximately 63% with an unacceptably high false-positive rate. Only useful if the cultures are negative.
- Increased rate of false-positives if the renal ultrasound is performed during acute phase of illness. Consider delaying until illness has defervesced.
- Refer babies < 3 mo with suspected UTI to pediatric specialty care.

Sources

–https://pubmed.ncbi.nlm.nih.gov/34281996/

–http://pediatrics.aappublications.org/content/early/2016/11/24/peds.2016-3026

–www.nice.org.uk/guidance/ng224

–https://www.sanfordguide.com/products/digital-subscriptions/sanford-guide-to-antimicrobial-therapy-mobile/

Management: Adults with Pyelonephritis

Recommendations from

> ACP 2021, ACR 2022

Evaluation

–Diagnosis: urinary symptoms plus fever and costovertebral tenderness.

–Obtain urine culture prior to the initiation of antibiotics.

–Complicated pyelonephritis: obstruction, male sex, immunosuppression, stone disease, and anatomic or functional urinary tract abnormality.

–Imaging (ACR):

- No imaging is needed for suspect pyelonephritis, first-time presentation, and uncomplicated history (ie, no history of pyelonephritis, diabetes, immunocompromise, stones or obstruction, prior renal surgery, advanced age, vesicoureteral reflux, lack of response to therapy, or pregnancy).
- CT abdomen and pelvis with IV contrast is usually appropriate if suspected acute pyelonephritis but complicated (see above).
- CT abdomen and pelvis with IV contrast (or with and without IV contrast) is usually appropriate if there is a history of renal stones or renal obstruction or with a history of pelvic renal transplant with native kidneys in situ and no other complication (see above).

Therapies

–Hospitalize patients with severe illness, elevated creatinine, severe pain, or who cannot tolerate oral intake.

–Obtain imaging, either ultrasound or CT scan, in patients with severe illness, new renal failure, history of stones, ureteral colic, concern for obstruction (ie, BPH), high urine pH > 7, or failure to respond to therapy.

–Men and women with uncomplicated pyelonephritis: prescribe fluoroquinolone × 5–7 d or TMP-SMX × 14 d.

–Ciprofloxacin 500 mg PO BID × 5 d, or 1000 mg PO daily × 5–7 d or levofloxacin 750 mg PO × 5–7 d.

–Ceftriaxone 1 g IV once with transition to oral therapy for patients who cannot take oral therapy initially.

–Second line:

- TMP-SMX 160/800 mg PO BID × 14 d.
- Cefixime 400 mg PO daily.
- Amoxicillin-clavulanate 875/125 mg PO BID.

–If high risk for resistance, may need inpatient parenteral therapy.

Sources

–Lee, R. Appropriate use of short-course antibiotics in common infections: best practice advice from the American College of Physicians. *Ann Intern Med.* 2021;174(6):822–827.

–https://www.sanfordguide.com/products/digital-subscriptions/sanford-guide-to-antimicrobial-therapy-mobile/

–American College of Radiology Appropriateness Criteria: Acute Pyelonephritis. 2022. https://acsearch.acr.org/docs/69489/Narrative/

Management: Women with Recurrent UTI

Recommendations from

› AUA 2022, EAU 2022

Evaluation

–Perform complete history and perform pelvic exam.

–Obtain results of previous cultures and microbial sensitivity.

–Ensure clean, noncontaminated sample with consideration for catheterized specimen.

–Avoid routine imaging and cystoscopy.

Therapies

–Do not treat asymptomatic bacteriuria and omit surveillance screening.

–Provide patient-initiated treatment while awaiting culture.

–Recommend cranberry prophylaxis.

–Use first-line therapy (ie, nitrofurantoin, TMP-SMX, fosfomycin) and tailor based on local antibiogram.

–Reserve fluoroquinolones only when culture data support the use and there are no alternative antimicrobials.

–Use short duration of therapy (≤7 d).

–Repeat culture if UTI only if symptoms persist following antimicrobial therapy. Do not perform test of cure if symptoms resolve.

–Prescribe vaginal estrogen in peri- and postmenopausal women.

–Prescribe antimicrobial prophylactic antibiotics with caution.

–Use antimicrobial prophylaxis when non-antimicrobial interventions have failed.

Sources

–https://www.auanet.org/guidelines-and-quality/guidelines/recurrent-uti

–https://uroweb.org/guidelines/urological-infections

MUSCULOSKELETAL DISORDERS

ANTERIOR CRUCIATE LIGAMENT (ACL) INJURIES

Management: Adults

Recommendations from

> AAOS 2022, ACR 2019

  –For prevention of primary ACL injuries, use training programs designed to prevent injury in athletes participating in high-risk sports.

  –Obtain a relevant history and focused musculoskeletal exam of the lower extremities to assess for an ACL injury.

  –When surgery is indicated for an acute isolated ACL tear, arrange early reconstruction surgery, as the risk of additional cartilage/meniscal injuries occurs at 3 mo.

  –Consider aspiration of painful, tense knee effusions after ACL injury.

  –Functional knee braces do not confer any clinical benefit in patients who have received isolated ACL reconstruction surgery.

Practice Pearl

- Although MRI should not be the initial imaging study, it is considered a highly sensitive option in diagnosing soft tissue injuries in those with negative plain radiographs. An accurate diagnosis can then guide surgical treatment, if indicated.

Sources

  –https://www.aaos.org/globalassets/quality-and-practice-resources/anterior-cruciate-ligament-injuries/aclcpg.pdf

  –https://acsearch.acr.org/docs/69419/Narrative/

BACK PAIN, LOW

Prevention: Adults

  –There are no current guidelines that address the primary or secondary prevention of low back pain.

Practice Pearls

- There is insufficient evidence to support physical activity for primary prevention of low back pain. (*J Sci Med Sport*. 2024;27:257–265)
- To prevent patients with acute low back pain who are at high risk of progressing to chronic low back pain, implement the STarT Back program. (*Am Fam Physician*. 2024;109(3):233–244)
- Screening tools to assess the risk of progression from acute to chronic low back pain include the PICKUP score, the Orebro Musculoskeletal Pain Screening Questionnaire, and STarT Back calculator.
- Exercise alone or exercise in combination with education is effective for secondary prevention of low back pain. Education alone, back belts, ergonomic interventions, and shoe insoles are likely not effective for both primary and secondary prevention. (*JAMA Intern Med*. 2016;176(2):199–208)

Management: Adults

Recommendations from

➤ ACP 2017, ICSI 2018, NICE 2020, ACR 2021, WHO 2023

Evaluation

–Exclude other specific causes of back pain such as cancer, infection, trauma, and inflammatory disease.

–Avoid routine imaging (X-ray, CT, MRI) in patients with nonspecific or radicular low back pain (LBP) without red flag symptoms.

–Obtain imaging in the following situations:
  - Persistent or progressive symptoms after 6 wk of optimal medical management.
  - History of prior lumbar surgery with new or worsening symptoms.
  - Presence of red flag symptoms.

Therapies

–For first-line management of acute and chronic LBP, consider nonpharmacologic treatments:
  - Superficial heat.
  - Massage.
  - Acupuncture.
  - Spinal manipulation.
  - Cognitive behavioral therapy.

–For second-line management of chronic LBP, consider pharmacologic treatments:
  - NSAIDs with or without oral acetaminophen.
  - Topical capsaicin.

–Offer pharmacologic treatments at the lowest effective dose for the shortest period of time.

–Do not offer SSRI, SNRI, tricyclic antidepressants, corticosteroids, muscle relaxants, or anticonvulsants.

–Do not offer therapeutic ultrasound, transcutaneous electric nerve stimulation, foot orthotics, and lumbar supports (ie, braces, belts).

–Consider behavioral health referral for patients with a high disability and/or who experience significant psychologic distress.

–Consider epidural steroid injections as an adjunct for acute and subacute LBP with a radicular component for short-term pain relief.

–Do not offer spinal fusion. (NICE)

–Consider surgery for persistent functional disabilities and pain due to progressive spinal stenosis, worsening spondylolisthesis, or herniated disk. (AAFP)

Guidelines Alert 9–1
GUIDELINES DISCORDANT: ROLE OF OPIOIDS IN LOW BACK PAIN

Organization	Guidance
ACP	Use only if patients have failed all other therapies and only if the potential benefits outweigh the risks of dependency, addiction, overdose, and misuse
NICE	Consider weak opioids only in the acute phase when NSAIDs are not effective
WHO	Consider only at the lowest effective dose for the shortest duration in conjunction with other modalities and never as monotherapy for chronic LBP
ICSI	Avoid opioids for acute and subacute LBP

Applying to Clinical Practice
• Opioids do not improve overall outcomes in chronic LBP. They have a limited role in patients at low risk for dependency and misuse who obtain significant functional improvement from them.
• Given the risk of dependence and adverse effects, choose therapies other than opioids for acute LBP.

Practice Pearls

• Exercise therapy:
   - For chronic LBP, exercise guided by a physical therapist produces the best long-term results (NNT 7 for pain relief). NSAIDs are also effective (NNT = 6). Duloxetine (NNT = 10) and opioids (NNT = 16) have benefits but also significant side-effect profiles. Other interventions do not show consistent long-term benefit. (*Can Fam Physician.* 2021;67(1):e20–e30)
   - For acute LBP, there is no clear benefit for exercise therapy.
• Pharmacologic therapy:
   - Consider and counsel the patients on potential side effects.
   - For acute LBP, NSAIDs and muscle relaxants provide small benefits on pain.
   - For chronic LBP, NSAIDs and topical lidocaine 5% are recommended as first-line treatment options. (*Am Acad Orthop Surg.* 2014;22(2):101–110)
   - Topical capsaicin has the highest quality evidence of all herbal medicines for reducing pain. (*SPINE.* 2016;41(2):116–133)
   - Magnesium is a reasonable option for those who have not responded to conventional treatment. (*Pain Ther* 2021;10:69–80)
   - When using opiates, restrict duration to 7 d or less.
   - Antidepressants (SSRIs, TCAs) have little to no benefit.

- Anticonvulsants (gabapentin, pregabalin) are ineffective for treatment of radicular and non-radicular LBP. (*CMAJ*. 2018;190(26):E786–E793)
- Thermal radiofrequency denervation is not effective for chronic LBP. (*Cochrane Database Sys Rev*. 2015;(10):CD008572–CD008572)
- Patients knowingly given placebo report improved pain and function. (*Pain*. 2019;160(12): 2891–2897)
- In the absence of red flag symptoms, immediate lumbar imaging does not improve clinical outcomes compared to those who received usual care. Imaging should be reserved for patients for whom noninvasive, conservative regimens have failed and surgery and/or injections are being considered. (*Lancet*. 2009;373(9662):463–472)
  - TUNA FISH mnemonic for red flag symptoms in chronic LBP: Trauma, Unexplained weight loss, Neurologic findings, Age > 50 y, Fever, Intravenous drug use, Steroid use, History of cancer. (*Am Fam Physician*. 2024;109(3):233–244)

Sources
–ACP. *Noninvasive Treatments for Acute, Subacute, and Chronic Low Back Pain: A Clinical Practice Guideline from the American College of Physicians*. 2017.
–ICSI. *Adult Acute and Subacute Low Back Pain*. 2018.
–NICE. *Low Back Pain and Sciatica in Over 16s: Assessment and Management*. 2020.
–ACR. *ACR Appropriateness Criteria: Low Back Pain*. 2021.
–WHO. *WHO Guideline for Non-surgical Management of Chronic Primary Low Back Pain in Adults in Primary and Community Care Settings*. 2023.

CLAVICLE FRACTURES

Management: Adults

Recommendations from
➤ AAOS 2022
–Immobilize with a sling rather than a figure-of-eight brace.
–Consider referring for surgery in the following scenarios:
  • Displaced lateral fracture with disruption of the coracoclavicular ligament.
  • Mid-shaft fracture with increasing displacement or comminution.
–Encourage smoking cessation.

Source
–AAOS. *Clinical Practice Guideline for the Treatment of Clavicle Fractures*. 2022.

HAND PAIN, CHRONIC

Management: Adults

Recommendations from

≫ ACR 2022, 2023

Evaluation

–Order radiographs as the initial imaging study for chronic (>3 mo) hand pain of unclear etiology to evaluate for osteoarthritis, static instability, chronic and nonunited fractures, soft tissue mineralization, erosions, and soft tissue swelling.
–For chronic hand pain with radiographs that are normal or inconclusive:
  • MRI hand without contrast is helpful in evaluating for pathology of the tendons (tendinopathy, tear, tenosynovitis) and injuries to the cartilage, pulleys, or ligaments.
  • Ultrasound of the affected area is equivalent to MRI for evaluating tendon pathology and a reasonable alternative for evaluating pulley injuries and palmar fibromatosis.
  • MRI without contrast and ultrasound are equivalent in evaluating for inflammatory arthropathy.

Sources

–ACR. *American College of Radiology Appropriateness Criteria Chronic Extremity Joint Pain-Suspected Inflammatory Arthritis, Crystalline Arthritis, or Erosive Osteoarthritis*. 2022.
–ACR. *American College of Radiology Appropriateness Criteria Chronic Hand and Wrist Pain*. 2023.

HIP PAIN, CHRONIC

Management: Adults

Recommendations from

≫ ACR 2022

–Thoroughly assess the patient through clinical history and physical exam prior to ordering imaging.
–Order radiography of the pelvis and hip as the initial imaging studies for the evaluation of chronic hip pain.
–For nondiagnostic or negative radiographs, the following imaging studies are usually appropriate depending upon the suspected pathology:
  • For suspected noninfectious extra-articular pathologies such as bursitis or tendinopathies, order US hip or MRI hip without IV contrast.
  • For suspected impingement or dysplasia, order MR arthrography hip or MRI hip without IV contrast.
  • For suspected labral tear, order MR arthrography hip or MRI hip without IV contrast.
–If the radiographs are equivocal or positive for mild hip osteoarthritis, recommend further imaging with MR arthrography hip or MRI hip without IV contrast as indicated to assess

articular cartilage integrity. CT arthrography hip may be an appropriate alternative if MRI is contraindicated.

–If the radiographs are concerning for intra-articular synovial hyperplasia or neoplasia, recommend further evaluation with MRI hip without and with IV contrast or MRI hip without IV contrast.

–For radiographs that demonstrate hip osteoarthritis and the patient has associated low back or knee pathology or pain that could be complicating the clinical picture, then it is usually appropriate to proceed with image-guided anesthetic with or without corticosteroid injection into a specific area of concern, such as hip joint or extra-articular peritendinous structures, to further quantify the amount of pain that particular structure is contributing to patient's symptoms.

Practice Pearls

- Do not routinely order imaging studies, as they should only be considered on an individual basis to help determine the etiology of pain if the diagnosis is uncertain and to further guide the treatment plan.
- Ultrasound is superior to other imaging modalities for dynamic evaluation of the hip, such as in cases of snapping hip syndrome, which may involve the iliopsoas tendon or iliotibial band.
- Perform radiographs when there is any concern for acute fractures, dislocation, or stress fracture.
- Publications differ in the superiority of CT arthrography vs. MRI without contrast vs. MR arthrography for evaluation of labral tears. However, MR arthrography remains the accepted standard for first-line imaging to rule out labral pathology.

Sources
–American College of Radiology. *ACR Appropriateness Criteria® Chronic Hip Pain*. 2022.
–*J Anaesthesiol Clin Pharmacol*. 2020;36(4):450–457.

HIP FRACTURES

Management: Adults

Recommendations from
➢ AAOS 2021
–Use preoperative pain control in patients with hip fractures.
–Perform hip fracture surgery within 48 h of admission.
–Consider hemiarthroplasty, internal fixation, or nonoperative management for nondisplaced femoral neck fractures.
–Perform unipolar or hemipolar hemiarthroplasty for displaced femoral neck fractures.
–Provide interdisciplinary care to co-manage patients with hip fractures to decrease complications and improve outcomes. Interdisciplinary care may include geriatric and orthopedic providers, nursing, dietary, and rehabilitation specialists such as occupational therapy and physical therapy. Co-management may include workup and treatment of osteoporosis, as well as addressing pain, fall mitigation, mental health, and nutrition.

Source
    –AAOS. *Management of Hip Fractures in Older Adults, Evidence-Based Clinical Practice Guideline.* The American Academy of Orthopaedic Surgeons Board of Directors. 2021.

LUMBAR DISC HERNIATION

Management: Adults

Recommendations from

> North American Spine Society 2012

–Offer transforaminal epidural steroid injection (ESI) for short-term (2–4 wk) pain relief in selected patients. Consider interlaminar epidural steroid injection as another option.

–There is insufficient evidence to recommend for or against the use of IV glucocorticoids, 5-HT receptor inhibitors, gabapentin, amitriptyline, and agmatine sulfate.

–There is insufficient evidence to recommend for or against PT/exercise programs as a stand-alone treatment modality, but it is an option for patients with mild-to-moderate symptoms. There is insufficient evidence for traction therapy.

–Consider spinal manipulation as an option for symptomatic relief.

–Do not use TNF-α inhibitors.

–Prior to surgery, assess patient for psychologic distress given association with poorer outcomes.

–Discectomy is recommended in patients with symptoms severe enough to warrant surgery. In patients with less severe symptoms, both surgery and medical/interventional strategies are effective for both short- and long-term relief.

Practice Pearls

• Earlier surgery (within 6 mo to 1 y) is associated with faster recovery and improved long-term outcomes.

• There is no explicit mention of what constitutes symptoms severe enough for surgery.

Source
    –North American Spine Society. *Clinical Guidelines for Multidisciplinary Spine Care Diagnosis and Treatment of Lumbar Disc Herniation with Radiculopathy.* 2022.

MUSCLE CRAMPS

Management: Adults

Recommendations from

> AAN 2010

–Consider vitamin B complex, naftidrofuryl, and calcium channel blockers (diltiazem), as they may be effective.

–Do not routinely recommend stretching for prevention of muscle cramps due to insufficient data.

–Although quinine is likely effective, do not recommend for routine treatment of cramps because of toxicity potential. Reserve quinine derivatives for disabling muscle cramps and monitor dosing carefully. Quinine derivatives are effective in reducing the frequency of muscle cramps, although the magnitude of benefit is smaller than the serious side effects.

Practice Pearls

- Thoroughly evaluate patient with recurrent cramps, paying particular attention to posture, biomechanical imbalances, and palpation of muscle tissue bilaterally to assess for homogeneity.
- The pathophysiology of exercise-associated muscle cramps is not fully understood with potential theories being (a) dehydration and electrolyte imbalance and (b) alterations in neuromuscular excitability.
- Static stretching is an effective treatment strategy for acute onset muscle cramps.
- Magnesium supplementation has not been shown to reduce cramp frequency, intensity, or duration.

Sources
–*Neurology.* 2010;74(8):691–696.
–*J Athl Train.* 2022;57(1):5–15.

OSTEOARTHRITIS (OA)

Management: Adults

Recommendations from

➤ ACR 2019, NICE 2022

Evaluation
–Diagnose OA clinically without imaging for patients who meet all of the following:
- Age ≥ 45 y.
- Have pain related to activity.
- Have no morning stiffness or morning stiffness lasts <30 min.

–Order imaging to diagnose OA if there are atypical features that suggest potential alternative diagnoses.

Therapies
–Strongly recommend individualized therapeutic exercises (eg, strength, aerobic, aquatic) for all people with OA.
–Recommend supervised exercise with physical therapy and/or occupational therapy over unsupervised exercise as this improves outcomes.
–Strongly encourage weight loss for overweight and obese patients to improve quality of life and physical function, as well as reduce pain, for all joint-related OA and particularly for lower extremity OA. Provide information regarding self-efficacy and self-management programs.
–Recommend the use of walking devices (such as canes) for lower extremity OA or hand orthoses for CMC OA if it is likely to improve function and reduce pain.
–Recommend tai chi for lower extremity OA.

- Consider balance exercises, yoga, cognitive behavioral therapy, thermal interventions, and kinesiotaping (only hand or knee OA).
- Approach to medications:
  - Offer topical NSAIDs for knee OA. Consider topical NSAIDs for other joints with OA.
  - If topical NSAIDs are ineffective, treat with oral NSAIDs if not contraindicated at lowest effective dose. If taken consistently, offer gastroprotective treatment, such as a PPI.
  - Consider duloxetine, topical capsaicin (except for hand OA), acetaminophen.
  - Do not offer opioids other than tramadol (see "Guidelines Alert 9-2" table below for additional information), chondroitin sulfate, or glucosamine.
  - Offer intra-articular steroid injections for short-term pain relief (2–10 wk) when other treatments are ineffective and/or to support therapeutic exercise.
  - Do not offer dry needling, intra-articular hyaluronic acid injections, prolotherapy, platelet-rich plasma (PRP), or stem cell therapies.
  - Do not offer transcutaneous electrical nerve stimulation (TENS) treatment.
- Consider walking aids (such as canes) for lower extremity OA.
- Consider referral for joint surgery for people with OA and severe joint symptoms refractory to nonsurgical treatments.

Sources

- American College of Rheumatology. *American College of Rheumatology/Arthritis Foundation Guideline for the Management of Osteoarthritis of the Hand, Hip, and Knee.* 2019.
- *BMJ.* 2023;380:24.

OSTEOARTHRITIS (OA), HIP

Management: Adults

Recommendations from

> AAOS 2023, NICE 2022

- Refer patients to physical therapy who have mild-to-moderate symptoms of hip OA to improve function and reduce pain.
- Unless contraindicated, offer NSAIDs for symptomatic hip OA for short-term pain relief.
- Offer intra-articular corticosteroid injections when other pharmacologic treatments are ineffective or contraindicated to reduce pain in the short term (2–10 wk) and improve function for symptomatic hip OA.
- Do not recommend intra-articular hyaluronic acid injections for improvement of function or reduction of pain in symptomatic hip OA.
- For mild-to-moderate symptomatic hip OA, consider referral for total hip arthroplasty if pain is significantly impacting quality of life and nonsurgical management is ineffective.
- For moderate-to-severe symptomatic hip OA, do not delay referral for total hip arthroplasty for additional nonsurgical management in those who have found nonsurgical management to be ineffective.

–Do not exclude patients from referral for total hip arthroplasty (THA) based on age, smoking, and obesity despite the possible association with increased risk of postoperative complications and poorer clinical outcomes.

–Screen for mental health disorders in patients with symptomatic hip OA who are undergoing total hip arthroplasty to improve outcomes.

–Recommend postoperative physical therapy to improve early function for those who have undergone total hip arthroplasty.

Guidelines Alert 9–2
GUIDELINES DISCORDANT: UTILITY OF SPECIFIC THERAPIES FOR OSTEOARTHRITIS

Intervention	ACR	NICE
Manual therapy (ie, manipulation and soft tissue techniques)	Do not recommend manual therapy in addition to exercise	Consider addition of manual therapy to exercise for hip and knee OA
Acupuncture	Consider for knee, hip, and/or hand OA	Do not recommend for any OA
Opioids	May consider tramadol when NSAIDs are contraindicated, other treatments have failed, or not a surgical candidate. All other opioids not recommended	May consider only "weak" opioids (codeine or dihydrocodeine) if used infrequently for short-term pain relief or all other pharmacologic treatments are contraindicated or ineffective

Applying to Clinical Practice
- The burdensome amount of functional impairment and the paucity of good outcomes data lead to many conditional recommendations for OA therapies.
- In the absence of good data, it is reasonable to consider therapies that the patient is motivated to pursue that do not carry high risk of adverse effect or cost.
- Overall, the decision of when to proceed with total joint arthroplasty should be made by the physician and patient in a shared decision-making process based on the unique patient factors.

Practice Pearls

- Do not routinely order imaging studies to monitor disease progression of OA, unless there has been an acute change in symptom quality or progression to evaluate for severity or rule out other diagnoses.
- The optimal timing for THA for symptomatic moderate-to-severe hip osteoarthritis:
  - Do not delay THA to pursue nonsurgical management.
  - Delay THA to achieve nicotine reduction or cessation.
  - Delay THA to achieve optimal DM control. The degree of DM control is not specified.
  - Do not delay THA due to obesity alone, nor to achieve a specific BMI or weight target, though weight loss should be strongly encouraged.
  - Do not delay THA due to deformity, bone loss, or presence of neuropathic joint.

Sources

  –*Ann Rheum Dis.* 2017;76:1484–1494.

  –*BMJ.* 2023;380:24.

  –American Academy of Orthopaedic Surgeons. *Management of Osteoarthritis of the Hip Evidence-Based Clinical Practice Guideline.* 2017. https://www.aaos.org/oahcpg

  –American College of Rheumatology and American Association of Hip and Knee Surgeons. *Clinical Practice Guideline for the Optimal Timing of Elective Total Hip or Knee Arthroplasty for Patients with Symptomatic Moderate to Severe Osteoarthritis or Osteonecrosis Who Have Failed Nonoperative Therapy.* 2023.

OSTEOARTHRITIS (OA), SHOULDER

Management: Adults

Recommendations from

> AAOS 2020, NICE 2022

- –Offer nonsurgical management prior to referring for surgical intervention, as patients with lower preoperative functioning experience higher postoperative functional improvement, and older age is associated with lower revision rates.
- –Refer for joint replacement if their OA-related pain is significantly interfering with quality of life and nonsurgical options are ineffective. The presence of night pain, pain flares, and joint instability symptoms are important indicators that surgery will likely be beneficial.
- –Do not offer hyaluronic acid injections or injectable biologics (such as PRP or stem cells).
- –Address concomitant depression in patients who are undergoing total shoulder arthroplasty (TSA) to improve postoperative outcomes.
- –Encourage smoking reduction or cessation in patients who are undergoing TSA.
- –May offer preoperative and postoperative physical therapy in select patients given potential benefit.

Practice Pearl

- • Anatomic TSA demonstrates better function and pain relief in the short- and mid-term follow-up when compared to hemiarthroplasty. Anatomic TSA and reverse TSA may both be considered for patients with shoulder OSA in the setting of excessive glenoid bone loss and/or rotator cuff dysfunction.

Sources

  –AAOS. *Management of Glenohumeral Joint Osteoarthritis, Evidence-Based Clinical Practice Guideline.* The American Academy of Orthopaedic Surgeons Board of Directors. 2020.

  –*BMJ.* 2023;380:24.

OSTEOARTHRITIS (OA), KNEE

Management: Adults

Recommendations from

> ACR 2018, ACR 2019, AAOS 2021

–Obtain knee X-ray as initial imaging for chronic knee pain, but do not order routinely.

–Use self-management and patient education programs to promote lifestyle habits aimed at preventing progression of knee OA.

–For overweight and obese patients with knee OA, encourage sustained weight loss.

–Recommend exercise programs to improve both function and pain, including:

- Neuromuscular training.
- Aquatic exercise.
- Strengthening.
- Walking.

–When not contraindicated, treat with topical/oral NSAIDs and acetaminophen to improve function and quality of life in those with knee OA.

–Injections:

- Offer intra-articular corticosteroid injections to provide short-term relief.
- Do not offer hyaluronic acid injections.

–External supports:

- Recommend canes and tibiofemoral braces if likely to improve function and pain.
- Consider short-term patellofemoral braces for patellofemoral OA if disease is significantly impacting ambulation and/or stability.

–Avoid arthroscopy with lavage and/or debridement for patients with primary diagnosis of knee OA.

–Consider arthroscopic partial meniscectomy to treat meniscal tears in patients with concomitant mild-to-moderate knee OA who have failed nonsurgical treatments.

–Consider referral for total knee arthroplasty for symptomatic knee osteoarthritis if pain is significantly impacting qualify of life and nonsurgical management is ineffective.

Practice Pearls

- Physical therapy is superior to intra-articular corticosteroids in improving both pain and function in the long term, but they similarly improve short-term pain and function. (*N Engl J Med*. 2020;382:1420–1429)
- ACR recommends against PRP for knee OA. AAOS recommends consideration of PRP to reduce pain and improve function.
- ACR recommends against the use of chondroitin, glucosamine, and vitamin D. AAOS recommends consideration of these agents due to potential to reduce pain based on limited evidence.
- The optimal timing for TKA for symptomatic moderate-to-severe knee OA is as follows:
  - Do not delay TKA to pursue nonsurgical management.

- Delay TKA to achieve nicotine reduction or cessation.
- Delay TKA to achieve optimal DM control. The degree of DM control is not specified.
- Do not delay TKA due to obesity alone, nor to achieve a specific BMI or weight target, though weight loss should be strongly encouraged.
- Do not delay TKA due to deformity, bone loss, or presence of neuropathic joint.

Sources

–American Academy of Orthopaedic Surgeons. *Management of Osteoarthritis of the Knee (Non-Arthroplasty) Evidence-Based Clinical Practice Guideline.* 2021.
–American College of Radiology. *ACR Appropriateness Criteria® Chronic Knee Pain.* 2018.
–American College of Rheumatology. *American College of Rheumatology/Arthritis Foundation Guideline for the Management of Osteoarthritis of the Hand, Hip, and Knee.* 2019.
–American College of Rheumatology and American Association of Hip and Knee Surgeons. *Clinical Practice Guideline for the Optimal Timing of Elective Total Hip or Knee Arthroplasty for Patients with Symptomatic Moderate to Severe Osteoarthritis or Osteonecrosis Who Have Failed Nonoperative Therapy.* 2023.

OSTEOPOROSIS, GLUCOCORTICOID-INDUCED

Prevention: Adults

Recommendations from

> ACR 2017

–Assess clinical fracture risk within 6 mo of starting GC treatment.
–Include history of dose and duration of steroids, falls, fractures, and frailty.
–High risk of fracture: malnutrition, weight loss/low body weight, hypogonadism, hyperparathyroidism, thyroid disease, family history of hip fracture, alcohol use, and smoking.
–For adults ≥ 40 y, use FRAX (https://www.shef.ac.uk/FRAX/tool.jsp)[1] to assess risk.
–For adults < 40 y with history of osteoporotic (OP) fracture or high risk, perform bone mineral density testing.
–For adults taking >.5 mg/d prednisone, FRAX risk increases by 15% for major OP fracture and 20% for hip fracture.
–High fracture risk: history of OP fracture, T-score ≤ −2.5 (postmenopausal or male ≥ 50 y), FRAX 10-y risk OP fracture ≥ 20% or hip fracture ≥ 3%.
–Moderate fracture risk: FRAX 10-y risk OP fracture 10%–19% or hip fracture 1%–3% (or if <40 y Z-score <−3 or ≥10% bone loss over 1 y and continued GC ≥ 7.5 mg/d for ≥6 mo).
–Low fracture risk: lower FRAX risk.
–Adults taking prednisone ≥ 2.5 mg/d for ≥3 mo: calcium (1000–1200 mg/d), vitamin D (600–800 U/d), healthy diet, normal weight, no smoking, exercise, alcohol ≤ 1–2 drinks/d.
–Adults at low risk for fracture: Ca, vitamin D, lifestyle as above.

---

[1] The FRAX calculator reports significantly lower fracture risk for female patients identified as Black, Asian, or Latina persons with identical risk factors to those of a White patient. This could have the effect of delaying intervention with osteoporosis therapy. (*N Engl J Med.* 2020;383(9):874–882)

–Adults at moderate or high risk for fracture: add oral bisphosphonate.

–If GC treatment continues, reassess risk every 12 mo.

–Continue bisphosphonate treatment for 5 y if continues to be at moderate-to-high risk or continues to take GC.

–Treat with another class of OP medication (teriparatide or denosumab) or IV bisphosphonate if malabsorption of oral form, if fracture after 18 mo of oral bisphosphonate, ≥10% bone loss after 1 y, or continue to be moderate-to-high risk after 5 y.

Source
–*Arthritis Rheumatol.* 2017:69(8):1521–1537.

Practice Pearls

- Clinical factors that may increase the risk of osteoporotic fracture estimated by FRAX calculator:
  - BMI < 21.
  - Parental history of hip fracture.
  - Current smoking.
  - ≥3 alcoholic drinks/d.
  - Higher glucocorticoid doses or cumulative dose.
  - IV pulse glucocorticoid use.
  - Declining central bone mineral density measurement.
- In women of childbearing potential, first line in those indicated for osteoporosis treatment is oral bisphosphonates. Second line is teriparatide.

ROTATOR CUFF TEARS

Management: Adults

Recommendations from

➢ AAOS 2019, ACR 2022

Evaluation

–Diagnose or stratify patients with suspected rotator cuff tears with a clinical examination. MRI without contrast, MR arthrography, and ultrasound are useful adjuncts to clinical exam.

–Order shoulder radiographs as initial imaging for chronic shoulder pain, including when rotator cuff disease is suspected.

Therapies

–Small-to-medium full thickness tears:
- Offer physical therapy and/or operative treatment, as both result in significant improvement in patient-reported outcomes. For patients who choose physical therapy, inform them that their tear size may progress over the next 5–10 y which could lead to a decrease in reported outcomes.
- Do not use routine acromioplasty as a concomitant treatment.

–Consider a single injection of corticosteroids with local anesthetic to provide short-term improvement in pain and function. Avoid multiple steroid injections, as they may compromise the rotator cuff integrity and affect subsequent repair attempts.

–Consider the use of hyaluronic acid injections for the treatment of rotator cuff tendinopathy.

–Do not routinely offer PRP for the treatment of rotator cuff tendinopathy.

–For high-grade partial thickness rotator cuff tears who fail conservative management, refer for orthopedic surgery consultation.

–Encourage early mobilization, as it improves postoperative clinical outcomes.

Practice Pearl

- Offer conservative management as first-line treatment for all partial thickness rotator cuff tears. Conservative management generally consists of a combination of rest, physical therapy, NSAIDs, and corticosteroid injections.

Sources

–AAOS. *Management of Rotator Cuff Injuries Evidence-Based Clinical Practice Guideline.* The American Academy of Orthopaedic Surgeons Board of Directors. 2019.

–*Eur Rev Med Pharmacol Sci.* 2021;25(2):609–619.

–American College of Radiology. *ACR Appropriateness Criteria Chronic Shoulder Pain.* 2022.

SHOULDER PAIN, CHRONIC

Management: Adults

Recommendations from

➤ ACR 2022

–Thoroughly assess the patient through clinical history and physical exam prior to ordering imaging.

–Order radiography of the shoulder as the initial imaging studies for the evaluation of chronic hip pain. Shoulder ultrasound may also be appropriate.

–For nondiagnostic or negative radiographs, the following imaging studies are usually appropriate depending upon the suspected pathology:

- For suspected rotator cuff disorders or subacromial subdeltoid bursitis (without prior surgery), may obtain ultrasound shoulder, MR arthrography shoulder, or MRI shoulder without IV contrast.

- For suspected labral pathology or shoulder instability, obtain MR arthrography shoulder or MRI shoulder without IV contrast.

- For suspected adhesive capsulitis, obtain MRI shoulder without IV contrast or pursue image-guided injection with anesthetic with or without corticosteroid into joint or surrounding structures for diagnosis.

- For suspected biceps tendon pathology, may obtain US shoulder, image-guided anesthetic $+/-$ corticosteroid injection into joint or surrounding structures, MR arthrography shoulder, or MRI shoulder without IV contrast.

- For suspected rotator cuff disorders or subacromial subdeltoid bursitis in setting of prior rotator cuff repair, may proceed with shoulder ultrasound, MR arthrography, MRI without IV contrast, or CT arthrography.

–If initial radiographs demonstrate calcific tendinopathy or calcific bursitis, consider image-guided diagnostic injection with anesthetic $+/-$ corticosteroid injection into shoulder or surrounding structures.

–If initial radiographs demonstrate osteoarthritis, order MRI shoulder without IV contrast.

Practice Pearls

- Do not routinely order imaging studies. They should only be considered on an individual basis to help determine the etiology of pain if the diagnosis is uncertain and to further guide treatment plan.
- Ultrasound is superior to other imaging modalities for dynamic evaluation of the shoulder, such as in cases of bicep tendon subluxation, subacromial impingement, or demonstration of joint effusion.

Source
–ACR. *American College of Radiology ACR Appropriateness Criteria, Chronic Shoulder Pain*. 2022.

VITAMIN D DEFICIENCY

Screening: Adults

Recommendations from

➤ USPSTF 2021, Endocrine Society 2011

–Insufficient evidence to screen for vitamin D deficiency in community dwelling, nonpregnant asymptomatic adults.

–Screen with serum 25-hydroxyvitamin D level in patients at risk[1] for deficiency.

Practice Pearls

- The USPSTF's review showed that treating vitamin D deficiency does not improve cancer risk, diabetes risk, fracture risk, or death in community-dwelling adults, and that other outcomes lacked sufficient data.
- Treating vitamin D deficiency has been considered in the care of other chronic disorders, but insufficient evidence exists. Vitamin D's effect on conditions including pregnancy, depression, diabetes, COPD, asthma, hypertension, and nonspecific pain has been assessed without definitive evidence of benefit.

Sources
–*J Clin Endocrinol Metab*. 2011;96(7):1911–1930.
–*JAMA*. 2021;325(14):1436–1442.
–*Am Fam Physician*. 2018;97(4):254–260.

---

[1] Indications for screening include rickets, osteomalacia, osteoporosis, CKD, hepatic failure, malabsorption syndromes, hyperparathyroidism, certain medications (anticonvulsants, glucocorticoids, AIDS drugs, antifungals, cholestyramine), Black and Latino persons, pregnancy, and lactation, older adults with history of falls or nontraumatic fractures, BMI > 30, and granulomatous diseases.

NEUROLOGIC DISORDERS

BELL PALSY

Management: Adults and Children

Recommendations from

⮞ AAO 2013, AAN 2012

Evaluation

–Do not routinely obtain lab studies, diagnostic imaging, or electrodiagnostic testing for Bell palsy.

–Consider Lyme disease (neuroborreliosis) testing in children of age < 15 y.

–Do not routinely obtain diagnostic imaging for straightforward Bell palsy.

Therapy

–If presenting within 72 h of symptoms, give steroids (prednisone 1 mg/kg PO daily × 7 d), with or without antiviral medications (eg, acyclovir or valacyclovir × 7 d) to patients 16 y and older.

–Do not use antiviral monotherapy.

–Arrange eye protection for patients with incomplete eye closure.

–Do not use physical therapy or acupuncture for Bell palsy.

Practice Pearls

- 2019 Cochrane analysis[1] found no benefit from adding antivirals to corticosteroids vs. corticosteroid monotherapy.
- Antivirals may have a marginal effect on facial nerve recovery when added to steroids, so counsel patients regarding the questionable benefit of antivirals if offered.

Sources

–https://pubmed.ncbi.nlm.nih.gov/24189771/

–https://n.neurology.org/content/79/22/2209.short

[1] https://doi.org/10.1002/14651858.CD001869.pub9

CONCUSSIONS AND HEAD INJURY

Management: Children, Young Adults, and Adults

Recommendations from

➤ CDC 2016, ACEP 2016, AAN 2013, NICE 2023

–Patients should receive medical evaluation for any of the following: loss of consciousness (even if now recovered), amnesia, persistent headache, any emesis, previous brain surgery, history of bleeding/clotting disorder, anticoagulation, antiplatelet therapy (besides aspirin alone), current intoxication (alcohol or other substances), behavioral alterations (ie, inattentive, not acting themselves), or concerns for safety/well-being (ie, vulnerable populations with unclear story).

–Obtain noncontrast CT for loss of consciousness or posttraumatic amnesia. There is no evidence for MRI over CT.

–Use standardized sideline assessment tools to assess athletes with suspected concussions.

–Educate all patients about concussions and postconcussive syndrome. Use tools such as the Acute Concussion Evaluation care plan developed by Gioia and Collins to guide follow-up management.

–Immediately remove from play any athlete with a suspected concussion.

–Do not permit an athlete to return to play until he/she has been cleared to play by a licensed health care professional.

Sources

–https://www.cdc.gov/traumaticbraininjury/pdf/tbi_clinicians_factsheet-a.pdf

–https://www.cdc.gov/headsup/pdfs/providers/ACE_care_plan_returning_to_work-a.pdf

–https://www.aan.com/Guidelines/home/GuidelineDetail/582

–www.nice.org.uk/guidance/ng232

DELIRIUM

Prevention: Adults in Hospital or Long-Term Care Settings

Recommendations from

➤ NICE 2010

–Identify risk factors including age ≥ 65, cognitive impairment and/or dementia, hip fracture, and severe illness.

–Minimize movement to new rooms/wards.

–Provide appropriate lighting, clear signage, clock, and calendar.

–Reorient patient by explaining where they are, who they are, and your role.

–Stimulate cognitive activity such as reminiscence.

–Facilitate regular visits from family and friends.

–Ensure adequate fluid intake.

–Assess for hypoxia and treat when appropriate.

–Assess for infection and treat; avoid unnecessary catheters.

–Encourage mobility including range-of-motion exercise.

–Assess for pain, including nonverbal signs, and treat appropriately.

–Support nutrition adequately.

–Ensure sensory function including hearing and visual aids.

–Promote healthy sleep patterns; minimize overnight interventions, medication administration, and noise.

Source

–www.nice.org.uk/guidance/cg103

Management: Adults in the Hospital or Long-Term Care Settings

Recommendations from

> ### NICE 2023

–Identify and manage underlying cause(s).

–Communicate, reorient, and reassure. Involve family and friends when possible. Revisit prevention recommendations.

–De-escalate agitation with verbal and nonverbal techniques.

–Consider short-term haloperidol when de-escalation techniques are unsuccessful and patient poses risk to self or others.

–For persistent delirium, reevaluate for underlying causes.

Practice Pearls

- Haloperidol carries a risk of QT prolongation and an FDA black-box warning related to an increase in all-cause mortality when patients with dementia are treated with atypical antipsychotics for behavioral problems. However, this is drawn from studies in the outpatient or long-term care settings.
- Short-term use of antipsychotics in the hospital may be associated with a minor increase in aspiration pneumonia events and cardiovascular events, but not an increase in mortality.
- Aripiprazole is an antipsychotic that does not affect the QT interval.

Sources

–www.nice.org.uk/guidance/cg103

–*Cleveland Clin J Med.* 2017;84(8):616–622. doi:https://doi.org/10.3949/ccjm.84a.16077

Management: Older Adults Undergoing Surgery

Recommendations from

> AGS 2021, APAPG 2024

–Enact multicomponent nonpharmacologic intervention programs to manage delirium for entire hospitalization, beginning at admission for at-risk patients.

–Consider regional anesthesia at the time of surgery to improve postoperative pain control and reduce delirium risk.

–Avoid inappropriate medications postoperatively in older adults. Optimize postoperative pain control, preferably with nonopioid pain medication.

–Do not routinely use antipsychotics for prevention or treatment of delirium. Consider use of time-limited therapy (3–5 d) for severe neuropsychiatric disturbance.

–Do not newly prescribe prophylactic cholinesterase inhibitors in the perioperative setting to prevent or treat delirium.

–Avoid benzodiazepines for postoperative delirium.

–Avoid pharmacologic therapy for hypoactive delirium.

–Avoid use of physical restraints.

–Ensure detailed medication reconciliation and indication reassessment during transitions of care.

Practice Pearls

- Older adults and people with dementia, severe illness, or a hip fracture are more at risk for developing delirium.
- Inappropriate medications include benzodiazepines, anticholinergics (eg, cyclobenzaprine, paroxetine, tricyclic antidepressants, diphenhydramine), H_2-receptor blockers, sedative-hypnotics, and meperidine.
- Pharmacologic treatment of hypoactive delirium has not shown to modify duration or severity of postoperative delirium; do not use antipsychotics in hypoactive delirium unless agitation threatens safety of patient or others and limit use to 3–5 d in this setting.
- The prevalence of delirium in people on medical wards in hospital is about 20%–30%, and delirium develops in 10%–50% of people having surgery. In long-term care, the prevalence is under 20%.
- Do not use physical restraints for behavioral control in older patients with delirium.
- Delirium can appear both hyperactive and hypoactive, with the above prevalence ensure vigilance when caring for hospitalized, surgical, and long-term care patients.

Source
–*J Am Geriatr Soc.* 2015;63(1):124–150.

DIZZINESS

Management: Adults

Recommendations from

> ACR 2023

Evaluation
–Vertigo
- For brief episodic vertigo triggered by specific head movements and suggestive of benign paroxysmal positional vertigo, do not routinely order imaging.
- When vertigo is persistent and neurologic examination is abnormal or HINTS examination suggests central etiology, order MRI head without IV contrast.
- When vertigo is persistent but neurologic examination is normal or HINTS examination suggests peripheral etiology, consider MRI head.
- When vertigo is associated with unilateral hearing loss or tinnitus, obtain MRI head and internal auditory canal with and without IV contrast or CT temporal bone without contrast. If there are other brainstem neurologic deficits, include imaging of the neck vessels.

–Disequilibrium
- When signs of cerebellar ataxia appear, order MRI head either without contrast or with and without contrast. Consider MRI of cervical and thoracic spine.
- When signs of sensory or proprioceptive ataxia appear, order MRI of cervical and thoracic spine.

–Nonspecific dizziness: when no vertigo, ataxia, or neurologic deficits, consider MRI head without contrast.

Source
–https://acsearch.acr.org/docs/69477/Narrative/

HEADACHE

Management: Adults

Recommendations from

> ICSI 2011, NICE 2022, ACR 2022, VA 2023

Evaluation
–Take a detailed history (characteristics of headache, functional impairment, past medical and family history, current and previous medications including over-the-counter used for headache, and social history and review of systems to help rule out systemic illness) and perform a focused physical and neurologic exam.

–Be alert for any causes for concern:
- Subacute and/or progressive over months.
- New or different headache.
- "Worst headache ever."

- Headache most severe at onset.
- Onset after age 50.
- Symptoms of systemic illness.
- Seizures.
- Any neurologic signs.

–Consider headache diary ×8 wk including frequency/duration/severity, any associated symptoms, medications taken, possible precipitants, and relationship to menstruation.

–Primary headaches can include migraine, tension-type, cluster, chronic daily headache, sinus-type,[1] or other.

- Tension-type: bilateral, pressing/tightening, mild-moderate, not aggravated by routine activities of daily life, variable duration.
- Migraine: unilateral or bilateral, pulsating/throbbing/banging, moderate-severe, aggravated by or causes avoidance of routine ADLs, photophobia or phonophobia, aura (flickering lights, spots/lines in vision, numbness/pins-needles, speech disturbance), lasts 4–72 h.
- Cluster headache: unilateral (around eye/above eye/alongside of face), variable quality, severe, causes restlessness/agitation, ipsilateral red/watery eye, nasal congestion, eyelid swelling, forehead/facial swelling, constricted pupil, lasts 15–180 min.

–Approach to imaging (ACR):

- No imaging:
  - Uncomplicated headaches.
  - New primary migraine or tension-type headache, normal neurologic exam.
  - Initial assessment of chronic headache, without new features or neurologic deficit.
- Urgent red flag symptoms require prompt evaluation:
  - Signs of systemic illness in the patient with new-onset headache.
  - New headache in patients over 50 y of age with symptoms of temporal arteritis.
  - Papilledema in an alert patient without focal neurologic signs.
  - An older patient with new headache and subacute cognitive change.
- Emergent red flag symptoms require immediate emergency department evaluation:
  - Onset of sudden, severe headache (seconds to a minute to a peak onset of intensity).
  - Headache with fever and neck stiffness.
  - Papilledema with altered level of consciousness and/or focal neurologic signs.
- Consider imaging or specialty consultation if:
  - Atypical headaches.
  - Changes in headache pattern.
  - Unexplained focal signs in the patient with a headache.
  - Headache precipitated by exertion, postural change, cough, or Valsalva.
  - New-onset cluster headache or another trigeminal autonomic cephalgia, hemicrania continua, or new daily persistent headache.

[1] Note on sinus-type headache: these are often migraine headaches misdiagnosed as sinus-type. Sinus-type headaches are defined by the International Classification of Headache Disorders (ICHD-II) as headache with purulent nasal discharge, pathologic sinus finding by imaging, and headache localized to specific facial and cranial areas of the sinuses.

- Specific neuroimaging recommendations for complicated headache. In patients with:
  - Sudden, severe headache reaching maximum severity within an hour, evaluate with CT head without IV contrast for initial imaging.
  - New headache and optic disc edema, evaluate with MRI head without and with IV contrast, MRI head without IV contrast, or CT head without IV contrast for the initial imaging. These procedures are equivalent alternatives.
  - New or progressively worsening headache with one or more of the following "red flags": subacute head trauma, related activity or event (sexual activity, exertion, positional), neurologic deficit, known or suspected cancer, immunosuppressed or immunocompromised state, age 50 y or older, evaluate with CT head without IV contrast, MRI head without and with IV contrast, or MRI head without IV contrast for the initial imaging. These procedures are equivalent alternatives. Pregnancy is also considered a "red flag" condition, with separate considerations for radiation and contrast exposure, typically avoiding CT scans.
  - New primary headache of suspected trigeminal autonomic origin (cluster headache), obtain MRI head without and with IV contrast for the initial imaging.
  - Chronic headache presenting with new features or increasing frequency, evaluate with MRI head without and with IV contrast or MRI head without IV contrast for the initial imaging. These procedures are equivalent alternatives.

Therapy

- If no cause for concern is found and headache meets criteria for primary headache disorder: initiate education, treatment, and lifestyle modification recommendations.
- If cause for concern is found, consider specialty consultation and perform any indicated diagnostic testing.
- Treatment of tension-type headache:
  - Give acetaminophen, aspirin, nonsteroidal anti-inflammatory drug (NSAID), or adjunctive therapy for acute headache.
  - If unsuccessful, consider other treatment, reconsider diagnosis, and consider medication overuse.
  - For frequent headaches, consider prophylactic treatments: amitriptyline or other TCA, venlafaxine. If prophylaxis unsuccessful, consider specialty referral.
- Treatment of cluster headache:
  - Acute: oxygen (100% FiO_2, ≥ 12 L/min), sumatriptan SQ, dihydroergotamine.
  - Bridging treatment: corticosteroids, ergotamine, occipital nerve block.
  - Maintenance treatment: verapamil. Avoid alcohol. Progress to high-dose verapamil, steroids, lithium, Depakote, or topiramate if needed.
- To prevent recurrent headaches, recommend for all patients:
  - Maintain regular sleep schedule, hydration, balanced diet, stress management.
  - Insufficient evidence for/against fluoxetine, venlafaxine.
  - Insufficient evidence for/against coenzyme q10, feverfew, melatonin, omega-3, vitamin B_2 or vitamin B_6.
- To prevent recurrent tension-type headaches:
  - Consider physical therapy interventions, aerobic exercise, and progressive strength training.

- Offer amitriptyline, though caution with side effects (cognitive impairments, dry mouth, weight gain, sedation, dizziness, blurred vision, gastrointestinal distress, nausea), effects on the elderly, and risk of overdose.
- Do not offer botulinum toxin injection.

Sources

–Beithon J et al. *Diagnosis and Treatment of Headache*. Updated 2011.

–www.nice.org.uk/guidance/cg150

–American College of Radiology. *Appropriateness Criteria Headache*. Revised 2022. http://www.choosingwisely.org/societies/american-college-of-radiology/

–https://www.healthquality.va.gov/guidelines/Pain/headache/index.asp

HEADACHE, MIGRAINE

Management: Adults

Recommendations from

➤ American Headache Society 2019, 2024, VA 2023

Evaluation

–Diagnose migraine using ICHD-3 criteria (Table 10–1).

Therapy

–Treat migraines at the first sign of pain.

–For mild-to-moderate attacks, use NSAIDs, nonopioid analgesics, acetaminophen, or combinations such as aspirin + acetaminophen + caffeine.

–For moderate or severe attacks or milder attacks that fail initial therapy, use triptans or ergotamine derivatives. Antiemetics and IV magnesium (in migraine with aura) are also likely effective.

TABLE 10–1 INTERNATIONAL CLASSIFICATION OF HEADACHE DISORDERS CRITERIA FOR MIGRAINE
Episodic
Five attacks with the following criteria, not explained by another condition:
–Duration 4–72 h untreated –≥2 of the following characteristics: unilateral location, pulsating quality, moderate or severe intensity, aggravated by (or causing avoidance of) routine physical activity –Nausea, vomiting, or photophobia and phonophobia
Chronic
≥15 d/mo for >3 mo of migraine or tension-type HA History of at least 5 episodic migraine attacks ≥8 d/mo with ≥2 of the following characteristics: unilateral location, pulsating quality, moderate or severe intensity, aggravated by (or causing avoidance of) routine physical activity plus duration of 4–72 h if migraine with aura or nausea, vomiting or photo/phonophobia if migraine without aura, that patient believes to be a migraine and gets relief from triptan or ergot derivative

–Offer prophylaxis if frequent attacks that interfere with regular routines and treatments fail or are overused (ie, used 10+ d/mo).
  • Frequency: offer prophylaxis if 6+ headache days per month, 4+ d per month with some disability, or 3+ d per month with severe disability. May consider for interested patients with lower headache frequency.
–Offer a prevention agent with established efficacy, starting at a low dose and titrate gradually to response or intolerance. Give a trial of at least 8 wk at target dose and set expectations that a 50% reduction in headache days or a decrease in severity are the goals of therapy. Consider combination therapy if there is an incomplete response. These agents include:
  • Antiepileptics: divalproex sodium, valproate sodium, topiramate.
  • Beta-blockers: metoprolol, propranolol, timolol.
  • Triptans: frovatriptan (only for short-term prevention of menstrual migraine). (AHS)
  • Onabotulinumtoxin A.
  • Calcitonin gene-related peptide-targeting therapies.
  • Candesartan or telmisartan (VA).
–Consider agents with probable effectiveness:
  • Antidepressants: nortriptyline, venlafaxine.
  • Beta-blockers: atenolol, nadolol.
  • Atogepant (VA).
  • Memantine (VA).
–If the above are ineffective or if the patient prefers, consider an agent with a single small study of effectiveness: lisinopril, clonidine, guanfacine, carbamazepine, nebivolol, pindolol, cyproheptadine.
–Data are insufficient to recommend novel injectable biologic agents for prophylaxis, as they lack long-term safety data and carry uncertain cost-effectiveness.

Sources
–*Headache.* 2019;59:1–18.
–*Headache.* 2024;64:333–341.
–https://www.healthquality.va.gov/guidelines/Pain/headache/index.asp

Management: Children and Adolescents

Recommendations from

➤ AAN 2019

Evaluation
–Diagnostic criteria for pediatric migraine:
  • At least 5 headaches over the past year that lasted 2–72 h when untreated.
  • Associated with nausea, vomiting, photophobia, or phonophobia.
  • 2 of 4 additional features:
    ○ Pulsatile quality.
    ○ Unilateral.

◦ Worsening with activity or limiting activity.

◦ Moderate-to-severe in intensity.

Therapy

–Treat migraine early (within <1 h of headache onset).

–Offer nonprescription oral analgesics like acetaminophen, ibuprofen, and naproxen.

–Consider triptans, though they are less commonly prescribed in children than in adults.

- Agents FDA-approved for children: almotriptan (age ≥ 12 y), rizatriptan (age 6–17 y), sumatriptan/naproxen (age ≥12 y), and zolmitriptan NS (age ≥ 12 y).
- If there is an incomplete response to triptan, add NSAID (ibuprofen or naproxen).
- Do not prescribe triptans to those with a history of ischemic vascular disease or accessory conduction pathway disorders, as the medication can exacerbate these disorders.
- Timing: taking triptan during a typical aura is safe, but it may be more effective if taken at onset of head pain.

–If HA is successfully treated with acute medication but recurs within 24 h, repeat the initial treatment.

–If prominent nausea or vomiting, offer antiemetics.

–Ergots have not been studied in children.

–Consider referral to headache specialist if hemiplegic migraine, migraine with brainstem aura who do not respond to initial treatments.

Source

–*Neurology.* 2019;93:487–499.

MULTIPLE SCLEROSIS (MS)

Management: Adults

Recommendations from

➤ AAN 2020

–Use corticosteroids (ie, 1000 mg/d methylprednisolone × 3 d) at time of initial presentation or relapse.

–Encourage smoking cessation.

–Refer to a specialist for disease-modifying therapy (DMT).

–Initiate disease-modifying therapy in patients with a single clinical demyelinating event and two or more brain lesions after discussing risks and benefits with patients with the goal to reduce the number of relapses or slow the progression of MS.

–Prescribe alemtuzumab, fingolimod, or natalizumab for people with highly active MS.

–Disease-modifying therapy can slow or stabilize disease; if disease activity resurfaces, change MS medication.

–Consider weekly home or outpatient physical therapy (8 wk) as it may improve balance, disability, and gait, but not upper-extremity dexterity.

–Consider motor and sensory balance training or motor balance training (3 wk) to improve static and dynamic balance.

–Consider oral cannabis extract and THC in patients with MS with spasticity and pain (excluding central neuropathic pain).

Practice Pearl

- Use 2017 McDonald Criteria for diagnosis.
  - ≥2 clinical attacks, ≥2 CNS lesions, or 1 lesion with clear evidence of prior attack involving a lesion in a distinct anatomical location.
  - ≥2 clinical attacks, 1 lesion, and dissemination in space demonstrated by an additional clinical attack implicating a different CNS site or by MRI.
  - 1 clinical attack, ≥2 lesions with objective clinical evidence, and dissemination in time[1] demonstrated by additional clinical attack or by MRI.
  - 1 clinical attack, 1 lesion with objective clinical evidence, dissemination in time and space demonstrated by additional clinical attack or by MRI.

Sources
–AAN. *Complementary and Alternative Medicine in Multiple Sclerosis.* 2014; Reaffirmed 2020.
–AAN. *Comprehensive Systemic Rehabilitation in Multiple Sclerosis.* 2015.
–AAN. *Practice Guideline: Disease-Modifying Therapies for Adults with Multiple Sclerosis.* 2018.

NORMAL PRESSURE HYDROCEPHALUS

Management: Adults

Recommendations from

➤ AAN 2015

–Consider shunting for normal pressure hydrocephalus with gait abnormalities.
–A positive response to a therapeutic lumbar puncture increases the chance of success with shunting.
–Patients with impaired cerebral blood flow reactivity to acetazolamide, measured by SPECT, are more likely to respond to shunting.

Source
–https://guidelines.gov/summaries/summary/49957

PAIN, CHRONIC

Management: Adults, Except Those with Cancer Pain or Undergoing End-of-Life Care

Recommendations from

➤ CDC 2016, ICSI 2017, ASIPP 2023

Evaluation
–Use validated tools to assess patient's functional status, pain, and quality of life.

---

[1] CSF-specific oligoclonal bands can substitute for "dissemination in time" for the purposes of these criteria.

–Assess for current or prior exposure to opioids and consider checking prescription drug monitoring program data before prescribing opioids.

–Assess for mental health comorbidities in patients with chronic pain.

–Screen all patients with chronic pain for substance use disorders.

–Before initiating opioids for chronic pain, seek a diagnostic cause of the pain and document objective findings on physical exam.

Therapy

–Prefer nonpharmacologic therapy and nonopioid medications for chronic pain.

–Prescribe NSAIDs and acetaminophen for dental pain.

–Use opioid therapy for both pain and function only if the anticipated benefits outweigh the risks.

–Attempt multimodal pain support (physical therapy, nonopioid medications, CBT, nonpharmacologic treatments) prior to initiation of opiate therapy for chronic pain.

–Establish treatment goals, including realistic benefits of opiate therapy and goals for pain and function, before starting opioid therapy for chronic pain. Plan how opioid therapy will be discontinued if benefits do not outweigh the risks.

–Discuss with patients the risks and benefits of opioid therapy before starting opioids and periodically during therapy.

–Access prescription drug monitoring program data initially and then intermittently for all patients receiving opiate therapy.

–Incorporate cognitive behavioral therapy or mindfulness-based stress reduction and exercise/physical therapy to pharmacologic therapy in chronic pain patients.

–When starting opioid therapy, use immediate-release opioids, and prescribe the lowest effective dose.

–Reserve long-acting opioids for patients with opioid tolerance and in whom the prescriber is confident of medication adherence.

–Carefully reassess benefits and risks when increasing daily dosage to >50 morphine milligram equivalents. Ensure patient has close access to naloxone in this setting.

–Avoid increasing daily dosage to >90 morphine milligram equivalents or carefully justify such doses.

–Reassess efficacy within 4 wk of starting opioid therapy for chronic pain and consider discontinuing opioids if benefits do not outweigh risks.

–Consider use of partial-agonist opiate therapy (buprenorphine) as initial treatment or as step-down therapy for patients with difficulty discontinuing opiate therapies.

Surveillance

–Evaluate risks of opioid-related harms.

–Advise patients who are initiating opioids or who have their opioid dose increased not to operate heavy machinery, drive a car, or participate in any activity that may be affected by the sedating effect of opioids.

–Prescribe naloxone emergency kit when patients have an increased risk of opioid overdose especially in patients who are taking ≥50 morphine milligram equivalents per day or concurrently using a benzodiazepine.

–Review prescription drug monitoring program data frequently.

–Obtain periodic urine drug testing to monitor diversion.

–Avoid concurrent opioid and benzodiazepine therapy whenever possible.

–Assess geriatric patients for their fall risk, cognitive impairment, respiratory function, and renal/hepatic impairment prior to initiation of opioids.

–Offer or arrange for medication-assisted treatment (eg, buprenorphine or methadone) for patients with opioid use disorders or those with difficulty weaning when benefits are outweighed by side effects.

Sources

–*MMWR Recomm Rep.* 2016;65(1):1–49.

–https://www.cdc.gov/drugoverdose/pdf/guidelines_at-a-glance-a.pdf

–Hooten M et al. *Pain: Assessment, Non-opioid Treatment Approaches and Opioid Management.* Bloomington, MN: Institute for Clinical Systems Improvement (ICSI); 2016:160.

–https://www.icsi.org/wp-content/uploads/2019/01/Pain.pdf

PAIN, NEUROPATHIC

Management: Adults

Recommendations from

➤ NICE 2013, 2019

–Offer a choice of amitriptyline, duloxetine, gabapentin, or pregabalin as initial treatment for neuropathic pain (except trigeminal neuralgia).

–Consider tramadol only as acute rescue therapy.

–Offer carbamazepine as initial treatment for trigeminal neuralgia.

–Consider capsaicin cream for localized neuropathic pain.

–Pregabalin and gabapentin carry a risk of dependence and abuse.

–Consider the following agents with expert supervision:
- Cannabidiol.
- Capsaicin patch.
- Lacosamide.
- Lamotrigine.
- Levetiracetam.
- Methadone.
- Morphine.
- Oxcarbazepine.
- Tapentadol.
- Topiramate.
- Tramadol (for long-term use).
- Venlafaxine.

–Spinal cord stimulation.

Sources

–http://www.guideline.gov/content.aspx?id=47701

–NICE guideline CG173. *Neuropathic Pain in Adults: Pharmacological Management in Non-specialist Settings*. 2013, updated 2019.

PROCEDURAL SEDATION

Management: Adults and Children

Recommendations from

> ACEP 2014

–Preprocedural fasting is not needed prior to procedural sedation.

–Use continuous capnometry and oximetry to detect hypoventilation.

–A nurse or other qualified individual must be present for continuous monitoring in addition to the procedural operator.

–Safe options for procedural sedation in children and adults include ketamine, propofol, and etomidate.

Practice Pearls

- The combination of ketamine and propofol is also deemed to be safe for procedural sedation in children and adults.
- Alfentanil can be safely administered to adults for procedural sedation.

Source

–http://www.guideline.gov/content.aspx?id=47772

RESTLESS LEGS SYNDROME AND PERIODIC LIMB MOVEMENT DISORDERS

Management: Adults

Recommendations from

> AAN 2016, American Academy of Sleep Medicine 2012

–Nonpharmacologic therapies:
  - Avoid or reduce caffeine, nicotine, and EtOH.
  - Perform evening stretches, massage, warm or cool baths, and light exercise.

–Recommendations for moderate-to-severe restless legs syndrome (RLS).
  - Strong evidence for the following meds:
    - Cabergoline.
    - Gabapentin.
    - Pramipexole.
    - Rotigotine.

- Moderate evidence for:
  - IV ferric carboxymaltose.
  - Pregabalin.
  - Ropinirole.
- For primary RLS with periodic limb movements of sleep:
  - Ropinirole.
- For primary RLS with concomitant anxiety or depression:
  - Gabapentin.
  - Pramipexole.
  - Ropinirole.
- For RLS and ferritin <75 mcg/mL:
  - Ferrous sulfate with vitamin C.
- For RLS with ESRD on hemodialysis:
  - Vitamin C and E supplementation.
  - Consider adding ropinirole, levodopa, or exercise.

Practice Pearls

- Potential for heart valve damage with pergolide and cabergoline.
- There is insufficient evidence to support any pharmacologic treatment for periodic limb movement disorder.

Sources

–Winkelman JW et al. Practice guideline summary: treatment of restless legs syndrome in adults: report of the Guideline Development, Dissemination, and Implementation Subcommittee of the American Academy of Neurology. *Neurology*. 2016;87(24):2585–2593. http://guidelines.gov/summaries/summary/50689/
–www.guidelines.gov/content.aspx?id=38320

SCIATICA

Management: Adults

Recommendations from

> NICE 2016

–Do not routinely offer imaging in a primary care setting to patient with low back pain with or without sciatica.
–Continue aerobic exercise program and referral to PT.
–Consider spinal manipulation or soft tissue massage as adjunct.
–Consider cognitive behavioral therapy.
–Promote return to work and normal activities.
–Consider NSAIDs and short-term, low-dose opioids for acute sciatica.
–Consider epidural steroid injection for acute, severe sciatica.

–Do not prescribe opioids or anticonvulsants for chronic low-back pain with sciatica.

–Consider the use of neuropathic agents such as gabapentin, pregabalin, and nortriptyline.

–Consider spinal decompression for people with disabling sciatica for neurologic deficits or chronic symptoms refractory to medical management, and spine imaging is consistent with sciatica symptoms.

–Belts, corsets, foot orthotics, rocker sole shoes, spine traction, acupuncture, ultrasound, transcutaneous electrical nerve stimulation (TENS), and interferential therapy have not proven to help patients with sciatica.

Source

–National Guideline Centre. *Low Back Pain and Sciatica in Over 16s: Assessment and Management*. London (UK): National Institute for Health and Care Excellence (NICE); 2016:18.

SEIZURES

Management: Adults, First Unprovoked Seizure

Recommendations from

> AAN 2015, ACR 2020, ACEP 2014

Evaluation

–Obtain initial imaging with a CT without contrast or an MRI without contrast. A CT is typically preferred if seizure is associated with trauma, though an MRI with or without may be appropriate. (ACR)

–Risk factors for a recurrent seizure include:

- Brain injury.
- Prior stroke.
- Abnormal EEG with epileptiform activity.
- Structural abnormality on brain imaging.
- Nocturnal seizure.

Therapy

–Start immediate antiepileptic therapy only if elevated risk of a recurrent seizure. (AAN)

–If known seizure disorder, give antiepileptic therapy in ED orally or by IV. (ACEP)

–For status epilepticus, give benzodiazepines and consider phenytoin, fosphenytoin, valproic acid, and levetiracetam as second-line agents. (ACEP)

Practice Pearl

- Recurrent seizures occur most frequently in the first 2 y. Over the long term (>3 y), immediate anti-epileptic drug (AED) therapy is unlikely to improve the prognosis for sustained seizure remission.

Sources

–https://guidelines.gov/summaries/summary/49218

–https://acsearch.acr.org/docs/69479/Narrative/

–https://www.acep.org/patient-care/clinical-policies/seizure/

Management: Children Age 6 mo to 5 y with Febrile Seizures

Recommendations from

➤ **AAP 2011**

–Perform a lumbar puncture if child presents with a fever and seizure and has meningeal signs or a history concerning for meningitis.

–Consider lumbar puncture for children 6–12 mo of age who present with a fever and seizure and are not up to date with their *Haemophilus influenzae* or *Streptococcus pneumoniae* vaccinations.

–Consider lumbar puncture in a child presenting with a fever and a seizure who has been pretreated with antibiotics.

–Do not perform EEG, neuroimaging, or routine labs (basic metabolic panel, calcium, phosphorus, magnesium, glucose, CBC) for a simple febrile seizure.

Practice Pearl

• A febrile seizure is a seizure accompanied by fever ($T \geq$ 100.4°F [38°C]) without CNS infection in a child age 6 mo to 5 y.

Source

–http://pediatrics.aappublications.org/content/127/2/389.full.pdf+html

STROKE, ACUTE ISCHEMIC

Management: Adults

Recommendations from

➤ **AHA/ASA 2018**

Evaluation

–Obtain noncontrast CT upon arrival at hospital, within 20 min of arrival.

–Obtain CT angiogram with initial imaging for patients who otherwise meet criteria for endovascular treatment (EVT), but do not delay IV alteplase if indicated. Do not delay for a serum creatinine measurement unless there is a history of renal impairment.

–See Table 10–2 for ACR guidance on further imaging modalities.

–In patients who are potential candidates for mechanical thrombectomy, consider imaging the extracranial carotid and vertebral arteries, in addition to the intracranial circulation for endovascular procedural planning.

–Measure blood glucose and treat hypoglycemia (<60 mg/dL).

–Obtain ECG and baseline troponin (but do not delay IV alteplase).

–Maintain O_2 saturation > 94%.

–Identify sources of hyperthermia (>38°C); give antipyretic medications.

–Correct hypotension and hypovolemia.

–Risk-stratify using NIH Stroke Scale Score (see Table 10–3).

TABLE 10–2 IMAGING MODALITIES IN STROKE	
Scenario	**"Usually Appropriate" Imaging Studies**
TIA, symptoms resolved	US duplex Doppler carotid artery, MRI head without IV contrast CT head without IV contrast, CTA head with IV contrast CTA neck with IV contrast MRA head without IV contrast
Adult, focal neuro deficit suggestive of acute stroke	MRI head without IV contrast, CT head without IV contrast, CT head with IV contrast, CT neck with IV contrast
Adult with ischemic CVA in past 24 h	US duplex Doppler carotid artery MRI head without IV contrast CT head without IV contrast CTA head with IV contrast CTA neck with IV contrast
Adult with ischemic CVA > 24 h ago	MRI head without IV contrast CT head without IV contrast CTA head with IV contrast CTA neck with IV contrast
Adult with known intraparenchymal hemorrhage	MRI head without and with IV contrast MRI head without IV contrast CT head without IV contrast CTA head with IV contrast

Source: ACR Appropriateness Criteria. https://acsearch.acr.org/docs/69478/Narrative/

TABLE 10–3 NATIONAL INSTITUTES OF HEALTH STROKE SCALE SCORE	
1a. Level of consciousness	0 = Alert; keenly responsive 1 = Not alert, but arousable by minor stimulation 2 = Not alert; requires repeated stimulation 3 = Unresponsive or responds only with reflex
1b. Level of consciousness questions: 　What is the month? 　What is your age?	0 = Answers two questions correctly 1 = Answers one question correctly 2 = Answers neither question correctly
1c. Level of consciousness commands: 　Open and close your eyes 　Grip and release your hand	0 = Performs both tasks correctly 1 = Performs one task correctly 2 = Performs neither task correctly
2. Best gaze	0 = Normal 1 = Partial gaze palsy 2 = Forced deviation

TABLE 10–3 NATIONAL INSTITUTES OF HEALTH STROKE SCALE SCORE *(continued)*	
3. Visual	0 = No visual loss 1 = Partial hemianopia 2 = Complete hemianopia 3 = Bilateral hemianopia
4. Facial palsy	0 = Normal symmetric movements 1 = Minor paralysis 2 = Partial paralysis 3 = Complete paralysis of one or both sides

5. Motor arm
  5a. Left arm
  5b. Right arm
	0 = No drift
	1 = Drift
	2 = Some effort against gravity
	3 = No effort against gravity; limb falls
	4 = No movement

6. Motor leg
  6a. Left leg
  6b. Right leg
	0 = No drift
	1 = Drift
	2 = Some effort against gravity
	3 = No effort against gravity
	4 = No movement

7. Limb ataxia	0 = Absent 1 = Present in one limb 2 = Present in two limbs
8. Sensory	0 = Normal; no sensory loss 1 = Mild-to-moderate sensory loss 2 = Severe to total sensory loss
9. Best language	0 = No aphasia; normal 1 = Mild-to-moderate aphasia 2 = Severe aphasia 3 = Mute, global aphasia
10. Dysarthria	0 = Normal 1 = Mild-to-moderate dysarthria 2 = Severe dysarthria
11. Extinction and inattention	0 = No abnormality 1 = Visual, tactile, auditory, spatial, or personal inattention 2 = Profound hemi-inattention or extinction
Total score = 0–42.	

Therapy: Thrombolytics

–For severe/disabling symptoms, give IV alteplase within 3 h from symptom onset, if ischemic stroke. Despite increased risk of hemorrhagic transformation, there is proven clinical benefit for patients with severe stroke symptoms.

–The benefit of IV alteplase between 3 and 4.5 h from symptom onset for patients with very severe stroke symptoms (NIHSS > 25) is uncertain. Give IV alteplase in this window for patients ≤ 80 y of age, without a history of both diabetes mellitus and prior stroke, NIHSS score ≤ 25, not taking any OACs, and without imaging evidence of ischemic injury involving more than one-third of the MCA territory.

–For mild/nondisabling symptoms, consider IV alteplase up to 4.5 h from symptom onset after discussion of risks and benefits.

–Do not give IV alteplase in the following scenarios:
- Ischemic stroke patients who have an unclear time and/or unwitnessed symptom onset and in whom last known normal (LKN) is >3 or 4.5 h.
- Ischemic stroke patients who awoke with stroke with time LKN > 3 or 4.5 h.
- Patients who have had a prior ischemic stroke within 3 mo.
- Recent severe head trauma (within 3 mo).
- Patients who have a history of intracranial hemorrhage.
- Patients with platelets < 100,000/mcL, INR > 1.7, aPTT > 40 s, or PT > 15 s (safety and efficacy are unknown). In patients without history of thrombocytopenia, treatment with IV alteplase can be initiated before availability of platelet count but should be discontinued if platelet count is <100,000/mcL.
- Patients who have received a treatment dose of LMWH within the previous 24 h. The use of IV alteplase in patients taking direct thrombin inhibitors or direct factor Xa inhibitors has not been firmly established but may be harmful.
- In patients with symptoms consistent with infective endocarditis, treatment with IV alteplase should not be administered because of the increased risk of intracranial hemorrhage.

–The following scenarios are not independent contraindications to IV alteplase:
- Age > 80.
- Warfarin use with INR ≤ 1.7.
- ESRD with normal aPTT.
- Seizure.
- Remote history of GI bleed.
- Recent non-STEMI.

–Special situations:
- Severely elevated BP: lower (to <185/110 mmHg) and assess stability before giving IV alteplase.
- Antiplatelet therapy (single or dual): proceed with IV alteplase, as the benefit outweighs the increased risk of symptomatic intracerebral hemorrhage.
- Major surgery in the prior 14 d: consider IV alteplase but weigh the risk of surgical-site hemorrhage against the anticipated benefits of reduced neurologic deficits.
- Concurrent stroke and acute MI: give IV alteplase at the dose appropriate for cerebral ischemia, then pursue percutaneous coronary angioplasty and stenting.

- Current malignancy: safety and efficacy of IV alteplase are not well established. Consider if reasonable (>6 mo) life expectancy and no other contraindications.
- Pregnancy/postpartum: consider when the anticipated benefits of treating moderate or severe stroke outweigh the anticipated increased risks of uterine bleeding.

–Obtain a follow-up CT or MRI scan at 24 h after IV alteplase before starting anticoagulants or antiplatelet agents.

Therapy: Mechanical Thrombectomy

–In selected patients with AIS within 6–24 h of LKN who have large vessel occlusion (LVO) in the anterior circulation, obtain CTP, DW-MRI, or MRI perfusion to aid in patient selection for mechanical thrombectomy.

–Offer mechanical thrombectomy with a stent retriever for patients with minimal prestroke disability, who have a causative occlusion of the internal carotid artery or proximal middle cerebral artery, have an NIHSS score of ≥6, have a reassuring noncontrast head CT (ASPECT score of ≥6), and if they can be treated within 6 h of LKN. No perfusion imaging (CT-P or MR-P) is required in these patients.

–Offer mechanical thrombectomy to selected patients with stroke within 6–16 h of LKN who have LVO in the anterior circulation and meet other DAWN[1] or DEFUSE 3[2] eligibility criteria.

–Some patients may be eligible for thrombectomy within 16–24 h of LKN per the DAWN eligibility criteria.

Therapy: Blood Pressure

–If otherwise eligible for acute reperfusion therapy but exhibit BP > 185/110 mmHg, use any of the following to lower BP:

- Labetalol 10–20 mg IV over 1–2 min, may repeat 1 time.
- Nicardipine 5 mg/h IV, titrate up by 2.5 mg/h every 5–15 min, maximum 15 mg/h; when desired BP reached, adjust to maintain proper BP limits.
- Clevidipine 1–2 mg/h IV, titrate by doubling the dose every 2–5 min until desired BP reached; maximum 21 mg/h.
- Other agents including hydralazine and enalaprilat may also be considered.

–If BP is not maintained ≤185/110 mmHg, do not administer alteplase.

–Maintain BP ≤ 180/105 mmHg during and after alteplase.

–Monitor BP every 15 min for 2 h from the start of alteplase therapy, then every 30 min for 6 h, and then every hour for 16 h.

–If systolic BP > 180–230 mmHg or diastolic BP > 105–120 mmHg, use one of the following:

- Labetalol 10 mg IV followed by continuous IV infusion 2–8 mg/min.
- Nicardipine 5 mg/h IV, titrate up to desired effect by 2.5 mg/h every 5–15 min, maximum 15 mg/h.
- Clevidipine 1–2 mg/h IV, titrate by doubling the dose every 2–5 min until desired BP reached; maximum 21 mg/h.
- If BP is not controlled or diastolic BP >140 mmHg, consider IV sodium nitroprusside.

[1] *N Engl J Med.* 2018;378(1):11–21. https://pubmed.ncbi.nlm.nih.gov/29129157/
[2] *N Engl J Med.* 2018;378:708–718. https://pubmed.ncbi.nlm.nih.gov/29364767/

–Treat hypertension early only when required by comorbid conditions (eg, concomitant acute coronary event, acute heart failure, aortic dissection, post-thrombolysis, symptomatic intracerebral hemorrhage, or preeclampsia/eclampsia). Lowering BP initially by 15% is probably safe.

–Consider lowering BP by 15% in the first 24 h after stroke in patients with BP $\geq$ 220/120 mmHg who did not receive IV alteplase or endovascular treatment and have no comorbid conditions requiring acute antihypertensive treatment, though the benefit of initiating or reinitiating treatment of hypertension within the first 48–72 h is uncertain.

–Start or restart antihypertensive therapy during hospitalization in patients with BP > 140/90 mmHg who are neurologically stable.

Therapy: Antiplatelets

–Give aspirin within 24–48 h after onset. For those treated with IV alteplase, delay until 24 h.

–In patients presenting with minor stroke, treat for 21 d with dual-antiplatelet therapy (aspirin and clopidogrel).

Therapy: Rehabilitation Poststroke

–Provide rehabilitation to stroke survivors at an intensity commensurate with anticipated benefit and tolerance.

–Provide a formal assessment of ADLs and IADLs, communication abilities, and functional mobility before discharge from acute care hospitalization and incorporate the findings into the care transition and the discharge planning process.

–Perform regular skin assessments with objective scales of risk such as the Braden scale.

–Consider resting ankle splints used at night and during assisted standing for prevention of ankle contracture in the hemiplegic limb.

–Continue regular turning, good skin hygiene, and use of specialized mattresses, wheelchair cushions, and seating until mobility returns.

–Use prophylactic-dose subcutaneous heparin (UFH or LMWH) for the duration of the acute and rehabilitation hospital stay or until the stroke survivor regains mobility.

–Remove a Foley catheter within 24 h of hospitalization. Assess urinary retention through bladder scanning or intermittent catheterization.

–Refer individuals discharged to the community to participate in exercise programs with balance training to reduce falls.

–Provide a formal fall prevention program during hospitalization.

–Administer a structured depression inventory such as the Patient Health Questionnaire-2 to routinely screen for poststroke depression.

–Evaluate individuals residing in long-term care facilities for calcium and vitamin D supplementation.

–Assess speech, language, cognitive communication, pragmatics, reading, and writing; assess vision and hearing for any contribution or deficits; identify communicative strengths and weaknesses; and identify helpful compensatory strategies.

–Start enteral diet within 7 d of admission after an acute stroke.

–For patients with dysphagia, consider using nasogastric tubes initially for feeding in the early phase of stroke (starting within the first 7 d) and to place percutaneous gastrostomy tubes in patients with longer anticipated persistent inability to swallow safely (>2–3 wk).

–Consider directing patients and families with stroke to palliative care resources. Caregivers should ascertain and include patient-centered preferences in decision-making, especially during prognosis formation and considering interventions or limitations in care.

Source
–*Stroke*. 2018;49(3):e46–e110.

Management: Adults with Stroke and Medical Comorbidities

Recommendations from

> ### AHA/ASA 2014, 2018

Atrial Fibrillation
–Start oral anticoagulation within 14 d after the onset of neurologic symptoms.
–If high risk for hemorrhagic conversion (ie, large infarct, hemorrhagic transformation on initial imaging, uncontrolled hypertension, or hemorrhage tendency), delay initiation of oral anticoagulation beyond 14 d.
–Choose VKA therapy (Class I; Level of Evidence A), apixaban (Class I; Level of Evidence A), or dabigatran (Class I; Level of Evidence B) for the prevention of recurrent stroke in patients with nonvalvular atrial fibrillation (AF), whether paroxysmal or permanent.
–If unable to take oral anticoagulants, aspirin alone is recommended. Consider the addition of clopidogrel to aspirin therapy.
–The closure of the left atrial appendage with the WATCHMAN device in patients with ischemic stroke or TIA and AF is of uncertain usefulness.

Hypertension
–Start BP therapy for previously untreated patients with ischemic stroke or TIA who after the first several days have an established SBP ≥ 140 mmHg or DBP ≥ 90 mmHg.
–In patients previously treated for HTN, resume BP therapy after the first several days for both prevention of recurrent stroke and other vascular events.
–Goals: <140/90 mmHg; for recent lacunar stroke reasonable SBP target < 130 mmHg.

Dyslipidemia
–Start intensive lipid-lowering therapy for patients with ischemic stroke or TIA presumed to be of atherosclerotic origin and an LDL-C ≥ 100 mg/dL, regardless of evidence of other clinical ASCVD.

Elevated Blood Glucose
–Screen all patients for DM with an HbA1c.

Obesity
–Calculate BMI for all patients and start weight-loss management when necessary.

Sleep Apnea
–Consider a sleep study for any patient with a history of CVA or TIA on the basis of very high prevalence in this population.

MI and Cardiac Thrombus
–Consider VKA therapy (INR: 2–3) for 3 mo in patients with ischemic stroke or TIA in the setting of acute anterior STEMI.

Cardiomyopathy

–In patients with ischemic stroke or TIA in sinus rhythm who have left atrial or left ventricular thrombus demonstrated by echocardiography or other imaging modality, give anticoagulant therapy with a VKA for ≥3 mo.

Valvular Heart Disease

–For patients with ischemic stroke or TIA who have rheumatic mitral valve disease and AF, use long-term VKA therapy with an INR target of 2.5 (range 2.0–3.0).

–For patients with ischemic stroke or TIA and native aortic or nonrheumatic mitral valve disease who do not have AF or another indication for anticoagulation, use antiplatelet therapy.

Prosthetic Heart Valve

–For patients with a mechanical aortic valve and a history of ischemic stroke or TIA before its insertion, use VKA therapy with an INR target of 2.5 (range 2.0–3.0).

–For patients with a mechanical mitral valve and a history of ischemic stroke or TIA before its insertion, use VKA therapy with an INR target of 3.0 (range 2.5–3.5).

–For patients with a mechanical mitral or aortic valve who have a history of ischemic stroke or TIA before its insertion and who are at low risk for bleeding, add aspirin 75–100 mg/d to VKA therapy.

–For patients with a bioprosthetic aortic or mitral valve, a history of ischemic stroke, or TIA before its insertion, and no other indication for anticoagulation therapy beyond 3–6 mo from the valve placement, use long-term therapy with aspirin 75–100 mg/d rather than long-term anticoagulation.

Aortic Arch Atheroma

–For patients with an ischemic stroke or TIA and evidence of aortic arch atheroma, use antiplatelet therapy.

Patent Foramen Ovale

–For patients with an ischemic stroke or TIA and a patent foramen ovale (PFO) who are not undergoing anticoagulation therapy, use antiplatelet therapy.

–For patients with an ischemic stroke or TIA and both a PFO and a venous source of embolism, anticoagulation is indicated, depending on stroke characteristics. When anticoagulation is contraindicated, an inferior vena cava filter is reasonable.

–For patients with a cryptogenic ischemic stroke or TIA and a PFO without evidence for DVT, available data do not support a benefit for PFO closure.

–In the setting of PFO and DVT, PFO closure by a transcatheter device might be considered, depending on the risk of recurrent DVT.

Patients <30

–Consider screening for hyperhomocysteinemia among young patients with a recent ischemic stroke or TIA. The most common concern is mutation in *MTHFR* gene. (*Circulation*. 2015; 132:e6–e9)

Hypercoagulable States

–Uncertain utility to screening for thrombophilic states in patients with ischemic stroke or TIA.

–Offer antiplatelet therapy to patients who are found to have abnormal findings on coagulation testing after an initial ischemic stroke or TIA if anticoagulation therapy is not administered.

Sickle Cell Disease

–For patients with sickle cell disease and prior ischemic stroke or TIA, use chronic blood transfusions to reduce hemoglobin S to <30% of total hemoglobin.

Pregnancy

–In the presence of a high-risk condition that would require anticoagulation outside of pregnancy, use one of the following options:

- LMWH twice daily throughout pregnancy, with dose adjusted to achieve the LMWH manufacturer's recommended peak anti-Xa level 4 h after injection, **OR**
- Adjusted-dose UFH throughout pregnancy, administered subcutaneously every 12 h in doses adjusted to keep the mid-interval aPTT at least 2× control or to maintain an anti-Xa heparin level of 0.35–0.70 U/mL, **OR**
- UFH or LMWH (as above) until the 13th wk, followed by substitution of a VKA until close to delivery, when UFH or LMWH is resumed.

–For pregnant persons receiving adjusted-dose LMWH therapy for a high-risk condition that would require anticoagulation outside of pregnancy, and when delivery is planned, discontinue LMWH ≥ 24 h before induction of labor or cesarean section.

–In the presence of a low-risk situation in which antiplatelet therapy would be the treatment recommendation outside of pregnancy, consider UFH or LMWH, or no treatment during the first trimester of pregnancy depending on the clinical situation.

Breastfeeding

–If anticoagulation is required, use warfarin, UFH, or LMWH.

–If antiplatelet therapy is required, use low-dose aspirin.

Sources

–*Stroke*. 2014;45.
–http://stroke.ahajournals.org
–*Stroke*. 2018;49:e46–e99.

Management: Adults Presenting to Primary Care After Acute Stroke

Recommendations from

➢ AHA/ASA 2022

–At first stroke follow-up visit.

- Obtain and review hospital records.
- Review patient's understanding of event, questions, fears, and psychologic consequences.
- Confirm that the evaluation for etiology is complete and, if needed, a treatment plan is in place.
- If carotid revascularization, antiplatelet therapy, or statin therapy is indicated, ensure implementation.

- If patient was a candidate for dual antiplatelet therapy, ensure that they are taking it and that they discontinue it at 21 d (or, 90 d if severe stenosis of intracerebral artery).
- If comorbidities that led to stroke, remediate them.

–Assess for functional impairments and address.

- Support individually tailored exercise program.
- Refer for balance training to reduce falls.
- Arrange other interventions if indicated.
  - Speech therapy.
  - Communication devices.
  - Enriched environments for cognitive needs.
  - Botulinum injection for spasticity.
  - Individualize pain pharmacotherapy.
  - Balance training.
  - Assistive devices for balance.
  - Mobility training.
  - AFO for foot drop, ankle instability.
  - Task practice.
  - ADL and IADL training.
  - Cane, walker, wheelchair.
  - Adaptive devices.
  - Eye exercises.
  - Audiovisual special exploration training.
  - Hearing amplification training.

Source
–*Stroke*. 2021;52:e558–e571.

SYNCOPE

Management: Adults

Recommendations from

> ACC/AHA 2017

–Evaluate syncope with a careful history and physical examination.

- Look for signs suggestive of cardiac syncope, especially when patient is aged >60 y, has known heart disease, had a brief or no prodrome, had syncope during exertion or while supine, and has had no more than 1–2 syncopal episodes.
- Consider noncardiac causes in younger patients without cardiac disease who had syncope while standing or rising to stand. Also consider noncardiac causes when there is a significant prodrome or situational triggers (coughing, laughing, micturating, defecating, swallowing), or when there is a pattern of similar episodes.

TABLE 10–4 EXAMPLE OF SERIOUS MEDICAL CONDITIONS THAT MIGHT WARRANT CONSIDERATION OF FURTHER EVALUATION AND THERAPY IN HOSPITAL SETTING

Cardiac Arrhythmic Conditions	Cardiac or Vascular Nonarrhythmic Conditions	Noncardiac Conditions
• Sustained or symptomatic VT • Symptomatic conduction system disease or Mobitz II or third-degree heart block • Symptomatic bradycardia or sinus pauses not related to neurally mediated syncope • Symptomatic SVT • Pacemaker, ICD malfunction • Inheritable cardiovascular conditions predisposing to arrhythmias	• Cardiac ischemia • Severe aortic stenosis • Cardiac tamponade • HCM • Severe prosthetic valve dysfunction • Pulmonary embolism • Aortic dissection • Acute HF • Moderate-to-severe LV dysfunction	• Severe anemia/gastrointestinal bleeding • Major traumatic injury due to syncope • Persistent vital sign abnormalities

Source: Reproduced with permission from Shen WK et al. 2017 ACC/AHA/HRS Guideline for the evaluation and management of patients with syncope: executive summary: a report of the American College of Cardiology/American Heart Association Task Force on Clinical Practice Guidelines and the Heart Rhythm Society. *Circulation.* 2017;136(5):e25–e59.

–Obtain the following studies routinely in the evaluation of syncope:
  • ECG.
  • Complete blood count, basic metabolic panel, and other targeted labs based on clinical assessment.
  • Echocardiogram if structural heart disease is suspected.
  • Stress test if exertional syncope of unclear etiology.
  • Continuous telemetry monitoring for patients admitted to hospital.
  • Prolonged cardiac monitoring if arrhythmic syncope is suspected.
  • Electrophysiologic study if syncope of suspected arrhythmic etiology with negative cardiac monitoring.
–See Table 10–4 for findings that warrant inpatient evaluation.

Source
–*Circulation.* 2017;135:e1159–e1195.

TINNITUS

Management: Adults

Recommendations from

➤ ACR 2023

–For pulsatile tinnitus without retrotympanic lesion, order MRA head with IV contrast, MRI head and internal auditory canal without and with IV contrast, CTA head and neck with IV contrast, or CTA head with IV contrast.
–For pulsatile tinnitus with a retrotympanic lesion, order CT temporal bone without IV contrast.

-For unilateral nonpulsatile tinnitus, with no hearing loss or neurologic deficit or trauma, order MRI head and internal auditory canal without and with IV contrast.

-For bilateral nonpulsatile tinnitus, with no hearing loss or neurologic deficit or trauma, do not order imaging studies.

Source

-https://acsearch.acr.org/docs/3094199/Narrative

TRANSIENT ISCHEMIC ATTACK (TIA)

Management: Adults

Recommendations from

➢ AHA 2022, NICE 2022

Guidelines Alert 10–1
GUIDELINES DISCORDANT: RISK STRATIFICATION IN TIA

Organization	Guidance
AHA/ASA	Risk scores such as ABCD^2 can help identify high-risk patients but are inadequate tools Obtain vessel imaging prior to disposition regardless of risk scores
	Obtain specialty evaluation within 24 h for all patients with suspected TIA Do not use ABCD^2 score to determine stroke risk or urgency of evaluation

Applying to Clinical Practice
- Symptoms of posterior stroke are excluded by ABCD^2 score.
- If large artery disease or AF is present, the risk score may underestimate risk.
- Obtain a cerebrovascular study promptly in all patients, regardless of risk score.

Guidelines Alert 10–2
GUIDELINES DISCORDANT: ROLE OF IMAGING IN SUSPECTED TIA

Organization	CT	MRI
AHA/ASA	Obtain noncontrast head CT routinely unless MRI is available promptly	MRI with diffusion-weighted imaging within 24 h of symptom onset
NICE	Do not obtain CT unless suspicion of alternative diagnosis	Consider MRI after consultation with specialist

Applying to Clinical Practice
- In the United States, the AHA/ASA guideline establishes the standard of care.

Evaluation

–To consider a TIA, the patient's neurologic evaluation must have returned to baseline. If continued neurologic signs or symptoms, ensure prompt evaluation for stroke or other cause.

–If TIA is suspected, factors suggestive of TIA vs. mimic include:

- Older age.
- Vascular risk factors (hypertension, diabetes, smoking, obesity, AF, previous stroke, obstructive sleep apnea).
- Short duration (<80 min).
- Abrupt onset.
- Minimal symptoms at onset.
- Preserved mentation.

–Routinely screen for carotid stenosis, unless the patient would not be a candidate for endarterectomy. CT angiography is more sensitive than MR angiography. Carotid Doppler ultrasound is another reasonable option.

Therapy

–Start antiplatelet agent immediately.

- NICE: aspirin 300 mg daily.
- AHA/ASA:
    - $ABCD^2$ < 4: aspirin 50–325 mg daily or clopidogrel 75 mg daily or aspirin/dipyridamole 25/200 mg daily.
    - $ABCD^2$ ≥ 4: aspirin 81 mg + clopidogrel 75 mg daily × 21–90 d, then monotherapy.
    - $ABCD^2$ ≥ 6: aspirin 81 mg + clopidogrel 75 mg daily ×21–90 d OR ticagrelor 180-mg load then 90-mg BID plus aspirin 75–100 mg daily ×30 d, then monotherapy.

–Statins: initiate or continue therapy.

–If HTN, antihypertensives with BP goal of <130/80 mmHg.

–If DM, appropriate glycemic management.

Sources

–*Stroke*. 2023;54:e109–e121.

–www.nice.org.uk/guidance/ng128

TRAUMATIC BRAIN INJURY

Management: Adults and Children

Recommendations from

> ACEP 2013

–Avoid CT scan of head for minor head trauma in patients who are low risk based on validated decision rules.

Source

–http://www.choosingwisely.org/societies/american-college-of-emergency-physicians/

TREMOR, ESSENTIAL

Management: Adults

Recommendations from

> AAN 2011

–Treat with propranolol or primidone.

–Alternative treatment options include alprazolam, atenolol, gabapentin, sotalol, or topiramate. Favor nonbenzodiazepine options due to risk of dependency and high side-effect profile.

–Do not use levetiracetam, pindolol, trazodone, acetazolamide, or 3,4-diaminopyridine.

Practice Pearls

- Essential tremor should be postural (occurs when body part is voluntarily maintained against gravity), symmetric, involving hands/wrists, lower extremities, and head/voice. It tends to improve with a small amount of alcohol intake. Patients with intention tremor, unilateral/symmetric tremor, or rest tremor should be evaluated for alternative diagnoses.
  - Propranolol or primidone for first-line therapy.
- Unilateral thalamotomy may be effective for severe refractory essential tremors.

Sources

–http://www.neurology.org/content/77/19/1752.full.pdf+html

–*Am Fam Physician.* 2018;97(3):180–186.

PREGNANCY AND PERINATAL CARE

ABORTION

Management: Women, Incomplete Abortion

Recommendations from

> WHO 2018, Society of Family Planning 2023

–Offer surgical or medical management vs. watchful waiting.

–If patient < 13-wk gestation elects medical management, give misoprostol 600 mcg orally or 400 mcg sublingually. Do not use vaginal misoprostol.

–If patient ≥ 13-wk gestation elects medical management, give repeated doses of misoprostol 400 mcg every 3 h sublingually, vaginally, or buccally.

Management: Women, Intrauterine Fetal Demise, 14–28-wk Gestation

Recommendations from

> WHO 2018

–Offer surgical or medical management vs. watchful waiting.

–If patient elects medical management, give 200-mg mifepristone[1] orally; 1–2 d later, give 400-mcg misoprostol sublingually or vaginally, and repeat every 4–6 h. Complete abortion expected at 24–48 h. If mifepristone is not available or not preferred by the patient, give misoprostol 400 mcg every 4–6 h as the initial treatment.

–Adjunctive osmotic dilators are of limited benefit and usually only effective at 24 and 0/7 wk of gestation and past and used in combination with misoprostol.

Management: Women, Elective Abortion

Recommendations from

> WHO 2018, ACOG/SFP 2020

–Options include vacuum aspiration (manual or electric), dilation, and evacuation or medical management.

---

[1] Mifepristone access is restricted by the FDA under the risk evaluation and mitigation strategy and approved through 70 d of gestation. Rules for its use are summarized here: https://www.fda.gov/drugs/postmarket-drug-safety-information-patients-and-providers/information-about-mifepristone-medical-termination-pregnancy-through-20-weeks-gestation

–For medical abortion, give mifepristone 200 mg once as initial dose. At least 24 h later, give misoprostol 800 mcg vaginally, sublingually, or buccally (WHO: If ≥12-wk gestation, give 400 mcg). Alternative regimen 24 h after mifepristone, give misoprostol 400 mcg vaginally, buccally, or sublingually q3 h × 4 doses between 14.0 and 23.6 GA. (*Contraception.* 2024)

–If mifepristone is not available, use misoprostol monotherapy (800 mcg, repeat q3 h up to 3 doses).

–Offer NSAIDs for pain management. (ACOG/SFP)

Sources

–*Contraception.* 2024;129.

–*Medical Management of Abortion.* Geneva: World Health Organization; 2018. License: CC BY-NC-SA 3.0 IGO.

–*Obstet Gynecol.* 2020;136.

–Society of Family Planning. *Clinical Recommendation (Society for Maternal Fetal Medicine): Medication Abortion.* 2023.

ANEMIA

Screening: Pregnant Persons

Recommendations from

➢ USPSTF 2015, ACOG 2021

–Consider screening all patients with hemoglobin or hematocrit at first prenatal visit.

Guidelines Alert 11–1 **GUIDELINES DISCORDANT: SCREENING FOR ANEMIA IN PREGNANCY**	
Organization	**Guidance**
ACOG	Screen all pregnant persons twice: In the first trimester At 24-0/7–27-6/7-wk EGA Evaluate first trimester Hct < 33% and second trimester Hct < 32% for etiology of anemia
USPSTF	Insufficient evidence to recommend for or against routine screening for iron deficiency anemia in pregnant patients to prevent adverse maternal or birth outcomes. Insufficient evidence to recommend for or against use of iron supplements for nonanemic pregnant patients

Applying to Clinical Practice
- The ACOG recommendation for screening is based on consensus/expert opinion rather than definitive evidence of benefit.
- Iron deficiency anemia is associated with low birth weight, preterm delivery, and perinatal mortality.
- While screening and supplementation have not been definitively proven to improve outcomes, the harms are minimal.
- ACOG's screening recommendations should be considered the standard of care until data suggest otherwise.

Practice Pearls

- An iron panel consistent with iron deficiency would reveal low iron level, increased total iron-binding capacity, decreased ferritin, and an iron/total iron-binding capacity ratio < 18%. Other patterns would warrant further evaluation for alternate etiologies.
- ACOG: supplement those with iron deficiency using low-dose iron starting in the first trimester or at diagnosis. Expect increasing reticulocyte index after 1 wk and increasing hematocrit after a few weeks. If there is no improvement, consider adherence, alternate dx, or escalate to IV iron.
- Oral iron is first-line therapy for iron deficiency anemia in pregnancy. IV iron is preferred choice (after 13th wk) for those who have oral iron intolerance. Cobalamin and folate deficiency should be excluded. (*Blood*. 2017;129:940–949)
- A growing body of evidence suggests that oral iron in single doses on alternating days is associated with better absorption and adherence (due to reduced side effects) compared to daily dosing or split doses on alternating days. (*Lancet Haematol*. 2017;4(11):e524; Tolkien et al. *PLoS One*. 2015;10(2):e0117383)
- Decision to transfuse should be based on the Hb, clinical context, and patient preferences. May be appropriate in severe anemia (<7 mg/dL according to WHO) in whom a 2-wk delay in Hb rise with oral iron may result in significant morbidity.

Sources
–USPSTF. https://www.uspreventiveservicestaskforce.org/
–*Ann Intern Med*. 2015;163:529–536.
–ACOG. *Obstet Gynecol*. 2021;138(2):e57.

ANXIETY

Screening: Pregnant Women

Recommendations from

➤ USPSTF 2023

–Screen for anxiety disorders in pregnant and postpartum persons.

Source
–JAMA. doi:10.1001/jama.2023.9301

BACTERIAL VAGINOSIS

Screening: Pregnant Women

Recommendations from

➤ USPSTF 2020

–Do not screen routinely.

–Insufficient evidence to recommend for or against routine screening for patients at high risk[1] for preterm delivery.

Source

–USPSTF. *Bacterial Vaginosis in Pregnant Persons to Prevent Preterm Delivery: Screening.* 2020.

BACTERIURIA, ASYMPTOMATIC

Screening: Pregnant Women

Recommendations from

> IDSA 2019, USPSTF 2019, ACOG/AAP 2017

–Screen for bacteriuria with urine culture at first prenatal visit or at 12–16-wk gestation.

–Treat pregnant patients who have asymptomatic bacteriuria with antimicrobial therapy for 4–7 d.

Practice Pearls

- Treating bacteriuria in pregnancy with antibiotics reduces the risk of pyelonephritis and low birth weight.
- A positive culture contains >100,000 CFU/mL of a single pathogen. Group B strep concentrations of >10,000 CFU/mL suggest vaginal colonization and would be an indication for intrapartum prophylaxis.

Sources

–USPSTF. *Asymptomatic Bacteriuria in Adults: Screening.* 2019.

–*Clin Infect Dis.* 2019;68(10):e83–e110.

–American Academy of Pediatrics, American College of Obstetricians and Gynecologists. *Guidelines for Perinatal Care.* 8th ed. Elk Grove Village, Illinois and Washington, DC: AAP/ACOG, 2017:159–160.

BREASTFEEDING CHALLENGES

Management: Women

Recommendations from

> ACOG 2021

–Recommend breastfeeding exclusively for 6 mo. Continue breastfeeding as complementary foods are introduced during the infant's first year of life or longer, as mutually desired by the woman and her infant.

–Provide proactive lactation support, including education on hand expression, in anticipation of potential breastfeeding difficulties.

---

[1] Risk factors: African-American race or ethnicity, BMI < 20, previous preterm delivery, vaginal bleeding, shortened cervix < 2.5 cm, pelvic infection, bacterial vaginosis.

–Manage engorgement expectantly if symptoms are mild and the infant has good latch.

–Perform a focused history and physical exam to distinguish the specific cause of persistent pain while breastfeeding or nipple injury. Treat as indicated.

–Reassure women that their milk supply is adequate if the average feeding frequency is 8–12 times per day, steady weight is gained by day 4 or 5, and 6–8 wet diapers occur on average per day. Counsel on signs of low milk supply or dehydration such as jaundice, insufficient wet or soiled diapers, lethargy, inconsolability, unchanged stool color (not bright yellow by day 5), and a lack of steady infant weight gain.

–Encourage breastfeeding in women who are stable on medication-assisted treatment for opioid use disorders who are not using illicit drugs and who have no other contraindications to breastfeeding.

–Do not use galactagogues as a first-line therapy.

Source
–ACOG. *Committee Opinion No. 820. Breastfeeding Challenges.* 2021.

BREECH PRESENTATION

Management: Pregnant Women Near Term

Recommendations from

➤ ACOG 2020

–Assess and document fetal presentation starting at 36 wk of gestation to allow for external cephalic version (ECV) when indicated and desired.

–Offer ECV to all women near term with breech presentations unless there are contraindications.

–Perform ECV after 37-0/7 wk, as spontaneous version is unlikely to occur after this gestational age, and the risk of spontaneous reversion is lower.

–For patients who are Rh-negative, give Rh-immune globulin unless known to have Rh-negative fetus, are already sensitized, or will be delivered in less than 72 h.

Practice Pearls

- Complications from ECV occur at rates less than 1% and include placental abruption, umbilical cord prolapse, rupture of membranes, stillbirth, and fetomaternal hemorrhage.
- Evidence supports the use of parenteral tocolysis to improve ECV success; adding neuraxial analgesia is reasonable.
- ECV is approximately 60% successful in achieving a cephalic vaginal birth.

Source
–*Obstet Gynecol.* 2020;135(5):e203–e212.

CESAREAN SECTION, PRIMARY

Prevention: Pregnant Women

Recommendations from

> ACOG 2012, WHO 2018

–Induce labor only for medical indications. If induction is performed for nonmedical reasons, ensure that gestational age is >39 wk and cervix is favorable. (ACOG)

–Do not diagnose failed induction or arrest of labor until sufficient time[1] has passed. (ACOG)

–Consider intermittent auscultation rather than continuous fetal monitoring if heart rate is normal. (ACOG)

–Implement prenatal education programs including childbirth training, nurse-led relaxation, couple-based support, and psychoeducation. (WHO)

–Consider mandatory second opinion for cesarean section decisions. (WHO)

–Give timely feedback to health care professionals regarding cesarean section decision-making. (WHO)

–Include in recovery counseling: wound care; pain management; assessing the wound for signs of infection, separation, or dehiscence; awareness of increased risk of thromboembolic disease; resuming activities (heavy lifting, formal exercise, sexual intercourse).

Practice Pearl

• If fetal heart rate variability is moderate, other factors have little association with fetal neurologic outcomes. For more on this and other related information on fetal monitoring, see Macones GA, Hankins GD, Spong CY, et al. The 2008 National Institute of Child Health and Human Development Workshop report on electronic fetal monitoring: update on definitions, interpretation, and research guidelines. *Obstet Gynecol.* 2008;112:661.

Sources

–*Obstet Gynecol.* 2012;120(5):1181.

–World Health Organization. *WHO Prevention Recommendations Non-Clinical Interventions to Reduce Unnecessary Cesarean Sections.* 2018.

–NICE. *Cesarean Birth.* 2024.

CESAREAN SECTION, REPEAT

Prevention: Pregnant Women, Prior Cesarean Delivery

Recommendations from

> AAFP 2014, ACOG 2017

–Attempting a vaginal birth after cesarean (VBAC) is safe and appropriate for most patients.

---

[1] Failed induction: inability to generate contractions every 3 min and cervical change after 24 h of oxytocin administration and rupture of membranes, if feasible. Arrest of labor, first stage: 6 cm dilation, membrane rupture, and 4 h of adequate contractions or 6 h of inadequate contractions without cervical change. Arrest of labor, second stage: no descent or rotation for 4 h (nulliparous woman with epidural), 3 h (nulliparous woman without epidural or multiparous woman with epidural), or 2 h (multiparous woman without epidural).

–Encourage and facilitate planning for VBAC. If necessary, refer to a facility that offers trial of labor after cesarean (TOLAC).

Practice Pearls

- Provide counseling, encouragement, and facilitation for a planned VBAC so that patients can make informed decisions. If planned VBAC is not locally available, offer patients who desire it referral to a facility or clinician who offers the service.
- Obtain informed consent for planned VBAC, including risk to patient, fetus, future fertility, and the capabilities of local delivery setting.
- Develop facility guidelines to promote access to planned VBAC and improve quality of care for patients who elect TOLAC.
- Assess the likelihood of planned VBAC as well as individual risks to determine who is an appropriate candidate for TOLAC.
- A calculator for probability for successful VBAC is available here[1]: https://mfmunetwork.bsc. gwu.edu/PublicBSC/MFMU/VGBirthCalc/vagbirth.html

Sources

–AAFP. *Clinical Prevention Recommendation: Vaginal Birth after Cesarean.* 2014.
–*Obstet Gynecol.* 2017;130(5):1167–1169.

CHLAMYDIA AND GONORRHEA

Screening: Pregnant Women

Recommendations from

> CDC 2021, AAFP 2021, AAP/ACOG 2017

–Screen all patients aged <25 y at first prenatal visit.
–Screen patients aged ≥25 y with risk factors.[2]
–Retest in the third trimester those <25 y or age ≥25 y with risk factors.
–If infection is detected, obtain test of cure 3–4 wk after treatment and retest again within 3 mo.

Sources

–CDC. *Sexually Transmitted Diseases Treatment Guidelines.* 2021. https://www.cdc.gov/std/ treatment-guidelines/screening-recommendations.htm
–*Am Fam Physician.* 2022;106(1):online.
–AAP & ACOG. *Guidelines for Perinatal Care.* 8th ed. 2017.

---

[1] Note that, while certain racial groups are documented to have poorer VBAC outcomes, the inclusion of race as a factor in the VBAC score may disproportionately dissuade women of color from attempting TOLAC because their clinician perceives their probability of success to be lower. As no biological basis for the difference has been identified, structural racism likely explains the disparity in outcomes, an effect that may be propagated by using the VBAC risk calculator to determine appropriateness of TOLAC. (*NEJM.* 2020;383(9):874–882)

[2] Risk factors per the CDC include new partner, more than one sex partner, a sex partner with concurrent partners, or a sex partner who has an STI; practice inconsistent condom use when not in a mutually monogamous relationship; have a previous or coexisting STI; have a history of exchanging sex for money or drugs; or have a history of incarceration.

CONTRACEPTION

Management: Women

Recommendations from

> CDC

–Recommend contraception with consideration of comorbidities according to Table 11–1.
–Contraceptive effectiveness is outlined in Table 11–2.

CONTRACEPTION, EMERGENCY

Management: Women

Recommendations from

> ACOG 2015, WHO 2016, Society for Family Planning 2023

–Offer emergency contraception to women who have had unprotected or inadequately protected sexual intercourse within the past 5 d and who do not desire pregnancy.
–Offer emergency contraceptive pills, copper intrauterine device (IUD) or LNG 52 IUD to patients who request it up to 5 d after unprotected or inadequately protected sexual intercourse.
–Advise use of barrier contraceptives to prevent pregnancy after using emergency contraception or abstain from sexual intercourse for 14 d or until next menses.
–Counsel regarding medication options: copper IUD is more effective than emergency contraceptive pills. If used within 5 d of unprotected intercourse, the levonorgestrel (LNG) 52 mg IUD is noninferior to the copper IUD for emergency contraception. Oral ulipristal acetate pills are more effective than oral LNG pills.

Practice Pearls

- Combined progestin-estrogen pills, the copper IUD, and LNG 52 IUD are not FDA approved for use as emergency contraception but have been shown to be safe and effective and can be used off-label for this indication.
- No clinician examination or pregnancy testing is necessary before provision or prescription of emergency contraception.
- The copper IUD is appropriate for use as emergency contraception for women who desire long-acting contraception.
- Information regarding effective long-term contraceptive methods should be made available whenever a woman requests emergency contraception.
- Ulipristal acetate is more effective than LNG-only regimen and maintains its efficacy for up to 5 d.
- The LNG-only regimen is more effective than combined hormonal regimen and is associated with less nausea and vomiting compared with the combined estrogen–progestin regimen.
- Insertion of copper IUD is the most effective method of emergency contraception.

TABLE 11–1 CDC MEDICAL ELIGIBILITY CRITERIA FOR CONTRACEPTIVE USE

Condition	Sub-Condition	Cu-IUD I	C	LNG-IUD I	C	Implant I	C	DMPA I	C	POP I	C	CHC I	C
Age		Menarche to <20 yrs:2 / ≥20 yrs:1		Menarche to <20 yrs:2 / ≥20 yrs:1		Menarche to <18 yrs:1 / 18-45 yrs:1 / >45 yrs:1		Menarche to <18 yrs:2 / 18-45 yrs:1 / >45 yrs:1		Menarche to <18 yrs:1 / 18-45 yrs:1 / >45 yrs:1		Menarche to <40 yrs:1 / ≥40 yrs:2	
Anatomical abnormalities	a) Distorted uterine cavity	4		4									
	b) Other abnormalities	2		2									
Anemias	a) Thalassemia	2		1		1		1		1		1	
	b) Sickle cell disease[1]	2		1		1		1		1		2	
	c) Iron-deficiency anemia	2		1		1		1		1		1	
Benign ovarian tumors	(including cysts)	1		1		1		1		1		1	
Breast disease	a) Undiagnosed mass	1		2		2*		2*		2*		2*	
	b) Benign breast disease	1		1		1		1		1		1	
	c) Family history of cancer	1		1		1		1		1		1	
	d) Breast cancer[1]												
	i) Current	1		4		4		4		4		4	
	ii) Past and no evidence of current disease for 5 years	1		3		3		3		3		3	
Breastfeeding	a) <21 days postpartum					2*		2*		2*		4*	
	b) 21 to <30 days postpartum												
	i) With other risk factors for VTE					2*		2*		2*		3*	
	ii) Without other risk factors for VTE					2*		2*		2*		3*	
	c) 30-42 days postpartum												
	i) With other risk factors for VTE					1*		1*		1*		3*	
	ii) Without other risk factors for VTE					1*		1*		1*		2*	
	d) >42 days postpartum					1*		1*		1*		2*	
Cervical cancer	Awaiting treatment	4	2	4	2	2		2		1		2	
Cervical ectropion		1		1		1		1		1		1	
Cervical intraepithelial neoplasia		1		2		2		2		1		2	
Cirrhosis	a) Mild (compensated)	1		1		1		1		1		1	
	b) Severe[1] (decompensated)	1		3		3		3		3		4	
Cystic fibrosis[1]		1*		1*		1*		2*		1*		1*	
Deep venous thrombosis (DVT)/Pulmonary embolism (PE)	a) History of DVT/PE, not receiving anticoagulant therapy												
	i) Higher risk for recurrent DVT/PE	1		2		2		2		2		4	
	ii) Lower risk for recurrent DVT/PE	1		2		2		2		2		3	
	b) Acute DVT/PE	2		2		2		2		2		4	
	c) DVT/PE and established anticoagulant therapy for at least 3 months												
	i) Higher risk for recurrent DVT/PE	2		2		2		2		2		4*	
	ii) Lower risk for recurrent DVT/PE	2		2		2		2		2		3*	
	d) Family history (first-degree relatives)	1		1		1		1		1		2	
	e) Major surgery												
	i) With prolonged immobilization	1		2		2		2		2		4	
	ii) Without prolonged immobilization	1		1		1		1		1		2	
	f) Minor surgery without immobilization	1		1		1		1		1		1	
Depressive disorders		1*		1*		1*		1*		1*		1*	

Key:

1 No restriction (method can be used)	3 Theoretical or proven risks usually outweigh the advantages
2 Advantages generally outweigh theoretical or proven risks	4 Unacceptable health risk (method not to be used)

TABLE 11–1 CDC MEDICAL ELIGIBILITY CRITERIA FOR CONTRACEPTIVE USE (*continued*)

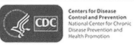

Centers for Disease Control and Prevention
National Center for Chronic Disease Prevention and Health Promotion

Condition	Sub-Condition	Cu-IUD I	Cu-IUD C	LNG-IUD I	LNG-IUD C	Implant I	Implant C	DMPA I	DMPA C	POP I	POP C	CHC I	CHC C
Diabetes	a) History of gestational disease	1		1		1		1		1		1	
	b) Nonvascular disease												
	i) Non-insulin dependent	1		2		2		2		2		2	
	ii) Insulin dependent	1		2		2		2		2		2	
	c) Nephropathy/retinopathy/neuropathy‡	1		2		2		3		2		3/4*	
	d) Other vascular disease or diabetes of >20 years' duration‡	1		2		2		3		2		3/4*	
Dysmenorrhea	Severe	2		1		1		1		1		1	
Endometrial cancer‡		4	2	4	2	1		1		1		1	
Endometrial hyperplasia		1		1		1		1		1		1	
Endometriosis		2		1		1		1		1		1	
Epilepsy‡	(*see also Drug Interactions*)	1		1		1*		1*		1*		1*	
Gallbladder disease	a) Symptomatic												
	i) Treated by cholecystectomy	1		2		2		2		2		2	
	ii) Medically treated	1		2		2		2		2		3	
	iii) Current	1		2		2		2		2		3	
	b) Asymptomatic	1		2		2		2		2		2	
Gestational trophoblastic disease‡	a) Suspected GTD (immediate postevacuation)												
	i) Uterine size first trimester	1*		1*		1*		1*		1*		1*	
	ii) Uterine size second trimester	2*		2*		1*		1*		1*		1*	
	b) Confirmed GTD												
	i) Undetectable/non-pregnant ß-hCG levels	1*	1*	1*	1*	1*		1*		1*		1*	
	ii) Decreasing ß-hCG levels	2*	1*	2*	1*	1*		1*		1*		1*	
	iii) Persistently elevated ß-hCG levels or malignant disease, with no evidence or suspicion of intrauterine disease	2*	1*	2*	1*	1*		1*		1*		1*	
	iv) Persistently elevated ß-hCG levels or malignant disease, with evidence or suspicion of intrauterine disease	4*	2*	4*	2*	1*		1*		1*		1*	
Headaches	a) Nonmigraine (mild or severe)	1		1		1		1		1		1*	
	b) Migraine												
	i) Without aura (includes menstrual migraine)	1		1		1		1		1		2*	
	ii) With aura	1		1		1		1		1		4*	
History of bariatric surgery‡	a) Restrictive procedures	1		1		1		1		1		1	
	b) Malabsorptive procedures	1		1		1		1		3		COCs: 3 / P/R: 1	
History of cholestasis	a) Pregnancy related	1		1		1		1		1		2	
	b) Past COC related	1		2		2		2		2		3	
History of high blood pressure during pregnancy		1		1		1		1		1		2	
History of Pelvic surgery		1		1		1		1		1		1	
HIV	a) High risk for HIV	2	2	2	2	1		1*		1		1	
	b) HIV infection					1*		1*		1*		1*	
	i) Clinically well receiving ARV therapy	1	1	1	1	If on treatment, see Drug Interactions							
	ii) Not clinically well or not receiving ARV therapy‡	2	1	2	1	If on treatment, see Drug Interactions							

Abbreviations: C=continuation of contraceptive method; CHC=combined hormonal contraception (pill, patch, and, ring); COC=combined oral contraceptive; Cu-IUD=copper-containing intrauterine device; DMPA = depot medroxyprogesterone acetate; I=initiation of contraceptive method; LNG-IUD=levonorgestrel-releasing intrauterine device; NA=not applicable; POP=progestin-only pill; P/R=patch/ring ‡ Condition that exposes a woman to increased risk as a result of pregnancy. *Please see the complete guidance for a clarification to this classification: www.cdc.gov/reproductivehealth/unintendedpregnancy/USMEC.htm.

TABLE 11–1 CDC MEDICAL ELIGIBILITY CRITERIA FOR CONTRACEPTIVE USE (continued)

Condition	Sub-Condition	Cu-IUD I	Cu-IUD C	LNG-IUD I	LNG-IUD C	Implant I	Implant C	DMPA I	DMPA C	POP I	POP C	CHC I	CHC C
Hypertension	a) Adequately controlled hypertension	1*		1*		1*		2*		1*		3*	
	b) Elevated blood pressure levels (properly taken measurements)												
	i) Systolic 140-159 or diastolic 90-99	1*		1*		1*		2*		1*		3*	
	ii) Systolic ≥160 or diastolic ≥100‡	1*		2*		2*		3*		2*		4*	
	c) Vascular disease	1*		2*		2*		3*		2*		4*	
Inflammatory bowel disease	(Ulcerative colitis, Crohn's disease)	1		1		1		2		2		2/3*	
Ischemic heart disease‡	Current and history of	1		2	3	2	3	3		2	3	4	
Known thrombogenic mutations‡		1*		2*		2*		2*		2*		4*	
Liver tumors	a) Benign												
	i) Focal nodular hyperplasia	1		2		2		2		2		2	
	ii) Hepatocellular adenoma‡	1		3		3		3		3		4	
	b) Malignant‡ (hepatoma)	1		3		3		3		3		4	
Malaria		1		1		1		1		1		1	
Multiple risk factors for atherosclerotic cardiovascular disease	(e.g., older age, smoking, diabetes, hypertension, low HDL, high LDL, or high triglyceride levels)	1		2		2*		3*		2*		3/4*	
Multiple sclerosis	a) With prolonged immobility	1		1		1		2		1		3	
	b) Without prolonged immobility	1		1		1		2		1		1	
Obesity	a) Body mass index (BMI) ≥30 kg/m²	1		1		1		1		1		2	
	b) Menarche to <18 years and BMI ≥ 30 kg/m²	1		1		1		2		1		2	
Ovarian cancer‡		1		1		1		1		1		1	
Parity	a) Nulliparous	2		2		1		1		1		1	
	b) Parous	1		1		1		1		1		1	
Past ectopic pregnancy		1		1		1		1		2		1	
Pelvic inflammatory disease	a) Past												
	i) With subsequent pregnancy	1	1	1	1	1		1		1		1	
	ii) Without subsequent pregnancy	2	2	2	2	1		1		1		1	
	b) Current	4	2*	4	2*	1		1		1		1	
Peripartum cardiomyopathy‡	a) Normal or mildly impaired cardiac function												
	i) <6 months	2		2		1		1		1		4	
	ii) ≥6 months	2		2		1		1		1		3	
	b) Moderately or severely impaired cardiac function	2		2		2		2		2		4	
Postabortion	a) First trimester	1*		1*		1*		1*		1*		1*	
	b) Second trimester	2*		2*		1*		1*		1*		1*	
	c) Immediate postseptic abortion	4		4		1*		1*		1*		1*	
Postpartum (nonbreastfeeding women)	a) <21 days							1		1		4	
	b) 21 days to 42 days												
	i) With other risk factors for VTE							1		1		3*	
	ii) Without other risk factors for VTE							1		1		2	
	c) >42 days							1		1		1	
Postpartum (in breastfeeding or non-breastfeeding women, including cesarean delivery)	a) <10 minutes after delivery of the placenta												
	i) Breastfeeding	1*		2*									
	ii) Nonbreastfeeding	1*		1*									
	b) 10 minutes after delivery of the placenta to <4 weeks	2*		2*									
	c) ≥4 weeks	1*		1*									
	d) Postpartum sepsis	4		4									

TABLE 11–1 CDC MEDICAL ELIGIBILITY CRITERIA FOR CONTRACEPTIVE USE *(continued)*

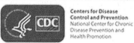

Centers for Disease Control and Prevention
National Center for Chronic Disease Prevention and Health Promotion

Condition	Sub-Condition	Cu-IUD I	Cu-IUD C	LNG-IUD I	LNG-IUD C	Implant I	Implant C	DMPA I	DMPA C	POP I	POP C	CHC I	CHC C
Pregnancy		4*		4*		NA*		NA*		NA*		NA*	
Rheumatoid arthritis	a) On immunosuppressive therapy	2	1	2	1	1		2/3*		1		2	
	b) Not on immunosuppressive therapy	1		1		1		2		1		2	
Schistosomiasis	a) Uncomplicated	1		1		1		1		1		1	
	b) Fibrosis of the liver†	1		1		1		1		1		1	
Sexually transmitted diseases (STDs)	a) Current purulent cervicitis or chlamydial infection or gonococcal infection	4	2*	4	2*	1		1		1		1	
	b) Vaginitis (*including trichomonas vaginalis and bacterial vaginosis*)	2	2	2	2	1		1		1		1	
	c) Other factors relating to STDs	2*	2	2*	2	1		1		1		1	
Smoking	a) Age <35	1		1		1		1		1		2	
	b) Age ≥35, <15 cigarettes/day	1		1		1		1		1		3	
	c) Age ≥35, ≥15 cigarettes/day	1		1		1		1		1		4	
Solid organ transplantation†	a) Complicated	3	2	3	2	2		2		2		4	
	b) Uncomplicated	2		2		2		2		2		2*	
Stroke†	History of cerebrovascular accident	1		2		2	3	3		2	3	4	
Superficial venous disorders	a) Varicose veins	1		1		1		1		1		1	
	b) Superficial venous thrombosis (acute or history)	1		1		1		1		1		3*	
Systemic lupus erythematosus†	a) Positive (or unknown) antiphospholipid antibodies	1*	1*	3*		3*		3*	3*	3*		4*	
	b) Severe thrombocytopenia	3*	2*	2*		2*		3*	2*	2*		2*	
	c) Immunosuppressive therapy	2*	1*	2*		2*		2*	2*	2*		2*	
	d) None of the above	1*	1*	2*		2*		2*	2*	2*		2*	
Thyroid disorders	Simple goiter/ hyperthyroid/hypothyroid	1		1		1		1		1		1	
Tuberculosis† (see also *Drug Interactions*)	a) Nonpelvic	1	1	1	1	1*		1*		1*		1*	
	b) Pelvic	4	3	4	3	1*		1*		1*		1*	
Unexplained vaginal bleeding	(suspicious for serious condition) before evaluation	4*	2*	4*	2*	3*		3*		2*		2*	
Uterine fibroids		2		2		1		1		1		1	
Valvular heart disease	a) Uncomplicated	1		1		1		1		1		2	
	b) Complicated†	1		1		1		1		1		4	
Vaginal bleeding patterns	a) Irregular pattern without heavy bleeding	1		1	1	2		2		2		1	
	b) Heavy or prolonged bleeding	2*		1*	2*	2*		2*		2*		1*	
Viral hepatitis	a) Acute or flare	1		1		1		1		1		3/4*	2
	b) Carrier/Chronic	1		1		1		1		1		1	1
Drug Interactions													
Antiretroviral therapy All other ARV's are 1 or 2 for all methods.	Fosamprenavir (FPV)	1/2*	1*	1/2*	1*	2*		2*		2*		3*	
Anticonvulsant therapy	a) Certain anticonvulsants (phenytoin, carbamazepine, barbiturates, primidone, topiramate, oxcarbazepine)	1		1		2*		1*		3*		3*	
	b) Lamotrigine	1		1		1		1		1		3*	
Antimicrobial therapy	a) Broad spectrum antibiotics	1		1		1		1		1		1	
	b) Antifungals	1		1		1		1		1		1	
	c) Antiparasitics	1		1		1		1		1		1	
	d) Rifampin or rifabutin therapy	1		1		2*		1*		3*		3*	
SSRIs		1		1		1		1		1		1	
St. John's wort		1		1		2		1		2		2	

Updated July 2016. This summary sheet only contains a subset of the recommendations from the U.S. MEC. For complete guidance, see: http://www.cdc.gov/reproductivehealth/unintendedpregnancy/USMEC.htm. Most contraceptive methods do not protect against sexually transmitted diseases (STDs). Consistent and correct use of the male latex condom reduces the risk of STDs and HIV.

CS266008-A

TABLE 11–2   PERCENTAGE OF WOMEN EXPERIENCING AN UNINTENDED PREGNANCY WITHIN THE FIRST YEAR OF TYPICAL USE AND THE FIRST YEAR OF PERFECT USE AND THE PERCENTAGE CONTINUING USE AT THE END OF THE FIRST YEAR: UNITED STATES

% of Women Experiencing an Unintended Pregnancy Within the First Year of Use

Method	Typical Use[a]	Perfect Use[b]	Women Continuing Use at 1 Y[c]
Male sterilization	0.15	0.10	100
Female sterilization	0.5	0.5	100
Nexplanon	0.1	0.1	89
Intrauterine contraceptives			
ParaGard (copper T)	0.8	0.6	78
Mirena/Liletta (LNG)	0.1	0.1	80
Depo-Provera	4	0.2	56
NuvaRing	7	0.3	67
Evra patch	7	0.3	67
Combined pill and progestin-only pill	7	0.3	67
Diaphragm	17	16	57
Condom			
Female (fc)	21	5	41
Male	13	2	43
Sponge			
Parous women	27	20	
Nulliparous women	14	9	
Withdrawal	20	4	46
Fertility awareness-based methods	15		47
Standard Days method[d]	12	5	
Two-Day method[d]	14	4	
Ovulation method[d]	23	3	
Symptothermal method[d]	2	0.4	
Spermicides[e]	21	16	42
No method[f]	85	85	

TABLE 11–2   PERCENTAGE OF WOMEN EXPERIENCING AN UNINTENDED PREGNANCY WITHIN THE FIRST YEAR OF TYPICAL USE AND THE FIRST YEAR OF PERFECT USE AND THE PERCENTAGE CONTINUING USE AT THE END OF THE FIRST YEAR: UNITED STATES *(continued)*

Emergency Contraceptive Pills: Treatment with COCs initiated within 120 h after unprotected intercourse reduces the risk of pregnancy by at least 60%–75%.[g] Pregnancy rates are lower if initiated in the first 12 h. Progestin-only EC reduces pregnancy risk by 89%.

Lactational Amenorrhea Method: LAM is a highly effective, temporary method of contraception.[h]

[a]Among typical couples who initiate use of a method (not necessarily for the first time), the percentage who experience an accidental pregnancy during the first year if they do not stop use for any other reason. Estimates of the probability of pregnancy during the first year of typical use for spermicides, withdrawal, fertility awareness-based methods, the diaphragm, the male condom, the oral contraceptive pill, and Depo-Provera are taken from the 1995 National Survey of Family Growth corrected for underreporting of abortion; see the text for the derivation of estimates for the other methods.

[b]Among couples who initiate use of a method (not necessarily for the first time) and who use it perfectly (both consistently and correctly), the percentage who experience an accidental pregnancy during the first year if they do not stop use for any other reason. See the text for the derivation of the estimate for each method.

[c]Among couples attempting to avoid pregnancy, the percentage who continue to use a method for 1 y.

[d]The ovulation and Two-Day methods are based on evaluation of cervical mucus. The Standard-Days method avoids intercourse on cycle days 8 through 19. The symptothermal method is a double-check method based on evaluation of cervical mucus to determine the first fertile day and evaluation of cervical mucus and temperature to determine the last fertile day.

[e]Foams, creams, gels, vaginal suppositories, and vaginal film.

[f]The percentages becoming pregnant in columns (2) and (3) are based on data from populations where contraception is not used and from women who cease using contraception in order to become pregnant. Among such populations, about 89% become pregnant within 1 y. This estimate was lowered slightly (to 85%) to represent the percentage who would become pregnant within 1 y among women now relying on reversible methods of contraception if they abandoned contraception altogether.

[g]ella (oral ulipristal acetate), oral levonorgestrel: Plan B One-Step, My Way, Take Action, and Next Choice are the only dedicated products specifically marketed for emergency contraception. The label for Plan B One-Step (1 dose is 1 white pill) says to take the pill within 72 h after unprotected intercourse. Research has shown that all of the brands listed here are effective when used within 120 h after unprotected sex. The label for Next Choice (1 dose is 1 peach pill) says to take 1 pill within 72 h after unprotected intercourse and another pill 12 h later. Research has shown that both pills can be taken at the same time with no decrease in efficacy or increase in side effects and that they are effective when used within 120 h after unprotected sex. The Food and Drug Administration has in addition declared the following 19 brands of oral contraceptives to be safe and effective for emergency contraception: Ogestrel (1 dose is 2 white pills), Nordette (1 dose is 4 light-orange pills), Cryselle, Levora, Low-Ogestrel, Lo/Ovral, or Quasence (1 dose is 4 white pills), Jolessa, Portia, Seasonale, or Trivora (1 dose is 4 pink pills), Seasonique (1 dose is 4 light-blue-green pills), Enpresse (1 dose is 4 orange pills), Lessina (1 dose is 5 pink pills), Aviane or LoSeasonique (1 dose is 5 orange pills), Lutera or Sronyx (1 dose is 5 white pills), and Lybrel (1 dose is 6 yellow pills).

[h]However, to maintain effective protection against pregnancy, another method of contraception must be used as soon as menstruation resumes, the frequency or duration of breastfeeds is reduced, bottle feeds are introduced, or the baby reaches 6 mo of age.

Source: Reproduced with permission from Zieman M, Hatcher RA., Allen AZ, Haddad L, 16th ed. *Managing Contraception;* 2021.

Sources

–*Contraception.* 2023; 121.

–*Obstet Gynecol.* 2015;126:e1–e11.

–Society of Family Planning Clinical Recommendation: emergency contraception. 2023.

CONTRACEPTION, EXTENDED USE OF LARC

Management: Women

Recommendations from

➤ SFP 2022

–See Table 11–3 for data on extended use of LARCs.

TABLE 11–3 EXTENDED USE OF LONG-ACTING REVERSIBLE CONTRACEPTION		
	FDA Approval	**Evidence for Extended Use?**
Copper 380-mm^2 IUD	10 y	Effective up to 12 y Likely effective up to 20 y for those age $\geq$ 30 y at insertion
Etonogestrel 68-mg implant	3 y	Effective to at least 5 y
LNG 19.5-, 13.5-mg IUDs	13.5 mg: 3 y 19.5 mg: 5 y	No data to evaluate extended use
LNG 52-mg IUD	Mirena: 7 y Liletta: 6 y	Effective at 8 y Data limited beyond 8–10 y, though likely effective

Source
    –*Contraception.* 2022;113:13–18.

DIABETES MELLITUS, GESTATIONAL (GDM)

Screening: Pregnant Women

Recommendations from

> USPSTF 2021, ACOG 2018, ADA 2023

–Screen for GDM in asymptomatic pregnant patients between 24 and 28 wk of gestational age, or at first presentation in those who present to care after 28 wk.

–Consider early screening for undiagnosed diabetes, preferably at the initiation of prenatal care, in overweight and obese patients with additional diabetic risk factors: physical inactivity, first-degree relative with diabetes, Black persons, American Indian, Asian American, Latino or Pacific Islander race, prior history of GDM or macrosomia (>4000 g), HTN, HDL $\leq$ 35 mg/dL, TG $\geq$ 250 mg/dL, PCOS, acanthosis nigricans, prior A1c $\geq$ 5.7%, or cardiovascular disease.

–Screen for prediabetes and diabetes in individuals who were diagnosed with GDM 4–12 wk postpartum using the 75-g oral GTT. Continue screening every 3 y for life.

Practice Pearl

• A1c screening has lower sensitivity than OGTT and is not recommended as a sole screening tool for GDM.

Sources
    –USPSTF. *Gestational Diabetes Mellitus: Screening.* 2021.
    –*Obstet Gynecol.* 2018;131:e49.
    –*Diabetes Care.* 2023;46(S1):S33.

Guidelines Alert 11–2	
GUIDELINES DISCORDANT: INITIAL PHARMACOTHERAPY IN GESTATIONAL DIABETES	
Organization	**Guidance**
ACOG, ADA	Use insulin as initial therapy (start at 0.7–1.0 U/kg/d)
NICE (UK), SMFM	Use metformin or insulin as initial therapy

Applying to Clinical Practice
- Many patients will require insulin.
- Metformin crosses the placenta leading to concern about sequelae in the child, though small studies have been reassuring.
- Insulin is a reasonable first step, though some scenarios may reasonably call for using metformin first.

Management: Pregnant Women

Recommendations from

> **ACOG 2018, SMFM 2018, NICE 2015, ADA 2023**

–Counsel regarding nutrition and exercise.

–Counsel those with an estimated fetal weight of 4500 g or more regarding the option of scheduled cesarean delivery vs. vaginal trial of labor.

–Instruct patients to record fasting and 1-h postprandial glucose levels. Target fasting blood glucose of 95 mg/dL and 1-h postprandial of 140 mg/dL or 2-h postprandial of 120 mg/dL.

–Use pharmacotherapy to achieve blood glucose goals when lifestyle modification is unsuccessful (see Guidelines Discordant table below).

–Start low-dose aspirin 100–150 mg/day (162 mg "may be acceptable") beginning between 12 and 16 wk to lower the risk of preeclampsia in every pregnant person with type 1 or type 2 diabetes.

–Unless otherwise indicated, do not induce those with well-controlled A1GDM before 39 wk. Expectant management until 40-6/7 wk is appropriate.

–For women with A2GDM, delivery is recommended at 39-0/7 to 39-6/7 wk of gestation.

–Start antepartum fetal testing at 32-wk gestational age in those requiring medication or under poor control and without other comorbidities. Consider starting surveillance earlier if other comorbidities are present. For those with A1GDM and no comorbidities, antepartum testing may not be necessary.

–Screen all women with GDM with a 75-g 2-h GTT 4–12 wk after delivery. Continue some form of screening q1–3 y lifelong.

–Advise postpartum weight loss to reduce future risk of type 2 diabetes mellitus (DM).

Sources

–ACOG Practice Bulletin No. 190: Gestational Diabetes Mellitus. *Obstet Gynecol.* 2018;131(2):e49–e64. https://www.scribd.com/document/371228843/190-Gestational-Diabetes-Mellitus-Agog

–NICE. Diabetes in pregnancy: management from preconception to the postnatal period (NG3). 2015.

–*Am J Obstet Gynecol.* 2018;218(5):B2–B4.

–*Diabetes Care.* 2023;46(suppl.1):S254–S266.

Guidelines Alert 11–3
GUIDELINES DISCORDANT: APPROACH TO SCREENING AND DIAGNOSIS OF GESTATIONAL DIABETES

Organization	Recommendation
ACOG	Screen using the 2-step strategy: 1. 1-h 50-g glucose tolerance test. Proceed to the second test if ≥135 mg/dL or ≥140 mg/dL 2. 3-h 100-g glucose tolerance test. Two elevated values = positive test (see Table 11–4)
ADA	Use either 2-step strategy (see above) or 1-step strategy: 1. 2-h 75-g glucose tolerance test. Positive if fasting ≥ 92 mg/dL, 1 h ≥ 180 mg/dL, or 2 h ≥ 153 mg/dL
USPSTF	Screen for gestational diabetes at 24 wk or after. One-step or two-step approach. Insufficient evidence for or against screening earlier

Applying to Clinical Practice
- The 2-step approach, while potentially more inconvenient, ultimately results in fewer diagnoses without an increase in adverse effects. It is plausible that the 2-step approach results in fewer false-positives and therefore fewer unnecessary treatments.

TABLE 11–4   ABNORMAL GLUCOSE TOLERANCE TEST VALUES

Criteria for GDM by 75-g 2-h OGTT if any of the following are abnormal:
  a. Fasting ≥ 92 mg/dL (5.1 mmol/L)
  b. 1 h ≥ 180 mg/dL (10.0 mmol/L)
  c. 2 h ≥ 153 mg/dL (8.5 mmol/L)
Criteria for GDM by 100-g 3-h OGTT:
  a. Carpenter–Coustan:
      i. Fasting ≥ 95 mg/dL (5.3 mmol/L)
      ii. 1 h ≥ 180 mg/dL (10.0 mmol/L)
      iii. 2 h ≥ 155 mg/dL (8.6 mmol/L)
      iv. 3 h ≥ 140 mg/dL (7.8 mmol/L)
  b. National Diabetes Data Group:
      i. Fasting ≥ 105 mg/dL (5.8 mmol/L)
      ii. 1 h ≥ 190 mg/dL (10.6 mmol/L)
      iii. 2 h ≥ 165 mg/dL (9.2 mmol/L)
      iv. 3 h ≥ 145 mg/dL (8.0 mmol/L)

COVID-19 VACCINATION

Prevention: Pregnant Women

Recommendations from

➢ ACOG 2023

–Recommend that all pregnant individuals receive a COVID-19 vaccine series, including a bivalent mRNA COVID-19 vaccine booster.

–Explain expected side effects during vaccine counseling, including those that are a normal immune reaction and part of developing antibodies to protect against COVID-19.

–Counsel pregnant and lactating patients to take acetaminophen if they have a fever after vaccination, as it is safe to take and does not affect antibody levels.

–Recommend bivalent mRNA COVID-19 booster at least 2 mo following their last primary dose or monovalent booster to all pregnant and recently pregnant (up to 6 wk postpartum) patients, due to waning immunity in pregnancy, and the potential for severe illness and death from SARS-CoV-2 during pregnancy.

–Recommend Novavax's monovalent COVID-19 vaccine as a booster to those individuals aged 18 and older who cannot or will not receive a bivalent mRNA COVID-19 booster.

–For primary vaccination, use an mRNA or Novavax COVID-19 series rather than the J&J/Janssen vaccine.

–For patients who do not receive the vaccine, document the discussion in the medical record. At subsequent visits, address ongoing questions and concerns about vaccination and offer vaccination again.

Practice Pearls

- In multiple reproductive developmental toxicity studies in animals, there have been no vaccine-related adverse effects on fertility, fetal, or postnatal development.
- Booster vaccination may occur in any trimester, and the emphasis should be on early administration to maximize maternal and fetal health.
- Vaccination with any product continues to be safer than remaining unvaccinated.

Source

–ACOG Clinical Practice Advisory. *COVID-19 Vaccination Considerations for Obstetric-Gynecologic Care.* 2020 (last updated January 2023).

DIABETES MELLITUS (DM), TYPE 2

Screening: Pregnant Women

Recommendations from

➢ ADA 2023, ACOG 2018

–Screen for undiagnosed DM type 2 at first prenatal visit if risk factors for DM are present.[1]

---

[1] Immigrants from Asia, Africa, South Pacific, Middle East (except Israel), Eastern Europe (except Hungary), the Caribbean, Malta, Spain, Guatemala, and Honduras.

–For all other patients, screen according to published guidelines (see section "Diabetes Mellitus, Gestational").

Practice Pearl

- Diagnose preexisting diabetes if:
  - Fasting glucose ≥ 126 mg/dL.
  - 2-h glucose ≥ 200 mg/dL after 75-g glucose load.
  - Random glucose ≥ 200 mg/dL with classic hyperglycemic symptoms.
  - A1c ≥ 6.5%.

Sources
–*Diabetes Care.* 2023;46(S1):S33.
–*Obstet Gynecol.* 2018;131(2):e49.

ECTOPIC PREGNANCY

Management: Women

Recommendations from

➤ NICE 2023, ACOG 2017

Evaluation
–Transvaginal ultrasound (TVUS) with a crown-rump length ≥ 7 mm but no cardiac activity.
- Repeat ultrasound in 7 d.
- Quantitative beta-hCG q 48 h × 2 levels.

–Transvaginal ultrasound with gestational sac ≥ 25 mm and no fetal pole.
- Repeat ultrasound in 7 d.
- Quantitative beta-hCG q 48 h × 2 levels.

Therapies
–Differentiate early intrauterine pregnancy loss from ectopic pregnancy.
–Consider uterine aspiration to identify the presence of chorionic villi (indicate intrauterine pregnancy).
–If chorionic villi are not confirmed, monitor hCG levels:
- Take first level 12–24 h after aspiration.
- Plateau/increase in hCG suggests incomplete evacuation or nonvisualized ectopic warranting further treatment.
- Decrease in hCG suggests failed intrauterine pregnancy; monitor with serial hCG measurements.

–Methotrexate candidates[1]:
- No significant pain.
- Adnexal mass < 3.5 cm.
- No cardiac activity on transvaginal ultrasound.

---

[1] Contraindications to methotrexate use include renal or hepatic disease, bone marrow dysfunction, and active gastrointestinal or respiratory disease. Asthma is not a contraindication.

- Beta-hCG < 5000 IU/L.
- Dose is 50 mg/m^2 IM.

–Laparoscopy if:

- Unstable patient.
- Severe pain.
- Adnexal mass ≥ 3.5 cm.
- Cardiac activity seen.
- Beta-hCG ≥ 5000 IU/L.

–Rhogam 250 IU to all Rh-negative women who undergo surgery for an ectopic.

Practice Pearls

- Ectopic pregnancy can present with:
  - Abdominal or pelvic pain.
  - Vaginal bleeding.
  - Amenorrhea.
  - Breast tenderness.
  - GI symptoms.
  - Dizziness.
  - Urinary symptoms.
  - Rectal pressure.
  - Dyschezia.
- Most normal intrauterine pregnancies will show an increase in beta-hCG level by at least 63% in 48 h.
- Intrauterine pregnancies are usually apparent by transvaginal ultrasound if beta-hCG > 1500 IU/L.

Sources

–www.guidelines.gov/content.aspx?id=39274
–NICE. Ectopic pregnancy and miscarriage: diagnosis and initial management (NG126). 2023.
–*Obstet Gynecol.* 2018;131(2):e65–e77.

FETAL ANEUPLOIDY

Screening: Pregnant Women

Recommendations from

➢ ACOG 2020

–Offer screening to all patients, ideally during the first prenatal visit. The decision should be reached through informed patient choice, including discussion of sensitivity, positive screening and false-positive rates, and risks/benefits of diagnostic testing (amniocentesis and chorionic villous sampling).
–Screening options include genetic screening ± nuchal translucency ultrasound and cell-free DNA. Choose one or the other.

–Cell-free DNA is the most sensitive and specific screening test for the common fetal aneuploidies. Nevertheless, it has the potential for false-positive and false-negative results and is not a substitute for diagnostic testing.

–Offer all patients a second-trimester ultrasound for structural defects, ideally between 18 and 22-wk EGA.

–For all patients with a positive screening test result for fetal aneuploidy, offer genetic counseling and a comprehensive ultrasound evaluation with an opportunity for diagnostic testing (chorionic villus sampling or amniocentesis) to confirm results.

–For patients with a positive serum analyte screening test result who want to avoid a diagnostic test, consider cell-free DNA screening as a follow-up test. Inform patients that this approach may delay definitive diagnosis and will fail to identify some fetuses with chromosomal abnormalities.

Practice Pearl

- Risk of chromosomal anomaly by maternal age at term:
    - 20-y-old: 1 in 525.
    - 30-y-old: 1 in 384.
    - 35-y-old: 1 in 178.
    - 40-y-old: 1 in 62.
    - 45-y-old: 1 in 18.

Source

–Screening for fetal chromosomal abnormalities. *ACOG Practice Bulletin 226.* 2020;136(4).

FETAL GROWTH RESTRICTION

Management: Pregnant Women

Recommendations from

> ACOG 2021

Evaluation

–Define as an estimated fetal weight < 10th percentile for gestational age, though fetuses < third percentile are at the highest risk of adverse outcomes.

–Monitor with serial umbilical artery assessments. Umbilical artery Doppler velocimetry used in conjunction with standard fetal surveillance, such as nonstress tests, biophysical profiles, or both, is associated with improved outcomes.

Therapies

–Optimal timing of delivery is unclear. Consider delivery at 38-0/7 to 39-0/7 wk for 3rd–10th percentile with normal umbilical artery Doppler, at 37-0/7 if <third percentile, and promptly at diagnosis regardless of EGA if umbilical artery flow is absent or reverse. When possible, reach these decisions in consultation with a maternal-fetal specialist.

–Offer antenatal corticosteroids if delivery is anticipated before 33-6/7 wk of gestation and between 34-0/7 and 36-6/7 wk of gestation if the risk of preterm delivery within 7 d and no previous course of corticosteroids.

–Consider magnesium sulfate for delivery before 32 wk of gestation for fetal and neonatal neuroprotection.

–Do not recommend nutritional and dietary supplemental strategies for the prevention of fetal growth restriction as they are not effective.

Source

–ACOG. Practice Bulletin No 227. Fetal Growth Restriction. 2021.

GROUP B STREPTOCOCCAL (GBS) DISEASE

Screening: Pregnant Women

Recommendations from

➢ AAP 2019, ACOG 2020

–Screen all patients between 36-0/7 and 37-6/7 wk of gestation for GBS colonization with a vaginal–rectal swab.

–Patients with GBS bacteriuria/UTI in the current pregnancy OR with prior infant affected by GBS disease are considered colonized and do not require further testing.

Practice Pearls

- Even patients planning a C-section benefit from GBS screening, in case of premature rupture of membranes (PROM).
- Culture results are valid for 5 wk and include births up to 41 and 0/7 wk.
- Repeat GBS screening is reasonable if the initial test was negative and gestation extends beyond 41 and 0/7 wk.

Sources

–ACOG committee opinion. *Prevention of Group B Streptococcal Early-Onset Disease in Newborns.* 2020.

–*Pediatrics.* 2019;144(2):e20191881; https://doi.org/10.1542/peds.2019-1881

Prevention: Pregnant Women

Recommendations from

➢ AAP 2019, ACOG 2020

–Give intrapartum antibiotic prophylaxis to prevent early-onset invasive GBS disease in high-risk pregnancies: positive GBS culture, GBS bacteriuria during pregnancy, or history of previous GBS-infected newborn.

–If a woman presents in labor with unknown GBS colonization status this pregnancy but has a history of GBS in a prior pregnancy or has gestational age less than 37 wk, offer intrapartum antibiotic prophylaxis.

–Do not give intrapartum antibiotic prophylaxis if a cesarean delivery is performed with intact membranes and before the onset of labor.

–Consider penicillin allergy testing for all patients with a history of penicillin allergy, particularly those that are suggestive of being IgE mediated, of unknown severity, or both.

Practice Pearls

- Penicillin G is the agent of choice for intrapartum antibiotic prophylaxis.
- Ampicillin is an acceptable alternative to penicillin G.
- Use cefazolin if the patient has a penicillin allergy that does not cause anaphylaxis, angioedema, urticaria, or respiratory distress.
- Use clindamycin[1] or vancomycin if the patient has penicillin allergy that causes anaphylaxis, angioedema, urticaria, or respiratory distress.

Sources
–ACOG committee opinion. *Prevention of Group B Streptococcal Early-Onset Disease in Newborns*. 2020.
–*Pediatrics*. 2019;144(2):e20191881; https://doi.org/10.1542/peds.2019-1881

HEADACHE

Management: Pregnant Women

Recommendations from

> ### ACOG 2022

Evaluation
–If a patient takes medications for headache prevention, review the necessity, as headache symptoms often decrease during pregnancy. If prevention medications are needed, first-line choices include calcium channel blockers and antihistamines. Several common choices (gabapentin, lisinopril, memantine, etc.) are contraindicated, and many others carry some fetal risk.
–If a headache includes severe pain, rapid onset, high blood pressure, visual changes, neurologic deficits, altered consciousness, vomiting, or fever, evaluate urgently for a secondary cause.
–In patients with preeclampsia and headache, consider alternative etiologies if altered level of consciousness, vomiting, or fever.

Therapies
–For headaches that occur during pregnancy, may be treated as before if not contraindicated if features are identical to prepregnancy headaches. If not, assess for "red flag" symptoms and consider preeclampsia if ≥20-wk EGA and BP ≥ 140/90 mmHg.
–If headache presents 24–48 h after spinal/epidural anesthesia with occipitofrontal pain and postural features, consult anesthesia for management of spinal headache.
–Treat migraine headaches with acetaminophen 1000 mg initially, or acetaminophen with caffeine (limit caffeine doses to 200 mg/d). Restrict NSAID use to the second trimester.
–Avoid butalbital, ergot alkaloids, and opioids. Use triptans, IV magnesium, and prednisolone with caution.
–For persistent headaches, use metoclopramide 10 mg with or without diphenhydramine 25 mg.

Source
–*Obstet Gynecol*. 2022;139(5):944.

---

[1] Use clindamycin if isolate is sensitive to both clindamycin and erythromycin. If not, use vancomycin.

HEPATITIS B VIRUS INFECTION

Screening: Pregnant Women

Recommendations from

> USPSTF 2019, CDC 2020, AAP 2017, ACOG 2023, AAFP 2010

  –Screen all patients with HBsAg at their first prenatal visit, regardless of history of testing or vaccination status.

  –Triple panel screen (HBsAg, anti-HBs, total anti-HBc) all pregnant patients who:
  - Do not have a documented negative triple screen result after the age of 18 y.
  - Have not completed an HBV vaccine series.
  - Have ongoing known risks, regardless of vaccination status or history of testing.

  –Retest at admission for delivery if >1 sex partner in the previous 6 mo, recent/current injection drug use, evaluation/treatment of STI.

Practice Pearls

- Breastfeeding is not contraindicated in patients with chronic HBV infection if the infant has received hepatitis B immunoglobulin-passive prophylaxis and vaccine-active prophylaxis.
- All pregnant patients who are HBsAg-positive should be reported to the local Public Health Department to ensure proper follow-up.
- Immunoassays for HBsAg have sensitivity and specificity > 98%. (*MMWR*. 1993;42:707)

Management: Pregnant Women

Recommendations from

> USPSTF 2019, CDC 2020, AAP 2017, ACOG 2023, AAFP 2010

  –Antepartum administration of hepatitis B immunoglobulin to HBV-infected pregnant people is not effective at reducing vertical transmission.

  –Offer treatment with antiviral therapy to pregnant patients with HBV infection and viral load greater than 200,000 IU/mL to decrease the risk of vertical transmission.
  - Tenofovir disoproxil fumarate is started at 24–28 wk gestation and continued up to 12 wk after delivery. Safe during breastfeeding.

  –Continue tenofovir treatment of pregnant people with chronic HBV infection and advanced cirrhosis.

  –The risk of vertical transmission of HBV associated with amniocentesis is low, but shared decision-making should be used.

  –Neonates of pregnant patients who are HBsAg-positive or status unknown at time of delivery should receive both hepatitis B immunoglobulin and hepatitis B virus vaccine within 12 h of birth.

  –Individuals with HBV infection are encouraged to breastfeed in the absence of other contraindications.

Sources

  –*Ann Intern Med.* 2009;150(12):874–876.
  –ACOG/CDC. *Screening and Referral Algorithm for Hepatitis B Virus (HBV) Infection Among Pregnant Patients.* 2020.

–ACOG. *Viral Hepatitis in Pregnancy.* 2023.
–AAP & ACOG. *Guidelines for Perinatal Care.* 8th ed. 2017.
–*Am Fam Physician.* 2010;81(4):502–504.
–CDC. *Sexually Transmitted Diseases Treatment Guidelines.* 2015.

HEPATITIS A VIRUS

Screening: Pregnant Women

Recommendations from

➤ ACOG 2023

–If at risk for hepatitis A infection, recommend vaccination with hepatitis A vaccine. Immunoglobulin and postexposure prophylaxis are also used.

Source
–*Obstet Gynecol.* 2023;142(3):745–759.

HEPATITIS C VIRUS (HCV) INFECTION

Screening: Pregnant Women

Recommendations from

➤ ACOG 2023, CDC 2020

–Screen all pregnant patients during each pregnancy for hepatitis C regardless of risk factors.[1]
–When possible, screen for and treat for hepatitis C virus infection prior to pregnancy.

Practice Pearls

- Route of delivery has not been shown to influence the rate of vertical transmission of HCV infection. Reserve cesarean sections for obstetric indications only.
- Breastfeeding is not contraindicated in patients with chronic HCV infection.
- Perform HCV RNA testing for:
  - Positive HCV antibody test result in a patient.
  - When antiviral treatment is being considered.
  - Unexplained liver disease in an immunocompromised patient with a negative HCV antibody test result.
  - Suspicion of acute HCV infection.
- Seroconversion may take up to 3 mo.
- Of persons with acute hepatitis C, 15%–25% resolve their infection; of the remaining, cirrhosis develops in 10%–20% within 20–30 y after infection, and hepatocellular carcinoma develops in 1%–5%.

[1] HCV risk factors: HIV infection; sexual partners of HCV-infected persons; persons seeking evaluation or care for STIs, including HIV; history of injection-drug use; persons who have ever been on hemodialysis; intranasal drug use; history of blood or blood component transfusion or organ transplant prior to 1992; hemophilia; multiple tattoos; children born to HCV-infected mothers; and health care providers who have sustained a needlestick injury.

- Patients testing positive for HCV antibody should receive a nucleic acid test to confirm active infection. A quantitative HCV RNA test and genotype test can provide useful prognostic information prior to initiating antiviral therapy. (*JAMA*. 2007;297:724)

Sources

–American College of Obstetricians and Gynecologists (ACOG) Practice Advisory. *Screening for Hepatitis C Infection*. 2021.
–CDC Screening Recommendations and Reports. *Hepatitis C Screening Among Adults*. 2020;69(2):1–17.

Management: Pregnant Women

Recommendations from

> AASLD 2020, EASL 2020, ACOG 2023

Evaluation

–Obtain HCV RNA and routine liver function tests at the start of pregnancy to help assess disease severity.
–In HCV-infected pregnant persons with pruritus or jaundice, evaluate for intrahepatic cholestasis of pregnancy.

Therapies

–Offer treatment to all women with HCV infection prior to becoming pregnant to reduce the risk of vertical transmission.
–Do not treat during pregnancy without a compelling indication and collaboration with obstetric and gastroenterology colleagues.
–If HCV-infected women with cirrhosis, consult a maternal-fetal medicine (ie, high-risk pregnancy) obstetrician.
–Do not restrict breastfeeding in HCV-infected mothers unless the mother has cracked, damaged, or bleeding nipples, or if coinfected with HIV, or infant has oral ulcers.
–Reassess women with HCV infection after delivery with an HCV-RNA assay to see if they have spontaneously cleared.

Practice Pearl

- There is no known way to reduce mother-to-child-transmission risk for HCV-infected women.
  - Offer pregnant people who are co-infected with HCV and HIV a planned cesarean delivery to reduce transmission.

Sources

–https://doi.org/10.1002/hep.31060
–https://doi.org/10.1016/j.jhep.2020.08.018

Management: Infants Exposed to HCV

Recommendations from

> AASLD 2020, EASL 2020

–Test all children born to HCV-infected women for HCV using an antibody-based test at or after 18 mo of age.

–HCV RNA assay testing can be used in the first year of life, but optimal timing is unknown.

–If HCV antibody is positive at 18 mo, test with HCV RNA assay at 3 y of age to confirm chronic HCV infection.

–If a child has HCV, test other siblings born from the same mother.

Sources
–https://doi.org/10.1002/hep.31060

–https://doi.org/10.1016/j.jhep.2020.08.018

HERPES SIMPLEX VIRUS (HSV), GENITAL

Screening: Pregnant Women

Recommendations from

> CDC 2015, USPSTF 2016

–Do not screen routinely for HSV with serologies.

Practice Pearls

- In patients with a history of genital herpes, routine serial cultures for HSV are not indicated in the absence of active lesions.
- Patients in whom primary HSV infection develops during pregnancy have the highest risk for transmitting HSV infection to their infants.

Sources
–*JAMA.* 2016;316(23):2525–2530.

–CDC. *Sexually Transmitted Diseases Treatment Guidelines.* 2015.

HUMAN IMMUNODEFICIENCY VIRUS (HIV)

Screening: Pregnant Women

Recommendations from

> AAFP 2019, USPSTF 2019, ACOG 2018, CDC 2021

–Screen all pregnant patients for HIV as early as possible during each pregnancy, using an opt-out approach.

–Repeat HIV testing in third trimester for patients in areas with high HIV incidence or prevalence.

–Offer rapid HIV screening to women during labor and delivery or during the immediate postpartum period who were not tested earlier in pregnancy or whose HIV is undocumented. If a rapid HIV test result in labor is reactive, antiretroviral prophylaxis should be immediately initiated while awaiting supplemental test results.

Practice Pearl

- Rapid HIV antibody testing during labor identified 34 HIV-positive patients among 4849 patients with no prior HIV testing documented (prevalence: 7 in 1000). Eighty-four percent of patients consented to testing. Sensitivity was 100%, specificity was 99.9%, positive predictive value was 90%. (*JAMA*. 2004;292:219)

Sources

–AAFP. *Screening for HIV Infection; Screening Recommendation Statement*. 2019.

–USPSTF. *Screening for HIV Infection*. 2019.

–CDC. *Sexually Transmitted Diseases Treatment Guidelines*. 2021.

–ACOG. Committee Opinion: Committee on Obstetric Practice and HIV Expert Work Group. *Obstet Gynecol*. 2018.

Management: Pregnant Women

Recommendations from

➤ ACOG 2018, IDSA 2020

Evaluation

–Include in initial prenatal labs a quantitative HIV RNA (viral load) level and CD4 cell count with percentage, HIV viral load, and HCV antibody. If HIV RNA is detectable, perform HIV genotypic resistance testing to help guide antepartum therapy.

–Monitor plasma HIV ribonucleic acid (RNA) levels at the initial prenatal visit, 2–4 wk after initiating (or changing) combined antiretroviral therapy (cART) drug regimens; monthly until RNA levels are undetectable; and then at least every 3 mo during pregnancy.

Therapies

–Treat with cART during the antepartum period.

–Women on ART that was initiated before pregnancy should continue their current regimen even if the agents are not one of the preferred antiretroviral drugs for use during pregnancy.

–Initiate ART for treatment-naïve women, as early as possible to reduce the risk of transmission at the time of delivery. Delaying ART beyond 28 wk of gestation may not fully suppress HIV RNA by the time of delivery, increasing the risk of perinatal transmission.

–Target sustained maternal viral loads of 1000 copies/mL or less to minimize the risk of perinatal transmission independent of the route of delivery or duration of ruptured membranes before delivery.

–Offer scheduled prelabor cesarean delivery at 38-0/7 wk of gestation if viral loads >1000 copies/mL to reduce the risk of perinatal transmission.

–Screen for hepatitis A virus, tuberculosis, and *Trichomonas vaginalis* in addition to standard prenatal testing.

–Offer primary or booster doses of adult-type tetanus and reduced diphtheria toxoids (Td or TdaP), inactivated influenza vaccine, pneumococcal vaccine, hepatitis A vaccine, and hepatitis B vaccine.

–Counsel women with HIV regarding the risk of breast milk transmission of HIV prior to delivery. In the United States, persons with HIV should avoid breastfeeding.

Practice Pearls

- Avoid methylergonovine for postpartum hemorrhage in women receiving a protease inhibitor or efavirenz.
- If women do not receive antepartum/intrapartum ART prophylaxis, infants should receive zidovudine for 6 wk.
- Infants born to women with HIV should have an HIV viral load checked at 14 d, at 1–2 mo, and at 4–6 mo.
- Screening for GDM is generally performed at the usual recommended gestational age of 24–28 wk. However, it is reasonable to perform testing earlier for women on protease inhibitors.

Sources
–*Obstet Gynecol.* 2018;132(3):e131–e137.
–*Clin Infect Dis.* 2020; ciaa1391.

LIVER DISEASE

Management: Pregnant Women

Recommendations from

> EASL 2023

Evaluation
–Differential: drug-induced liver disease, autoimmune diseases (PBC, PSC), viral hepatitis, intrahepatic cholestasis of pregnancy.
–Ultrasound: safe at any gestation in pregnancy. In the case of worsening cholestasis, recommend ultrasound to exclude obstruction by gallstones or progression of strictures.
–MRCP: safe at any gestation in pregnancy.
–ERCP: ideally performed in 2nd/3rd trimester, fetal radiation estimated <0.1–0.5 mGy.[1]
–To assess for drug-induced liver disease: take a careful history of previous and current prescribed and over-the-counter medications and herbal products.

Intrahepatic Cholestatic Diseases[2]
–Advise that 50% have worsening or de novo pruritus during pregnancy but stable serum hepatic liver tests. Perform repeated measurements of total serum bile acids. Higher serum bile acids are associated with preterm birth. Live birth rates are reduced in primary biliary cholangitis and primary sclerosing cholangitis.
–Postnatally, 70% have worsening of serum liver tests.
–Monitor serum bile acid concentration weekly after 32-wk gestation to aid with identifying pregnancies at increased risk for spontaneous preterm birth, fetal anoxia, meconium-stained amniotic fluid, and stillbirth (at concentrations > 40 micromol/L).
  - Postprandial serum bile acid concentration > 100 micromol/L is associated with increased risk of stillbirth after 35-wk gestation. Delivery must be urgently planned.

---

[1] Threshold radiation for malformation is 50 mGY.
[2] Approximately of one-third of new diagnoses of primary biliary cholangitis are made during pregnancy and misdiagnosed with intrahepatic cholestasis of pregnancy. Primary sclerosing cholangitis is in the differential as well. Most females diagnosed with PSC are in their childbearing years and have concurrent inflammatory bowel disease.

Treatment

–Ursodeoxycholic acid is treatment of choice as safe in pregnancy and breastfeeding. While having small effect on symptoms of maternal pruritus, it reduces the risk of spontaneous preterm birth and may be protective against stillbirth.

–Obeticholic acid use is currently not recommended. If combining ursodeoxycholic acid and cholestyramine, ensure administration is 4 h apart.

–Correct vitamin K deficiency with anion exchange resins (cholestyramine 4–8 g/d or colestipol 5–10 g/d) or rifampicin (300–600 mg daily). Monitor coagulation tests.

  • Administer vitamin K to neonates of pregnant people treated with rifampicin.

–Recommend emollients and cooling gels to prevent dryness of skin, avoid hot baths or showers, and keep nails shortened.

Hepatic Tumors

–Majority of liver masses detected in pregnancy are benign, due to widespread use of abdominal ultrasound.

  • Hepatocellular adenoma: regularly image to monitor size. Manage conservatively if <5 cm diameter, no risk of complications related to the tumor. If >5 cm, close surveillance is recommended. Limited data suggests preventing prolonged second stage or labor and considering assisted delivery to reduce the risk of hemorrhage.

  • Hemangioma: large (>4 cm), peripherally located, and exophytic hemangiomas are at higher risk of rupture. Manage conservatively. Resection can be performed if rapidly enlarging or rupture.

  • Focal nodular hyperplasia: imaging is not routinely recommended during pregnancy. There is no increased risk with vaginal delivery.

–Hepatocellular carcinoma: perform close surveillance with abdominal ultrasound or MRI each trimester. Treatment is individualized per a multidisciplinary team.

–Cholangiocarcinoma, metastatic lesions to the liver: survey with ultrasound for hepatic metastasis from extrahepatic cancers. Multidisciplinary treatment is recommended with adherence to oncological management for nonpregnant people.

Autoimmune Hepatitis; Transplant Recipients

–Continue therapy with prednisolone, budesonide, thiopurines, and immunosuppressive drugs with good safety data for improved fetal/maternal outcomes. Consider an increase in dose postpartum due to increased risk of flares.

–Increased risk of GDM, hypertensive disorders, preterm birth, and fetal growth restriction. Consider low dose aspirin therapy initiation in first trimester.

–Adrenal suppression risk: consider increasing glucocorticoid dose at the time of delivery and during any perinatal infection or period of hyperemesis.

–Immunosuppressive drugs:

  • Azathioprine, cyclosporine, tacrolimus, and prednisolone are safe.

  • Mycophenolate mofetil is teratogenic and should be stopped >12 wk prior to conception.

–Metabolic dysfunction-associated steatosis liver disease:

  • Thorough preconception counseling is important of the risks of maternal and fetal risks associated.

- During pregnancy, treat metabolic comorbidities and screen for GDM and hypertensive disease in pregnancy including tests of liver function.
  –Wilson disease:
- Continue treatment with zinc, D-penicillamine, and trientine. Reduce dose of chelators in second and third trimesters.
  –Cirrhosis
  –Portal hypertension: recommend screening endoscopy within 1 y prior to conception to assess for clinically significant varices. Initiate or continue beta-blockers for primary or secondary prophylaxis of variceal bleeding (unless contraindications present). High-risk varices should undergo endoscopic band ligation.

Source

–European Association for the Study of the Liver. *Clinical Practice Guidelines on the Management of Liver Diseases in Pregnancy*. 2023.

HYPERBILIRUBINEMIA, NEONATAL

Management: Newborns, EGA ≥ 35 wk

Recommendations from

> AAP 2022

Evaluation

–If maternal antibody screen is positive or unknown, collect a direct antiglobulin test from the newborn as soon as possible to assess for risk of hyperbilirubinemia from hemolysis.
–For all newborns, promote breastfeeding support. Do not routinely supplement with formula.
–When hyperbilirubinemia is present, do not treat with water or dextrose supplementation. If feeding is thought to be inadequate, consider supplementation with formula or donor breast milk.
–Risk factors for significant hyperbilirubinemia include:

- Lower gestational age.
- Jaundice in the first 24 h of life.
- Bilirubin close to phototherapy threshold or phototherapy prior to discharge.
- Hemolysis (verified or suspected by rate of rise ≥ 0.3 mg/dL/h in first 24 h, ≥0.2 mg/dL/h after).
- Parent or sibling requiring treatment for hyperbilirubinemia.
- Family history suggesting inherited RBC disorder such as G6PD deficiency.
- Exclusive breastfeeding with inadequate intake.
- Scalp hematoma or significant bruising.
- Down syndrome.
- Macrosomia, infant of diabetic mother.

–Risk factors for neurotoxicity from hyperbilirubinemia include:
  • Gestational age < 38 wk.
  • Albumin < 3.0 g/dL.
  • Hemolysis (isoimmune hemolytic disease, G6PD deficiency, etc.).
  • Sepsis.
  • Clinical instability in prior 24 h.
–Monitor all infants for hyperbilirubinemia.
  • 0–24 h of life: assess visually for jaundice at least every 12 h and measure total serum bilirubin (TSB) or transcutaneous bilirubin (TcB) immediately for infants with jaundice.
  • 24–48 h of life: screen all infants for hyperbilirubinemia with either TSB or TcB.
  • If TcB is ≥15 mg/dL or within 3 mg/dL of phototherapy threshold, measure TSB.
  • Use TSB (not TcB or visual assessment) to guide treatment decisions.
  • If the rate of rise is rapid (≥0.3 mg/dL/h in first 24 h, ≥0.2 mg/dL/h after), suspect hemolysis. If not already done, collect a direct antiglobulin test.
–Prolonged jaundice: if a breastfed infant remains jaundiced after 3–4 wk of age, or formula-fed infant after 2 wk of age, measure total and direct bilirubin levels to evaluate for pathologic cholestasis and review the newborn screening test results.

Therapies
–Use the published nomogram to identify phototherapy thresholds based on gestational age and neurotoxicity risk factors. A free online tool is available at: https://bilitool.org/
–If TSB exceeds phototherapy threshold, treat with intensive phototherapy.
–If an infant who has already been discharged exceeds the threshold, consider home LED-based therapy rather than readmission if the following criteria are met:
  • EGA ≥ 38 wk.
  • ≥48-h old.
  • Clinically well, feeding adequately.
  • No neurotoxicity risk factors (see above).
  • No prior phototherapy.
  • TSB no more than 1 mg/dL above treatment threshold.
  • Immediate availability of in-home device.
  • Ability to measure TSB daily.
–If electing home LED-based therapy, admit for inpatient therapy if the TSB is ≥1 mg/dL above the phototherapy threshold.
–Maintain feeding routines. Interrupting therapy for breastfeeding does not decrease the therapy's effectiveness. Consider formula supplementation, which may cause TSB to fall more quickly, though the risk of interfering with breastfeeding may outweigh the benefit.
–Provide lactation and feeding support to breastfeeding mothers. Encourage mothers of breastfed babies with jaundice to wake the baby for feeds if necessary.
–Monitoring during phototherapy: monitor baby's temperature and ensure thermoneutral environment, monitor hydration by daily weighing of the baby and assessing wet diapers, and give baby eye protection and routine eye care.

–For infants in the hospital on phototherapy, measure TSB in the first 4–6 h after initiating phototherapy. Repeat every 6–12 when serum bilirubin level is stable or falling. The timing and frequency of TSB checks should be guided by the age of child, neurotoxicity risk factors, and TSB level and trajectory.

–For all infants on phototherapy, measure hemoglobin and/or hematocrit to assess for anemia and provide a baseline. Obtain direct antiglobulin test when mother had positive Ab screen, blood group O, or Rh(D)−. Measure G6PD activity if TSB increases despite intensive therapy, increases suddenly, or rises after an initial decline.

–Consider concluding phototherapy when TSB is at least 2 mg/dL below the threshold level at the initiation of therapy. Consider longer duration of treatment when risk factors for prolonged hyperbilirubinemia (EGA < 38 wk, age < 48 h at the start of therapy, hemolytic disease).

–Intensify phototherapy by adding another light source or increasing the irradiance of the initial light source used if any of the following apply: TSB rising rapidly (>8.5 mm/L/h); TSB is within 50 mm/L below threshold for exchange transfusion after 72 h+ since birth; TSB fails to respond to initial phototherapy within 6 h of starting phototherapy.

–Escalate to intensive care emergently if TSB is >2 mg/dL below exchange transfusion threshold despite phototherapy.

–After concluding therapy, measure bilirubin again at 12–18 h later to evaluate for rebound hyperbilirubinemia. Consider TcB instead of TSB if >24 h after phototherapy. Use phototherapy thresholds described above to decide whether to reinitiate treatment.

–At hospital discharge, use the difference between the most recent bilirubin level and the phototherapy threshold to determine the timing of follow-up.

- 0.1–1.9 mg/dL. If age < 24 h, delay discharge and measure TSB in 4–8 h. If >24 h, measure TSB in 4–24 h and either delay discharge or discharge with close follow-up or phototherapy.
- 2.0–3.4 mg/dL. TSB or TcB in 4–24 h.
- 3.5–5.4 mg/dL. TSB or TcB in 1–2 d.
- 5.5–6.9 mg/dL. F/u 2 d (or, as needed if >72 h age); TSB or TcB according to clinical judgment.
- ≥7.0 mg/dL. F/u 3d (or, as needed if >72 h age); TSB or TcB according to clinical judgment.

Sources
–*Pediatrics.* 2022;150(3):e2022058859.
–NICE. Jaundice in newborn babies under 28 d. CG98. 2023.

HYPERTENSION, GESTATIONAL AND PREECLAMPSIA

Screening: Pregnant Women

Recommendations from

> USPSTF 2023, NICE 2023

–Screen with blood pressure measurements throughout pregnancy, even among asymptomatic pregnant persons at every prenatal care visit.

–Urine dipstick screen is considered positive if 1+ or more. Follow up with albumin:creatinine ratio (8 mg/mmol is threshold) or protein:creatinine ratio (30 mg/mmol is threshold) to assess for significant proteinuria.

Practice Pearls

- Screening for protein with urine dipstick has low accuracy.
- Diagnose preeclampsia if blood pressure is ≥140/90 ×2, 4 h apart, after 20 wk gestation AND there is proteinuria (≥300 mg/dL in 24 h or protein:creatinine ratio ≥ 0.3, or protein dipstick ≥ 1+), thrombocytopenia, renal insufficiency, impaired liver function, pulmonary edema, or cerebral/visual symptoms.

Sources
–*JAMA*. 2023;330(11):1074–1082.
–NICE. Hypertension in pregnancy: diagnosis and management. 2023.

Prevention: Pregnant Women

Recommendations from

➤ USPSTF 2023, ACOG 2020

–Start aspirin 81[1] mg/d after 12 of gestation if ≥1 major risk factor for preeclampsia. Continue until delivery.

Practice Pearls

- Major risk factors: personal history of preeclampsia, multifetal gestation, chronic hypertension, DM, renal disease, and autoimmune disease.
- In patients at high risk for preeclampsia, ACOG recommends initiating aspirin as late as 28 wk and continuing until delivery.

Sources
–*Ann Intern Med*. 2014;161:819–826.
–*Obstet Gynecol*. 2020;135(6):1492.

Management: Pregnant and Postpartum Women

Recommendations from

➤ ACOG 2020

–Initiate low-dose (81 mg/d) aspirin for preeclampsia prophylaxis, between 12 and 28 wk of gestation (ideally before 16 wk of gestation) and continue until delivery in:
  - Women with any high-risk factors for preeclampsia (previous pregnancy with preeclampsia, multifetal gestation, renal disease, autoimmune disease, type 1 or type 2 diabetes mellitus, chronic kidney disease, and chronic hypertension).
  - Women with more than one of the moderate-risk factors (first pregnancy, maternal age of 35 y or older, a body mass index of >30 at first visit, family history of preeclampsia, sociodemographic characteristics, and personal history factors).

[1] NICE 2023 recommendation is for 75 mg to 150 mg aspirin daily from 12 wk until delivery of baby.

–Initiate antihypertensive treatment for acute-onset severe hypertension (SBP ≥ 160 or DBP ≥ 110 mmHg) that is confirmed as persistent (15 min or more). Antihypertensive options included hydralazine, labetalol, and nifedipine. Goal blood pressure is 135/85 mmHg or less.

–Induce labor at 37-0/7 wk of gestation (or beyond upon diagnosis).

–Proceed toward delivery at 34-0/7 wk of gestation or beyond when gestational hypertension or preeclampsia with severe features is diagnosed.

–Magnesium sulfate should be used for seizure prophylaxis in women with gestational hypertension and preeclampsia with severe features.

–Use nonsteroidal anti-inflammatory medications preferentially over opioid analgesics in postpartum patients, even if on magnesium.

–For outpatient management:

- Once or twice weekly dipstick proteinuria.
- Once or twice a week blood pressure measurement until sustained below 135/85 mmHg.
- Measure full blood count, liver function, and renal function at presentation and then weekly.
- Fetal heart auscultation at every antenatal appointment.
- Ultrasound of fetus at diagnosis; repeat every 2–4 wk if clinically indicated.

–Postnatal management:

- Evaluate blood pressure daily for the first 2 d after birth, then at least once between day 3 and day 5, thereafter as clinically indicated.
- If no antihypertensive treatment is started (due to BP < 140/90 sustained), but postpartum blood pressure readings are 150/100 mmHg or higher, start antihypertensive treatment.

Source
–ACOG. Practice Bulletin No. 222. *Gestational Hypertension and Preeclampsia.* 2020.

HELLP SYNDROME

Management: Pregnant Women

Recommendations from
> ACOG, Journal of Hepatology CPG

–If symptoms suggestive of hepatic hematoma (right shoulder, abdominal, or epigastric pain): recommend abdominal ultrasound.

–Recommend platelet transfusion if the platelet count < 100 × 10⁹/L.

–Nonsevere hypertension (systolic BP 140–159 mmHg or diastolic 90–109 mmHg): initiate treatment with oral labetalol, nifedipine, or methyldopa.

–Severe hypertension (systolic > 160 mmHg or diastolic > 110 mmHg):

- Treat urgently in monitored setting with oral or IV labetalol, nifedipine, or oral methyldopa.
- Give magnesium sulfate to prevent eclamptic seizures and as neuroprotective agent for preterm preeclampsia if delivery is required before 32 wk of gestation.

–Recommend delivery once maternal coagulopathy and severe hypertension are controlled.

Source
–European Association for the Study of the Liver. *Clinical Practice Guidelines on the Management of Liver Diseases in Pregnancy*. 2023.

HYPERTENSION, CHRONIC IN PREGNANCY

Management: Pregnant Women

Recommendations from

➤ **ACOG 2019, 2023**

Evaluation

–Diagnose chronic hypertension in pregnancy when elevated blood pressure is present before pregnancy or 20 wk of gestation.

–Obtain baseline evaluation of LFTs, serum creatinine, serum electrolytes, BUN, CBC, spot urine protein/creatinine ratio, or 24-h urine for total protein and creatinine. Consider ECG for women with longstanding hypertension (HTN > 4-y duration or age > 30 y).

–In cases of diagnostic uncertainty between chronic HTN and superimposed preeclampsia, admit patient for inpatient surveillance with assessment of hematocrit, platelets, creatinine, LFTs, and new-onset proteinuria.

Therapies

–Initiate antihypertensive medications when SBP > 160 mmHg or DBP > 110 mmHg.

–When using medication to treat hypertension, aim for target blood pressure of 135/85 mmHg.

- Labetalol is first line.
- Nifedipine is second line.
- Methyldopa is third line.

–Initiate low-dose aspirin (81 mg) between 12 and 28 wk of gestation and continue through delivery.

–Consider placental growth factor-based testing to help rule out preeclampsia between 20 wk and 36 wk and 6 d of pregnancy if available and high risk of developing preeclampsia.

–Schedule antenatal appointments weekly if hypertension is poorly controlled, or every 2–4 wk if well controlled.

–Fetal assessment: ultrasound for fetal growth and amniotic fluid volume assessment, umbilical artery doppler velocimetry at 28 wk, 32 wk, and 36 wk.

–Advise delivery according to Table 11–5.

TABLE 11–5 TIMING OF DELIVERY IN PREGNANT PATIENTS WITH CHRONIC HYPERTENSION	
	ACOG Recommended Timing of Delivery (wk of Gestation)
cHTN not requiring medication	≥38+0 to 39+6
cHTN controlled with medication	≥37+0 to 39+0
Severe HTN, difficult to control	34+0 to 36+6

–Monitor blood pressure after delivery, with goal BP > 140/90 mmHg:
  - Daily for the first 2 d after birth.
  - At least once between day 3 and day 5 after birth.
  - As clinically indicated thereafter.

Practice Pearls

- Risks of chronic hypertension in pregnancy include maternal death, stroke, pulmonary edema, renal insufficiency/failure, myocardial infarction, preeclampsia, placental abruption, GDM, post-partum hemorrhage, and cesarean delivery.
- Risks of chronic hypertension in pregnancy also include stillbirth/perinatal death, growth restriction, preterm birth, and congenital anomalies.

Source
–*Obstet Gynecol.* 2019;133(1):e26–e50.

INTIMATE PARTNER VIOLENCE

Screening: Pregnant Women

Recommendations from

> USPSTF 2018, ACOG 2012

–Screen all pregnant patients for intimate partner violence.

Practice Pearls

- Screening for intimate partner violence has the most robust evidence during pregnancy and the postpartum period.
- Pregnant patients may be at increased risk for intimate partner violence compared to their non-pregnant peers.
- Validated interventions include home-visit interventions for psychosocial supports and brief counseling and referral to violence prevention organizations.

Sources
–*JAMA.* 2018;320(16):1678–1687.
–*Obstet Gynecol.* 2012;119(2):412–417.

LABOR AND DELIVERY: DELAYED UMBILICAL CORD CLAMPING

Management: Pregnant Women, Third Stage of Labor

Recommendations from

> ACOG 2020

–Delay umbilical cord clamping for at least 30–60 s in term and preterm infants, except when immediate clamping is necessary because of neonatal or maternal indications (ie, resuscitation).

–Do not perform cord milking for extremely preterm infants (<28 wk of gestation).

–There is insufficient evidence to support or refute umbilical cord milking in infants born at 32 wk of gestation or more, including term infants.

Practice Pearl

- A 2019 study of umbilical cord milking was halted early because extremely preterm infants (23–27 wk of gestation) in the cord milking arm more often developed intraventricular hemorrhage compared with similar infants in the delayed cord clamping group.

Source

–ACOG. Committee Opinion No. 814. *Delayed Umbilical Cord Clamping After Birth*. 2020.

LABOR AND DELIVERY: INDUCTION OF LABOR

Management: Pregnant Women

Recommendations from

➢ **NICE 2021, ACOG 2009**

–Review risks and benefits prior to deciding on induction. Benefits will vary by indication. Risks (vs. spontaneous labor) include an increased number of vaginal exams, limitations on the birth setting, uterine hyperstimulation, increased discomfort, and a longer hospital stay.

–Verify gestational age prior to induction. A term gestation is confirmed if an ultrasound completed <20-wk EGA supports current EGA ≥39 wk, fetal heart tones have been documented for >30 wk, or if 36 wk have passed since positive pregnancy test.

–Use prostaglandin (eg, misoprostol, dinoprostone) or[1] mechanical cervical dilator (eg, Foley catheter balloon) before oxytocin induction in patients with an unfavorable cervix (typically: Bishop score ≤ 6).

–Dosing of prostaglandin for ripening:

- Misoprostol: 25 mcg q3–6 h (may consider 50 mcg q6). (ACOG: vaginal; NICE: oral) Start oxytocin <4 h after the last misoprostol dose.
- Dinoprostone. Give second dose 6–12 h after the initial dose if inadequate cervical change; maximum 3 doses in 24 h.

–Oxytocin dosing for induction.

- Low dose: start 0.5–2 mU/min, increase by 1–2 mU/min every 15–40 min.
- High dose: start 6 mU/min, increase by 3–6 mU/min every 15–40 min.
- If uterine tachysystole occurs, decrease or discontinue oxytocin; consider repositioning or administering oxygen and/or IV fluids. If persists, consider tocolytics such as terbutaline.

Practice Pearl

- A 2021 Cochrane Review suggests oral misoprostol may be the best method for cervical ripening. It leads to fewer cesarean deliveries than vaginal dinoprostone or Foley catheter and higher

---

[1] Do not use both together. Combining misoprostol and a Foley bulb does not improve vaginal delivery rates but does lead to more chorioamnionitis (*Obstet Gynecol*. 2020;136(5):953–961).

rates of vaginal birth than dinoprostone. Oral and vaginal misoprostol result in similar vaginal birth rates, but oral has lower rates of uterine hyperstimulation and fewer cesarean deliveries for fetal distress. Ideal misoprostol dosing is poorly defined—25 mcg regimens are likely to be best; dosing intervals from q1 h–q6 h have been studied without conclusive superiority (https://doi.org/10.1002/14651858.CD014484).

Sources
–*Obstet Gynecol*. 2009:114(2):386.
–www.nice.org.uk/guidance/ng207

LABOR AND DELIVERY: ROUTINE LABOR

Management: Pregnant Women

Recommendations from

> NICE 2022, ACOG 2024, WHO 2018

–Allow mother to choose her birth setting (eg, home, midwifery unit, or hospital obstetric unit). Home birth has a small increase (1 in 250) in serious medical problems for the newborn vs. birth in a midwifery unit or hospital. (NICE)

–Encourage support from birth companion(s). Communicate clearly and respectfully.

–Suggest relaxation techniques such as mindfulness, breathing exercises, water immersion, and massage for pain control during latent labor. Encourage mobility and an upright position unless high risk.

–Latent phase of labor (up to 6 cm dilation) widely varies among individuals. The median latent-phase duration in nulliparous patients ranges from 0.6 to 6.0 h. Prolonged latent phase is defined as longer than 16 h.

–Avoid continuous external fetal monitoring in routine/low-risk situations.[1] Offer continuous external fetal monitoring (and, transfer to obstetrics-led care if not already there) if any of the following:
  - Maternal HR > 120 or BP > 160/110 (or >140/90 ×2).
  - Maternal urine protein ≥ 2+ with BP > 140/90 ×1.
  - Vaginal bleeding.
  - ROM > 24 prior to labor.
  - Meconium.
  - Atypical pain.
  - High-risk maternal comorbidities.
  - Fetal abnormal lie.
  - High or free-floating head in nulliparous woman.

[1] This is the recommendation from NICE and WHO. ACOG does not take an official position on continuous monitoring vs. intermittent auscultation. They note that continuous external fetal monitoring does not affect perinatal death and cerebral palsy outcomes in low-risk pregnancies and cite a higher risk of c-section and operative vaginal deliveries with continuous external fetal monitoring. They also recognize the need to adequately train staff in intermittent monitoring and the effect on staffing that the two approaches have.

- Suspected fetal growth restriction or macrosomia.
- Suspected oligohydramnios or polyhydramnios.
- FHR < 110 or > 160.
- Fetal deceleration was heard on intermittent auscultation.
- Reduced fetal movement.

–During labor, support maternal choice for breathing/relaxation techniques, massage, immersion in water, and music.

–Offer nitrous oxide for analgesia.

–Offer opioids for anesthesia (limited pain relief; may cause drowsiness/nausea/vomiting in mom and respiratory depression and drowsiness in baby).

–If receiving care in an obstetric unit, offer epidural/ neuraxial anesthesia for pain relief during any stage of labor (no increase in first stage of labor or cesarean birth; longer second stage of labor and increased vaginal instrumental birth; more intense monitoring and reduced mobility).

–Refer to Table 11–6 for criteria for labor dystocia by stage of labor, and recommended interventions when arrest is diagnosed.

–Recommend early amniotomy for patients undergoing augmentation or induction of labor (see Guidelines Discordant table).

–Consider use of either low dose or high dose oxytocin strategies in the active management of labor to reduce operative deliveries. The AHRQ 2020 systematic review determined that high dose oxytocin is associated with a lower cesarean delivery rate among nulliparous pregnant people, with no difference in maternal hemorrhage.

–In patients with ruptured membranes and protracted active labor or contractions that cannot be accurately monitored externally, place intrauterine pressure catheter.

–When diagnosing second-stage arrest, include clinical factors that may affect the likelihood of vaginal delivery, a discussion of risks and benefits, and individual patient preference. Evidence supports decreased duration of the first stage of labor and rates of cesarean delivery for upright positioning and ambulation.

TABLE 11–6   CRITERIA FOR LABOR DYSTOCIA AND RECOMMENDED MANAGEMENT STEPS

Term	Definition	Arrest of Labor	Management
Active phase of labor	Cervical dilation of 6 cm and greater The first stage of labor typically progresses at 1-cm dilation per hour, but does not intervene solely for a progression rate at <1 cm/h (WHO)	No progression in cervical dilation in patients who are at least 6 cm dilated with rupture of membranes despite: 4 h of adequate uterine activity OR 6 h of inadequate uterine activity with oxytocin augmentation	Perform cesarean delivery in patients with active phase arrest of labor
Second stage of labor	10 cm dilated and 100% effaced Pushing commences at this point when cervical dilation is achieved	Lack of fetal rotation or descent despite adequate contractions, pushing efforts, and time (>3 h of pushing in nulliparous, >2 h of pushing in multiparous)	Assess for operative vaginal delivery before performing cesarean delivery for second-stage arrest

Guidelines Alert 11–4
GUIDELINES DISCORDANT: EARLY AMNIOTOMY IN AUGMENTATION OR INDUCTION OF LABOR

Organization	Guidance
ACOG	Consider early amniotomy in patients undergoing augmentation or induction of labor. It decreases time to delivery without increasing cesarean delivery rate or other maternal or neonatal complications
WHO	Do not routinely perform amniotomy to prevent a delay in labor. No specific guidance related to amniotomy early in induction

Applying to Clinical Practice
• ACOG relies on several studies that show benefits without significant harm. When induction is definitively indicated, recommend early amniotomy when it is technically feasible.

–Offer nonpharmacologic supportive care measures to assist labor progression: continuous emotional support, peanut ball, hydration (PO or IV), perineal massage, water immersion, acupuncture, ambulation, and positioning strategies.

–Reduce perineal trauma using either "hands on" (guarding perineum and flexing baby's head) or "hands poised" (hands off perineum and baby's head but in readiness) technique. Avoid perineal massage, lidocaine spray, and routine episiotomy during labor.

–Perform cervical examinations as often as needed when clinically indicated.

–Manage third stage of labor:
- Administer 10 IU oxytocin immediately after birth of anterior shoulder.
- Clamp and cut cord after 1 min (unless FHR < 60) but before 5 min.
- Use controlled cord traction until delivery of placenta.
- Remove the placenta actively if hemorrhage or placenta is not delivered within 1 h.

Sources
–www.nice.org.uk/guidance/cg190
–*WHO Recommendations: Intrapartum Care for a Positive Childbirth Experience.* Geneva: World Health Organization; 2018. License: CC BY-NC-SA 3.0 IGO.
–*Obstet Gynecol.* 2019;133(2):e164.
–ACOG. *First and Second Stage Labor Management.* CPG 8. 2024.

LABOR AND DELIVERY: PRELABOR RUPTURE OF MEMBRANES (PROM)

Management: Pregnant Women

Recommendations from

➤ ACOG 2020, Cochrane Database of Systematic Reviews 2013, NICE 2021

–Diagnose PROM based on history and physical exam. Avoid digital examinations unless patient appears to be in active labor or delivery seems imminent (ACOG). Sterile speculum exam is preferred.

–In all patients with PROM, initial period of electronic fetal heart monitoring and uterine activity monitoring should be done. Non-reassuring fetal status and clinical chorioamnionitis are indications for delivery.

–<23–24 wk of gestation at risk for imminent delivery:
- Expectant management or induction of labor.
- Consider antibiotics as early as 20-0/7 wk of gestation.
- Do not use GBS prophylaxis before viability.
- Do not use corticosteroids, tocolysis, or magnesium sulfate before viability; consider as early as 23-0/7 wk of gestation.

–24-0/7 to 33-6/7 wk of gestation at risk for imminent delivery:
- Use IV magnesium sulfate for its fetal neuroprotective effect < 32-0/7 wk of gestation, if there are no contraindications.
- Consider trial of expectant management.
- Use antibiotics to prolong latency if there are no contraindications.
- Give a single course of corticosteroids. Consider at 23-0/7 wk gestation if the risk of preterm birth within 7 d.
- Treat intra-amniotic infection if present (and proceed to delivery).
- GBS screening and prophylaxis as indicated.

–34-0/7 to 36-6/7 wk of gestation:
- Expectant management (NICE) or proceed toward delivery.
- Consider a single course of corticosteroid. Do not delay delivery for steroids.
- GBS screening and prophylaxis as indicated. If positive, proceed toward delivery.
- Treat intra-amniotic infection if present (and proceed toward delivery).

–≥37-0/7 wk of gestation:
- GBS screening and prophylaxis as indicated.
- Treat intra-amniotic infection if present.
- Proceed toward delivery.

–There is not enough evidence to show that removal of cerclage after preterm PROM diagnosis has been made. If cerclage remains in place with preterm PROM, prolonged antibiotics prophylaxis beyond 7 d is not recommended.

–Outpatient management of preterm PROM is not recommended.

Practice Pearls

- Twenty-two studies involving over 6800 pregnant persons with PROM prior to 37 gestational weeks were analyzed. Routine antibiotics decreased the incidence of chorioamnionitis (RR 0.66), prolonged pregnancy by at least 7 d (RR 0.79), and decreased neonatal infection (RR 0.67), but had no effect on perinatal mortality compared with placebo.
- Between 34-0/7 and 36-6/7 wk of gestation, NICE recommends expectant management until 37 wk of gestation in the absence of other contraindications. ACOG does not make an explicit recommendation. Either expectant management (with close monitoring) or delivery is reasonable.

Sources
–*Obstet Gynecol.* 2020;135(3):e80–e97.

–NICE. Inducing labour (NG207). 2021.

–http://www.cochrane.org/CD001058/PREG_antibiotics-for-preterm-rupture-of-membranes

LABOR AND DELIVERY: PRETERM LABOR

Prevention: Pregnant Women

Recommendations from

⮞ ACOG 2021

–Do not use maintenance tocolytics to prevent preterm birth.

–Do not give antibiotics for the purpose of prolonging gestation or improving neonatal outcomes in preterm labor with intact membranes.

–In patients with prior spontaneous preterm delivery, start progesterone therapy between 16 and 24 wk of gestation.

–Consider cerclage placement to improve preterm birth outcomes in patients with prior spontaneous preterm delivery < 34 wk, current singleton pregnancy, and short cervical length (<25 mm) before 24 wk of gestation.

–Consider antenatal corticosteroids at 22-0/7 wk to 23-6/7 wk of gestation if neonatal resuscitation is planned and after appropriate counseling.

–Give antenatal corticosteroids between 24-0/7 wk and 25-6/7 wk.

Practice Pearls

- There is no evidence to support the use of prolonged tocolytics for patients with preterm labor.
- There is no evidence to support strict bed rest for the prevention of preterm birth.
- The positive predictive value of a positive fetal fibronectin test or a short cervix for preterm birth is poor in isolation.
- Do not give antenatal corticosteroids if less than 22 wk gestational age due to lack of evidence to suggest benefit.

Sources

–*Obstet Gynecol.* 2012;120(4):964–973.

–ACOG Practice Advisory. *Use of Antenatal Corticosteroids at 22 Weeks of Gestation.* 2021.

Management: Pregnant Women ≥20-wk EGA

Recommendations from

⮞ ACOG 2016, Cochrane Database of Systematic Reviews 2013, NICE 2015

Evaluation

–Consider fetal fibronectin testing and/or the cervical length measurement as part of a diagnosis of preterm labor and to predict preterm birth in symptomatic women, but do not rely exclusively on these tests to direct management as the positive predictive value is poor.

- Cervical length: if >1.5 cm, preterm labor is unlikely; if ≤1.5 cm and the clinical situation suggests it, diagnose and manage preterm labor. (NICE)

- Fetal fibronectin: use to determine the likelihood of birth within 48 h if cervical length measurement is not available. (NICE)

Therapies

–Give a single dose of corticosteroids for pregnant persons between 24 and 34 gestational weeks or women with ROM or multiple gestations who may deliver within 7 d.

- Consider corticosteroids at earlier gestation (ACOG: starting at 23 wk; NICE: starting at 22 wk) if risk of delivery within 7 d.
- Consider corticosteroids between 34 and 35-6/7 wk if at risk of delivery within 7d.
- Betamethasone or dexamethasone IM are the most widely studied options.

–Consider second course of corticosteroids for women < 34-wk EGA who are >7 d remote from their first course and are at very high risk of giving birth within 48 h.

–Give magnesium sulfate (4 g IV ×1, then 1 g/h ×24 h) for neuroprotection.

- ACOG: give if possible preterm delivery prior to 32 wk.
- NICE: give between 24 and 29-6/7 wk; consider as early as 23 wk and as late as 33-6/7 wk.
- Indomethacin is a potential option for use in conjunction with magnesium sulfate.

–Consider tocolysis for up to 48 h. Do not use after 34-wk gestation. Do not recommend maintenance therapy. Options include:

- Beta-agonists.
- Nifedipine (NICE: first line).
- Indomethacin.

–Do not use tocolytics for women with preterm contractions without cervical change, especially if <2 cm.

–Do not use antibiotics in preterm labor with intact membranes.

–Do not routinely recommend bedrest and hydration, as they have not been shown to prevent preterm birth.

Practice Pearls

- Magnesium sulfate administered prior to 32 wk reduces the severity and risk of cerebral palsy.
- Cochrane analysis found no difference in the incidence of preterm delivery comparing hydration and bedrest with bedrest alone.

Sources

–*Obstet Gynecol.* 2016;128:e155–e164.

–http://www.cochrane.org/CD003096/PREG_hydration-for-treatment-of-preterm-labour

LABOR AND DELIVERY: POSTPARTUM HEMORRHAGE (PPH)

Prevention: Pregnant Women

Recommendations from

> ACOG 2017, WHO 2023

–Give uterotonic medications to all patients during the third stage of labor.

- Oxytocin 10 IU, IV, or IM is the first choice.
- Methylergometrine or oral/rectal misoprostol is an alternative.

–Promptly perform uterine massage.

–Use controlled cord traction to remove the placenta.

–Use objective methods to quantify blood loss to detect postpartum hemorrhage earlier.

–Monitor for signs of excessive blood loss (tachycardia, hypotension).

Practice Pearl

- Routinely use objective measurement of postpartum blood loss to improve the detection and prompt treatment of postpartum hemorrhage.
  - Initiate the PPH treatment bundle when measured blood loss is >500 mL or >300 mL with early warning signs of excessive blood loss.
  - First-line PPH treatment bundle should include rapid uterine massage, administration of an oxytocic agent and tranexamic acid, IVF, examination of the genital tract, and escalation of care.
  - ACOG defines maternal hemorrhage as cumulative blood loss of ≥1000 mL or blood loss accompanied by signs or symptoms of hypovolemia within 24 h after birth.
  - Guidelines recommend consideration and investments made into the use of sustainable and climate-friendly drapes. Objective methods to measure postpartum blood loss must ensure the birthing parent's customary and cultural requirements are respected and maintained.

Sources

–*Obstet Gynecol.* 2017;183(130):e168–e186.

–WHO. 2023 Recommendations on the assessment of blood loss and use of a treatment bundle for postpartum hemorrhage. 2023.

Management: Pregnant Women

Recommendations from

➤ WHO 2012, ACOG 2017, ACR 2020, NICE 2022

–Uterotonics for the treatment of PPH:
  - Intravenous oxytocin is the recommended agent.
  - Alternative uterotonics:
    ◦ Misoprostol 800-mcg sublingual.
    ◦ Methylergonovine 0.2-mg IM.
    ◦ Carboprost 0.25-mg IM.

–Administer tranexamic acid.

–Additional interventions for PPH:
  - Isotonic crystalloid resuscitation.
  - Bimanual uterine massage.

–Therapeutic options for persistent PPH:
  - Uterine artery embolization.
  - B-Lynch suture.
  - Balloon tamponade.
  - Hysterectomy (most extreme, last resort).

–Therapeutic options for a retained placenta:
  - Controlled cord traction with oxytocin 10 IU IM/IV.
  - Manual removal of placenta.
    ○ Give single dose of first-generation antibiotic for prophylaxis against endometritis.
  - Recommend against methylergonovine, misoprostol, or carboprost (Hemabate) for retained placenta.
–Role of imaging: (ACR)
  - Most of the causes of PPH can be diagnosed clinically, but imaging may play a role in diagnosis.
  - Pelvic ultrasound (transabdominal and transvaginal with Doppler) is the imaging modality of choice for the initial evaluation of PPH.
  - Contrast-enhanced CT of the abdomen and pelvis and CT angiogram of the abdomen and pelvis may be appropriate to determine if active ongoing hemorrhage is present, to localize the bleeding, and to identify the source of bleeding.

Practice Pearl

- Misoprostol 800–1000 mcg can also be administered as a rectal suppository for PPH related to uterine atony.

Sources
–*Obstet Gynecol.* 2017;130:e168–e186.
–*J Am Coll Radiol.* 2020;17:S459–S471.
–*WHO Recommendations for the Prevention and Treatment of Postpartum Haemorrhage.* Geneva: World Health Organization; 2023.
–www.nice.org.uk/guidance/cg190

LABOR AND DELIVERY: TRIAL OF LABOR AFTER CESAREAN (TOLAC)

Management: Pregnant Women, Previous Cesarean Delivery

Recommendations from

➢ ACOG 2019

–Most women with 1 previous cesarean delivery and a low-transverse incision should be counseled about and offered TOLAC.
–In patients who have had a cesarean delivery or major uterine surgery, misoprostol should not be used for cervical ripening.
–Epidural analgesia may be used as a part of TOLAC during labor.

Practice Pearl

- The benefits of a VBAC include avoiding major abdominal surgery, lower rates of hemorrhage, thromboembolism, and infection, and a shorter recovery period. VBAC may also decrease maternal risks associated with cesarean sections, including hysterectomy, bowel/bladder injury, and future abnormal placentation.

Source
  −*Obstet Gynecol.* 2019;133(2):e110−e127.

LABOR AND DELIVERY: VAGINAL LACERATIONS

Prevention: Women Undergoing Vaginal Delivery

Recommendations from

➤ ACOG 2018

  −Insufficient evidence to recommend a specific mode of manual perineal support at delivery:
  - Consider applying warm perineal compresses during pushing to reduce the incidence of third-degree and fourth-degree lacerations.
  - Consider perineal massage during the second stage of labor to help reduce the incidence of third-degree and fourth-degree lacerations.
  - Do not routinely perform episiotomy. Perform episiotomy only when needed in high-risk cases such as shoulder dystocia, vaginal breech, or instrumental deliveries. When necessary, prefer mediolateral episiotomy over midline episiotomy.

Source
  −ACOG Practice Bulletin No. 198: Prevention and management of obstetric lacerations at vaginal delivery. *Obstet Gynecol.* 2018;132(3):e87−e102.

Management: Women Immediately Postpartum

Recommendations from

➤ ACOG 2018

  −For full-thickness external anal sphincter lacerations, either end-to-end repair or overlap repair is acceptable.
  −There are limited data to support a single dose of antibiotic at the time of anal sphincter repair, though administration is reasonable.

Source
  −*Obstet Gynecol.* 2018;132(3):e87−e102.

LEAD POISONING

Screening: Pregnant Women

Recommendations from

➤ USPSTF 2019, CDC 2000, AAP 2000, ACOG 2012

  −Do not screen universally.

–There is insufficient evidence to recommend for or against routine screening for patients at increased risk.[1]

–For pregnant patients with blood levels of 5 mcg/dL or higher, identify sources of lead exposure and offer counseling. Measure maternal or umbilical cord blood lead levels at delivery.

Practice Pearl

- Symptoms of lead poisoning are generally nonspecific: constipation, abdominal pain, anemia, headache, fatigue, myalgias and arthralgias, anorexia, sleep disturbance, difficulty concentrating, and hypertension, among others. Test blood lead levels if these symptoms are present in the setting of increased risk.

Sources

–USPSTF. *Screening for Elevated Blood Lead Levels in Children and Pregnant Patients.* 2019.

–Ettinger A, Wengrovitz A, eds. *Guidelines for the Identification and Management of Lead Exposure in Pregnant and Lactating Women.* US Dept of Health and Human Services; 2010.

–*Obstet Gynecol.* 2012;120:416–420.

MACROSOMIA

Management: Pregnant Women

Recommendations from

➢ ACOG 2020

–Diagnose macrosomia using ultrasound. Prediction of birth weight is imprecise by ultrasonography or clinical measurement. Accuracy of EFW by ultrasound biometry is no better than abdominal palpation.

–Recommend aerobic and strength-conditioning exercise during pregnancy to reduce the risk of macrosomia.

–Optimize maternal glycemic control.

–Discuss the risks and benefits of vaginal births and cesarean births based on the degree of suspected macrosomia.

- Scheduled cesarean birth may be beneficial for newborns with suspected macrosomia with an EFW of >5000 g in women without diabetes and an EFW of ≥4500 g in women with diabetes.

- Suspected fetal macrosomia is not an indication for induction of labor before 39 wk of gestation. There is insufficient evidence that benefits of reducing shoulder dystocia risk outweigh harms of early delivery.

Practice Pearl

- Historically, macrosomia has been defined as >4000 g or 4500 g. No universally accepted definition exists.

---

[1] Important risk factors for lead exposure in pregnant patients include recent immigration, pica practices, occupational exposure, nutritional status, culturally specific practices such as the use of traditional remedies or imported cosmetics, and the use of traditional lead-glazed pottery for cooking and storing food.

Source
–ACOG. Practice Bulletin No 216. Macrosomia. 2020.

NEURAL TUBE DEFECTS

Prevention: Pregnant Women

Recommendations from

> USPSTF 2023, AAFP 2016, ACOG 2017

–Recommend a daily supplement containing 400–800 mcg of folic acid for anyone planning or capable of pregnancy.

Sources
–*Obstet Gynecol.* 2017;130:e279–e290 (lww.com).
–*JAMA.* 2023;330(5):454–459. USPSTF. *Folic Acid Supplementation to Prevent Neural Tube Defects.* 2023.
–AAFP. *Clinical Prevention Recommendation.* https://www.aafp.org/patient-care/clinical-Prevention Recommendations/all/neural-tube-defects.html

PERINATAL MENTAL HEALTH

Management: Anxiety and Depression

Recommendations from

> ACOG 2023

–Risk counseling for perinatal anxiety and depression is part of every obstetrician's care:
- Initiate psychopharmacotherapy as indicated in equitable manner. Psychotherapy is the first-line treatment for mild-to-moderate perinatal depression. Refer patients to appropriate behavioral health resources.
- Provide education surrounding self-care and the roles of adequate sleep, exercise, balanced nutrition, minimizing stressors, and building a community of support.
- Use validated screening tool to monitor response to treatment and guide up-titration of medication to achieve goal remission of symptoms (defined as improvement of symptoms by 50% or more from baseline).
  - Validated screening instruments:
    - Depression: EPDS.
    - Anxiety: GAD-7, EPDS anxiety subscale (subitems 3,4,5), STAI.
  - Recommended up-titrating schedule: at 4 d, 7 d, reassess monthly. If antidepressant naïve, can consider slower titration of every 10–14 d.
- Pharmacotherapy plays an important role. See Table 11–7 for list of risks and benefits.
  - Overlying principles: 1) use the lowest effective dose that achieves the clinical goal; 2) avoid switching medications, and 3) avoid polypharmacy.

TABLE 11–7 RISKS AND BENEFITS OF ANTIDEPRESSANT THERAPY DURING PREGNANCY	
Risks of Undertreatment for Depression and Anxiety During Pregnancy	**Risks of Antidepressant Use During Pregnancy**
Limited engagement in medical and self-care Substance use Preterm birth Low birth weight Preeclampsia Impaired infant attachment and related long-term developmental effects Suicide	Persistent pulmonary hypertension of the newborn Transient neonatal aspiration syndrome Preeclampsia (SNRI) Spontaneous pregnancy loss

- First line: selective serotonin reuptake inhibitors (escitalopram 5–20 mg qAM or sertraline 25–200 mg qAM, unless history of successful pharmacotherapy with other agents).
- Avoid benzodiazepines for anxiety. Serotonin-norepinephrine reuptake inhibitors are reasonable alternatives.
- Avoid downtitration during third trimester. Doing so does not improve neonatal outcomes.
- Continue effective psychopharmacotherapy during early postpartum period.

Source
– ACOG. Screening and Diagnosis of Mental Health Conditions During Pregnancy and Postpartum. Number 4,5. 2023.

Management: Bipolar Disorder

Recommendations from

➢ ACOG 2023
– Validated screening tools: MDQ, CIDI.
– Women are at highest lifetime risk in perinatal period of developing bipolar disorder.
– Principles of treatment:
  - Do not discontinue mood stabilizers (exception: valproic acid) during pregnancy. Risks of recurrence or exacerbation of mood symptoms outweigh risks of medication.
  - Continue routine prenatal screening for GDM.
  - Monitor dosing closely. Postpartum dosing for lithium and lamotrigine is important to avoid toxicity.
– Lithium use in first trimester: order detailed cardiac ultrasound examination in second trimester.

Source
– ACOG. Screening and Diagnosis of Mental Health Conditions During Pregnancy and Postpartum. Number 4,5. 2023.

POSTPARTUM DEPRESSION

Prevention: Postpartum Women

Recommendations from

> USPSTF 2019, Canadian Task Force on Preventative Health Care 2022, ACOG 2023

Evaluation

–Refer those at increased risk for perinatal depression to counseling interventions.

–There is no accurate screening tool to identify those at risk. Consider providing counseling to patients with 1 or more of the following risk factors: history of depression, current depressive symptoms, certain socioeconomic risk factors such as low income or adolescent or single parenthood, recent intimate partner violence, or mental health–related factors.

–These recommendations do not apply to pregnant or postpartum patients with a personal history of depression, or those already receiving assessment or treatment for other mental disorders.

–When clinically indicated, consider using the Edinburgh Postnatal Depression Scale Questionnaire as part of the assessment and to aid clinical monitoring.

Therapies

–Moderate-to-severe postpartum depression with onset in third trimester or within 4 wk postpartum:

- Choose selective serotonin reuptake inhibitors as first-line psychopharmacotherapy.
- Consider brexanolone given rapid onset. Disadvantages: limited access, high cost, lack of lactation safety data, and requirement for inpatient monitoring during infusion.
- Lactation and breastfeeding while using pharmacologic treatment are encouraged.

–Avoid abrupt discontinuation of SSRIs/SNRIs. Recommend 2–4 wk progressive taper to avoid discontinuation symptoms (anxiety, gastrointestinal upset, dizziness, headaches, agitation, sleep disruption, tremors).

–Postpartum psychosis: psychiatric emergency that must be managed with a psychiatrist; 66% recurrence rate in the absence of pharmacotherapy.

- Recommended pharmacotherapy while connecting to psychiatrist includes:
  - Sedating antipsychotic medication (olanzapine, haloperidol).
  - Benzodiazepine (lorazepam).
  - Consider addition of benztropine or diphenhydramine to prevent extrapyramidal symptoms and dystonia.

Sources

–https://jamanetwork.com/journals/jama/fullarticle/2724195
–*CMAJ*. 2022;194:981–989. doi: 10.1503/cmaj.220290

Guidelines Alert 11–5	
GUIDELINES DISCORDANT: SCREENING FOR POSTPARTUM DEPRESSION	
USPSTF	Screen for depression in the general adult population, including pregnant and postpartum patients
CTFPHC	Do not screen all individuals for depression during pregnancy and the postpartum period using questionnaires, if usual care during these periods involves regular inquiry and attention to mental health and well-being

Applying to Clinical Practice
- Postpartum depression is common and responds well to treatment.
- Routine assessment is warranted, whether via formal screening tools or attentive clinical assessments.

Sources
–https://jamanetwork.com/journals/jama/fullarticle/2724195
–CMAJ. 2022;194:981–989. doi: 10.1503/cmaj.220290

Rh D ALLOIMMUNIZATION

Screening: Pregnant Women

Recommendations from

> AAFP 2014, USPSTF 2007, ACOG 2017

–Order ABO type and Rh D antibody testing for all pregnant patients at their first prenatal visit.
–Repeat Rh D antibody testing for all unsensitized Rh D-negative patients at 24–28 wk of gestation.

Practice Pearl

- Rh D antibody testing at 24–28 wk can be skipped if the biologic father is known to be Rh D negative.

Sources
–AAFP. *Update on Prenatal Care.* 2014.
–*Obstet Gynecol.* 2017;13:e57–e70.
–http://www.uspreventiveservicestaskforce.org/3rduspstf/rh/rhrs.htm

Prevention: Pregnant Women

–For unsensitized Rh D-negative patients, give anti-D immune globulin at 28 wk of gestation.
- Repeat after delivery, within 72 h, if infant is confirmed to be Rh D positive.
- Other situations to give anti-D immune globulin to an unsensitized Rh D-negative patient:
  - External cephalic version.
  - Uterine evacuation for molar pregnancy.

      ◦ First trimester pregnancy loss with instrumentation.[1]

      ◦ Ectopic pregnancy.

      ◦ Antenatal hemorrhage after 20 wk of gestation.

      ◦ Abdominal trauma.

      ◦ Fetal death in second or third trimester.

      ◦ First trimester miscarriage ("consider").

   –Repeat antibody screen before giving anti-D immune globulin.

Source

   –*Obstet Gynecol.* 2018;131:e8.

ROUTINE PRENATAL CARE

Management: Pregnant Women

Recommendations from

> AAFP, USPSTF, NICE, ACOG

   –See Table 11–8 for routine prenatal care guidance and Table 11–9 for perinatal recommendations.

SUBSTANCE USE DISORDERS IN PREGNANCY

Management: Pregnant Women

Recommendations from

> WHO 2014, ASAM 2020, CMQCC 2020, ABM 2023

   –Ask all pregnant persons about their use of alcohol and other illicit drugs at prenatal visits. Alcohol use in pregnancy is associated with an increased risk of preterm birth and small for gestational age in infants.

   –Offer a brief intervention and individualized care to all pregnant persons using alcohol or drugs.

   –Refer pregnant persons with alcohol, cocaine, or methamphetamine use disorder to a detoxification center.

     • Women with opioid use disorder should continue a structured opioid maintenance program with either methadone or buprenorphine.

     • Women with a benzodiazepine use disorder should gradually wean the dose.

     • Women with alcohol use disorder during pregnancy should have an individualized treatment plan. Psychosocial treatment is a first-line intervention. Avoid disulfiram (associated with fetal abnormalities). Naltrexone and acamprosate should be carefully considered given the possible risks of medication exposure (limited data) vs. risks of alcohol use.

---

[1] ACOG suggests that clinicians "consider" giving immune globulin in any first trimester miscarriage in a patient who is unsensitized and Rh D negative. While the risk of alloimmunization is quite low, the consequence is great.

TABLE 11–8 COMPILED RECOMMENDATIONS FOR ROUTINE PRENATAL CARE

Preconception visit

1. Measure height, weight, and blood pressure.
2. Assess immunization status for tetanus toxoid, reduced diphtheria toxoid, and acellular pertussis (Tdap); measles–mumps–rubella; hepatitis B; rubella, and varicella. Immunize as indicated. Live vaccines should be administered at least 1 mo prior to pregnancy.
3. Assess all patients for pregnancy risk: substance abuse, domestic violence, sexual abuse, psychiatric disorders, risk factors for preterm labor, exposure to chemicals or infectious agents, hereditary disorders, gestational diabetes, or chronic medical problems. Initiate interventions to optimize maternal, fetal, and pregnancy outcomes.
4. Educate patients about proper nutrition; offer weight reduction strategies for patients with obesity.
5. With the exception of universal HIV and hepatitis C screening, screening lab tests should be considered selectively in appropriate high-risk groups.
6. Initiate folic acid 400–800 mcg/d; 4 mg/d for a history of a child affected by a neural tube defect.

Initial prenatal visit

1. Confirm pregnancy.
2. Assess medical, surgical, obstetric, psychosocial, and family history, and perform a complete physical examination. Record baseline blood pressure, height, weight, and calculate BMI.
3. Order CBC, blood type (ABO and Rh D) and antibody screen, rubella titer, varicella titer, HIV, syphilis screening, hepatitis B surface antigen, hepatitis C antibody, urine NAAT for gonorrhea and chlamydia, urinalysis (proteinuria, glucosuria), urine culture. Pap smear if not up to date. Other selective screening tests as indicated.
4. Order an obstetrical ultrasound for dating if any of the following: beyond 16-wk gestational age, unsure of last menstrual period, size/date discrepancy on examination, or for inability to hear fetal heart tones by 12 gestational weeks.
5. Discuss fetal aneuploidy screening and counseling regardless of maternal age.
6. Prenatal testing for sickle cell anemia (African descent), thalassemia (African, Mediterranean, Middle Eastern, Southeast Asians), Canavan disease and Tay-Sachs (Jewish patients), cystic fibrosis (White and Ashkenazi Jew individuals), and fragile X syndrome (family history of nonspecified mental retardation) when indicated.
7. Test for tuberculosis in medium- to high-risk patients.[a]
8. Consider a 1-h 50-g glucose tolerance test for certain high-risk groups.[b]
9. Obtain an operative report in all women who have had a prior cesarean section.
10. Psychosocial risk assessment for mood disorders, substance abuse, or domestic violence.

Frequency of visits for uncomplicated pregnancies

1. Every 4 wk until 28 gestational weeks; q2 wk from 28 to 36 wk; weekly >36 wk.
2. Offer a single ultrasound examination at 18- to 20-wk gestation if not indicated earlier (ACOG). Consider offering routine ultrasonography between 11- and 14-wk gestation even if not medically indicated (NICE). There is no evidence to support routine ultrasonography in uncomplicated pregnancies.

TABLE 11–8   COMPILED RECOMMENDATIONS FOR ROUTINE PRENATAL CARE (*continued*)

Routine checks at follow-up prenatal visits

1. Assess weight, blood pressure, and urine for glucose and protein.
2. Exam: edema, fundal height, and fetal heart tones at all visits; fetal presentation starting at 36 wk.
3. Ask about regular uterine contractions, leakage of fluid, vaginal bleeding, or decreased fetal movement.
4. Discuss labor precautions.

Antepartum lab testing

1. Offer first trimester, second trimester, or combined testing to screen for fetal aneuploidy; invasive diagnostic testing for fetal aneuploidy should be available to all women regardless of maternal age.
   a. First trimester.
   b. Second trimester screening options: amniocentesis at 14 wk; a Quad Marker Screen at 16–18 wk; and/or a screening ultrasound with nuchal translucency assessment.
2. Consider serial transvaginal sonography of the cervix every 2–3 wk to assess cervical length for patients at high risk for preterm delivery starting at 16 wk.
3. No role for routine bacterial vaginosis screening.
4. 1-h 50-g glucose tolerance test in all women between 24 and 28 wk.
5. Screen for GBS colonization between 36- and 38-wk gestation with rectovaginal swab.
6. Recommend weekly amniotic fluid assessments and twice weekly nonstress testing starting at 41 wk.

Prenatal counseling

1. Cessation of smoking, drinking alcohol, or use of any illicit drugs.
2. Avoid cat litter boxes, hot tubs, certain foods (ie, raw fish or unpasteurized cheese).
3. Proper nutrition and expected weight gain: National Academy of Sciences advises weight gain 28–40 lb (prepregnancy BMI < 20), 25–35 lb (BMI 20–26), 15–25 lb (BMI 26–29), and 15–20 lb (BMI ≥ 30).
4. Inquire about domestic violence and depression at initial visit, at 28 wk, and at postpartum visit.
5. Recommend regular mild-to-moderate exercise 3 or more times a week.
6. Avoid high-altitude activities, scuba diving, and contact sports during pregnancy.
7. Benefits of breastfeeding vs. bottle-feeding.
8. Discuss postpartum contraceptive options (including tubal sterilization) during third trimester.
9. Discuss analgesia and anesthesia options and offer prenatal classes at 24 wk.
10. Discuss repeat C-section vs. VBAC (if applicable).
11. Discuss the option of circumcision if a boy is delivered.
12. Avoid air travel and long train or car trips beyond 36 wk.
13. Discuss the uncertain benefit of kick counting in the prevention of stillbirth. Kick counting may be associated with increased risk of iatrogenic preterm birth, induction of labor, and cesarean birth.

TABLE 11–8 COMPILED RECOMMENDATIONS FOR ROUTINE PRENATAL CARE (*continued*)

Prenatal interventions

1. Suppressive antiviral medications starting at 36 wk for women with a history of genital herpes.
2. Cesarean delivery is indicated for women who are HIV positive or have active genital herpes and are in labor.
3. For patients who report a history of abuse, offer interventions and resources to increase their safety during and after pregnancy.
4. For patients with severe depression, consider treatment with an SSRI (avoid paroxetine if possible).
5. Rh immune globulin 300 mcg IM for all Rh-negative women with negative antibody screens between 26 and 28 wk.
6. Refer for nutrition counseling at 10–12 wk for BMI < 20 or at any time during pregnancy for inadequate weight gain.
7. Start prenatal vitamins with iron and folic acid 400–800 mcg/d and 1200 mg elemental calcium/d starting at 4-wk preconception (or as early as possible during pregnancy) and continued until 6-wk postpartum.
8. Give inactivated influenza vaccine IM to all pregnant persons during influenza season.
9. Give Tdap vaccine during each pregnancy between 27- and 36-wk of gestation.
10. Consider progesterone therapy IM weekly or intravaginally daily to women at high risk for preterm birth.
11. Recommend an external cephalic version at 37 wk for all noncephalic presentations.
12. Offer labor induction to women at 41 wk by good dates.
13. Treat all women with confirmed syphilis with penicillin G during pregnancy.
14. Treat all women with gonorrhea with ceftriaxone; follow treatment with a test of cure.
15. Treat all women with chlamydia with azithromycin; follow treatment with a test of cure. Doxycycline is contraindicated during the second and third trimesters of pregnancy.
16. Treat all GBS-positive women with penicillin G when in labor or with spontaneous rupture of membranes.
17. Offer group prenatal care as an alternative to traditional prenatal care if available and involve partners.
18. Discuss and document preferences about mode of birth early on and confirm toward the end of pregnancy, as preferences may have changed.

Postpartum interventions

1. Treat all infants born to HBV-positive women with hepatitis B immunoglobulin and initiate HBV vaccine series within 12 h of life.
2. All women with a positive tuberculosis skin test and no evidence of active disease should receive a postpartum chest X-ray; treat with isoniazid 300 mg PO daily for 9 mo if chest X-ray is negative.
3. Administer a Tdap booster if tetanus status is unknown or the last Td (tetanus-diphtheria) vaccine was >10 y ago.
4. Administer an MMR vaccine to all rubella nonimmune women.
5. Offer HPV vaccine to all women ≤ 26 y who have not been immunized.
6. Initiate contraception.
7. Repeat Pap smear at 6-wk postpartum check.

TABLE 11–8 COMPILED RECOMMENDATIONS FOR ROUTINE PRENATAL CARE (*continued*)

[a]Post gastrectomy, gastric bypass, immunosuppressed (HIV-positive, diabetes, renal failure, chronic steroid/immunosuppressive therapy, head/neck or hematologic malignancies), silicosis, organ transplant recipients, malabsorptive syndromes, alcoholics, intravenous drug users, close contacts of persons with active pulmonary tuberculosis, medically underserved, low socioeconomic class, residents/employees of long-term care facilities and jails, health care workers, and immigrants from endemic areas.

[b]Overweight (BMI ≥ 25) and an additional risk factor: physical inactivity; first-degree relative with DM; high-risk ethnicity (eg, Black, Latina, American Indian, Asian American, Pacific Islander persons); history of gestational diabetes mellitus (GDM); prior baby with birthweight > 9 lb; unexplained stillbirth or malformed infant; HTN on therapy or with BP ≥140/90 mmHg; HDL cholesterol level < 35 mg/dL (0.90 mmol/L) and/or a triglyceride level > 250 mg/dL (2.82 mmol/L); polycystic ovary syndrome; history of impaired glucose tolerance or HgbA1c ≥ 5.7%; acanthosis nigricans; cardiovascular disease; or ≥2+ glucosuria.

Sources: Adapted from http://www.icsi.org/prenatal_care_4/prenatal_care_routine_full_version_2.html;
Am Fam Physician. 2014;89(3):199–208.
USPSTF. *Hepatitis C Virus Infection in Adolescents and Adults: Screening.* 2020.
NICE. *Antenatal Care (NG201).* 2021.
NICE. *Inducing Labour (NG207).* 2021.
NICE. *Postnatal Care (NG194).* 2021.
ACOG. Practice Bulletin No 229. *Antepartum Fetal Surveillance.* 2021.

TABLE 11–9 AAP AND AFP PERINATAL AND POSTNATAL GUIDELINES

Breastfeeding	Strongly recommends education and counseling to promote breastfeeding
Hemoglobinopathies	Strongly recommends ordering screening tests for hemoglobinopathies in neonates
Hyperbilirubinemia	Perform ongoing systematic assessments during the neonatal period for the risk of an infant developing severe hyperbilirubinemia
Phenylketonuria	Strongly recommends ordering screening tests for phenylketonuria in neonates
Thyroid function abnormalities	Strongly recommends ordering screening tests for thyroid function abnormalities in neonates

Sources: Pediatrics. 2004;114:297–316; 2005;115:496–506.

–Encourage mothers with a substance use disorder history to breastfeed unless the risks outweigh the benefits. Make an individualized care plan in partnership with the patient and a multidisciplinary team. In general, recommend breastfeeding to mothers who stop nonprescribed substance use by the time of delivery. Continue to support them with lactation support and substance use disorder treatment.

–Carefully monitor and treat infants of mothers with substance use disorder(s).

Practice Pearls

- Support pregnant people who discontinue nonprescribed substance use by delivery hospitalization to breastfeed, unless there is another contraindication.
- Target perinatal dyadic breastfeeding support to facilitate breastfeeding continuation. This includes multidisciplinary substance use disorder treatment, prenatal education, and postpartum lactation support.
- Use of toxicology testing to guide breastfeeding decision-making has limitations. If used, it must be interpreted within clinical contexts including patient history and collateral information.

Sources

    –*The ASAM National Practice Guideline for the Treatment of Opioid Use Disorder.*

    –California Maternal Quality Care Collaborative Opiate Use Disorder Toolkit.

    –*ABM Clinical Protocol #21: Breastfeeding in the Setting of Substance Use and Substance Use Disorder*; revised 2023.

SURGICAL SITE INFECTIONS (SSI)

Prevention: Pregnant Women

Recommendations from

> Cochrane Database of Systematic Reviews 2014, ACOG 2018

    –Treat remote infections prior to elective operations.

    –Do not shave incision site unless hair interferes with operation. If necessary, remove hair immediately before operation with clippers.

    –Control serum blood glucose levels and avoid perioperative hyperglycemia.

    –Instruct patients to shower or bathe (full body) at least the night before abdominal surgery.

    –Prepare the surgical site preoperatively with an alcohol-based agent unless contraindicated.

    –Use a vaginal preparation with povidone-iodine solution immediately prior to uterine or vaginal surgery.

    –Give prophylactic IV antibiotics preoperatively within 60 min of skin incision as opposed to administration after cord clamping.

Practice Pearls

- A vaginal prep prior to cesarean section reduces the incidence of postpartum endometritis. This benefit was especially true for patients in active labor or with ruptured membranes.
- The incidence of maternal infectious morbidity is decreased (RR 0.54) when prophylactic antibiotics are administered preoperatively as opposed to after cord clamping.

Sources

    –*Obstet Gynecol.* 2018;131:e172–e189.

    –http://www.cochrane.org/CD007892/PREG_vaginal-cleansing-before-cesarean-delivery-to-reduce-post-cesarean-infections

SYPHILIS

Screening: Pregnant Women

Recommendations from

> CDC 2015, AAFP 2019, USPSTF 2018, WHO 2017, AAP/ACOG 2017

    –Screen all pregnant patients at the first prenatal visit.

–Screen again at 28 gestational weeks if high risk[1] or previously untested.

- Use a nontreponemal test (Venereal Disease Research Laboratory [VDRL] test or rapid plasma reagent [RPR] test) for initial screening.

Practice Pearls

- Confirm all reactive nontreponemal tests with a fluorescent treponemal antibody absorption (FTA-ABS) test.
- If high risk, consider testing a third time at the time of delivery.
- Syphilis is a reportable disease in every state.

Sources

–CDC. *Sexually Transmitted Diseases Treatment Guidelines*. 2015.

–USPSTF. *JAMA*. 2018;320(9):911–917.

–WHO. *Syphilis Screening and Treatment for Pregnant Woman*. 2017.

–https://www.aafp.org/patient-care/clinical-Screening Recommendations/all/syphilis.html

–American Academy of Pediatrics; American College of Obstetricians and Gynecologists. *Guidelines for Perinatal Care*. 8th ed. Elk Grove Village, IL: American Academy of Pediatrics; American College of Obstetricians and Gynecologists; 2017.

THYROID DISEASE

Screening: Pregnant Women

Recommendations from

> ATA 2017, AAFP 2014

–There is insufficient evidence to recommend for or against routine screening of all patients.

–Obtain TSH levels at confirmation of pregnancy if:

- A history or current symptoms of thyroid dysfunction.
- Known thyroid antibody positivity or presence of a goiter.
- History of head or neck radiation or prior thyroid surgery.
- Age > 30 y.
- Autoimmune disorders.
- History of pregnancy loss, preterm delivery, or infertility.
- Multiple prior pregnancies.
- Family history of thyroid disease.
- BMI ≥ 40.
- Use of amiodarone or lithium, or recent administration of iodinated radiologic contrast.
- Residing in an area of known moderate-to-severe iodine insufficiency.

---

[1] High-risk features include elevated community prevalence, concomitant HIV infection, and past incarceration or sex work.

Sources
   –*Thyroid.* 2017;27(3):315.
   –*Am Fam Physician.* 2014;89(4):273–278.

Management: Pregnant and Postpartum Women

Recommendations from

➢ **ATA 2017, ACOG 2020**

Evaluation

–Hypothyroidism in pregnancy is defined as:

   • An elevated TSH (>2.5 mIU/L) and a suppressed free thyroxine (FT_4).
   • TSH ≥ 10 mIU/L (irrespective of FT_4).

–If a thyroid nodule is found, arrange thyroid ultrasound and TSH testing.

Therapies

–Do not treat subclinical hypothyroidism (TSH 2.5–9.9 mIU/L and a normal FT_4) in pregnancy.

–If hypothyroid, treat with levothyroxine, starting with 1–2 mcg/kg or 100 mcg daily. Goal of therapy is to normalize TSH levels (between the lower limit of reference range and 2.5 mU/L). Monitor TSH levels every 4 wk when treating thyroid disease in pregnancy.

–Measure a TSH receptor antibody level at 20–24 wk for any history of Graves disease.

–Patients found to have thyroid cancer during pregnancy would ideally undergo surgery during the second trimester.

–Do not treat transient hCG-mediated TSH suppression in early pregnancy with antithyroid drug therapy.

–If hyperthyroid, use propylthiouracil or methimazole. Avoid methimazole in the first trimester.

–Treat Graves disease during pregnancy with the lowest possible dose of antithyroid drug needed to keep the mother's thyroid hormone levels at or slightly above the reference range for total T_4 and T_3 values in pregnancy (1.5 times above nonpregnant reference ranges in the second and third trimesters), and the TSH below the reference range for pregnancy.

–Pregnancy is a relative contraindication to thyroidectomy and should only be used when medical management has been unsuccessful or ATDs cannot be used.

Practice Pearl

• Surgery for well-differentiated thyroid carcinoma can often be deferred until postpartum period.

Sources
   –*Thyroid.* 2016;26(10):1343–1421.
   –*Thyroid.* 2017;27(3):315–390.
   –http://thyroidguidelines.net/sites/thyroidguidelines.net/files/file/thy.2011.0087.pdf
   –*Obstet Gynecol.* 2020; 135(6):e261–e274.

TOBACCO USE

Screening: Pregnant Women

Recommendations from

> AAFP 2015, USPSTF 2015, ICSI 2014

–Screen all pregnant patients for tobacco use and provide pregnancy-directed counseling and literature for those who smoke.

Practice Pearl

- The "5-A" framework is helpful for smoking cessation counseling:
  - Ask about tobacco use.
  - Advise to quit through clear, individualized messages.
  - Assess willingness to quit.
  - Assist in quitting.
  - Arrange follow-up and support sessions.

Sources

–AAFP. *Clinical Preventive Service Screening Recommendation: Tobacco Use.* 2015.

–USPSTF. *Tobacco Smoking Cessation in Adults, Including Pregnant Patients: Behavioral and Pharmacotherapy Interventions.* 2015.

–ICSI. *Preventive Services for Adults.* 20th ed. 2014.

WEIGHT GAIN IN PREGNANCY

Prevention: Pregnant Women

Recommendations from

> USPSTF 2021

–Provide behavioral counseling interventions aimed at promoting healthy weight gain and preventing excess gestational weight gain in pregnancy to all pregnant patients.

Practice Pearl

- The Institute of Medicine recommends the following for weight gain in pregnancy: 1.1–4.4 lbs are expected in the first trimester, with the rest of the gain to follow.
  - BMI < 18.5: 28–40 lbs.
  - BMI 18.5–24.9: 25–35 lbs.
  - BMI 25–29.9: 15–25 lbs.
  - BMI ≥ 30: 11–20 lbs.

Sources

–*JAMA.* 2021;325(20):2087–2093. doi:10.1001/jama.2021.6949

–Institute of Medicine. *Weight Gain During Pregnancy: Reexamining the Guidelines.* Washington, DC. National Academies Press; 2009.

VENOUS THROMBOEMBOLISM

Prevention: Pregnant Women

Recommendations from

> ACOG 2018
>> −Consider thromboprophylaxis for patients at increased risk for thromboembolism.
>> −There is not sufficient evidence for routine prophylaxis in pregnancy.
>> −No risk assessment tool has been sufficiently validated, but risk factors include personal history of thrombosis, thrombophilia, cesarean delivery, obesity, hypertension, autoimmune disease, heart disease, sickle cell disease, multiple gestations, and preeclampsia.

PULMONARY DISORDERS

ASTHMA

Prevention: Children and Adolescents

Recommendations from

> Global Initiative for Asthma (GINA) 2021
  - Advise pregnant persons and parents of young children not to smoke.
  - Treat vitamin D deficiency in pregnant persons.
  - Encourage vaginal delivery.
  - Minimize use of broad-spectrum antibiotics during the first year of life.

Practice Pearls

- Environmental exposures such as automobile exhaust and dust mites are associated with higher rates of asthma, while others (household pets and farm animals) may be protective. Avoiding tobacco smoke and air pollution is protective, but allergen avoidance measures have not been shown to be effective in primary prevention.
- Public health interventions to reduce childhood obesity, increase fruit and vegetable intake, improve maternal-fetal health, and reduce socioeconomic inequality would address major risk factors. (*Lancet*. 2015;386:1075–1085)
- Maternal intake of allergenic food likely decreases the risk of allergy and asthma in offspring.
- Breastfeeding is generally advisable, but not for the specific purpose of preventing allergies and asthma.
- Obesity in pregnancy is associated with asthma development in children, but data is lacking on the safety and efficacy of weight loss efforts during pregnancy.

Source
  - Global Initiative for Asthma. *Global Strategy for Asthma Management and Prevention*. 2021. www.ginasthma.org

Management: Children > 5 y and Adults, Acute Exacerbation

Recommendations from

> GINA 2022

–Consider alternative causes for the patient's respiratory symptoms, including anaphylaxis, foreign body, bronchiectasis, congenital heart disease/cardiac failure, pulmonary embolism, and chronic obstructive pulmonary disease (COPD).

–If in the clinic, assess the severity of asthma exacerbation while starting short-acting beta agonist (SABA) and supplemental oxygen as needed. Transfer to acute care facility if altered mentation, silent chest, or signs of severe exacerbation (agitated, accessory muscle use, HR > 120, 90% O_2 saturation on room air) are observed. Give inhaled SABA, inhaled ipratropium bromide, oxygen, and systemic corticosteroids as soon as possible.

–If in the ED, start treatment with repeated doses of inhaled SABA, early oral corticosteroids, and supplemental oxygen. Titrate oxygen to maintain O_2 saturation 93%–95% in adults, and 94%–98% in children aged 6–12 y.

–Consider IV magnesium if patient is not responding to initial SABA, ipratropium bromide, oxygen, and systemic steroids.

–No role for routine antibiotics, chest X-ray (CXR), or blood gases in asthma exacerbation. Use antibiotics only for suspected bacterial infections.

–After stabilization:

- Initiate inhaled corticosteroid (ICS) before hospital discharge or step-up ICS treatment for 2–4 wk. Stress daily use.
- Prescribe 5–7 d course oral corticosteroid for adults and 3–5 d course for children. Follow-up within 2–7 d to ensure symptoms are well controlled and that the treatment is continued.
- Use the exacerbation as an opportunity to review the patient's chronic medication regimen, identify misunderstandings, and review the asthma action plan.

Practice Pearl

- Corticosteroids dosing:
  - For children: prednisolone 1–2 mg/kg/d to max 40 mg/d.
  - For adults: methylprednisolone 1 mg/kg IV q6 h initially for severe exacerbations. Prednisolone 40–50 mg PO for mild to moderate.
  - Magnesium dosing: magnesium sulfate 2 g IV.
  - Rapid-acting beta-agonists (SABA) dosing: 4–10 puffs albuterol pMDI with spacer or 2.5–5 mg nebulized q20 min for 1 h.

Source

–Global Initiative for Asthma. *Global Strategy for Asthma Management and Prevention 2022 Update.* http://www.ginasthma.org

Management: Children Age > 5 y, Adolescents, Chronic Asthma

Recommendations from

> GINA 2022, NICE 2017

Evaluation

–Diagnose asthma by history: typical symptoms are a combination of shortness of breath, cough, wheezing, and chest tightness; variability over time and in intensity; frequent triggers.

–Use spirometry with bronchodilators to confirm diagnosis, determine the severity of airflow limitation and its reversibility. Repeat spirometry at least every 1–2 y for asthma monitoring. FEV_1 and FEV_1/FVC ratio are reduced in asthma and increase by more than 12% after a bronchodilator challenge.

–Obtain a CXR at the initial visit to exclude alternative diagnoses.

–Consider allergy testing for history of atopy, rhinitis, rhinorrhea, and seasonal variation or specific extrinsic triggers.

Therapies

–Assess tobacco use and advise smokers to quit.

–Encourage allergen and environmental or occupational trigger avoidance.

–Recommend an asthma action plan based on peak expiratory flow monitoring for all patients.

–Educate patients, assist them in self-management, develop goals of treatment, create an asthma action plan, and regularly monitor asthma control.

–Major independent risk factors for exacerbations:

  • Uncontrolled asthma.

  • Frequent asthma exacerbations (>1 in the past year).

  • History of ICU admission or intubation for asthma exacerbation.

–Potentially modifiable risk factors:

  • Medications: high SABA use, lack of ICS, inadequate ICS.

  • Comorbidities: obesity, chronic rhinosinusitis, gastroesophageal reflux disease (GERD), pregnancy, food allergies, blood eosinophilia.

–See Tables 12–1 and 12–2 for treatment recommendations.

Source

–Global Initiative for Asthma. *Global Strategy for Asthma Management and Prevention.* 2022. www.ginasthma.org

TABLE 12–1 STEP THERAPY IN ASTHMA MANAGEMENT, AGES 12+

	Start Here If	Preferred	Alternative
Step 1	Symptoms < 2×/mo	Low-dose ICS-formoterol as needed	SABA + ICS as needed
Step 2	Symptoms < 4–5 d/wk	Low-dose ICS-formoterol as needed	Low-dose ICS daily
Step 3	Symptoms most days, or waking with asthma ≥ 1×/wk	Low-dose ICS-formoterol daily	Low-dose ICS-LABA daily
Step 4	Daily symptoms, or waking with asthma ≥ 1×/wk	Medium-dose ICS-formoterol daily Consider short-course OCS if presenting with severely uncontrolled asthma	Medium-/high-dose ICS-LABA daily
Step 5		Add on LAMA Refer for assessment of phenotype Consider high-dose daily ICS-formoterol, biologics	Add on LAMA Refer for assessment of phenotype Consider high-dose daily ICS-LABA, biologics

Review response q2–3 mo, or sooner if clinically indicated.
If symptoms are uncontrolled on preferred strategy, trial the alternative. If remains uncontrolled on alternative, escalate to next higher step.
If good control is maintained for 3 mo, step down treatment to the next lower step.
ICS, inhaled corticosteroid; SABA, short-acting beta-agonist; LABA, long-acting beta-agonist; LAMA, long-acting muscarinic antagonist; OCS, oral corticosteroid.

TABLE 12–2 STEP THERAPY IN ASTHMA MANAGEMENT, AGES 6–11

	Start Here If	Preferred	Alternative
Step 1	Symptoms < 2×/mo	SABA plus low-dose ICS as needed	Daily low-dose ICS
Step 2	Symptoms > 2×/mo, <1×/d	Daily low-dose ICS	Daily LTRA, or SABA plus low-dose ICS as needed
Step 3	Symptoms most days, or waking with asthma ≥ 1×/wk	Low-dose ICS-LABA, OR Medium-dose ICS, OR Budesonide/formoterol 100/6 mcg MART	Low-dose ICS + LTRA
Step 4	Daily symptoms, or waking with asthma ≥ 1×/wk	Medium-dose ICS-LABA, OR Budesonide/formoterol 200/6 mcg MART Refer for expert advice	Add tiotropium or LTRA
Step 5		Refer for phenotypic assessment Consider higher-dose ICS-LABA or add-on therapy with biologics	Add-on anti-IL5, or consider low-dose OCS with attention to risk of side effects

Review response q2–3 mo, or sooner if clinically indicated.
If symptoms are uncontrolled on preferred strategy, trial the alternative. If remains uncontrolled on alternative, escalate to next higher step.
If good control is maintained for 3 mo, step down treatment to the next lower step.
ICS, inhaled corticosteroid; SABA, short-acting beta-agonist; LABA, long-acting beta-agonist; OCS, oral corticosteroid; LTRA, leukotriene receptor antagonist; MART, maintenance and reliever therapy.

BRONCHIOLITIS, ACUTE

Management: Infants and Children

Recommendations from

> **NICE 2015, AAP 2023**

Evaluation

–Consider diagnosis in children under 2 y of age, especially in the first year of life. Incidence peaks between 3 and 6 mo.

–Symptoms typically peak between 3 and 5 d. Cough resolves in 90% of infants within 3 wk.

–Diagnose bronchiolitis if the patient has a coryzal prodrome lasting 1–3 d, followed by all of the following:

- Persistent cough.
- Either tachypnea or chest recession (or both).
- Either wheeze or crackles on chest auscultation (or both).

–Other common symptoms include fever (30% of cases, usually <39°C) and poor feeding (typically after 3–5 d of illness).

–Consider alternate diagnosis of pneumonia if the patient has high fever (>39°C) and/or persistently focal crackles.

–Admit to hospital if any of the following:

- Apnea (observed or reported).
- Persistent room air O_2 saturation < 90% (age ≥ 6 wk) or < 92% (age < 6 wk or any age with underlying health conditions).
- Inadequate oral fluid intake.
- Persisting severe respiratory distress (ie, grunting, marked chest recession, or respiratory rate > 70 breaths/min).

–Do not routinely perform specific viral testing, radiography, or laboratory studies (changes on X-ray may mimic pneumonia but do not require antibiotics).

Therapies

–Do not perform chest physiotherapy unless relevant comorbidities (ie, spinal muscular atrophy, severe tracheomalacia).

–Do not use any of the following to treat bronchiolitis in babies or children:

- Antibiotics.
- Hypertonic saline.
- Epinephrine (nebulized).
- Salbutamol.
- Montelukast.
- Ipratropium bromide.
- Systemic or ICS/a combination of systemic corticosteroids and nebulized adrenaline.

–Give oxygen supplementation to babies and children with bronchiolitis if their O_2 saturation is <90% (age ≥ 6 wk) or <92% (age < 6 wk or any age with underlying health conditions).

–Ensure adequate hydration by oral or nasogastric feeding.

–Do not routinely perform upper airway suctioning in babies or children with bronchiolitis. Consider upper airway suctioning in babies and children who have respiratory distress or feeding difficulties because of upper airway secretions.

Sources
–https://www.nice.org.uk/guidance/ng9
–https://doi.org/10.1542/aap.ppcqr.396139

BRONCHITIS, ACUTE

Management: Adults

Recommendations from

➤ CDC 2017
   –Avoid CXR if all the following are present:
   - Heart rate < 100 beats/min.
   - Respiratory rate < 24 breaths/min.
   - Temperature < 100.4°F (38°C).
   - No exam findings consistent with pneumonia (consolidation, egophony, fremitus).
   –Colored sputum does not predict bacterial infection.
   –Avoid routine use of antibiotics regardless of duration of cough.
   –Treat symptomatically, as necessary:
   - Cough suppression (codeine, dextromethorphan).
   - Antihistamines (first or second generation).
   - Pharyngeal drainage with decongestants (phenylephrine).

Practice Pearls

- Primary clinical goal is to exclude pneumonia.
- Consider antitussive agents for short-term relief of coughing.
- Avoid routine beta-2-agonists or mucolytic agents to alleviate cough.

Source
–https://www.cdc.gov/antibiotic-use/community/for-hcp/outpatient-hcp/adult-treatment-rec.html

CHRONIC OBSTRUCTIVE PULMONARY DISEASE (COPD)

Screening: Adults

Recommendations from

➤ USPSTF 2022
   –Do not screen asymptomatic adults for COPD.

Practice Pearls

- Neither screening for COPD in asymptomatic adults nor treatment of asymptomatic COPD has been shown to reduce morbidity/mortality or improve quality of life.
- This does not apply to very high-risk populations such as patients with alpha-1-antitrypsin deficiency or those who have known occupational exposures.
- Symptom-based questionnaires have high sensitivity (67%–90%) but poor specificity (25%–73%) for COPD.
- In symptomatic patients (ie, dyspnea, chronic cough, or sputum production with a history of exposure to cigarette smoke or other toxic fumes), diagnostic spirometry to measure FEV_1/FVC ratio is indicated.

Source
–*JAMA*. 2022;327(18):1806–1811.

Management: Adults, Acute Exacerbation

Recommendations from

➤ GOLD 2023, ERS/ATS 2017

Evaluation

–Diagnose exacerbation when dyspnea and/or cough and sputum worsen over less than 14 d. (GOLD)

–Consider alternate diagnoses: pneumonia, heart failure, and pulmonary embolism are most frequent, followed by pneumothorax, pleural effusion, MI, and/or cardiac arrhythmias.

–Classify severity (see Table 12–3).

Therapies

–Consider admission to hospital if classified as severe, acute respiratory failure, new physical signs (cyanosis, peripheral edema, etc.), failure to respond to initial management, serious comorbidities (HF, new arrhythmia, etc.), or insufficient support at home.

–Treat according to severity: (GOLD)
- Mild: short-acting bronchodilators.

TABLE 12–3 CLASSIFYING THE SEVERITY OF COPD EXACERBATIONS

Signs	Mild	Moderate (Meets 3 of 5)	Severe
Dyspnea	VAS < 5	VAS ≥ 5	Same as moderate, PLUS ABG with new/worsening hypercapnia ($PaCO_2$ > 45 mmHg) and acidosis (pH < 7.35)
RR	<24 bpm	≥24 bpm	
HR	<95 bpm	≥95 bpm	
SaO_2	≥92% room air AND change ≤3%	<92% room air AND/OR change >3%	
CRP	<10 mg/L	≥10 mg/L	

VAS, visual analog dyspnea scale.
Source: Adapted from Fig. 5.1 in Global Initiative for Chronic Obstructive Lung Disease. *Global Strategy for the Diagnosis, Management, and Prevention of Chronic Obstructive Pulmonary Disease (2023 Report).* https://goldcopd.org/2023-gold-report-2/

- Moderate: SABA +/− SAMA and oral glucocorticoids and/or antibiotics.
- Severe (acute respiratory failure): hospitalization or ED.

–Use noninvasive positive pressure ventilation for moderate-to-severe hypercapnic respiratory failure. Bi-PAP improves survival and decreases need for intubation, infectious complications, and hospital length of stay in moderate-to-severe COPD exacerbations.

–Use bronchodilators for acute treatment despite lack of high-quality evidence (GOLD). Deliver by nebulizer or metered-dose inhalers.[1] Inhale 1–2 puffs q1 h for 2–3 doses and then q2–4 h. Do not use continuous nebulizer.

–Continue controller long-acting inhalers (long-acting beta-agonist [LABA], LAMA, ICS) during the exacerbation or start as soon as feasible. (GOLD)

–Do not use methylxanthines due to side-effect profiles.

–Postexacerbation care:

- Before 1 mo, review discharge therapy and inhaler technique. Assess for need for long-term oxygen treatment through a new ABG and O_2 saturation. Document symptoms via CAT or mMRC and document capacity for ADLs. (GOLD)
- At 3–4 mo, reassess lung function by spirometry and prognosis (ie, BODE index[2]). Reassess inhaler techniques and need for oxygen. (GOLD)
- Enroll in pulmonary rehabilitation within 3 wk of hospital discharge. (ERS/ATA)

Guidelines Alert 12–1
GUIDELINES DISCORDANT: THERAPY FOR COPD EXACERBATIONS IN THE AMBULATORY SETTING

	GOLD	ERS/ATS
Corticosteroids	Use glucocorticoids for moderate or severe exacerbations: prednisone 40 mg PO daily × 5 d or prednisolone 40 mg PO or IV daily × 5 d	≤14 d corticosteroid course
Antibiotics	Treat with antibiotics for 5–7 d if exacerbation is associated with sputum color change, increased volume, or thickness. Choose an aminopenicillin with clavulanic acid, macrolide, or a tetracycline, depending on local bacterial resistance patterns	Administer antibiotics

Applying to Clinical Practice
- The more specific GOLD recommendations are a reasonable pathway for treating most patients.

[1] MDI with spacer may work as well as nebulizers, but nebulizers may be preferred in sicker patients due to ease of use.
[2] *N Engl J Med.* 2004;350:1005–1012. http://www.nejm.org/doi/full/10.1056/NEJMoa021322#t=article

Practice Pearls

- The scope of the ERS/ATS guidelines is much narrower, owing to the lack of conclusive evidence for much of the detail in the GOLD recommendations.
- Short courses of oral antibiotics and oral corticosteroids are the only evidence-based therapies that improve outcomes in COPD exacerbations. There are insufficient data to guide choice of antibiotic or treatment duration. (*Ann Intern Med*. 2020;172:413–422)
- Use antibiotics for three cardinal symptoms:
    - Increased dyspnea.
    - Increased sputum volume.
    - Increased sputum purulence.
    - Any two of the above if one of the two includes increased purulent sputum. (GOLD)
- Procalcitonin-based determination of antibiotic benefit is controversial with conflicting findings in studies. (GOLD)

Sources

–*Eur Respir J*. 2017;49:1600791.

–Global Initiative for Chronic Obstructive Lung Disease. *Global Strategy for the Diagnosis, Management, and Prevention of Chronic Obstructive Pulmonary Disease (2023 Report)*. https://goldcopd.org/2023-gold-report-2/

Management: Adults, Chronic Stable COPD

Recommendations from

> GOLD 2023, ATS 2020, CHEST 2023

Evaluation

–Establish diagnosis with spirometry using FEV_1/FVC ratio ($FEV_1/FVC < 0.7$).

–Classify severity based on FEV_1.

- GOLD 1 (mild): $FEV_1 \geq 80$
- GOLD 2 (moderate): FEV_1 50–79
- GOLD 3 (severe): FEV_1 30–49
- GOLD 4 (very severe): $FEV_1 < 30$

–Group patients by symptom history using GOLD ABE system and use this to dictate therapy (see Fig. 12–1). Evaluate symptoms using either COPD Assessment Tool (CAT)[1] or Modified British Medical Research Council Dyspnea Scale (mMRC).[2]

Therapies

–Counsel for smoking cessation. Smoking cessation has the greatest capacity to influence the natural history of COPD. Nicotine replacement products, bupropion, and nortriptyline may be effective with a supportive intervention program.

–Consider updated vaccinations such as influenza, SARS-Cov-2, pneumococcal vaccines, Tdap, and zoster.

---

[1] Available online at: https://www.catestonline.org/patient-site-test-page-english.html
[2] Available online at: https://www.pcrs-uk.org/mrc-dyspnoea-scale

FIG. 12–1   GOLD APPROACH TO SYMPTOM GROUPING AND INITIAL THERAPY IN COPD.

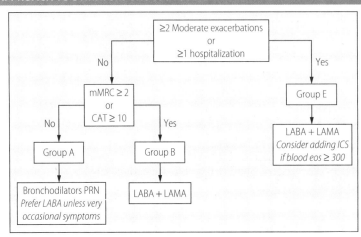

Source: Adapted from Figs. 2.3 and 4.2 in Global Initiative for Chronic Obstructive Lung Disease. *Global Strategy for the Diagnosis Management, and Prevention of Chronic Obstructive Pulmonary Disease [2023 Report]*.

–Review at follow-ups: symptoms, exacerbations, smoking status, exposure to other risk factors,[1] inhaler technique and adherence, physical activity and exercise, need for pulmonary rehabilitation, self-management skills, need for oxygen/NIV/lung volume reduction/palliative approaches, vaccinations, management of comorbidities, and spirometry at least annually.

–Initial therapy:
  • CAT < 10, mMRC 1: start monotherapy LAMA or LABA. (CHEST)
  • CAT ≥ 10, mMRC ≥ 2: start dual LAMA-LABA and do not de-escalate. (CHEST)

–If persistent dyspnea despite initial therapy:
  • Check adherence, inhaler technique, and comorbidities.
  • Consider switching inhaler device or molecules.
  • Escalate nonpharmacologic treatments.
  • Investigate other causes of dyspnea.

–If persistent exacerbations despite initial therapy:
  • Check adherence, inhaler technique, and comorbidities.
  • If on LABA or LAMA monotherapy, escalate to LABA + LAMA. Add ICS if blood eosinophil count (eos) > 300.
  • If on LABA+LAMA (eos < 300) or LABA+LAMA+ICS, add azithromycin (preferable in former smokers) or roflumilast (if FEV_1 < 50% and chronic bronchitis).
  • If on ICS and develops pneumonia or blood eos are <100, de-escalate.

–Escalate to triple therapy with LAMA/LABA/ICS in those with persistent symptoms and do not de-escalate. (CHEST)

–If persistent exacerbations despite triple therapy, add macrolide therapy or roflumilast or N-acetylcysteine. (CHEST)

[1] Risk factors: smoking, alpha-1-antitrypsin deficiency, occupational dust/agent/fume exposure, asthma, and factors that affect lung growth.

–Arrange pulmonary rehabilitation for symptomatic patients with moderate-to-severe COPD ($FEV_1 < 50\%$ of predicted).

–Prescribe continuous oxygen therapy for COPD patients with room air hypoxemia ($PaO_2 \leq 55$ mmHg, $PaO_2 \leq 60$ mmHg with right heart failure or erythrocytosis, or $SpO_2 \leq 88\%$). Titrate to keep $SaO_2 \geq 90\%$. Reassess every 60–90 d to see if supplemental oxygen is still indicated or if titration is needed.

–Screen COPD patients for osteoporosis and depression.

–Offer nutritional support for patients with severe COPD with malnutrition.

–Calculate the BODE index (BMI, airflow obstruction, dyspnea, and exercise capacity on a 6-min walk test) to assess the risk of death in severe COPD.[1]

Guidelines Alert 12–2 GUIDELINES DISCORDANT: STEPWISE MEDICATION APPROACH TO CHRONIC COPD	
GOLD	**ATS**

1. A bronchodilator PRN
2. If persistent symptoms, add LABA + LAMA
3. If persistent symptoms, frequent and/or severe exacerbations:
  a. Blood eosinophils ≥ 100 cells/mcL: LAMA + LABA + ICS
  b. Blood eosinophils < 100 cells/mcL or still has exacerbations with LAMA + LABA + ICS:
    – Add roflumilast (if $FEV_1 < 50\%$, chronic bronchitis, ≥1 exacerbation/year)
    – Add macrolide (if not current smoker, use azithromycin 250 mg/d or 500 mg 3 times/week up to 1 y)
    – Stop ICS (esp. if PNA or side effects develop)
	1. LABA + LAMA if dyspnea and exercise intolerance
	2. If persistent symptoms and 1+ exacerbation requiring treatment in the past year: ICS + LABA + LAMA
	3. If a patient taking ICS + LABA + LAMA goes a year without an exacerbation, stop the ICS

Other suggestions: –Tiotropium improves exercise performance and increases effectiveness of pulmonary rehabilitation –Phosphodiesterase-4 inhibitors improve lung function and reduce moderate-to-severe exacerbations for patients with severe COPD	Other suggestions: –Avoid maintenance oral corticosteroids for frequent severe exacerbations –In patients with severe refractory dyspnea, consider opiates to manage the symptom
Applying to Clinical Practice • Both pathways start with a foundation of LABA + LAMA and build to therapy with LABA + LAMA + ICS. • ATS cites a study showing that the LABA + LAMA combination improved symptom scores and reduced exacerbations more than monotherapy without additional adverse effects. This is consistent with recommendations from GOLD 2023. • Triple therapy ICS/LABA/LAMA is superior in reducing exacerbations compared to ICS/LABA, LABA/LAMA, or LAMA alone (NNT 16), so escalate quickly when indicated.	

[1] See http://www.nejm.org/doi/full/10.1056/NEJMoa021322#t=article

Practice Pearls

- Available LABA + LAMA combinations include formoterol/aclidinium, formoterol/glycopyrronium, indacaterol/glycopyrronium, vilanterol/umeclidinium, and olodatreol/tiotropium.
- Available LABA + LAMA + ICS combination devices include fluticasone/umeclidinium/vilanterol, beclomethasone/formoterol/glycopyrronium, and budesonide/formoterol/glycopyrrolate.
- Confirm suspected COPD with postbronchodilator spirometry. Perform spirometry in patients with symptoms and/or risk factors.
- Repeat spirometry at least annually to assess severity in patients with COPD.
- Can consider lung volume reduction surgery in patients with severe upper lobe emphysema and low post-pulmonary rehab exercise capacity.
- Consider roflumilast, a phosphodiesterase-4 inhibitor, to reduce exacerbations for patients with severe chronic bronchitis and frequent exacerbations.

Sources

–Global Initiative for Chronic Obstructive Lung Disease. *Global Strategy for the Diagnosis, Management and Prevention of Chronic Obstructive Pulmonary Disease 2020 Report.* https://goldcopd.org/
–*Am J Respir Crit Care Med.* 2020;201(9):e56–e69.
–https://www.cdc.gov/pneumococcal/vaccination.html
–2023 Canadian Thoracic Society guideline on pharmacotherapy in patients with stable COPD. *CHEST.* 2023; 164(5):1159–1183.

COUGH, CHRONIC

Management: Adults and Children > 14 y, Cough > 8-wk Duration

Recommendations from

> ACCP 2020, ERS 2020

Evaluation

–Determine the duration of the cough as acute (<3 wk), subacute (3–8 wk), or chronic (>8 wk), as this can guide the differential diagnosis.

–Evaluate for red flag symptoms, occupational/environmental exposures, travel exposures, physical exam, and CXR.

–Consider the common causes of chronic cough with a normal CXR:
- Smoking.
- ACE inhibitor use.
- Upper airway cough syndrome (formerly known as postnasal drip syndrome).
- Asthma (classic, cough-variant, or nonasthmatic eosinophilic bronchitis).
- Gastroesophageal reflux disease.
- Nonasthmatic eosinophilic bronchitis.
- Cough hypersensitivity.

Therapies

–Oral prednisolone ×1 wk helps in classic asthma in adults, but systemic leukotriene antagonists (montelukast) are more effective in all groups.

–Consider 2–4 wk of ICS, though it may not be superior to placebo. ·

–Avoid using bronchodilators alone as maintenance treatment for cough in asthma.

–Avoid empiric therapy for gastroesophageal reflux disease if there are no peptic/esophageal symptoms.

–Diagnose "unexplained chronic cough" if lasting >8 wk without an identifiable cause after investigation and supervised therapeutic trials.

–Consider cough hypersensitivity and treat with speech therapy or cough neuromodulators: morphine 5 mg BID has strong evidence, while gabapentin and pregabalin have moderate evidence.

–Do not routinely perform chest CT scans on patients with chronic cough, normal CXR, and normal physical exam.

Practice Pearls

- If a specific etiology is not evident, it is reasonable to treat empirically for upper airway cough syndrome/postnasal drip (decongestant + first-generation antihistamine, +/− intranasal steroids, intranasal antihistamines, saline nasal rinses, nasal anticholinergics), gastroesophageal reflux disease (lifestyle modifications, H_2-blocker, baclofen), asthma (ICS) or nonasthmatic eosinophilic bronchitis (ICS).
- If no etiology is evident and empiric therapies fail to resolve the cough, consider referral to pulmonology, ENT, or further testing such as chest CT, bronchoscopy, and screening for OSA. ·
  - Red flag symptoms for cough:
    - Hemoptysis.
    - Smoker age > 45 with new cough, change in cough, or coexisting voice disturbance.
    - Adults age 55–80 with a 30 pack-year history or who have quit less than 15 y ago.
    - Dyspnea, especially at rest or at night.
    - Hoarseness.
    - Systemic symptoms: fever, weight loss, peripheral edema with weight gain.
    - Dysphagia.
    - Vomiting.

- Recurrent pneumonia.
- Abnormal physical exam or CXR.
- The quality of evidence surrounding cough suppressants is poor. None routinely outperform placebo, but placebo improves symptoms in >50% of patients in many studies. Few have serious adverse effects, but antihistamines and dextromethorphan have a higher rate of nonserious adverse effects.[1]

Sources
–*Eur Respir J.* 2020;55:1901136.
–*Chest.* 2018;153(1):196–209.
–*Am Fam Physician.* 2017;96(9):575–580.

Management: Children < 14 y, Cough > 4-wk Duration

Recommendations from

> ACCP 2020

–Evaluate cough > 4-wk for signs/symptoms such as productive cough, wheezing, recurrent infections, hemoptysis, growth failure, facial pain, dyspnea, chest pain, and digital clubbing.
–Order CXR and spirometry if >6 y.
–"Specific cough" has signs/symptoms and/or spirometry/CXR findings. Indicates underlying disorder like bronchiectasis, retained foreign body or large airway obstruction, aspiration, cardiac anomalies, cystic fibrosis, asthma, TB, and tracheomalacia.
–"Protracted bacterial bronchitis" is a chronic wet cough w/o other specific symptoms or findings on imaging/spirometry. Prescribe 2–4 wk of antibiotics following local antibiograms.
–"Nonspecific cough" is a dry cough without signs/symptoms and with normal CXR and spirometry:
  • Usually postviral cough or acute viral bronchitis.
  • Watch, wait, and review every 2–4 wk evaluating for specific signs or symptoms.
  • Discuss with parents the trial of therapy with ICS (400 mcg/d budesonide equivalent). Follow up in 2 wk; if cough resolves, may be asthma.
–Do not recommend OTC medications for symptomatic relief of cough.

Sources
–*Eur Respir J.* 2020;55:1901136.
–*Chest.* 2020;158(1):P303–P329.
–*Chest.* 2018;153(1):196–209.

Management: Adults and Children > 12 y, Chronic Cough Due to Asthma or Nonasthmatic Eosinophilic Bronchitis (NAEB)

Recommendations from

> ACCP 2020

–Use noninvasive measurement of airway inflammation. Eosinophilic airway inflammation is likely to be associated with a more favorable response to ICS.

---

[1] *Cochrane Database Syst Rev.* 2014;2014(11). https://www.ncbi.nlm.nih.gov/pmc/articles/PMC7061814/

–Use ICS as first-line therapy.

–If response to ICS is incomplete, step up the ICS dose and consider a therapeutic trial of a leukotriene inhibitor after reconsideration of alternative causes of cough.

–In cough-variant asthma (but not NAEB), consider beta-agonist in combination with ICS.

Practice Pearl

- Evidence is much greater for trial of leukotriene inhibitor in chronic cough due to asthma than NAEB due to the smaller amount of trials for NAEB.

Source
   –*Chest.* 2020;158(1):68–96.

INTERSTITIAL LUNG DISEASE (ILD)

Screening: Adults

Recommendations from

> ACR 2023

   –Screen for ILD in those with Systemic Autoimmune Rheumatic Diseases at risk for ILD, ie, rheumatoid arthritis, systemic sclerosis, idiopathic inflammatory myositis, mixed connective lung tissue disease, and Sjögren disease.

   –Screen with pulmonary function test and high-resolution computed tomography. Monitor with repeat pulmonary function test, high-resolution computed tomography intermittently, and ambulatory pulse oximetry.

Source
   –American College of Rheumatology (ACR). *Guideline for the Screening and Monitoring of Interstitial Lung Disease in People with Systemic Autoimmune Rheumatic Disease.* 2023. https://rheumatology.org/interstitial-lung-disease-guideline#2023-ild-guideline

Management: Adults

Recommendations from

> ACR 2023

   –Systemic Autoimmune Rheumatic Diseases-ILD (not systemic sclerosis-ILD): use glucocorticoids as first line, followed by mycophenalation, azathioprine, rituximab, and cyclophosphamide.

   –Systemic sclerosis-ILD and mixed connective lung tissue disease-ILD: use tocilizumab as first line.

   –Systemic sclerosis-ILD: use nintedanib as first line.

   –Idiopathic inflammatory myositis-ILD: use JAK inhibitors or calcineurin inhibitors as first line.

   –Optimize medical management prior to referral for stem cell or lung transplant.

Source
   –American College of Rheumatology (ACR). *Guideline for the Screening and Monitoring of Interstitial Lung Disease in People with Systemic Autoimmune Rheumatic Disease.* 2023. https://rheumatology.org/interstitial-lung-disease-guideline#2023-ild-guideline

LUNG CANCER

Screening: Adults

Recommendations from

> USPSTF 2021, ACCP 2021, NCCN 2020, ACR 2022, ACS 2023

–For patients aged 50–80 with ≥20 pack-year smoking history, screen for lung cancer annually with low-dose chest CT (USPSTF) or CT chest without IV contrast (ACR) after discussion of benefits, limitations, and harms of lung cancer screening.

–Time since quitting has been removed as criterion.

–Use the Tammemagi lung cancer risk calculator[1] when weighing risk factors other than smoking history. Screen those with >1.3% 6-y risk. (NCCN)

–Stop screening if a significant medical problem develops that would limit ability to receive treatment for an early-stage lung cancer or a life expectancy < 5 y.

–Do not screen routinely with CXR and/or sputum cytology.

–Only screen if a highly skilled support team is available to evaluate CT scans, schedule appropriate follow-up, and perform lung biopsies safely when indicated.

Practice Pearls

- Risk assessment for lung cancer:
  - Cigarette smoking (20-fold increased risk). Medication and counseling together are better than either alone to increase cessation rates.
  - Second-hand smoke exposure, according to NCCN, is not a sufficient risk factor for lung cancer to warrant a screening recommendation with LDCT. It is a highly variable exposure risk. However, it should be considered in conjunction with other risk factors.
  - Family history of lung cancer in first-degree relatives.
  - Pulmonary disease history (COPD or pulmonary fibrosis).
  - Documented radon gas exposure (can be measured in the home), severe air pollution. Air pollution increases risk of lung cancer by 40% with highest pollution exposure. (*Am J Respir Crit Care Med*. 2006;173:667)
  - Occupational exposures (silica, asbestos, arsenic, nickel, chromium, coal smoke, soot, diesel fumes).
- If a pulmonary nodule is found on LDCT, the characterization of the nodule—solid, part-solid, nonsolid, multiple nonsolid—will determine what size nodule screens positive. NCCN guidelines discuss appropriate follow-up imaging, procedures, and referrals.
- If coronary arterial calcification is detected on chest CT, its presence may be a marker of atherosclerosis. Further evaluation is recommended if it is reported as severe. (*J Am Coll Radiol*. 2018;15:1087–1096)
- Reducing overall risk:
  - Smokers who quit gain 13% reduction in risk of all-cause mortality and 21% reduction in risk of lung cancer mortality in first 5 y. The excess risk decreases to that of a

[1] https://brocku.ca/lung-cancer-screening-and-risk-prediction/risk-calculators/

never-smoker ~20 y after quitting on average; however, for lung cancer it takes ~30 y. (*JAMA. 2008;299(17):2037–2047*)

- No evidence that vitamin E, tocopherol, retinoids, vitamin C, or beta-carotene in any dose reduces the risk of lung cancer. (*Ann Intern Med.* 2013;159:824)
- Minimize indoor exposure to radon (can be measured in home), especially if smoker. Avoid occupational exposures (asbestos, arsenic, nickel, chromium, beryllium, and cadmium).

Sources

–https://www.uspreventiveservicestaskforce.org/Page/Document/Update SummaryFinal/lung-cancer-screening

–*J Natl Compr Canc Netw.* 2018;16:412–441.

–https://www.cancer.org/health-care-professionals/american-cancer-society-prevention-early-detection-guidelines/lung-cancer-screening-guidelines.html

–*Chest.* 2018;153(4):954–985. https://www.ncbi.nlm.nih.gov/pubmed/29374513

–*National Comprehensive Cancer Network Guidelines Version 1.2020*, Lung Cancer Screening. https://www.nccn.org/professionals/physician_gls/

–*PLOS Med.* 2014;11:1–13.

–https://acsearch.acr.org/docs/3102390/Narrative

–Screening for lung cancer: 2023 guideline update from the American Cancer Society. *CA Cancer J Clin.* 2024;74:50–81.

OBESITY HYPOVENTILATION SYNDROME

Management: Adults

Recommendations from

> ATS 2019

Evaluation

–Diagnose obesity hypoventilation syndrome (OHS) in the setting of:
- BMI > 30.
- Sleep-disordered breathing.
- Awake daytime hypercapnia, awake resting $PaCO_2$ > 45 mmHg at sea level.

–In high pretest probability of OHS, screen with $PaCO_2$.

–In low-to-moderate probability of OHS (BMI 30–40 with sleep-disordered breathing), a serum bicarbonate level < 27 mmol/L can rule out OHS. If ≥27, screen with a $PaCO_2$.

–Follow up elevated $PaCO_2$ with both a sleep study (polysomnography or respiratory polygraph) and awake ABG.

Therapies

–Use CPAP, regardless of concomitant OSA.

–If CPAP is inadequate, change to noninvasive ventilation.

–If hospitalized adults are suspected to have OHS w/o prior formal sleep study diagnosis, discharge on noninvasive ventilation and refer to sleep laboratory within 3 mo after hospital discharge due to high-risk short-term mortality w/o therapy.

–Pursue weight-loss interventions that produce sustained 25%–30% weight loss of actual body weight. This is the level of weight loss that may be required to resolve hypoventilation.

–Even multifaceted weight-loss lifestyle programs may not produce these results.

–If patient has no contraindications, evaluate for bariatric surgery.

Practice Pearl

- Of obese patients referred to sleep centers for OSA or sleep-disordered breathing, 8%–20% are diagnosed with OHS. Ninety percent of OHS patients have coexistent OSA, and 70% of total OHS patients have severe OSA. The other 10% have nonobstructive, sleep-dependent hypoventilation.

Source
–*Am J Resp Crit Care Med.* 2019;200(3):e6–e24.

OBSTRUCTIVE SLEEP APNEA (OSA)

Screening: Adults

Recommendations from

> USPSTF 2022, AAFP 2017

–Insufficient evidence to recommend for or against routine screening in the general adult population.

–Test for OSA in conjunction with a comprehensive sleep evaluation such as STOP-BANG or Epworth Sleepiness Scale.

–Diagnose OSA when apnea-hypopnea index is ≥5 events/h. Severe OSA is apnea-hypopnea index ≥ 30 events/h.

–Use a polysomnogram or home sleep apnea testing to diagnose OSA in uncomplicated adult patients presenting with signs and symptoms that indicate risk of OSA.

–Use a polysomnogram, rather than home sleep apnea testing, to diagnose OSA in patients with significant cardiorespiratory disease, potential respiratory muscle weakness due to neuromuscular condition, awake hypoventilation or suspicion of sleep-related hypoventilation, chronic opioid medication use, and history of stroke or severe insomnia.

–If a single home sleep apnea testing is negative, inconclusive, or technically inadequate, a polysomnogram be performed for the diagnosis or exclusion of OSA.

Practice Pearls

- This applies to adults 18 y or older who do not have signs or symptoms of OSA, those with unrecognized symptoms of OSA, or those who do not report their symptoms as a concern.
- This does not apply to patients who have symptoms or concerns about OSA, or those with conditions that can trigger the development of OSA such as stroke.
- Current screening questionnaires have been developed mostly on populations with higher prevalence of OSA and are not adequately validated in general populations.

Sources

–USPSTF. *JAMA.* 2022;328(19):1945–1950.

–*Am Fam Phys.* 2017;96(2):122A–122C.

Management: Adults

Recommendations from

➤ AASM 2017, 2019

Therapies

–Treat OSA with positive airway pressure (PAP), either continuous (CPAP) or autoadjusting. (APAP)

–Choose CPAP and APAP rather than bi-level PAP (BPAP) because BPAP is more costly and does not prevent obstructive breathing events at low expiratory pressure levels. Patients with a PAP requirement over 20 cm H_2O will require BPAP because of the limitation of settings on CPAP.

–Alternatives to PAP include weight loss, positional therapy, oral appliance therapy, surgical management of anatomical nasal obstruction, or maxillomandibular advancement.

–To improve adherence, choose nasal or intranasal mask interface rather than oronasal or oral, use heated humidification (reduces sleepiness, dry mouth/throat/nose, nasal congestion, hoarseness, headache, epistaxis), and offer educational, behavioral, and other troubleshooting interventions particularly in the setting of PTSD/anxiety.

Practice Pearls

- Excessive daytime sleepiness: PAP, when compared to no treatment, shows significant improvement in sleepiness.
- Impaired sleep: mixed data that PAP will alleviate this symptom.
- HTN: PAP therapy causes a clinically significant BP reduction. But, if PAP is burdensome to sleep cycle, patients without sleep symptoms may be treated with standard anti-HTN treatment in lieu of PAP.
- CV events/mortality: insufficient evidence to recommend PAP as a means to reduce CV events or CV mortality.

Sources

–*J Clin Sleep Med.* 2019;15(2):335–343.

–VA/DoD. *CPG for the Management of Chronic Insomnia Disorder and Obstructive Sleep Apnea,* Version 1.0-2019.

–USPSTF. *JAMA.* 2022;328(19):1945–1950.

–*Am Fam Phys.* 2017;96(2):122A–122C.

PLEURAL EFFUSION

Management: Adults, Nonmalignant

Recommendations from

> BTS 2010; ACR 2023

–Initial imaging: CXR or CT with IV contrast is preferred, with consideration for chest ultrasound or CT without IV contract in patients with suspected parapneumonic effusion or empyema or minor blunt trauma with suspected effusion or dyspnea, cough, or chest pain with suspected effusion.

–Use ultrasound or a posteroanterior CXR to detect a pleural effusion. Consider a lateral decubitus CXR to differentiate pleural liquid from pleural thickening.

–CT scans detect very small effusions (<10 mL of fluid). Use CT scan to evaluate undiagnosed exudative pleural effusions prior to complete pleural fluid drainage. Obtain CT scan in the setting of pleural infection which has not responded to initial chest tube drainage.

–Thoracic ultrasound is more sensitive than CT scan to distinguish loculations.

–Perform thoracentesis for any undiagnosed effusions of >1 cm from the chest wall on lateral decubitus CXR. Do not perform thoracentesis on bilateral pleural effusions in a setting which is strongly suggestive of a transudative process, unless there are atypical features or a failure to respond to therapy. In patients with advanced cancer, do not perform thoracentesis for small effusions.

–Perform diagnostic thoracentesis for all patients with a pleural effusion in the setting of sepsis or pneumonic illness.

–During thoracentesis, bedside ultrasound guidance improves the likelihood of successful aspiration and reduces risk of organ puncture.

–Send pleural fluid for cell count and differential, Gram stain and culture, protein, lactate dehydrogenase, and cytology. A minimum of 50–60 mL of pleural fluid should be withdrawn for analysis. Assess pleural fluid pH in nonpurulent effusions when pleural infection is suspected. Check pleural fluid glucose when pleural fluid pH is not available and pleural infection is suspected.

–Involve a chest physician or thoracic surgeon in the care of all patients who require chest tube drainage for pleural infection.

Sources

–*BTS Pleural Disease Guideline.* 2010.

–*Thorax.* 2010;65(suppl 2):ii1–76.

–American College of Radiology. *Workup of Pleural Effusion or Pleural Disease.* 2023. https://acsearch.acr.org/docs/3158179/Narrative

Management: Adults, Malignant Etiology

Recommendations from

> BTS 2010, ACCP 2014

Evaluation

–If MPE is suspected, send pleural fluid for cytology (minimum 50 mL; ideally 200 mL to allow for cell block and molecular testing).

–Refer all patients with MPE to pulmonologist and/or thoracic surgeon for treatment options.

Therapies

–Asymptomatic patients require frequent follow-up but no treatment.

–Treat symptomatic patients initially with therapeutic thoracentesis (1000–1500 mL) to relieve symptoms.

–Consider recurrent outpatient therapeutic thoracentesis for patients with expected survival less than 1 mo and/or poor performance status and/or slow reaccumulation of the pleural effusion (ie, >1 mo).

–Otherwise, pursue definitive intervention after first or second thoracentesis. Choice of therapy depends on projected survival and availability of resources. Individualize management and present to a multidisciplinary Tumor Board for advice. (*JAMA*. 2012;307:2432)

–Treatment options:

- Indwelling (tunneled) pleural catheter (considered for patients with trapped lung who experience some relief following thoracentesis): for patients who want to avoid hospitalization or discomfort of pleurodesis.

- Talc pleurodesis (Talc poudrage) via thoracoscopy: consider for patients with longer projected survival and those who don't want an indwelling catheter. Contraindicated for patients with trapped lung.

- Talc pleurodesis (slurry) via chest tube: consider for patients with longer projected survival or contraindication to thoracoscopy. Contraindicated for patients with trapped lung.

- Consider chemotherapy as an adjunct treatment option. Patients undergoing first-line systemic therapy for tumors with high response rates (small-cell lung cancer and lymphoma) may avoid definitive treatments.

Practice Pearl

- Indwelling pleural catheter (IPC-pleurX catheter) requires a regular outpatient drainage schedule. Address potential burden for the patient or caregiver. Complications from IPCs are uncommon. The infection rate is 5%, with more than half the patients responding to antibiotics without removing the catheter (*Chest*. 2013;144:1597). Other problems with IPCs include pneumothorax (5.9%), cellulitis (3.4%), obstruction/clogging (3.7%), and unspecified catheter malfunction (9.1%). The most common adverse events with talc pleurodesis include fever, pain, and GI symptoms. Less common are cardiac arrhythmia, dyspnea, systemic inflammatory response, empyema, and talc dissemination.

Sources

–https://www.guideline.gov/summaries/summary/49355/management-of-malignant-pleural-effusion

–*Chest*. 2012;142:394.

–*Chest*. 2013;143(5):e4555–e4975.

–*J Natl Compr Canc Netw*. 2012;10:975.

–*Thoracic Society Pleural Disease Guideline*. 2010.

–*Thorax*. 2010;65(suppl 2):132.

PNEUMOTHORAX, SPONTANEOUS

Management: Adults

Recommendations from

> BTS 2010

–Use standard standing CXR for the initial diagnosis; expiratory films are not necessary. Reserve CT scan for uncertain or complex cases.

–Tension pneumothorax is a medical emergency. Suspect in the setting of respiratory distress or hypotension. Treat with oxygen supplementation and needle decompression.

–Symptoms including dyspnea are more important than the size of pneumothorax in determining the management strategy.

–If the patient has spontaneous[1] pneumothorax size <2 cm and minimal symptoms, consider discharge with outpatient follow-up and return precautions.

–If the patient has significant dyspnea or pneumothorax size >2 cm, recommend needle aspiration with 16–18 G needle. If pneumothorax is then >2 cm and symptoms improved, consider discharge with outpatient follow-up. For pneumothorax <2 cm with minimal symptoms, consider conservative management/observation. If after needle aspiration, the patient is still symptomatic, or size still <2 cm, recommend chest drain size 8–14 Fr and admission.

–Use needle aspiration and small-bore chest drains (<20 Fr) rather than large-bore chest drains for reduced hospitalization and length of stay.

–If there is a persistent air leak at 48 h, consult with chest physician.

–Smoking cessation counseling is recommended to prevent recurrence.

Practice Pearl

• Ultrasound with attention to pleural interface for lung sliding (seashore sign on M-mode) is highly sensitive for pneumothorax. While the guidelines are yet to be updated, ultrasound has proven more sensitive than CXR for pneumothorax. (*Acad Emerg Med.* 2010;17(1):11–17) (*Am J Emerg Med.* 2019. https://doi.org/10.1016/j.ajem.2019.02.028)

Sources

–*Thoracic Society Pleural Disease Guideline.* 2010.
–*Thorax.* 2010;65(suppl 2):ii18–31.
–*Acad Emerg Med.* 2010;17(1):11–17.

---

[1] These recommendations do not apply for secondary pneumothorax, or pneumothorax in the setting of underlying lung disease. For patients with underlying lung disease, admit at a minimum for observation and oxygen, even if not actively managed.

PULMONARY HYPERTENSION

Management: Adults

Recommendations from

> ACCP 2019

Evaluation

–Refer all patients with pulmonary arterial hypertension (PAH) to a center with expertise in diagnosis before therapy is started.

–Evaluate severity consistently. WHO Functional Classification for PAH has ranking I–IV based on progression of symptoms of dyspnea, fatigue, and weakness on exertion and not on exertion. Evolution of symptoms includes lower extremity edema, angina, or syncope which would indicate right heart dysfunction/failure.

Therapies

–Treat contributing causes such as sleep apnea and systemic hypertension aggressively.

–Arrange a supervised exercise activity.

–Keep patient up-to-date on influenza and pneumococcal PNA immunization schedules.

–Avoid pregnancy and nonessential surgery in PAH. When these do occur, refer to a multidisciplinary PAH center.

–Avoid exposure to high altitude. Supplemental oxygen may be needed to keep O_2 saturation > 91% in air travel.

–Incorporate palliative care services.

–If acute vasoreactivity testing is positive, start calcium channel blockers unless contraindicated (ie, right heart failure).

–Otherwise, use combination therapy (ambrisentan + tadalafil) or monotherapy (bosentan, macitentan, ambrisentan, riociguat, sildenafil, or tadalafil).

–If rapid disease progression or poor prognosis, initiate parenteral prostanoids such as IV epoprostenol, IV treprostinil, or SC treprostinil. If parenteral prostanoids are not tolerated, the patient can take inhaled prostanoids with oral PDE-5 inhibitors and oral endothelin receptor antagonists. The patient can take up to 3 classes of PAH pharmacotherapy until consideration for lung transplant.

Source

–*Chest*. 2019;15(3):565–586.

PULMONARY NODULES

Management: Adults

Recommendations from

> Fleischner Society 2017, ACR 2023

–Adult ≥ 35 y, incidental nodule on CXR, perform chest CT without IV contrast.

–Adult ≥ 35 y, incidental nodule on < 6 mm on chest CT. No further acute testing.

–Adult ≥ 35 y, incidental nodule on ≥6 mm on chest CT. Plan for repeat chest CT without IV contract or FDG-PET/CT while body scan.

–Adult ≥ 35 y, incidental nodule not fully captured on thoracic CT, perform chest CT without IV contrast.

–Categorize nodules by size, solid or subsolid, single or multiple, low or high[1] risk.

–See Fig. 12–2 for management algorithm.

–Do not follow up solid nodules 6 mm or less in diameter in low-risk adults >35-y-old, even if multiple nodules are present.

–Use the Brock model[2] for initial risk assessment of pulmonary nodules larger than 8 mm in patients who have ever smoked.

–Do not follow up diffuse, central, or laminated pattern of calcification or fat.

FIG. 12–2 FLEISCHNER SOCIETY 2017 GUIDELINES FOR MANAGEMENT OF INCIDENTALLY DETECTED PULMONARY NODULES IN ADULTS.

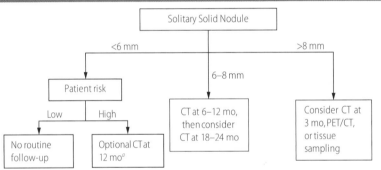

a Certain patients at high risk with suspicious nodule morphology, upper lobe location or both may warrant 12 mo f/u.

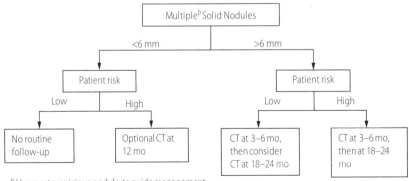

b Use most suspicious nodule to guide management.

[1] These guidelines do not apply to immunocompromised patients, patients with cancer, or for lung cancer screening.
[2] An online calculator is available at https://www.uptodate.com/contents/calculator-solitary-pulmonary-nodule-malignancy-risk-in-adults-brock-university-cancer-prediction-equation

FIG. 12-2 (*continued*)

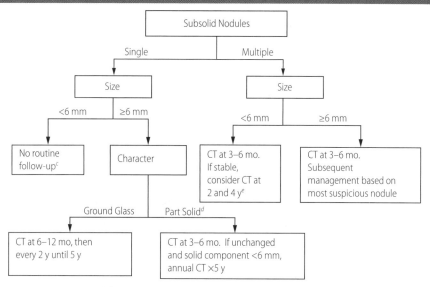

[c] In certain suspicious nodules <6 mm, consider follow-up at 2 and 4 y. If solid component(s) or growth develops, consider resection (recommendations 3A and 4A).

[d] In practice, part-solid nodules cannot be defined as such until >6 mm, and nodules <6 mm do not usually require follow-up. Persistent part-solid nodules with solid components >6 mm should be considered highly suspicious (recommendations 4A–4C).

[e] Multiple <6 mm pure ground-glass nodules are usually benign, but consider follow-up in selected patients at high risk at 2 and 4 y (recommendation 5A).

Note: These recommendations do not apply to lung cancer screening, patients with immunosuppression, or patients with known primary cancer.

–Consider a PET-CT scan for patients with a pulmonary nodule and an initial risk of malignancy > 5%.

–Suggestions for pulmonary nodules management:

- Serial CT scans when the malignancy risk is <5%.
- CT-guided biopsy when the risk of malignancy is 5%–65%.
- Video-assisted thoracoscopic surgery when the chance of malignancy exceeds 65%.
- Consider bronchoscopy when a bronchus sign is present on CT scan.

Sources

–*Radiology.* 2017;284:228–243.

–American College of Radiology. *Incidentally Detected Indeterminate Pulmonary Nodule.* 2023. https://acsearch.acr.org/docs/69455/Narrative

SUDDEN INFANT DEATH SYNDROME

Prevention: Infants

Recommendations from

> AAP 2016

–Place infants on their backs to sleep.
–Use a firm sleep surface without soft objects or loose bedding.
–Breastfeed.
–For the first 6–12 mo, infants should sleep in parents' room (but not in parents' bed).
–Avoid smoke exposure, alcohol and illicit drug use, overheating.

Practice Pearls

- Stomach and side sleeping have been identified as major risk factors for sudden infant death syndrome.
- Pacifiers may be protective.

Source
–*Pediatrics*. 2016;138(5):e20162938.

RENAL DISORDERS

KIDNEY INJURY, ACUTE (AKI)

Prevention: Adults, Acute Illness

Recommendations from

> NICE 2023, VA/DoD 2019, KDIGO 2012

–General care of the acutely ill patient.

- In the absence of hemorrhagic shock, use isotonic crystalloids rather than colloids for intravascular volume expansion.
- Do not use diuretics to prevent or treat AKI except in the management of volume overload.
- Do not use low-dose dopamine in either the prevention or treatment of AKI.
- Use vasopressors in addition to fluids for management of vasomotor shock with or at risk for AKI. Avoid the combination of ACE/ARB, diuretics, and nonsteroidal anti-inflammatory drugs. This combination is more likely to cause AKI, especially in those >75 y of age and with preexisting renal impairment.

Practice Pearls

- AKI is defined as any of the following:
  - The increase in SCr by ≥0.3 mg/dL over 48 h.
  - Increase in SCr to ≥1.5 times baseline within the past 7 d.
  - Urine volume < 0.5 mL/kg/h for 6 h.
- Stages of AKI and corresponding lab values (Table 13–1).

TABLE 13–1 STAGES OF ACUTE KIDNEY INJURY			
	Stage 1	**Stage 2**	**Stage 3**
Creatinine increase over 48 h	0.3 mg/dL or 1.5–2 × above baseline	2–3 × baseline	3 × baseline, or Cr > 4.0 mg/dL with acute rise of 0.5 mg/dL
Urine output: less than 0.5 mg/kg/h for at least	6 h	12 h	24 h (or, anuria > 12 h)
Adapted from KDIGO 2012, Table 3.			

Sources

- –NICE. *Acute Kidney Injury: Prevention, Detection and Management.* London, UK: National Institute for Health and Care Excellence (NICE); 2023. https://www.nice.org.uk/guidance/ng148
- –VA/DoD. *Clinical Practice Guideline for the Management of Chronic Kidney Disease in Primary Care.* Washington, DC: Department of Veterans Affairs, Department of Defense; 2019.
- –Kidney Disease Improving Global Outcomes (KDIGO). *KDIGO Clinical Practice Guideline for Acute Kidney Injury: Kidney International Supplements.* 2012;2(1).

Prevention: Adults Receiving Intravenous Iodine-Based Contrast

Recommendations from

> NICE 2023, VA/DoD 2019, KDIGO 2012

- –Encourage oral hydration before and after contrast administration if increased risk[1] of kidney injury.
- –Consider temporarily stopping ACE inhibitors and ARBs if eGFR < 40 mL/min/1.73 m^2.
- –For patients receiving renal replacement therapy, involve the nephrologist before administering contrast.
- –Measure estimated GFR prior to contrast only in patients at increased risk for kidney injury.
- –Consider IV volume expansion to at-risk adults, including those with:
  - Chronic kidney disease (CKD) with eGFR < 30 mL/min/1.73 m^2.
  - Heart failure.
  - Age 75 y or older.
  - History of renal transplant.
  - Use of a large volume of contrast medium.
  - Intra-arterial administration of contrast medium with first-pass renal exposure.
  - Consider temporarily stopping ACE inhibitors and ARBs in adults having iodine-based contrast media if they have CKD with an eGFR < 40 mL/min/1.73 m^2.
  - Inconsistent evidence for N-acetylcysteine use to prevent contrast-induced nephropathy.
- –Consult a pharmacist to assist with drug dosing in adults or children at risk for AKI.

Sources

- –NICE. *Acute Kidney Injury: Prevention, Detection and Management of Acute Kidney Injury up to the Point of Renal Replacement Therapy.* London, UK: National Institute for Health and Care Excellence (NICE); 2013. https://www.nice.org.uk/guidance/ng148
- –VA/DoD. *Clinical Practice Guideline for the Management of Chronic Kidney Disease in Primary Care.* Washington, DC: Department of Veterans Affairs, Department of Defense; 2019.
- –Kidney Disease Improving Global Outcomes (KDIGO). *KDIGO Clinical Practice Guideline for Acute Kidney Injury: Kidney International Supplements.* 2012;2(1).

---

[1] High risk features include eGFR < 30 mL/min/1.73 m^2, history of renal transplant, large volume of contrast material, or intra-arterial administration of contrast medium with first-pass renal exposure.

Management: Children and Adults with AKI

Recommendations from

> NICE 2013, 2019

–Perform a urinalysis in all patients with AKI. Consider checking urine electrolytes (ie, urine sodium, urine creatinine, urine urea, and urine osmolarity) to calculate a FENa or FEUrea.

–Do not routinely obtain a renal ultrasound when the cause of the AKI has been identified.

–Detect AKI with any of the following criteria:

- Rise in serum creatinine ≥ 0.3 mg/dL in 48 h.
- Fifty percent or more rise in creatinine in the last 7 d.
- Urine output < 0.5 mL/kg/h.

–Refer for renal replacement therapy patients with any of the following refractory to medical management:

- Hyperkalemia.
- Metabolic acidosis.
- Uremia.
- Fluid overload.

Sources

–https://doi.org/10.1016/0002-9343(84)90368-1

–https://www.nice.org.uk/guidance/ng148

KIDNEY DISEASE, CHRONIC (CKD)

Screening: Adults

Recommendations from

> USPSTF 2012, ACP 2013, AAFP 2014, NICE 20121, VA/DoD 2019, KDIGO 2024

Guidelines Alert 13–1	
GUIDELINES DISCORDANT: WHO TO SCREEN FOR CKD	
Organization	**Guidance**
USPSTF	Insufficient evidence to recommend for or against routine screening
ACP, AAFP, NICE, KDIGO, VA/DoD	Evaluate patients who are at risk[a] with assessment of GFR and urine albumin.

Applying to Clinical Practice

- Most society guidelines find reason to screen certain higher-risk populations, especially those with DM or HTN.
- USPSTF notes that more study is needed to show that universal screening for CKD improves clinical outcomes and notes the potential for adverse effects from medications used to treat early CKD.

[a]Risk factors vary by organization, but generally include DM, HTN, CVD, structural renal disease, nephrolithiasis, benign prostatic hyperplasia (BPH), multisystem diseases with potential kidney involvement (eg, systemic lupus erythematosus [SLE]), family history of Stage 5 CKD or hereditary kidney disease, or personal history of hematuria or proteinuria, age > 60 y.

Practice Pearls

- Diagnose CKD if either of the following present for >3 mo:
  - Markers of kidney damage such as albuminuria > 30 mg/g, urinary sediment abnormalities, electrolyte abnormalities due to tubular disorders, histologic abnormalities, structural abnormalities by imaging, or kidney transplantation.
  - GFR < 60 mL/min/1.73 m^2.
- Monitor GFR at least annually in people who are prescribed drugs known to be nephrotoxic.[1]
- Do not test for proteinuria in adults taking an ACE inhibitor or ARB, regardless of diabetes status.

Sources

–USPSTF. *Chronic Kidney Disease (CKD): Screening.* 2012.

–AAFP. *Clinical Recommendations: Chronic Kidney Disease.* 2014.

–*Ann Intern Med.* 2013;159(12):835.

–NICE. https://www.nice.org.uk/guidance/ng203

–*Kidney Int.* 2024;105(suppl 4S):S117–S314.

Management: Adults

Recommendations from

> KDIGO 2021, NKF-KDOQI 2014, NICE 2021, VA/DoD 2019

Evaluation

–Establish CKD stage by eGFR and presence of albuminuria with abnormalities being present for at least 3 mo. In patients with a new finding of eGFR of <60 mL/min/1.73 m^2, repeat the study in 2 wk to confirm this finding.

–Establish etiology. Refer to urology or nephrology if appropriate.[2]

- Etiology: assign probable cause of CKD based on absence or presence of systemic disease and the location within the kidney of observed or presumed pathologic-anatomic abnormalities.
- GFR category[3]:
  - G1: GFR > 90 (mL/min/1.73 m^2).
  - G2: GFR 60–89.
  - G3a: GFR 45–59.
  - G3b: GFR 30–44.
  - G4: GFR 15–29.
  - G5: GFR < 15.

---

[1] Examples: calcineurin inhibitors, lithium, or nonsteroidal anti-inflammatory drugs.

[2] Possible indications for urology consultation: isolated or gross hematuria, renal masses or complex cysts, symptomatic or obstructing nephrolithiasis, hydronephrosis or bladder abnormalities, urinary symptoms.

Possible indications for nephrology consultation: eGFR < 30 mL/min/1.73 m^2, decline in eGFR > 5 mL/min/1.73 m^2 per year, non-DM with heavy proteinuria or hematuria, unclear cause of CKD, complications of CKD (anemia, acidosis, hyperphosphatemia, hyperparathyroidism, electrolyte abnormalities), DM with heavy proteinuria or hematuria, management of nephrolithiasis, autosomal dominant polycystic kidney disease.

[3] Use serum creatinine-based eGFR for initial assessment. If eGFR < 60 mL/min/1.73 m^2, consider 1 time serum cystatin C-based eGFR to confirm diagnosis and refine staging of CKD.

- Albuminuria category by urine albumin-to-creatinine ratio (ACR): (ACR is recommended over protein-to-creatinine ratio (PCR) because of its sensitivity for low levels of proteinuria).
  - A1: ACR < 3 (mg/mmol).
  - A2: ACR 3–30.
  - A3: ACR > 30.

−Evaluate for chronicity.

- In those with GFR < 60 mL/min/1.73 m^2 (GFR categories G3a–5), evaluate history of prior indicators for kidney disease and prior measurements.
- If duration is >3 mo, then CKD is confirmed. If not >3 mo, CKD is not confirmed or is unclear.

Therapies

−Treat the underlying cause of the CKD.

−Control BP and individualize BP targets based on age, coexisting comorbidities, presence of retinopathy, and tolerance of treatment. *See Ch 2: Cardiovascular Disorders – Hypertension for discussion of BP targets.*

−Use ACE-I or ARB in these scenarios:

- GFR ≥ 15, ACR > 30 (consider down to ACR > 3).
- GFR ≥ 15, ACR > 3, DM2.

−Do not combine ACE-I and ARB.

−Use SGLT2i in patients with CKD, eGFR ≥ 20 mL/min/1.73 m^2, and any of the following (KDIGO):

- DM2.
- ACR ≥ 200 mg/g.
- Heart failure.
- Consider: eGFR 20–45 mL/min/1.73 m^2 and ACR < 200 mg/g.

−Lower protein intake to 0.8 g/kg/d in adults with diabetes and nondiabetics with GFR categories G3–5.

−Recommend salt intake of <2 g/d.

−Supplement bicarbonate in CKD with metabolic acidosis.

−Give oral iron therapy every other day for Stage 3 or worse CKD with anemia.

−Use erythropoietic-stimulating agents only if hemoglobin < 10 g/dL.

−Refer to nephrology for consideration of renal replacement therapy after shared decision-making if 5-y risk of RRT is >5%, if ACR > 70, or on >4 antihypertensives. (NICE)

−Use caution with nephrotoxic medications, including over-the-counter medicines and herbal remedies.

−Recommend immunizations for influenza, Tdap, 13-valent pneumococcal conjugate vaccine, hepatitis B virus, zoster, and MMR.

Surveillance

−Monitor for CKD progression with annual GFR and ACR. Assess more frequently if there is higher risk for progression based on GFR and ACR.

−Monitor for complications in CKD Stage 3a–5 with hemoglobin, electrolytes, calcium, phosphate, intact parathyroid hormone, and 25-OH vitamin D.

Practice Pearls

- Recommendation for low protein (0.6–0.8 g/kg/d) diet: if offered to CKD Stage 3 and 4 patients, it may slow progression to ESRD, but also may be associated with risk of calorie malnutrition; thus, multidisciplinary support is recommended with use (VA/DoD). Alternate committees recommend to not offer low-protein diets (dietary protein intake less than 0.6–0.8 g/kg/d). (NICE)
- eGFR calculators that incorporate race are based on flawed data and may exacerbate health inequities. Use caution when adjusting eGFR calculations based on race. (*N Engl J Med*. 2020;383(9):874–882)

Sources

- –https://www.ajkd.org/article/S0272-6386(14)00491-0/pdf
- –*Kidney Int*. 2020;98:S1–S115.
- –*Kidney Int*. 2021;99:S1–S87.
- –NICE. Chronic kidney disease: assessment and management. *NICE Guideline*. 2021. www.nice.org.uk/guidance/ng203
- –VA/DoD. *VA/DoD Clinical Practice Guideline for the Management of Chronic Kidney Disease*. 2019. https://www.healthquality.va.gov/guidelines/CD/ckd/VADoDCKDCPGProviderSummaryFinal5082142020.pdf
- –*Kidney Int*. 2024;105(suppl 4S):S117–S314.

Management: Adults and Children, CKD-Related Mineral or Bone Disorders

Recommendations from

➤ **KDIGO 2017**

- –Monitor serum calcium, phosphorus, immunoreactive parathyroid hormone, and alkaline phosphatase levels:
  - Beginning with Stage G3a CKD (adults).
  - Beginning with Stage G2 CKD (children).
- –Measure 25-OH vitamin D levels beginning in Stage G3a CKD.
- –Treat all vitamin D deficiency with vitamin D supplementation with standard recommended dosing. Decisions to treat should be based on trends of vitamin D levels, not a single level.
- –In Stages G3–5 CKD, consider a bone biopsy before bisphosphonate therapy if a dynamic bone disease is a possibility.
- –In Stages G3–5 CKD, aim to normalize calcium and phosphorus levels.
- –In Stage G5 CKD, seek to maintain a PTH level of approximately 2–9 times the upper normal limit for the assay.

Practice Pearl

- Options for oral phosphate binders:
  - Calcium acetate.
  - Calcium carbonate.
  - Calcium citrate.
  - Sevelamer carbonate.
  - Lanthanum carbonate.

Source

–https://kdigo.org/wp-content/uploads/2017/02/KDIGO_CKD_MBD_Guideline_r6.pdf

NEPHROLITHIASIS

Management: Adults

Recommendations from

➤ AUA 2019, EAU 2024

Evaluation

–At time of diagnosis, take a detailed medical and dietary history (intake of fluid, protein, calcium, sodium, high oxalate-containing foods, fruits/vegetables, and over-the-counter supplements).

–Lab analysis to include electrolytes, calcium, creatinine, uric acid, and urinalysis with microscopy.

–If primary hyperparathyroidism is suspected, obtain intact parathyroid hormone level.

–Where available, obtain a stone analysis at least once.

–Obtain imaging studies to quantify stone burden. Choose CT urogram for initial diagnosis of acute flank pain. See Table 13–2 for recommendation on selection of imaging studies.

–In patients with recurrent stones, obtain metabolic testing: 24-h urine for total volume, pH, calcium, oxalate, uric acid, citrate, sodium, potassium, and creatinine.

Therapies

–Advise dietary approaches per Table 13–3.

–Offer medications to prevent recurrence per Table 13–4.

Surveillance

–Obtain 24-h urine for stone risk factors within 6 mo of initiation of therapy, then at least annually.

Sources

–*J Urol.* 192(2):316–324. https://doi.org/10.1016/j.juro.2014.05.006

–https://uroweb.org/guidelines/urolithiasis/

TABLE 13–2 SELECTION OF IMAGING STUDIES FOR KIDNEY STONE DISEASE	
Clinical Scenario	**Most Appropriate Imaging Modality**
Acute flank pain suspicious for stone disease	CT abdomen and pelvis without IV contrast
Acute flank pain suspicious for stone disease; pregnant patient	Ultrasound of kidneys and bladder
Acute flank pain, suspicious for stone disease, inconclusive CT scan	Consider MR urogram, CT with IV contrast, or CT urogram with and without IV contrast
Source: American College of Radiology. *ACR Appropriateness Criteria.* https://acsearch.acr.org/docs/69362/Narrative/	

TABLE 13–3 DIETARY INTERVENTIONS FOR KIDNEY STONES

Clinical Scenario	Intervention
All with stones	Advise fluid intake to achieve ≥2.5 L urine output daily
High urinary calcium	Limit sodium intake Consume 1000–1200 mg/d of dietary calcium
Calcium oxalate stones, relatively high urinary oxalate	Limit oxalate-rich foods[a] Maintain normal calcium consumption
Calcium stones, relatively low urinary citrate	Increase intake of fruits and vegetables Limit nondairy animal protein
Uric acid or calcium stones, relatively high urinary uric acid	Limit nondairy animal protein
Cystine stones	Limit sodium and protein

[a]Examples of oxalate-rich foods: vegetables: spinach, beet greens, rhubarb, Swiss chard, okra; nuts and seeds: almonds, cashews, peanuts, sesame seeds; grains: wheat bran, buckwheat, quinoa; fruits: raspberries, figs; legumes: soybeans and soy products, navy beans; other foods: cocoa powder, dark chocolate, tea (black and green), sweet potatoes.
Source: AUA 2019

TABLE 13–4 MEDICATION INTERVENTIONS FOR KIDNEY STONES

Clinical Scenario	Intervention
Recurrent calcium stones, high urine calcium	Thiazide diuretics (hydrochlorothiazide 50 mg/d or chlorthalidone 25 mg/d)
Recurrent calcium stones, low urine citrate	Potassium citrate
Recurrent calcium oxalate stones, hyperuricosuria,[a] normal urinary calcium	Allopurinol
Recurrent calcium stones, no other metabolic abnormalities or persistent stone formation despite interventions	Thiazide diuretics and/or potassium citrate
Uric acid stones	Potassium citrate; goal urine pH > 6.0 Do not use allopurinol as first-line therapy
Cystine stones	Potassium citrate; goal urine pH > 7.0
Cystine stones, unresponsive to diet and urine alkalization	Cystine-binding thiol drugs (ie, alpha-mercaptopropionyl glycine)
Struvite stones, residual or recurrent after surgical intervention	Consider acetohydroxamic acid

[a]Hyperuricosuria: urinary uric acid > 800 mg/day.
Source: AUA 2019.

RENAL MASSES, SMALL

Management: Adults

Recommendations from

> ASCO 2017, AUA 2021

–Based on tumor-specific findings and competing risks of mortality, consider renal tumor biopsy for all patients with a small renal mass (SRM) (<4 cm in size).

–Manage initially with active surveillance for patients who have significant comorbidities and limited life expectancy (end-stage renal disease, SRM < 1 cm, life expectancy < 5 y).

–Offer partial nephrectomy for SRM to all patients for whom an intervention is indicated and who have a tumor that is amenable to this approach.

–Consider percutaneous thermal ablation for patients whose tumors can be ablated completely. Obtain a biopsy before or at the time of ablation.

–Reserve radical nephrectomy only for patients whose tumor is of significant complexity that is not amenable to partial nephrectomy or where partial nephrectomy may result in unacceptable morbidity even when performed at centers of excellence. Consider referral to experienced surgeon and a center with experience.

–Consider referral to a nephrologist if CKD (GFR < 45 mL/min/1.73 m^2) or progressive CKD develops after treatment, especially if associated with proteinuria.

Practice Pearls

- SRMs are commonly discovered incidentally during diagnostic evaluation for other medical conditions. A significant number of SRMs are benign. As the size increases (especially >4 cm), the likelihood of malignancy increases. Imaging with MRI, CT scans, and ultrasound cannot make an absolute diagnosis of malignancy, necessitating a core biopsy if possible. About 10%–15% of patients will have a nondiagnostic biopsy and must be monitored closely and rebiopsied if the mass is growing. Radiofrequency ablation (RFA) is commonly used to ablate small cancers but should have a biopsy done first to document malignancy.

- Decision regarding therapy in patients with significant comorbidities is difficult. The Charleston Comorbidity Index (CCI) is a tool that can predict 1-y mortality. In patients with a short life expectancy, surveillance and supportive care is the best approach for this population. Partial nephrectomy is the treatment of choice for SRM that are amenable to nephron-sparing surgery. Radical nephrectomy in the past has been the procedure of choice in managing small RCC. Today partial nephrectomy is preferred and radical nephrectomy now is the treatment of choice in <30% of patients with SRM.

Sources

–*J Clin Oncol.* 2017;35:668–680.
–*N Engl J Med.* 2010;362–624.
–*Eur Urol.* 2016;69:116.
–*JAMA.* 2015;150:664.
–*Eur Urol.* 2015;67.

14

RHEUMATOLOGIC DISORDERS

ANKYLOSING SPONDYLITIS AND SPONDYLOARTHRITIS

Management: Adults

Recommendations from

> ACR/Spondylitis Association of America/Spondyloarthritis Research and Treatment Network 2019

–Treat with scheduled NSAIDs and tumor necrosis factor inhibitor (TNFi) therapy.

–Add slow-acting antirheumatic drugs when TNFi medications are contraindicated. Do not coadminister.

–Do not discontinue/taper biologic with stable disease.

–Use local parenteral corticosteroids for active sacroiliitis, active enthesitis, or peripheral arthritis for symptoms refractory to NSAIDs. Avoid systemic corticosteroid use.

–Refer to an ophthalmologist for concomitant iritis.

–Use TNFi monoclonal antibody therapy for ankylosing spondylitis with inflammatory bowel disease.

–Refer for a physical therapy program: active and weight-bearing; avoid spine manipulation.

–Do not routinely perform surveillance imaging of spine.

–Screen for fall risk, osteoporosis.

Sources

–*Arthritis Rheumatol.* 2016;68(2):282–298.

–rheumatology.org; 2019 Update of the American College of Rheumatology/Spondylitis Association of America/Spondyloarthritis Research and Treatment Network Recommendations for the Treatment of Ankylosing Spondylitis and Nonradiographic Axial Spondyloarthritis.

GOUT

Management: Adults, Acute Gouty Attack

Recommendations from

> NICE 2022, ACR 2020, ACP 2017

–Start NSAIDs, colchicine, or short course of oral steroid (ACP: prefer corticosteroids unless contraindications; prednisolone 35 mg/d × 5 d).

–If using NSAIDs, consider concurrent PPI. (NICE)

–If NSAIDs/colchicine contraindicated or ineffective, consider intra-articular or intramuscular corticosteroid.

–Consider ice to the affected joint as adjunct.

Sources

–*2020 American College of Rheumatology Guideline for the Management of Gout.* rhumatology. org/Portals/0/Files/Gout-Guideline-Final-2020.pdf

–http://guidelines.gov/summaries/summary/50608/management-of-acute-and-recurrent-gout-a-clinical-practice-guideline-from-the-american-college-of-physicians?q=gout

–www.nice.org.uk/guidance/ng219

–*Ann Intern Med.* 2017;166(1):58–68.

Management: Adults, Chronic Gout

Recommendations from

➤ **ACR 2020, NICE 2022**

Evaluation

–Confirm clinical diagnosis with a serum urate level ≥ 6 mg/dL. If serum urate < 6 mg/dL and gout is strongly suspected, repeat in >2 wk after flare. (NICE)

–If diagnosis remains uncertain or unconfirmed, consider joint aspiration and evaluation for crystals. (NICE)

–If joint aspiration cannot be performed, consider imaging with X-ray, ultrasound, or CT. (NICE)

Therapies

–Advise dietary restrictions: limit purine, high-fructose corn syrup, and EtOH intake. Weight loss is beneficial. Do not offer vitamin C supplementation.

–Initiate urate lowering therapy (ULT) in the patients who have:

- Frequent or troublesome gout flares (ACR ≥ 2/y).
- Tophi.
- CKD Stages 3–5.
- Arthritis/evidence of radiographic damage (ie, bony erosions).
- Serum urate > 9 mg/dL (ACR, conditional).
- Urolithiasis (ACR, conditional).

–Do not lower uric acid in asymptomatic hyperuricemia. (ACR)

–When initiating ULT, use an anti-inflammatory (colchicine, NSAID, steroid) to prevent flares and continue for 3–6 mo. (ACR)

–When initiating ULT, wait 2–4 wk after flare has subsided, unless flares are very frequent. (NICE)

–Medications used in ULT:

- Use allopurinol or febuxostat first line (avoid febuxostat if cardiovascular disease).
- If cardiovascular disease, choose allopurinol.
- Start with low dose (allopurinol ≤ 100 mg/d, febuxostat ≤ 40 mg/d).

- Titrate up to achieve serum urate < 6 mg/dL, or <5 mg/dL if tophi/arthritis/ongoing flares despite urate < 6 (max doses: allopurinol 800 mg/d, febuxostat 80 mg/d).
- Probenecid is another option in patients without CKD, but less effective.
- Pegloticase is an expensive IV medication with adverse effects so is not a first-line option.
- Avoid interleukin-1 agents unless last resort, and only consider with guidance of rheumatologist.

–Once target serum uric acid level is achieved, monitor serum urate annually.

–Consider continuing ULT indefinitely to prevent recurrence. (ACR)

–If on hydrochlorothiazide for hypertension, change to an alternate antihypertensive, perhaps losartan. In HLD, do not add fenofibrate to treatment plan. Continue aspirin if indicated for other diagnoses.

Practice Pearls

- Consider HLA-B*5801 prior to initiating allopurinol for patients of Southeast Asian and African descent. Do not test others.
- In patients with prior allopurinol allergy, start allopurinol desensitization.
- In patients taking febuxostat for gout who have CVD or have had new CV event, switch to alternative ULT agent.

Sources

–*2020 American College of Rheumatology Guideline for the Management of Gout*; rhumatology. org/Portals/0/Files/Gout-Guideline-Final-2020.pdf

–National Institute for Health and Care Excellence. *Gout: Diagnosis and Management. NICE guideline.* 2022. www.nice.org.uk/guidance/ng219

RHEUMATOID ARTHRITIS (RA)

Management: Adults

Recommendations from

> ACR 2021

Evaluation

–TB screening prior to use of disease-modifying antirheumatic drugs (DMARDs) and biologics:
- Check a TB skin test or IGRA before initiating these medications.
- If latent TB, treat for at least 1 mo prior to the initiation of a biologic or tofacitinib.

Therapies

–Symptomatic early rheumatoid arthritis:
- If the disease activity is low, and the patient is naïve to DMARD therapy, use DMARD monotherapy (methotrexate [MTX] preferred) over double or triple therapy.
- If the disease activity is moderate or high, and the patient is naïve to DMARD therapy, use DMARD monotherapy over double or triple therapy.

- Methotrexate is strongly recommended over hydroxychloroquine, sulfasalazine, bDMARD, or tsDMARD monotherapy for DMARD-naïve patients with moderate-to-high disease activity.
- If the disease activity remains moderate or high despite DMARD monotherapy (with or without glucocorticoids), use combination DMARDs, a TNFi, or a nontumor necrosis factor (TNF) biologic (all with or without MTX).
- If disease flares, add short-term glucocorticoids at the lowest dose and for the shortest duration possible.

–Established rheumatoid arthritis:
- If disease activity is low and the patient is naïve to DMARD, use DMARD monotherapy (MTX preferred) over TNFi.
- If disease activity is moderate to high and the patient is naïve to DMARD, use DMARD monotherapy (MTX preferred) over tofacitinib and combination DMARD therapy.
- If disease activity remains moderate or high despite DMARD monotherapy, use combination DMARDs, add a TNFi, non-TNF biologic, or tofacitinib (all with or without MTX).

–Vaccination recommendations for patients with rheumatic and musculoskeletal diseases (RMD):
- For RMD patients aged ≥65 y and RMD patients aged >18 and <65 y who are on immunosuppressive medication, give high-dose or adjuvanted influenza vaccination over regular-dose influenza vaccination.
- For RMD patients aged <65 y who are on immunosuppressive medication, pneumococcal vaccination is strongly recommended.
- For RMD patients aged >18 y who are on immunosuppressive medication, recombinant zoster vaccine is strongly recommended.
- For RMD patients aged >26 and <45 y who are on immunosuppressive medication and not previously vaccinated, vaccination against HPB is conditionally recommended.

Practice Pearl

- Anti-TNFα agents, abatacept, and rituximab all contraindicated in:
  - Serious bacterial, fungal, and viral infections, or with latent TB.
  - Acute viral hepatitis or Child-Pugh score B or C.
  - Instances of a lymphoproliferative disorder treated ≤5 y ago, decompensated heart failure, or any demyelinating disorder.
  - CBCD, LFTs, and Cr should be monitored every 2–4 wk during the first 3 mo, every 8–12 wk during the next 3–6 mo, and every 12 wk thereafter for patients on leflunomide, MTX, and sulfasalazine. Only baseline levels are recommended for hydroxychloroquine.
  - Live attenuated vaccines, if indicated, can be given prior to initiating therapy with TNFi biologics or non-TNF biologics. A 2-wk waiting period is recommended before starting biologics. Live attenuated vaccines are not recommended during therapy with biologics.

Source
–ACR. American College of Rheumatology Guideline for the treatment of rheumatoid arthritis. *Arthritis Care Res.* 2021.

POLYMYALGIA RHEUMATICA

Management: Adults

Recommendations from

> ACR 2015

–Choose glucocorticoid therapy over NSAIDs to treat PMR.

–Initiate glucocorticoids at a minimum dose of 12.5–25 mg prednisone equivalent daily as initial treatment. Avoid doses ≤ 7.5 mg/d or >30 mg/d.

–Duration of glucocorticoids will be individualized, but a minimum of 12 mo of therapy is assumed. Tapering schedules should be customized based on regular monitoring of disease activity, lab markers, and adverse effects.

–Consider addition of MTX in patients at high risk for relapse, prolonged therapy, or glucocorticoid-related adverse events (due to comorbidities, concomitant medications).

–Avoid TNFα-blocking agents.

–Consider an individualized exercise program targeting the maintenance of muscle mass/function and reducing fall risk.

–Avoid the use of Chinese herbal preparations Yanghe and Biqi.

Source

–ACR. Recommendations for the management of polymyalgia rheumatica. *Arthritis Rheumatol.* 2015(67):2569–2580.

SYSTEMIC LUPUS ERYTHEMATOSUS (SLE, LUPUS)

Management: Adults

Recommendations from

> British Society for Rheumatology (BSR) 2017, EULAR/ACR 2019

Evaluation

–Diagnose lupus in patients with 4 or more of the following symptoms/findings, with at least 1 serologic finding and 1 clinical finding, either contemporaneously or sequentially at any time:

- Malar rash.
- Discoid rash.
- Photosensitivity.
- Oral or nasal ulcers.
- Inflammatory arthritis.
- Serositis (ie, pleural effusion, pericardial effusion, pericarditis).
- Renal dysfunction (ie, proteinuria > 500 mg/d, cellular casts, lupus nephritis).
- Neurologic dysfunction (ie, severe headache, altered mental status, seizures, psychosis, mononeuritis multiplex, myelitis, peripheral or cranial neuropathy).
- Hematologic dysfunction (ie, hemolytic anemia, WBC < 4000, lymphocytes < 1500, platelets $< 100,000$).

- Autoimmune dysfunction (ie, positive anti-dsDNA Ab, anti-Sm Ab, lupus anticoagulant test, anticardiolipin, or false-positive syphilis FTA, lowered C3/C4).
- Antinuclear antibody (ANA) positivity with elevated titer.

Therapies

–Mild disease (SLEDAI-2K < 6, BILAG C) is characterized by fatigue, malar rash, diffuse alopecia, oral ulcers, arthralgias, myalgias, or platelets 50,000–150,000.
  - Acute treatment: prednisone ≤ 20 mg daily, hydroxychloroquine ≤ 6.5 mg/kg/d, MTX 7.5–15 mg/wk, and/or NSAIDs.
  - Maintenance treatment: prednisone ≤ 7.5 mg/d, hydroxychloroquine 200 mg/d, and/or MTX 10 mg/wk.

–Moderate disease (SLEDAI-2K 6–12, BILAG B) represents potential permanent damage, with fever, rash up to 22% of body surface area, cutaneous vasculitis, alopecia with scalp inflammation, arthritis, pleurisy, pericarditis, hepatitis, or platelets 25,000–50,000.
  - Acute treatment: prednisone ≤ 0.5 mg/kg/d AND (azathioprine 1.5–2.0 mg/kg/d OR MTX 10–25 mg/wk OR mycophenolate mofetil 2–3 g/d OR cyclosporin ≤2.0 mg/kg/d).
  - Maintenance treatment: prednisone ≤ 7.5 mg/d AND azathioprine 50–100 mg/d OR MTX 10 mg/wk OR mycophenolate mofetil 1 g/d OR (cyclosporin 50–100 mg/d AND hydroxychloroquine 200 mg/d).

–Severe disease (SLEDAI-2K > 12 or BILAG A) represents organ- or life-threatening disease, with rash involving more than 22% of body surface area, myositis, severe pleurisy, and/or pericarditis with effusion, ascites, enteritis, myelopathy, psychosis, acute confusion, optic neuritis, or platelets < 25,000.
  - Acute treatment: prednisone ≤ 0.5 mg/kg/d and/or IV methylprednisolone 500 mg × 1–3 OR prednisone ≤ 0.75–1 mg/kg/d and azathioprine 2–3 mg/kg/d OR mycophenolate mofetil 2–3 g/d OR cyclosporin 2.5 mg/kg/d.
  - Maintenance treatment: prednisone 7.5 mg/d AND mycophenolate mofetil 1.0–1.5 g/d OR azathioprine 50–100 mg/d OR cyclosporin 50–100 mg/d and hydroxychloroquine 200 mg/d.

–Consider rituximab and belimumab in patients who do not respond to the regimens above. Consider rituximab especially for patients with severe renal or CNS flare (SLEDAI ≥ 10). Belimumab is specifically approved for use with antibody positive SLE (anti-dsDNA).

–IVIG and plasmapheresis may be considered in patients with refractory cytopenias, thrombotic thrombocytopenia purpura, rapid deteriorating acute confusional state, and catastrophic antiphospholipid antibody syndrome.

–Aim to reduce and stop drugs except hydroxychloroquine eventually when in stable remission.

–Test for TPMT (thiopurine S-methyltransferase) activity prior to starting azathioprine:
  - Very low levels of TPMT activity are associated with life-threatening bone marrow toxicity.

–Encourage high-SPF UV-A and UV-B sunscreen use for patients with photosensitivity symptoms.

Surveillance

–Assess blood counts weekly as azathioprine doses are increased.

–Measure serum immunoglobulins prior to starting mycophenolate mofetil, cyclosporin, and rituximab, 3–6 mo later and then annually.

–Screen for chronic infections (tuberculosis, hepatitis B, hepatitis C, HIV, and HPV) prior to starting immunosuppressive therapy.

–In patients with stable/low-activity disease, assess the following every 6–12 mo:

- Vital signs, vaccination status, modifiable risk factors (hypertension, hyperlipidemia, diabetes, obesity, tobacco use).
- Blood count, renal function, liver function, vitamin D_3, anti-dsDNA titer, C3/C4 level, urinalysis.
- Disease activity using standardized questionnaire (eg, BILAG, SLEDAI, or SLICCC/ACR scores).
- Quality of life using standardized questionnaire (eg, Short-form 36 or LupusQoL).

–In patients with active disease, assess the following every 1–3 mo:

- Blood count, renal function, liver function, creatinine, anti-dsDNA titer, C3/C4 level, urinalysis.

–Check anti-Ro and anti-La antibodies prior to pregnancy as these are associated with neonatal lupus/conduction defects.

Practice Pearls

- Five percent of the general population will have a positive ANA; 95% of patients with SLE will have a positive ANA.
- Do not routinely test for ANA or other autoimmune antibodies unless the patient has other signs/symptoms of SLE and a positive result would therefore be diagnostically helpful as nonspecific ANA positivity is not uncommon in the general population.
- Be aware that leukopenia and neutropenia are common in SLE and may therefore be indicative of active disease or a medication side effect.
- Cyclosporin and tacrolimus may be particularly useful in patients with cytopenias as these medications exhibit this side effect less frequently.
- Infections, cardiovascular disease, and malignancy are the leading causes of death in patients with SLE.
- Consider the etiology of an acute flare when treating it. Common causes include medication nonadherence, exposure to sunlight, concurrent or recent infection, hormonal changes, or recent medication changes.
- CRP is often normal or only mildly elevated in SLE, even with arthritis or serositis. ESR is more sensitive but also not specific.
- Rising anti-dsDNA antibodies and falling, low complement levels are associated with an acute flare.
- Forty percent of patients with SLE, however, do not have positive anti-dsDNA antibodies.
- ANA, anti-Sm, and anti-RNP antibodies do not fluctuate with disease intensity.

Source

–*Rheumatology*. 2018;57(1):e1–e45. https://doi.org/10.1093/rheumatology/kex286

SKIN DISORDERS

ACNE

Management: Adolescents and Young Adults

Recommendations from

> AAD 2024, NICE 2023

–See Table 15–1 for treatment recommendations based on severity.
–Use topical therapies as initial treatment as monotherapy (except topical antibiotics—do not use as monotherapy) or in combination with other topical or oral therapies.
  • Topical retinoids (tretinoin, adapalene, tazarotene, trifarotene).
  • Benzoyl peroxide.
  • Topical antibiotics (erythromycin, clindamycin, minocycline, dapsone).
–Consider clascoterone (topical antiandrogen), salicylic acid, and azelaic acid.
–Use oral antibiotics (doxycycline has the strongest data) as an adjunct to benzoyl peroxide and other topicals, not as monotherapy. Limit to shortest duration possible, typically <4 mo.

TABLE 15–1 TREATMENT OPTIONS FOR ACNE	
Acne Severity	**Therapy Approach**
Mild	Use multimodal combination therapy with >1 of: –Topical retinoids –Benzoyl peroxide –Topical antibiotics Use fixed dose combinations to facilitate adherence: –Topical antibiotic + benzoyl peroxide –Topical retinoid + benzoyl peroxide –Topical retinoid + antibiotic
Moderate to severe	Begin with topical treatments as above Add systemic antibiotics as needed for the shortest time possible. Consider hormonal agents (combined oral contraceptives, spironolactones) Consider intralesional corticosteroids for patients at risk for scarring Consider isotretinoin

–Consider combined oral contraceptives and/or spironolactone in female patients without contraindications.

–Consider intralesional corticosteroids for patients with larger papules or nodules who are at risk for scarring.

–Insufficient evidence to recommend for/against oral steroids, metformin for acne.

–Consider oral isotretinoin for severe recalcitrant nodular acne. Monitor LFTs and lipid panel during therapy. Pregnancy prevention is mandatory, and patients must enroll in FDA-mandated iPLEDGE program.

–Insufficient data for comedone extraction, chemical peels, laser devices, microneedle radiofrequency device, or photodynamic therapy.

–Insufficient data for low-glycemic-load diet, low dairy diet, low whey diet, omega 3 fatty acids, or chocolate.

–Skin care advice: (NICE)

- Use skin pH neutral or slightly acidic wash twice daily.
- Do not use oil-based or comedogenic skin care products, sunscreens, and makeup.
- No picking or scratching lesions.

Practice Pearls

- Benzoyl peroxide helps prevent bacterial resistance. Improvement may be seen within days. It causes burning, dryness, stinging, erythema, peeling, hypersensitivity, and bleaching of hair and clothing.
- Tretinoin comes in a range of strengths; increasing the potency gradually will minimize skin irritation. Retinoids can cause photosensitivity, erythema, dryness, pruritus, and stinging.
- Clindamycin is the favored topical antibiotic. Limit duration to 12 wk.
- Do not use topical antibiotics as monotherapy because of the risk of bacterial resistance.
- Topical adapalene, tretinoin, and BP are safely used in preadolescent children.
- Use systemic antibiotics for shortest duration and do not use as monotherapy without topicals.
- Remember that contraceptives have several medical contraindications.

Sources
–https://doi.org/10.1016/j.jaad.2023.12.017
–www.nice.org.uk/guidance/ng198
–*Am Fam Physician.* 2019;100(8):475–484.

ACTINIC KERATOSIS (AK)

Management: Adults

Recommendations from

> AAD 2021

–Protect from exposure to UV light with sunscreen and sun-protective clothing.
–Treat with topical 5-fluorouracil, topical imiquimod, or cryosurgery.
–Consider diclofenac gel and photodynamic therapy.

–Consider combination therapy: 5-fluorouracil and cryosurgery or imiquimod plus cryosurgery.

–Do not use the following combination therapies: diclofenac gel and cryosurgery, topical adapalene and cryosurgery, or imiquimod following ALA-blue light PDT.

–Follow up to assess treatment success, recurrence, or development of new actinic keratosis.

–Consider nontreatment vs. observation in patients with limited life expectancy or morbidity outweighs potential benefits.

Practice Pearls

- 5-Fluorouracil offers better success rates than imiquimod or photodynamic therapy, though dosing and adverse effects make adherence challenging. (*N Engl J Med*. 2019;380(10):935–946)
- Dosing recommendations for fluorouracil vary, but typically 1–2 applications daily for 2–6 wk. (*Am Fam Physician*. 2010;81(10):1186–1188)
- Definition: actinic keratosis are keratinocyte neoplasms found on skin from long-term UV exposure.
- Choice of optimal therapy ideally involves shared decision-making between clinician and patient.
- Selection of treatment options based on location of lesion, efficacy, tolerability, burden, and patient preferences.
- NSAIDs such as diclofenac gel carry black box warning for cardiovascular and gastrointestinal side effects.

Source
–AAD. Guideline care for the management of actinic keratosis. *J Am Acad Dermatol*. 2021.

ATOPIC DERMATITIS (AD) AND ECZEMA

Management: Adults and Children

Recommendations from

➤ AAD 2022, AAI 2024, NICE 2023

Evaluation

–Do not use skin prick tests or blood tests (eg, radioallergosorbent test) for the routine evaluation of atopic dermatitis.

–Consider alternate diagnoses such as contact dermatitis, psoriasis, seborrheic dermatitis, photodermatoses, primary immunodeficiency disorders, infestations (ie, scabies), and infections.

–In children, diagnose eczema when there is itchy skin with ≥3 of the following: (NICE)
  - Active flexural dermatitis involving skin creases (ie, bends of the elbows or knees) or on the cheeks or extensor areas.
  - Prior flexural dermatitis.
  - Dry skin in past 12 mo.
  - Asthma or allergic rhinitis in patient or first-degree relative < 4-y-old.
  - Onset of signs/symptoms under age 2 y.

Therapies

–Apply skin moisturizers after bathing with hypoallergenic neutral to low pH nonsoap cleansers. Prescription moisturizers bring minimal additional benefit compared with over-the-counter emollients.

–Use topical corticosteroids as first-line therapy.

–Consider wet-wrap therapy with topical corticosteroids for moderate-to-severe atopic dermatitis during flares that are refractory to medium-to-high potency corticosteroids. Limit duration to 4–7 d and application from 1 h to overnight.

- In patients using higher potency steroids or calcineurin inhibitors, offer the option of once-a-day application vs. twice-a-day depending on patient preferences. (AAI)

–Consider topical calcineurin inhibitors (tacrolimus or pimecrolimus) as an alternative to corticosteroids.[1]

–Use medium potency topical corticosteroids intermittently as maintenance therapy.

- In patients who have frequent flares, treat areas prone to flares proactively with mid-potency steroids or calcineurin inhibitors. Consider treating for 2 d a week for several months after inducing remission to prevent future flares. (AAI)

–Consider topical crisaborole 2% or ruxolitinib cream 1.5% as a corticosteroid alternative for mild-to-moderate atopic dermatitis.

- Consider topical ruxolitinib for short-term treatment. Do not exceed 20% body surface area. Maximum 60 g/wk.

–Consider dilute bleach baths in patients with moderate-to-severe disease as an adjunct to other therapies for patients who find them tolerable and helpful.

–Consider phototherapy for acute and chronic atopic dermatitis in both adults and children. NB-UVB is mostly used due to low-risk profile.

–Consider systemic immunomodulating agents for severe cases that are refractory to topical agents and phototherapy such as cyclosporine or methotrexate. Systemic steroids should be avoided except as bridge to another therapy.

- Avoid elimination diets unless there are other signs of a serious food allergy.
- In patients with moderate-to-severe disease refractory to topical therapies, refer for allergen immunotherapy.
- In patients refractory to topical therapies, consider specialty referral for systemic immune modulating therapies.

–Do not use oral antibiotics unless there is clinical evidence of infection.

- Do not use systemic corticosteroids.

–Do not use topical antimicrobials, topical antihistamines, or topical antiseptics.

- If topical corticosteroids have not controlled the eczema within 1–2 wk in children, exclude secondary bacterial infection, consider short course of high potency steroids (<14 d, not on face or neck), and then refer for specialty care if still not controlled. (NICE)
- Do not routinely use oral antihistamines. If severe eczema, consider 1 mo trial. (NICE)

[1] Combining steroids and calcineurin inhibitors has not been shown to bring additional benefit vs. either agent alone. Some use corticosteroids for general body application and calcineurin inhibitors for more sensitive areas like the face and skin folds where the adverse effects of steroids are more relevant.

- Refer to specialist if severe and not responding after 1 wk, if treatment of superinfected eczema has failed, if the diagnosis is uncertain, inadequate control, suspected contact allergic dermatitis, or significant social or psychological implications.

Practice Pearls

- Emollients are the foundation of therapy. Educate patients and families extensively about their use:
  - Use a large quantity, and use daily regardless of visible symptoms.
  - Apply by smoothing onto skin rather than rubbing in.
  - If using multiple topicals, apply 1 product at a time with several minutes in between applications. The order of application is not important.
- As atopic dermatitis is an immune-driven disease, nearly all patients will require prescription anti-inflammatories.
- Skin prick tests and RAST-type blood tests are useful to identify causes of allergic reactions, but not for diagnosing dermatitis or eczema. When testing for suspected allergies is indicated, patch testing with ingredients of products that come in contact with the patient's skin is recommended.

Sources

–AAD. *Atopic Dermatitis Clinical Guideline.* 2020. aad.org/clinical-quality/guidelines

–American Academy of Dermatology. *Choosing Wisely.* 2020.

–AAD. *Guidelines on Comorbidities Associated with Atopic Dermatitis.* 2022.

–JAAD. *Guidelines of Care for the Management of Atopic Dermatitis in Adults with Topical Therapies.* 2022.

–*Ann Allerty Asthma Immunol.* 2024;132:274–312.

–www.nice.org.uk/guidance/cg57

PRESSURE ULCERS

Prevention: Adults with Impaired Mobility

Recommendations from

➤ NICE 2014, ACP 2015

–In adults with impaired mobility, assess risk in both outpatient and inpatient settings (eg, the Braden Scale in adults and the Braden Q Scale in children).

–Educate patient, family, and caregivers regarding the causes and risk factors of pressure ulcers.

–Use compression stockings cautiously in patients with lower extremity arterial disease. Avoid thigh-high stockings when compression stockings are used.

–Move patients with caution. Avoid dragging patient when moving and lubricate or powder bed pans prior to placing under patient.

–Minimize pressure on skin, especially areas with bony prominences.

- Turn patient side-to-side every 2 h.
- Pad areas over bony prominences.
- Pad skin-to-skin contact.

- Use heel protectors or place pillows under calves.
- Consider a bariatric bed for patients weighing over 300 lb.
- Consider high-specification foam (not air) mattress for high-risk patients admitted to secondary care or who are undergoing surgery.

–Manage moisture.

- Moisture barrier protectant on skin.
- Frequent diaper changes.
- Scheduled toileting.
- Treat candidiasis if present.
- Consider a rectal tube for stool incontinence with diarrhea.

–Maintain adequate nutrition and hydration.

–Keep the head of the bed at or >30-degree elevation.

Practice Pearl

- Outpatient risk assessment for pressure ulcers:
  - Is the patient bed or wheelchair bound?
  - Does the patient require assistance for transfers?
  - Is the patient incontinent of urine or stool?
  - Any history of pressure ulcers?
  - Does the patient have a clinical condition placing the patient at risk for pressure ulcers?
    o DM.
    o Peripheral vascular disease.
    o Stroke.
    o Polytrauma.
    o Musculoskeletal disorders (fractures or contractures).
    o Spinal cord injury.
    o Guillain–Barré syndrome.
    o Multiple sclerosis.
    o Cancer.
    o Chronic obstructive pulmonary disease.
    o Coronary heart failure.
    o Dementia.
    o Preterm neonate.
    o Cerebral palsy.
  - Does the patient appear malnourished?
  - Is equipment in use that could contribute to ulcer development (eg, oxygen tubing, prosthetic devices, urinary catheter)?

Sources

–National Clinical Guideline Centre. *Pressure Ulcers: Prevention and Management of Pressure Ulcers*. London, UK: National Institute for Health and Care Excellence; 2014.

–*Ann Intern Med*. 2015;162(5):359–369.

Management: Adults

Recommendations from

> NICE 2014, ACP 2015

–Regularly document ulcer size.

–Debride any necrotic tissue if present with sharp debridement or autolytic debridement.

–Use hydrocolloid or foam dressings to reduce wound size.

–Provide nutritional supplementation for patients who are malnourished.

–Recommend a pressure-redistributing foam mattress.

–Consider electrical stimulation as adjunctive therapy to accelerate wound healing.

–Do not routinely use negative pressure wound therapy, electrotherapy, or hyperbaric oxygen therapy.

–Only use antibiotics for superimposed cellulitis or underlying osteomyelitis.

Practice Pearl

- Moderate-quality evidence supports the addition of electrical stimulation to standard therapy to accelerate healing of Stage II–IV ulcers.

Sources

–http://www.guideline.gov/content.aspx?id=48026

–https://guidelines.gov/summaries/summary/49050

PSORIASIS, PLAQUE-TYPE

Management: Adults

Recommendations from

> AAD 2009, AAD-NPF 2009, 2019

–Use topical therapies for mild-to-moderate disease.

–Recommend emollients applied 1–3 times daily.

–Use topical corticosteroids daily or BID as the cornerstone of therapy. Limit Class I (ie, high potency) topical steroids to 4 wk maximum.

–Topical agents that have proven efficacy when combined with topical corticosteroids:

- Topical vitamin D analogs.
- Topical tazarotene.
- Topical salicylic acid.

–Reserve systemic therapies for severe, recalcitrant, or disabling psoriasis.

- Methotrexate:
  - Dose: 7.5–30 mg PO weekly (common 10–20 mg).
  - Monitor CBC and liver panel monthly (every 4 wk initially, while on higher doses and space to 8 wk for duration of treatment).

- Cyclosporine:
  - Initial dose: 2.5–3 mg/kg divided BID (narrow therapeutic window).
  - Monitor for nephrotoxicity, HTN, and hypertrichosis.
- Acitretin:
  - Dose: 10–50 mg PO daily.
  - Monitor: liver panel.

–Considerations for comorbidities:
- Consider early and more frequent cardiovascular screening (obesity, HTN, HLD, DM, metabolic syndrome) in patients with psoriasis requiring systemic or phototherapy treatments, or psoriasis involving >10% of BSA.
- Recommend screening for anxiety and depression in patients with psoriasis.
- Recommend smoking cessation and limiting alcohol intake.
- If a concern for comorbid IBD arises, refer the patient back to their PCP or to a gastroenterologist. Avoid IL-17 inhibitor therapy in patients with IBD.

Practice Pearls

- Approximately 2% of population has psoriasis.
- Eighty percent of patients with psoriasis have mild-to-moderate disease.
- Topical steroid toxicity:
  - Local: skin atrophy, telangiectasia, striae, purpura, or contact dermatitis.
  - Hypothalamic–pituitary–adrenal axis may be suppressed with prolonged use of medium- to high-potency steroids.
- Methotrexate contraindications: pregnancy, breastfeeding, alcohol use disorder, chronic liver disease, immunodeficiency syndromes, cytopenias, hypersensitivity reaction.
- Cyclosporine contraindications: CA, renal impairment, uncontrolled HTN.
- Acitretin contraindications: pregnancy, chronic liver or renal disease.

Sources
–http://www.aad.org/File%20Library/Global%20navigation/Education%20and%20quality%20care/Guidelines-psoriasis-sec-3.pdf

–http://www.aad.org/File%20Library/Global%20navigation/Education%20and%20quality%20care/Guidelines-psoriasis-sec-4.pdf

–*J Am Acad Dermatol.* 2019;90:1073–1113.

SKIN CANCER

Screening: Adults and Adolescents

Recommendations from

➢ USPSTF 2023

–Insufficient evidence to assess the balance of benefits and harms of visual skin examination by a clinician to screen for skin cancer.

Practice Pearls

- Clinicians must use their clinical judgment in deciding whether to screen for skin cancer. History of frequent sunburns, older age, and male sex are risk factors.
- Melanoma is 30 times more common in White persons than Black persons, but persons with darker skin are often diagnosed at later stages. The most common type of melanoma among Black persons occurs on skin not frequently exposed to sunlight (ie, palms of hands, soles of feet, under nails).
- Benefits and harms:
  - *Benefits:* basal and squamous cell carcinomas are the most common types of cancer in the United States and represent the vast majority of all cases of skin cancer; however, they rarely result in death or substantial morbidity, whereas melanoma has notably higher mortality rates.
  - *Harms:* potential for harm clearly exists, including a high rate of unnecessary biopsies, possibly resulting in cosmetic or, more rarely, functional adverse effects, and the risk of overdiagnosis and overtreatment.
- Twenty-eight million people in the United States use UV indoor tanning salons, increasing the risk of squamous, basal cell cancer, and malignant melanoma. (*J Clin Oncol.* 2012;30:1588)
- Clinical features of increased risk of melanoma (family history, multiple nevi previous melanoma) are linked to sites of subsequent malignant melanoma, which may be helpful in surveillance. (*JAMA Dermatol.* 2017;153:23)
- There are no guidelines for patients with familial syndromes (familial atypical mole and melanoma [FAM-M]), although systematic surveillance is warranted.[1]

Source
–*JAMA.* 2023;329(15):1290.

Prevention: Adults and Children

Recommendations from

> USPSTF 2018, National Cancer Institute 2019

–Counsel to minimize UV exposure for people aged 6 mo to 24 y with light skin types. (USPSTF)

–Offer selective counseling to adults over 24 y with light skin types. (USPSTF)

–Insufficient evidence to recommend skin self-exam. (USPSTF)

–Avoid sunburns and tanning booths,[2] especially severe blistering sunburns at a younger age. (NCI)

Practice Pearls

- Use sunscreen (SPF 15) and protective clothing, spend limited time in the sun, avoid indoor tanning and blistering sunburn in adolescents and young adults.
- Phenotypic risk factors (fair skin) include ivory or pale skin color, light eye color, red or blond hair, freckles, or easily sunburned skin.

---

[1] Consider dermatologic risk assessment if family history of melanoma in ≥2 blood relatives, presence of multiple atypical moles, or presence of numerous actinic keratoses.

[2] Indoor tanning may account for 450,000 cases of skin cancer and 10,000 melanomas each year. (*JAMA Dermatol.* 2014;150:390)

- Nicotinamide (vitamin B$_3$) shows promise in preventing skin cancers but further studies are required. (*J Invest Dermatol*. 2012;132:1498)
- Chemopreventive agents (beta-carotene, isotretinoin, selenium, and celecoxib) have not shown prevention of new skin cancers in randomized clinical trials. (*Arch Dermatol*. 2000;136:179)

Sources
–*JAMA*. 2018;319(11):1134–1142.
–http://www.cancer.gov/types/skin/hp/skin-prevention-pdq

SKIN CANCER, BASAL CELL CARCINOMA (BCC)

Management: Adults

Recommendations from

> AAD 2018

Evaluation
–Biopsy suspicious lesions using punch, shave, or excisional biopsy.
–Stratify lesions based on risk of recurrence. These qualities carry higher risk of recurrence:

- Any lesion on face, temple, ear, genitalia, hands, feet.
- Lesions ≥ 10 mm on cheeks, forehead, scalp, neck, shin.
- Lesions ≥ 20 mm on trunk and extremities.
- Poorly defined borders.
- Recurrent lesion.
- Patient with immunosuppression or prior radiation therapy.
- Aggressive growth pattern (not nodular or superficial).
- Perineural involvement.

Therapies
–Curettage and electrodessication or Mohs micrographic surgery.
–Excise low-risk lesions with 4 mm margin of uninvolved skin and to the depth of mid-subcutaneous adipose tissue.
–For high-risk lesions, consider standard excision or Mohs micrographic surgery.
–Consider nonsurgical options for low-risk lesions. Head-to-head studies of effectiveness are not available.

- Curettage and electrodessication, particularly on trunk and extremities where cosmetic outcome is less important.
- Cryosurgery, primarily when surgical options are contraindicated or impractical.
- Topical imiquimod, for superficial basal cell carcinoma of trunk, neck, and extremities. Dose once-a-day 5 times a week for 6 wk, and council about likelihood of local adverse effects.
- Topical 5-FU, twice daily for 3–6 wk. Council about likelihood of local adverse effects.
- Photodynamic therapy, for small, well-demarcated nodular basal cell carcinoma.

–Radiation therapy is a second-line option when surgery is not feasible.

Surveillance

–After diagnosis, screen annually for skin cancers as the subsequent risk of basal cell carcinoma, squamous cell carcinoma, and melanoma is high.

–Do not recommend retinoids, selenium, or beta-carotene for prevention of subsequent skin cancers.

–There is insufficient evidence around nicotinamide, alpha-difluoromethylornithine, or celecoxib.

Source

–*J Am Acad Dermatol.* 2018;78:540–559.

SKIN CANCER, MELANOMA

Management: Adults

Recommendations from

➤ NICE 2022

–Measure vitamin D level and replete if levels are low.

–Excise melanoma with margins.

- Stage 0: 0.5-cm margin.
- Stage I: 1-cm margin.
- Stage II: 2-cm margin.

–Consider topical imiquimod to treat Stage 0 if excision would lead to unacceptable disfigurement or morbidity. Consider repeat skin biopsy after topical treatment.

–Refer people with incurable melanoma to palliative care services.

Source

–NICE. *Melanoma: Assessment and Management.* 2022.

SKIN CANCER, SQUAMOUS CELL CARCINOMA

Management: Adults

Recommendations from

➤ AAD 2018

Evaluation

–Biopsy concerning lesions using punch, shave, or excisional biopsy.

–Stratify lesions as low vs. high risk. High-risk features include:

–Large size.

- ≥20 mm on trunk and extremities.
- ≥10 mm on cheeks, forehead, scalp, pretibial.
- Any size on central face, eyelids, eyebrows, periorbital skin, nose, lips, chin, mandible, preauricular and postauricular skin, temple, ear, genitalia, hands, and feet.

–Poorly defined borders.

–Recurrent.

–Patient with immunosuppression.

–Cancer on site of prior radiation therapy or chronic inflammatory process.

–Rapidly growing tumor.

–Neurologic symptoms.

–Pathologic findings.

- Poorly differentiated.
- High-risk histologic subtype (adenoid, adenosquamous, desmoplastic, or metaplastic).
- Depth ≥ 2 mm or Clark level IV–V.
- Perineural, lymphatic, or vascular involvement.

Therapies

–Treat most lesions with surgical excision using 4- to 6-mm margins and depth to mid-subcutaneous adipose tissue.

–For tumors with high-risk features, obtain assessment of surgical margins.

–For patients with low-risk lesions who prefer not to or who are unable to undergo surgical excision, consider curettage and excision or cryotherapy as alternatives, though the cure rate may be lower than with surgical excision.

–For patients with high-risk lesions, microscopic controlled excision ("Mohs procedure") is an acceptable alternative to standard excision.

–Do not use topical therapies such as 5-fluorouracil or imiquimod.

–There is insufficient evidence to recommend laser therapies or electronic surface brachytherapy.

Surveillance

–Perform annual total body skin exam for anyone with a prior history of squamous cell carcinoma.

–Encourage sun protection (eg, sunscreens), sun avoidance, and tanning bed avoidance.

–Do not recommend retinoids, celecoxib, DMFO, nicotinomide, or dietary supplementation with selenium or beta-carotene to prevent recurrence of skin cancers.

Source

–*J Am Acad Dermatol.* 2018;78:560–578.

PEDIATRICS: SCREENINGS AND DEVELOPMENTAL CARE

THE MANAGEMENT OF MEDICAL CONDITIONS IN THE PEDIATRIC POPULATION IS ADDRESSED IN THOSE CONDITIONS' RESPECTIVE CHAPTERS.

ALCOHOL ABUSE AND DEPENDENCE

Screening: Children and Adolescents

Recommendations from

> AAFP 2010, USPSTF 2018, ICSI 2010

–There is insufficient evidence to recommend for or against screening or counseling interventions to prevent or reduce alcohol misuse by adolescents.

Practice Pearls

- AUDIT and CAGE questionnaires have not been validated in children or adolescents.
- Screen using a tool designed for adolescents, such as the CRAFFT, BSTAD, or S2BI.
- Reinforce not drinking and driving or riding with any driver under the influence.
- While behavioral counseling has been proven to be beneficial in adults, data do not support its benefit in adolescents.
- Ask about friends' alcohol use.

Sources

–USPSTF. *Unhealthy Alcohol Use in Adolescents and Adults: Screening and Behavioral Counseling Interventions.* 2018.
–https://www.icsi.org/guidelines__more/catalog_guidelines_and_more/catalog_ guidelines/
–*Ann Fam Med.* 2010;8(6):484–492.

ANEMIA

Screening: Newborns, Infants, and Children

Recommendations from

‣ USPSTF 2015, AAFP 2015, AAP 2017

–See Guidelines Alert 16–1 for discussion of screening for pediatric anemia.

Guidelines Alert 16–1 GUIDELINES DISCORDANT: WHETHER TO SCREEN ROUTINELY FOR ANEMIA	
Organization	**Guidance**
AAFP, USPSTF	Insufficient evidence to recommend for or against screening infants and newborns Consider selective screening in high-risk children[a] with malnourishment, low birth weight, or symptoms of anemia
AAP	Universal screening of Hgb at 12 mo

Applying to Clinical Practice
- The AAP recommends screening because iron deficiency anemia can lead to neurodevelopmental harm.
- USPSTF notes that more study is needed to identify ideal screening tests and show that iron supplementation improves clinical outcomes in those who screen positive.
- Harms of screening include false-positive results, discomfort to patient, and cost.
- Harms of treatment with oral iron include GI upset, staining of teeth and gums, and the potential for drug interactions or iron overdose.
- Given the manageable harms and potential for poor outcomes, it is reasonable to screen universally until better data are available, especially in higher-risk settings.

[a]Includes infants living in poverty, Black persons, Alaska Native persons, immigrants from developing countries, preterm and low-birth-weight infants, infants whose principal dietary intake is unfortified cow's milk or soy milk, bottle feeding beyond 1 y, having a mom who is currently pregnant, living in an urban area and having less than 2 servings per day of iron-rich foods (iron-fortified breakfast cereals or meats).

Practice Pearls

- If anemic, measure ferritin, C-reactive protein, and reticulocyte hemoglobin content. Reticulocyte hemoglobin content is a more sensitive and specific marker than serum hemoglobin level for iron deficiency.
- One-third of patients with iron deficiency will have a hemoglobin level > 11 g/dL.
- Use of transferring receptor 1 (TfR$_1$) assay as screening for iron deficiency is under investigation.

Sources

–AAFP. *Clinical Recommendations: Iron Deficiency Anemia.* 2015.

–USPSTF. *Iron Deficiency in Young Children: Screening.* 2015.

–Hagan JF, Shaw JS, Duncan PM, eds. *Bright Futures: Guidelines for Health Supervision of Infants, Children, and Adolescents.* 4th ed. American Academy of Pediatrics; 2017.

–*Pediatrics.* 2010;126(5):1040–1050.

ANXIETY

Screening: Children and Adolescents

Recommendations from

> USPSTF 2022

–Screen for anxiety in children and adolescents aged 8–18 y.

–Current evidence is insufficient to assess the balance of benefits and harms of screening for anxiety in children 7 y or younger.

Practice Pearls

- Available screening tools for children include Screen for Child Related Anxiety Disorders (SCARED), Patient Health Questionnaire—Adolescent (GAD and panic disorder), and Social Phobia Inventory.
- Effective treatments for anxiety include psychotherapy (cognitive behavioral therapy) and/or pharmacotherapy (SSRI/SNRI).
- It is possible that by diagnosing and treating anxiety disorders at a young age, chronic mental illness later in life can be prevented.

Source

–*JAMA*. 2022;328(14):1438–1444. doi:10.1001/jama.2022.16936

ATTENTION-DEFICIT/HYPERACTIVITY DISORDER (ADHD)

Screening: Children and Adolescents

Recommendations from

> AAFP 2016, AAP 2019, NICE 2018

–Do not screen routinely.

–Initiate an evaluation for ADHD for any child 4–18 y who presents with academic or behavioral problems and symptoms of inattention, hyperactivity, or impulsivity. Diagnosis requires that the child meet *DSM-5* criteria[1] and direct supporting evidence from parents or caregivers and classroom teacher.

–Screen for comorbid conditions, including emotional or behavioral conditions (eg, anxiety, depression, oppositional defiant disorder, conduct disorders, substance use), developmental conditions (eg, learning and language disorders, autism spectrum disorders), and physical conditions (eg, tics, sleep apnea).

---

[1] The *DSM-5* criteria define 4 dimensions of ADHD: (1) attention-deficit/hyperactivity disorder primarily of the inattentive presentation (ADHD/I) (314.00 [F90.0]); (2) attention-deficit/hyperactivity disorder primarily of the hyperactive-impulsive presentation (ADHD/HI) (314.01 [F90.1]); (3) attention-deficit/hyperactivity disorder combined presentation (ADHD/C) (314.01 [F90.2]); and (4) other specified and unspecified ADHD (314.01 [F90.8]).

Practice Pearls

- Stimulant prescription rates continue to rise. (*Lancet*. 2016;387(10024):1240–1250)
- Current estimates are that 7.2% of children/adolescents meet criteria for ADHD. (*Pediatrics*. 2015;135(4):e994)
- The U.S. Food and Drug Administration (FDA) approved a "black box" warning regarding the potential for cardiovascular side effects of ADHD stimulant drugs. (*N Engl J Med*. 2006;354:1445)

Sources

–AAFP. *Clinical Recommendation: ADHD in Children and Adolescents*. 2016.

–AAP. *Clinical Practice Guideline for the Diagnosis, Evaluation, and Treatment of Attention-Deficit/Hyperactivity Disorder in Children and Adolescents*. 2019.

–NICE. *Attention Deficit Hyperactivity Disorder: Diagnosis and Management*. 2018. nice.org.uk/guidance/ng87

AUTISM SPECTRUM DISORDER

Screening: Children and Adolescents

Recommendations from

➤ USPSTF 2016, AAP 2014

Guidelines Alert 16–2	
GUIDELINES DISCORDANT: WHETHER TO SCREEN ROUTINELY FOR AUTISM	
Organization	**Guidance**
USPSTF	Insufficient evidence for or against routine screening
AAP	Screen with autism-specific tool at 18 mo and 24 mo

Applying to Clinical Practice
- Good data support a benefit for interventions when a caregiver raises concern for autism spectrum disorder.
- There are few data regarding asymptomatic screening.
- It is reasonable to follow AAP's recommendation for routine screening while awaiting better data, given the plausible benefit and minimal potential harm.

Practice Pearls

- M-CHAT is the most commonly used screening tool (see Appendix).
- Listen and respond to concerns raised by caregivers; signs may be identifiable by 9 mo of age.
- Prevalence is 1 in 68; 4.5:1 male:female ratio. (*MMWR Surveill Summ*. 2016;65(3):1–23)

Sources

–*JAMA*. 2016;315(7):691–696.

–*Pediatrics*. 2006;118(1):405.

–*Pediatrics*. 2014;135(5):e1520.

CELIAC DISEASE

Screening: Children and Adolescents Without Diagnosis or Symptoms of Celiac Disease

Recommendations from

> ➤ USPSTF 2017, AAFP 2017, NICE 2015

–Do not screen the asymptomatic general population, as insufficient evidence exists regarding screening of asymptomatic people.

–Screen first-degree relatives of people with celiac disease. (NICE)

–Rule out celiac disease using serologic testing as part of the evaluation of the following signs, symptoms, or associated conditions: persistent unexplained abdominal or gastrointestinal symptoms, faltering growth, prolonged fatigue, unexpected weight loss, severe or persistent mouth ulcers, unexplained iron, vitamin B_{12}, or folate deficiency, type 1 diabetes, autoimmune thyroid disease, and irritable bowel syndrome (in adults). (NICE)

Practice Pearls

- Patients must continue a gluten-containing diet during diagnostic testing.
- IgA tissue transglutaminase (TTG) is the test of choice (>90% sensitivity/specificity), along with total IgA level.
- IgA endomysial antibody test is indicated if the tissue transglutaminase test is equivocal.
- Avoid antigliadin antibody testing.
- Consider serologic testing for any of the following: Addison disease; amenorrhea; autoimmune hepatitis; autoimmune myocarditis; chronic immune thrombocytopenic purpura; dental enamel defects; depression; bipolar disorder; Down syndrome; Turner syndrome; epilepsy; lymphoma; metabolic bone disease; chronic constipation; polyneuropathy; sarcoidosis; Sjögren syndrome; or unexplained alopecia.

Sources

–AAFP. *Clinical Recommendation: Screening for Celiac Disease.* 2017.

–*JAMA.* 2017;317(12):1252.

–NICE. *Coeliac Disease: Recognition, Assessment and Management.* 2015.

CHOLESTEROL AND LIPID DISORDERS

Screening: Children and Adolescents

Recommendations from

> ➤ USPSTF 2023, NLA 2011, AAP 2017, AHA 2007, NHLBI 2012

–In familial hypercholesterolemia, screen at age 9–11 y with a fasting lipid panel or nonfasting non-HDL-C. If non-HDL-C $\geq$ 145 mg/dL, perform fasting lipid panel. (USPSTF)

–Genetic screening for familial hypercholesterolemia is generally not needed for diagnosis or clinical management.

–Cascade screening: testing lipid levels in all first-degree relatives of diagnosed familial hypercholesterolemia patients.

Guidelines Alert 16–3
GUIDELINES DISCORDANT: WHETHER TO SCREEN CHILDREN FOR DYSLIPIDEMIA

Organization	Guidance
USPSTF	Insufficient evidence to recommend for or against routine universal lab screening
AHA, NHLBI, AAP	Selectively screen with fasting lipid panel patients age > 2 y with concerning personal or family history[a] Universal screening in adolescents regardless of FH between age 9 and 11 y and again between age 18 and 21 y

Applying to Clinical Practice
- Lifelong dyslipidemia leads to cardiovascular disease. It is plausible that screening children will lead to interventions that prevent ASCVD in adulthood.
- Studies have not yet been completed to demonstrate that lifestyle modifications or starting statins at a young age will prevent ASCVD.
- Universal screening is reasonable, though if a family would be reluctant to start statins at a young age the benefits may be minimal.

[a]Obesity, hypertension, diabetes, smoking history, or parent aged <55 y with coronary artery disease, peripheral arterial disease, cerebrovascular disease, or hyperlipidemia.

Practice Pearls

- Childhood drug treatment of dyslipidemia lowers lipid levels, but the effect on childhood or adult outcomes is uncertain.
- Lifestyle approach is recommended starting after age 2 y.
- Fasting lipid profile is the recommended screening tool. If within normal limits, repeat testing in 3–5 y is recommended.

Sources
–*J Clin Lipidol.* 2011;5:S1–S8.
–*JAMA.* 2023;330(3):253–260.
–*Circulation.* 2007;115:1947–1967.
–NHLBI. *Expert Panel on Integrated Guidelines for Cardiovascular Health and Risk Reduction in Children and Adolescents.* 2012.
–Hagan JF, Shaw JS, Duncan PM, eds. *Bright Futures: Guidelines for Health Supervision of Infants, Children, and Adolescents.* 4th ed. 2017.

CONGENITAL HEART DISEASE

Screening: Newborns

Recommendations from

➢ AAP 2011

–Screen all newborns with pulse oximetry for critical congenital heart disease at ≥24 h of life but prior to discharge home from the hospital.

Practice Pearl

- Obtain oxygen saturations in the right hand and in 1 foot.

Source

–AAP. *Endorsement of HHS Recommendation for Pulse Oximetry Screening for CCHD.* 2012.

CRYPTORCHIDISM

Screening: Newborns, Infants, and Children

Recommendations from

➢ AUA 2014

–Screen all young children at each well child visit for undescended testes.

Source

–AUA. *Evaluation and Treatment of Cryptorchidism: AUA Guideline.* 2014.

Management: Newborns, Infants, and Children

Recommendations from

➢ EAU 2016, CUA 2017

–Do not routinely obtain imaging, as it is not cost-effective and may delay referral and treatment.
–Refer to surgical specialist if persists after 3–6 mo of age.
–Treat with orchiopexy between 6 and 18 mo of age to prevent infertility and testicular cancer.

Sources

–*J Pediatr Urol.* 2016;12:335–343.
–AUA. *Evaluation and Treatment of Cryptorchidism: AUA Guideline.* 2014.
–*Can Urol Assoc J.* 2017;11(7):E251–E260.

Practice Pearls

- Fertility rates are reduced to 33%–65% for men who have bilateral undescended testes but are essentially normal (90%) for unilateral.
- Orchiopexy prior to puberty reduces rates of testicular cancer, but the rates remain higher than that of the general population.

DENTAL CARIES

Screening: Children and Adolescents

Recommendations from

> USPSTF 2021, AAP 2014, AAFP 2014, Bright Futures Oral Health Guide

–Current evidence is insufficient to assess the balance of benefits and harms of routine screening examinations for dental caries performed by primary care clinicians in children younger than 5 y.

Practice Pearl

- Caries risk assessment tool can be found at: https://www.aapd.org/globalassets/media/policies_guidelines/bp_cariesriskassessment.pdf

Sources

–USPSTF. *Screening and Interventions to Prevent Dental Caries in Children Younger than 5 Years.* 2021.

–AAFP. *Clinical Recommendation.* 2014.

–*Pediatrics.* 2014;133(5):s1–s10.

DEPRESSION

Screening: Children and Adolescents

Recommendations from

> USPSTF 2022, AAP 2021

–There is insufficient evidence to recommend for or against routine screening of children 11 y of age or younger.

–Screen all adolescents (age 12+) for major depressive disorder.

–Have systems in place to ensure accurate diagnosis, appropriate psychotherapy, and adequate follow-up.

Practice Pearls

- Screen in primary care clinics with the Patient Health Questionnaire for Adolescents (PHQ-A) (73% sensitivity; 94% specificity) or the Beck Depression Inventory-Primary Care (BDI-PC) (91% sensitivity; 91% specificity). See Appendix.
- Treatment options include pharmacotherapy (fluoxetine and escitalopram are FDA approved for this age group), psychotherapy, collaborative care, psychosocial support interventions, and complementary alternative medicine approaches.
- Patients who have started taking antidepressants should be monitored closely for suicidality, clinical worsening, or unusual changes in behavior.

Sources

–*Ann Intern Med.* 2016;164(5):360–366.

–Hagan JF, Shaw JS, Duncan PM, eds. *Bright Futures: Guidelines for Health Supervision of Infants, Children, and Adolescents.* 4th ed. American Academy of Pediatrics; 2017; updated 2021.

–USPSTF. *Screening for Depression and Suicide Risk in Children and Adolescents.* 2022.

DEVELOPMENTAL DYSPLASIA OF THE HIP (DDH)

Screening: Newborns

Recommendations from

> AAP 2017, AAFP 2017

–Examine newborn and continue periodic surveillance physical exam for developmental dysplasia of the hip including length discrepancy, asymmetric thigh or buttock creases, performing Ortolani test, and observing for limited abduction.

–Obtain ultrasound for "high-risk" infants 6 wk to 6 mo of age: history of breech presentation, family history, parental concern, history of clinical hip instability on exam, or history of lower extremity swaddling.

–Consider radiography after 4 mo of age in high-risk infants without physical exam findings or any child with positive physical exam findings.

–Refer to orthopedics if unstable or dislocated hip in physical exam. Referral does not require imaging.

Practice Pearl

• There is evidence that screening leads to earlier identification; however, 60%–80% of the hips of newborns identified as abnormal or suspicious for developmental dysplasia of the hip by physical examination, and >90% of those identified by ultrasound in the newborn period, resolve spontaneously, requiring no intervention.

Sources

–*Pediatrics.* 2016;138(6):e20163107.

–*Am Fam Physician.* 2017;96(3):196–197.

DIABETES

Screening: Children and Adolescents

Recommendations from

> USPSTF 2022, AAP 2021, ADA 2012

–See table for discordant screening recommendations.

–Repeat screening every 3 y if negative.

Guidelines Alert 16–4
GUIDELINES DISCORDANT: WHETHER TO SCREEN CHILDREN FOR DIABETES

Organization	Guidance
ADA, AAP	Screen all children at risk[a] for type 2 diabetes beginning at age 10 or the start of puberty
USPSTF	Current evidence is insufficient to assess the balance of benefits and harms of screening for type 2 diabetes in asymptomatic children and adolescents

"At risk[a]" groups:
- Overweight or obese.
- Family history of DM type 2 in a first- or second-degree relative.
- Asian, Black, Latino, Alaska Native, or Pacific Islander.
- History of maternal gestational or preexisting DM during the pregnancy.
- History of being small for gestational age.
- Signs of insulin resistance (acanthosis nigricans, hypertension, dyslipidemia, polycystic ovary syndrome, central adiposity).

Applying to Clinical Practice
- Potential harms from screening include labeling, overdiagnosis, and overtreatment leading to hypoglycemia and gastrointestinal issues.
- Diabetes is the third most common childhood chronic disease, and many of the complications can begin in childhood.
- Up to half of children and adolescents diagnosed with prediabetes will return to normal glycemia within 2 y.

Sources
- *Diabetes Care.* 2021;44(suppl. 1):S15–S33.
- USPSTF. *Screening for Prediabetes and Type 2 Diabetes in Children and Adolescents.* 2022.
- *JAMA.* 2022;328(10):963–967. doi:10.1001/jama.2022.14543
- Koren D, Levitsky L. Type 2 diabetes mellitus in childhood and adolescence. *AAP.* 2021;42(4):167–179.

EATING DISORDERS

Screening: Children and Adolescents

Recommendations from

➤ USPSTF 2022

- There is insufficient evidence to assess the balance of benefits and harms of screening for eating disorders in adolescents and adults.
- Consensus from AAP is that it is worthwhile to screen for eating disorders by inquiring about exercise and eating patterns.

Practice Pearls

- All providers should be aware of physical and behavioral signs and symptoms associated with disordered eating and *DSM-5* diagnostic criteria for eating disorders. Knowledge of local resources to refer patients to is imperative.
- Bright Futures has sample screening tools for screening for eating disorders.

Sources
–USPSTF. *Screening for Eating Disorders in Adolescents and Adults.* 2022.
–Identification and management of eating disorders in children and adolescents. *J Pediatr.* 2021.

FAMILY VIOLENCE AND ABUSE

Screening: Children and Adolescents

Recommendations from

> **USPSTF 2018, AAFP 2013, AAP 2010**

–There is insufficient evidence to recommend for or against routine screening of parents or guardians for the physical abuse or neglect of children.

Practice Pearls

- All providers should be aware of physical and behavioral signs and symptoms associated with abuse and neglect, including burns, bruises, and repeated suspect trauma.
- CDC publishes a toolkit of assessment instruments: https://www.cdc.gov/violenceprevention/pdf/ipv/ipvandsvscreening.pdf
- Prevention interventions with possible but not proven efficacy include:
  - School-based programs that teach children to recognize and avoid sexually abusive situations.
  - Empowerment and relationship skills training for women.
  - Programs that change social and cultural gender norms.

Sources
–*JAMA.* 2018;320(20):2122–2128.
–Kodner C, Wetherton A. Diagnosis and management of physical abuse in children. *Am Fam Physician.* 2013;88(10):669–675.
–*Pediatrics.* 2010;126(4):833–841. doi:10.1542/peds.2010-2087

GROWTH ABNORMALITIES

Screening: Newborns and Infants < 2 y

Recommendations from

> **CDC 2010, AAP 2010**

–Use the 2006 World Health Organization (WHO) international growth charts for children age < 24 mo.

Practice Pearls

- The Centers for Disease Control and Prevention (CDC) and American Academy of Pediatricians (AAP) recommend the WHO as opposed to the CDC growth charts for children of age < 24 mo.
- The CDC growth charts should still be used for children of age 2–19 y.
- This recommendation recognizes that breastfeeding is the recommended standard of infant feeding, and therefore the standard against which all other infants are compared.

Sources
  –CDC. Use of World Health Organization and CDC growth charts for children aged 0–59 mo in the United States. *MMWR*. 2010;59(no. RR-9):1–15.
  –*AAP News*. 2010;31(11).

HEARING IMPAIRMENT

Screening: Newborns

Recommendations from

▷ AAP 1999, USPSTF 2008
  –Universal screening of all newborn infants for hearing loss.

Practice Pearls

- Screen before 1 mo of age. Refer infants who do not pass the initial screening for audiologic and medical evaluation before 3 mo of age.
- Screening involves either a 1-step or a 2-step process. The 2-step process includes otoacoustic emissions (OAEs) followed by auditory brainstem response (ABR) in those who fail the OAE test. The 1-step process uses either OAE or ABR testing.

Sources
  –*Pediatrics*. 1999;103(2).
  –*Pediatrics*. 2008;122(1).

HEMOGLOBINOPATHIES

Screening: Newborns

Recommendations from

▷ AAFP 2010, USPSTF 2007
  –Screen all newborns for hemoglobinopathies (including sickle cell disease).

Practice Pearls

- Screening for sickle cell disease is mandated in all 50 states and the District of Columbia.
- Infants with sickle cell anemia should receive prophylactic penicillin starting at 2 mo of age and pneumococcal vaccinations at recommended intervals.

Source
    –*Am Fam Physician.* 2008;77(9):1300–1302.

HEPATITIS B VIRUS (HBV) INFECTION

Screening: Children and Adolescents

Recommendations from

➤ **USPSTF 2020, CDC 2018, 2020**

    –Screen high-risk individuals using HBV surface antigen (HBsAg):
    • Foreign-born persons from countries where HBV prevalence ≥ 2%.[1]
    • US-born persons not vaccinated at birth whose parents were born in countries where HBV prevalence ≥ 8%.[2]
    • HIV-positive persons.
    • Household contacts or sexual partners of persons with HBV infection.
    • Men who have sex with men.
    • Persons with injection drug use.
    • Hemodialysis patients. (CDC)
    • Persons needing immunosuppressive therapy, immunosuppression related to organ transplantation, and immunosuppression for rheumatologic or gastroenterologic disorders. (CDC)
    • Blood, organ, plasma, semen, or tissue donors. (CDC)
    • People with elevated alanine aminotransferase levels (≥19 IU/L for women and ≥30 IU/L for men). (CDC)
    • Infants born to HBV-infected mothers (HBsAg and antibody to hepatitis B surface antigen [anti-HBs] only are recommended). (CDC)

Sources
    –USPSTF. *JAMA.* 2020;324(23):2415–2422.
    –CDC. *MMWR Recomm Rep.* 2018;67(1):1–31.
    –CDC. 2020. www.cdc.gov/hepatitis/hbv/hbvfaq.htm

HUMAN IMMUNODEFICIENCY VIRUS (HIV)

See Chapter 8: Infectious Disease for screening recommendations that include adults and adolescents.

---

[1] HBV prevalence ≥ 2% in Africa, Asia, South Pacific, Middle East (except Cyprus and Israel), Eastern Europe (except Hungary), Malta, Spain, indigenous populations of Greenland, Alaska Natives, indigenous populations of Canada, Caribbean, Guatemala, Honduras, and South America.
[2] HBV prevalence ≥ 8% in Angola, Benin, Burkina Faso, Burundi, Cameroon, Central African Republic, Congo, Côte d'Ivoire, Djibouti, Equatorial Guinea, Gabon, Gambia, Ghana, Guinea, Liberia, Malawi, Mali, Mauritania, Mozambique, Namibia, Niger, Nigeria, Senegal, Sierra Leone, Somalia, South Sudan, Sudan, Swaziland, Togo, Uganda, Zimbabwe, Haiti, Kiribati, Nauru, Niue, Papua New Guinea, Solomon Islands, Tonga, Vanuatu, Kyrgyzstan, Laos, Vietnam, Mongolia, and Yemen.

HYPERTENSION (HTN), CHILDREN AND ADOLESCENTS

Screening: Children and Adolescents

Recommendations from

➢ AAP 2017, NHLBI 2012, AAFP 2018, USPSTF 2020

Guidelines Alert 16–5 GUIDELINES DISCORDANT: SCREENING FOR BLOOD PRESSURE	
Organization	**Guidance**
USPSTF	Insufficient evidence to support screening for high blood pressure in children and adolescents, as balance of benefits and harms cannot be determined
AAP, AAFP, NHLBI	Measure BP only at preventative visits for children of age ≥ 3[a] y Measure BP at each encounter for children of age ≥ 3 y who have obesity, renal disease, history of aortic arch obstruction or coarctation, diabetes, or are taking medications known to raise blood pressure

Applying to Clinical Practice
- BP readings are less reliable in children, the link between pediatric hypertension and future cardiovascular events has not been well established, and long-term antihypertensive therapy beginning in childhood has not been well studied for adverse effects.
- Obesity in children has much clearer links to adult morbidity; use BP readings as part of an overall assessment that addresses weight, diet, exercise, and other modifiable environmental factors.
- Secondary causes of HTN are more common in children than adults, so a screening program may identify these.

[a]In children of age <3 y, conditions that warrant BP measurement include prematurity, very low birth weight, or neonatal complications; congenital heart disease; recurrent urinary tract infections (UTIs), hematuria, or proteinuria; renal disease or urologic malformations; familial hypercholesterolemia of congenital renal disease; solid-organ transplant; malignancy or bone marrow transplant; drugs known to raise BP; systemic illnesses; and increased intracranial pressure.

Practice Pearls

- Hypertension: average systolic blood pressure (SBP) or diastolic blood pressure (DBP) ≥ 95th percentile for sex, age, and height on 3 or more occasions. See Table 16–1 and the Appendix for more detail.
- Counsel children and adolescents who have been diagnosed with hypertension regarding lifestyle modifications including diet and physical activity.
- Prescribe pharmacologic therapy to children and adolescents who fail lifestyle modifications.
- USPSTF concludes that the evidence to support screening for high BP in children and adolescents is insufficient and that the balance of benefits and harms cannot be determined.

TABLE 16–1 CUTOFFS FOR PEDIATRIC STAGE 1 HYPERTENSION

	Age	1	2	3	4	5	6	7	8	9	10	11	12	13+	14	15	16	17
Female	SBP	105	109	110	112	113	114	115	117	118	120	124	126	127	127	128	128	128
	DBP	62	66	69	71	73	74	75	75	75	76	77	79	81	82	82	82	82
Male	SBP	105	108	109	110	112	114	116	117	119	121	128	128	131	134	135	137	138
	DBP	57	61	64	68	71	73	74	75	77	78	78	79	81	84	85	86	87

Source: Am AssocPediatr. 140(3):e20171904.

Sources

–*Pediatrics.* 2017;140(3):e2017–e1904.

–NHLBI. *Expert Panel on Integrated Guidelines for Cardiovascular Health and Risk Reduction in Children and Adolescents.* 2012.

–NHLBI. *A Pocket Guide to Blood Pressure Management in Children.* 2012.

–AAFP. *High Blood Pressure in Children and Adolescents.* 2018.

–USPSTF. *Screening for High Blood Pressure in Children and Adolescents.* 2020.

ILLICIT DRUG USE

Screening: Children and Adolescents

Recommendations from

> **USPSTF 2020, ICSI 2014, AAP 2021**

–There is insufficient evidence to recommend for or against routine screening for illicit drug use.

Guidelines Alert 16–6 **GUIDELINES DISCORDANT: WHETHER TO SCREEN FOR PEDIATRIC ILLICIT DRUG USE**	
Organization	**Guidance**
USPSTF	Insufficient evidence to recommend for or against routine screening for illicit drug use
AAP	Perform risk assessment beginning at age 11 using CRAFFT tool[a] and take appropriate follow-up action if positive
Applying to Clinical Practice	
• While illicit drug use is a significant issue for adolescents, it is not clear which, if any, interventions are effective when someone screens positive. • If effective interventions are available, screening is reasonable.	
[a]http://crafft.org/	

Sources

–*ICSI Preventive Services for Adults.* 20th ed. 2014.

–USPSTF. *Screening for Unhealthy Drug Use.* 2020.

–Hagan JF, Shaw JS, Duncan PM, eds. *Bright Futures: Guidelines for Health Supervision of Infants, Children, and Adolescents.* 4th ed. American Academy of Pediatrics; 2017, updated 2021.

LEAD POISONING

Screening: Children and Adolescents

Recommendations from

> AAFP 2006, USPSTF 2019, CDC 2000, AAP 2000

–Insufficient evidence to recommend for or against routine screening in asymptomatic children at increased risk.[1]

–Do not screen asymptomatic children at average risk.

Practice Pearls

- CDC recommends that children who receive Medicaid benefits should be screened unless high-quality, local data demonstrates the absence of lead exposure among this population.
- Screen at ages 1 and 2 y, or by age 3 y if a high-risk child has never been screened.
- The threshold for elevated blood lead is 5 mcg/dL. (CDC. *Low Level Lead Exposure Harms Children: A Renewed Call for Primary Prevention.* 2012)
- CDC personal risk questionnaire (http://www.cdc.gov/nceh/lead/publications/screening.htm):
  - Does your child live in or regularly visit a house (or other facility, eg, daycare) that was built before 1950?
  - Does your child live in or regularly visit a house built before 1978 with recent or ongoing renovations or remodeling (within the last 6 mo)?
  - Does your child have a sibling or playmate who has or did have lead poisoning?

Sources

–USPSTF. *Elevated Blood Lead Levels in Childhood and Pregnancy: Screening.* 2019.

–*Pediatrics.* 1998;101(6):1702.

–Advisory Committee on Childhood Lead Poisoning Prevention. Recommendations for blood lead screening of young children enrolled in Medicaid: targeting a group at high risk. *CDC MMWR.* 2000;49(RR14):1–13.

–AAFP. *Clinical Recommendations: Lead Poisoning.* 2006.

---

[1] Child suspected by parent, health care provider, or Health Department to be at risk for lead exposure; sibling or playmate with elevated blood lead level; recent immigrant, refugee, or foreign adoptee; child's parent or caregiver works with lead; household member uses traditional folk or ethnic remedies or cosmetics or who routinely eats food imported informally from abroad; residence near a source of high lead levels.

MOTOR VEHICLE INJURY

Screening: Children and Adolescents

Recommendations from

➤ ICSI 2013

–Ask about car seats, booster seats, seat belt use, and helmet use while riding motorcycles.

Practice Pearls

- One study demonstrated a 21% reduction in mortality with the use of child restraint systems vs. seat belts in children of age 2–6 y involved in motor vehicle collisions. (*Arch Pediatr Adolesc Med.* 2006;160:617–621)
- Head injury rates are reduced by approximately 75% in motorcyclists who wear helmets compared with those who do not.
- Properly used child restraint systems can reduce mortality up to 21% compared with seat belt usage in children of age 2–6 y.
- All infants and toddlers should ride in a rear-facing car safety seat until they are of age 2 or until they have met the max height or weight allowed by car seat manufacturer.

Source

–ICSI. *Preventive Services for Children and Adolescents*. 19th ed. 2013.

NEWBORN METABOLIC SCREENING

Screening: Newborns

Recommendations from

➤ ICSI 2013

–Perform a metabolic screening test prior to hospital discharge for all newborns.

Practice Pearls

- Perform the newborn screen after 24 h of age. Infants who receive their newborn screen before 24 h of age should have it repeated before 2 wk of age.
- Optimal screening time for premature infants and infants with illnesses is within 7 d of birth, and in all cases before discharge from nursery.
- If screening is positive, implement phenylalanine restrictions immediately after birth to prevent the neurodevelopmental effects of PKU.

Sources

–Advisory Committee on Heritable Disorders in Newborns and Children. 2015.
–ICSI. *Preventive Services for Children and Adolescents*. 19th ed. 2013.
–USPSTF. *Phenylketonuria in Newborns: Screening*. 2008.

OBESITY

Screening: Children and Adolescents

Recommendations from

⯈ AAP 2023, USPSTF 2017

Guidelines Alert 16–7	
GUIDELINES DISCORDANT: SCREENING FOR OBESITY IN CHILDREN AND ADOLESCENTS	
Organization	**Guidance**
USPSTF	Screen ages 6+ with BMI Frequency: undetermined Threshold: age- and sex-specific BMI ≥ 95th percentile Intervention: refer to comprehensive, intensive behavioral interventions to promote weight loss
AAP	Screen ages 2+ with BMI Frequency: at least annually Threshold: age- and sex-specific BMI > 85th percentile Intervention: evaluate for obesity-related comorbidities using a comprehensive patient history, mental and behavioral health screening, SDoH evaluation, physical exam, and diagnostic studies

Applying to Clinical Practice
- Availability of interventions varies across communities. Screen at the youngest age for which behavioral interventions are available.

Sources
–AAP. Clinical practice guideline for the evaluation and treatment of children and adolescents with obesity. *Pediatrics*. 2023;151(2).
–USPSTF. *Obesity in Children and Adolescents: Screening*. 2017.

RETINAL ASSESSMENT

Screening: Newborns

Recommendations from

⯈ AAO 2022
–Screen all newborns in the newborn nursery with red reflex and refer urgently for detected abnormality.

Source
–https://www.aao.org/education/clinical-statement/vision-screening-infants-children-2022

SCOLIOSIS

Screening: Children and Adolescents

Recommendations from

➢ AAFP 2013, USPSTF 2017

–There is insufficient evidence to assess the balance of benefits and harms of screening for adolescent idiopathic scoliosis in children and adolescents of age 10–18.

Sources
–AAFP. *Choosing Wisely: Scoliosis in Adolescents.* 2013.
–USPSTF. *Screening for Adolescents Idiopathic Scoliosis.* 2017.

SEXUALLY TRANSMITTED INFECTIONS

Screening: Children and Adolescents

Recommendations from

➢ USPSTF 2021

–Screen for chlamydia and gonorrhea in all sexually active women 24 y or younger.
–Current evidence is insufficient to assess the balance of benefits and harms of screening for chlamydia and gonorrhea in men.

Source
–USPSTF. *Screening for Chlamydia and Gonorrhea.* 2021.

SPEECH AND LANGUAGE DELAY

Screening: Children and Adolescents

Recommendations from

➢ AAFP 2015, USPSTF 2024

Guidelines Alert 16–8
GUIDELINES DISCORDANT: SCREENING FOR SPEECH AND LANGUAGE DELAY

AAFP, USPSTF	Evidence is insufficient to recommend for or against routine use of brief, formal screening instruments in primary care to detect speech and language delay in children up to age 5 y
AAP	Screen using validated test during well child checks at 9, 18, and 24/30 mo

Applying to Clinical Practice
- Fair evidence suggests that interventions can improve the results of short-term assessments of speech and language skills; however, no studies have assessed long-term outcomes.
- Studies have not fully addressed the potential harms of screening or interventions for speech and language delays, such as labeling, parental anxiety, or unnecessary evaluation and intervention.
- Screening is reasonable if effective interventions are available.

Practice Pearls

- In a study of 9000 toddlers in the Netherlands, 2-time screening for language delays reduced the number of children who required special education (2.7% vs. 3.7%) and reduced deficient language performance (8.8% vs. 9.7%) at age 8 y. (*Pediatrics*. 2007;120:1317)
- There is insufficient evidence to recommend a specific test, but parent-administered tools are best (eg, Communicative Development Inventory, Infant-Toddler Checklist, Language Development Survey, Ages and Stages Questionnaire).

Sources
–AAFP. *Clinical Recommendation: Speech and Language Delay*. 2015.
–*JAMA*.2024;331(4): 329–334.
–*Pediatrics*. 2015;136(2):e474–e481.
–*Pediatrics*. 2006;118(1):405.
–*Pediatrics*. 2015;136(2):e448.

SUICIDE RISK

Screening: Children and Adolescents

Recommendations from

> AAP 2016

–Ask questions about suicidal thoughts in routine history taking throughout adolescence.

Source
–Suicide and suicide attempts in adolescents. *Pediatrics*. 2016;138(1):e20161420.

THYROID DISEASE

Screening: Newborns

Recommendations from

> AAFP 2015, ATA 2020, AACE 2012, ASRM 2015, CTF 2019

–Screen all newborns for congenital hypothyroidism.

Sources
  –Advisory Committee on Heritable Disorders in Newborns and Children. 2015.
  –*Am Fam Phys.* 2015;91(11).
  –*Endocr Pract.* 2012;18(6):988.
  –*Ann Intern Med.* 2015;162(9):641–650.
  –*ASRM.* 2015;104(3):545–553.
  –*CMAJ.* 2019;191:E1274–E1280.
  –*Thyroid.* 2021;31(3):387–419.

TOBACCO USE

Screening: Children and Adolescents

Recommendations from

➤ USPSTF 2020

  –Provide interventions including education or brief counseling to prevent the initiation of tobacco use.

Practice Pearls

- The efficacy of counseling to prevent tobacco use in children and adolescents is uncertain.
- Screen for use of any tobacco product including but not limited to cigarettes, cigars, hookah tobacco, smokeless tobacco products, vapes, e-cigarettes, hookah pens, and other electronic nicotine delivery systems.

Source
  –USPSTF. *JAMA.* 2020;323(16):1590–1598.

TUBERCULOSIS, LATENT

Screening: Children and Adolescents

Recommendations from

➤ USPSTF 2023, CDC 2010

  –Screen by tuberculin skin test or interferon-gamma release assay (IGRA) if increased risk of tuberculosis. Frequency of testing is based on likelihood of further exposure to TB and level of confidence in the accuracy of the results.

Practice Pearls

- Risk factors include birth or residence in a country with increased TB prevalence and residence in a congregate setting (shelters, correctional facilities).
- Typically, a tuberculin skin test is used to screen for latent TB.
- Interferon-gamma release assay is preferred if:
  - Testing persons who have a low likelihood of returning to have their tuberculin skin test read.
  - Testing persons who have received a Bacille Calmette–Guérin vaccination.

Sources
–*JAMA*. 2023;329(17):1487–1494.
–*CDC MWWR*. 2010;59(RR-5).

VISUAL IMPAIRMENT

Screening: Children and Adolescents

Recommendations from

> USPSTF 2017

–Screen vision for all children of age 3–5 y at least once to detect amblyopia.
–There is insufficient evidence for vision screening in children < 3 y of age.

Practice Pearl

- May screen with a visual acuity test, a stereoacuity test, a cover–uncover test, and the Hirschberg light reflex test.

Sources
–USPSTF. *Vision Screening in Children Aged 6 Months to 5 Years*. 2017.
–*JAMA*. 2017;318(9):836–844.
–https://www.aao.org/education/clinical-statement/vision-screening-infants-children-2022

WOMEN'S HEALTH

ABNORMAL UTERINE BLEEDING

Management: Women, Reproductive Age

Recommendations from

> ACOG 2012, NICE 2018

Evaluation

–Classify bleeding using the PALM (structural) and COEIN (nonstructural) acronyms:

- Polyp.
- Adenomyosis.
- Leiomyoma.
- Malignancy and hyperplasia.
- Coagulopathy.
- Ovulatory dysfunction.
- Endometrial.
- Iatrogenic.
- Not yet classified.

–History: age of menarche, bleeding patterns, severity of bleeding, pain, medical/surgical history, medications, signs and symptoms of bleeding disorder, impact on quality of life.

–Physical: pelvic exam including external, bimanual, and speculum exam including Pap if needed.

–Labs: pregnancy test, CBC, TSH, chlamydia, and perhaps a coagulation panel and/or von Willebrand testing.

–Order transvaginal ultrasound (TVU) if there is an abnormal physical examination or if symptoms persist despite treatment.

–Perform endometrial biopsy in all patients older than 45 y and patients younger than 45 y with history of unopposed estrogen exposure (including obesity, PCOS), failed medical management, and persistent bleeding. Do not obtain ultrasound measurement of endometrial thickness to rule out malignancy.

Therapies

–Offer levonorgestrel IUD as first-line therapy for women with no identified pathology, fibroids < 3 cm, or suspected adenomyosis. (NICE)

–If levonorgestrel is not used, consider trial of therapies in patients without risk of endometrial hyperplasia, neoplasia, or structural abnormalities (ie, adolescents). Therapy options include NSAIDs, progestins, combination oral contraceptives, or tranexamic acid.

–Structural anatomical causes such as fibroids > 3 cm or polyps may require procedural intervention such as endometrial ablation, myomectomy, uterine artery embolization, or hysterectomy.

Sources
–*Obstet Gynecol.* 2012;120(1):197–206.
–www.nice.org.uk/guidance/ng88

BREAST CANCER

Screening: Women

Recommendations from

> **USPSTF 2024, ACS 2016, NCCN 2019, ACP 2019, ACOG 2017, WHO 2014, ACR 2023**
  –See below.

Guidelines Alert 17–1
GUIDELINES DISCORDANT: SCREENING AGE AND INTERVAL FOR BREAST CANCER SCREENING

	Consider Screening[a]	Screen Regularly	Screening Frequency	Stop Screening	Include Breast Exam?
USPSTF 2024		40–74 y	Every 2 y	Inconclusive data age > 75 y	Screen "with or without"
ACS 2016	40–44 y	≥45 y	Every year until 54 y, then every 1–2 y	Life expectancy < 10 y	"Do not use"
NCCN 2023		40–80 y	Every year	>80 y	Yes
ACP 2019	40–49 y	50–74 y	Every 2 y	≥75 y or life expectancy <10 y	"Should not use"
ACOG 2017	40–49 y	50–75 y	Every 1–2 y	>75 y with shared decision-making	"May be offered"
WHO 2014	40–49 only in well-resourced settings	50–75 y	Every 2 y	75 y	Only in low-resource settings

Applying to Clinical Practice
• Screening at 40 rather than 50 does increase overdiagnosis and unnecessary biopsies, but also reduces cancer-related deaths, particularly in marginalized groups such as Black women.
• Screening every 2 y seems to confer the same benefit as annual screening, with a somewhat lower burden of interventions.
• Screening every 2 y beginning at age 40 has become the standard of care. Patients who are at low risk and have a strong preference to avoid the risk of overdiagnosis/additional testing may opt to wait until age 45 or 50.

[a]Guidelines within this column make statements for this age group supporting an assessment of risk, often relying heavily upon family history, and eliciting patient preference to guide a discussion of risks and benefits to determine whether to screen.

Practice Pearls

- Harms and benefits of mammography screening:
  - *Benefits:* Based on fair evidence, screening mammography in women age 40–70 y decreases breast cancer mortality. The benefit is higher in older women (reduction in risk of death in women age 40–49 y = 15%–20%, 25%–30% in women age ≥ 50 y) but still remains controversial. (*BMJ.* 2014;348:366) (*Ann Intern Med.* 2009;151:727)
  - *Harms:* Based on solid evidence, screening mammography may lead to potential harm by overdiagnosis (indolent tumors that are not life threatening) and unnecessary biopsies for benign disease. It is estimated that 20%–25% of diagnosed breast cancers are indolent and unlikely to be clinically significant. (*CA Cancer J Clin.* 2012;62:5) (*Ann Intern Med.* 2012;156:491)
  - Clinical breast exam does not improve breast cancer mortality (*Br J Cancer.* 2003;88:1047) and increases the rate of false-positive biopsies. (*J Natl Cancer Inst.* 2002;94:1445)
  - Twenty-five percent of breast cancers diagnosed before age 40 y are attributable to *BRCA1* or *2* mutations.
  - The sensitivity of annual screening of young (age 30–49 y) high-risk women with magnetic resonance imaging (MRI) and mammography is superior to either alone, but MRI is associated with a significant increase in false-positives. (*Lancet.* 2005;365:1769) (*Lancet Oncol.* 2011;378:1804)
  - Computer-aided detection in screening mammography appears to reduce overall accuracy (by increasing false-positive rate), although it is more sensitive in women age < 50 y with dense breasts. (*N Engl J Med.* 2007;356:1399)
  - Digital mammography and film screen mammography have equal accuracy in women 50- to 79-y-old, but digital is more accurate in women 40- to 49-y-old. (*Ann Intern Med.* 2011;155:493)
  - It is estimated that 1.6 million breast biopsies are performed each year in the United States with the overwhelming majority having benign disease. (*JAMA.* 2015;313:1122)
  - Racial disparities in breast cancer outcomes persist.
- Continued controversy over screening:
  - The Canadian National Breast Screening study that began in 1980 found no survival benefit for mammography in 40- to 59-y-old women, but many experts in the United States consider the study to be flawed because of its design. (*BMJ.* 2014;348:g366) (*N Engl J Med.* 2014;370:1965)
  - A meta-analysis (*JAMA.* 2014;311:1327) found an overall reduction of 19% in breast cancer mortality (15% for women in their 40s and 32% for women in their 60s). They were concerned about overdiagnosis and other potential harms of screening including false-positive findings and unnecessary biopsies. (*N Engl J Med.* 2016;375:1438)
  - Recent trials have led to an increase in further screening studies based on the predicted individual risk of breast cancer occurrence. These also include a history of lobular carcinoma in situ, atypical hyperplasia, or history of breast cancer (invasive and DCIS). (*Ann Intern Med.* 2016;165:700, 737)

Sources

–https://uspreventiveservicestaskforce.org/uspstf/draft-recommendation/breast-cancer-screening-adults

–http://www.cancer.org

–*Ann Intern Med.* 2016;164:279.

–*Ann Intern Med.* 2019;170:547.

–*CA Cancer J Clin.* 2016;66:95.

–*JAMA.* doi:10.1001/jama.2024.5534

–*Obstet Gynecol.* 2017;130:241.

–https://www.who.int/cancer/publications/mammography_screening/en/

–Guidelines Version 1.2019. www.nccn.org

–Expert Panel on Breast Imaging: Mainiero MB, Moy L, et al. ACR appropriateness criteria® breast cancer screening. *J Am Coll Radiol.* 2017;14(11S):S383–S390. doi:10.1016/j.jacr.2017.08.044

Screening: Women, High Risk

Recommendations from

➤ ACS 2017, NCCN 2019

–Annual mammogram and MRI.

–Clinical encounter every 6–12 mo to begin when identified as being at increased risk; referral to genetic counseling if not already done.

Guidelines Alert 17–2 GUIDELINES DISCORDANT: WHEN TO START SCREENING FOR BREAST CANCER IN HIGH-RISK PATIENTS	
Recommendations from:	**Population**
ACS	Start at age 30 y
NCCN	Start 10 y prior to the youngest family member; not prior to 30 y for mammogram and 25 y for MRI

Applying to Clinical Practice
- While there are subtle differences in the age to start screening, the higher priority is identifying the patients for whom this recommendation applies.
- If family history (FH) for women in their 20s–30s suggests a high-risk feature, use a risk-calculating model (ie, Gail, BRCAPRO, Tyrer-Cuzic) to identify those with a >20% lifetime risk.

Practice Pearls

- ACS considers high risk to be one of the following: lifetime risk of breast cancer 20%–25% or greater (according to risk assessment tools), known as *BRCA1* or 2 mutation, first-degree relative (parent, brother, sister, or child) with a *BRCA1* or *BRCA2* gene mutation and unknown personal BRCA status, history of radiation therapy to the chest between the ages of 10 and 30 y, Li–Fraumeni syndrome, Cowden syndrome, or Bannayan–Riley–Ruvalcaba syndrome, or first-degree relatives with one of these syndromes.
- NCCN considers high risk to be a lifetime risk of breast cancer > 20% based on personal and FH and genetic predisposition (*BRCA1* or 2), PALB 2, CHEK 2 (http://www.cancer.gov/bcrisktool/).

- *BRCA2*-related breast cancer is more like sporadic BC with 75% of patients with hormonal receptor positivity and a significant decrease in aggressive growth. Ovarian cancer will develop in only 15% of *BRCA2* patients with the average time of onset being in the mid-50s.
- One in 40 Ashkenazi Jewish men and women carry a deleterious *BRCA1* or *2* gene (BRCA1 185del AG, 5382inse mutations, and BRCA2 6174delT mutation).
- Some experts believe all men and women of Ashkenazi descent should be tested for these 3 genes, even with no personal or FH of malignancy. (*N Engl J Med.* 2016;374:454)
- Risk-reducing bilateral mastectomy in *BRCA1* and *2* mutation carriers results in a 90% risk reduction in incidence of breast cancer and a 90% rate of satisfaction among patients who underwent risk-reducing surgery at 10-y follow-up. (*N Engl J Med.* 2001;345:159) (*JAMA.* 2010;304:967)

Sources

-*CA Cancer J Clin.* 2015;65:30.
-*N Engl J Med.* 2015;372:2353.
-*J Clin Oncol.* 2016;34:1882.
-*JAMA.* 2012;307:1394.
-*J Clin Oncol.* 2016;34:1840.
-*JAMA.* 2019;322:652.

Screening: Women, High Risk, Considering BRCA Testing

Recommendations from

> ### USPSTF 2019, NCCN 2023

–Use a risk assessment tool to establish risk for women with family or personal history of breast, ovarian, tubal, or peritoneal cancer or *BRCA1* or *2* gene mutation. (USPSTF)
–Suggested screening tools include:
- Ontario Family History Assessment Tool.
- Manchester Scoring System (https://jmg.bmj.com/content/42/7/e39).
- Referral Screening Tool (https://www.breastcancergenescreen.org/).
- Pedigree Assessment Tool.
- 7-Question Family History Screening Tool (https://pubmed.ncbi.nlm.nih.gov/19682358/).
- International Breast Cancer Intervention Study instrument (https://ibis.ikonopedia.com/).
- BRCAPRO.

–Refer for genetic counseling if risk is increased.
–Do not screen with a risk assessment tool in the absence of suggestive history.
–Screen patients without cancer who have an FH of a deleterious *BRCA1* and *2* gene mutation. (NCCN)
- Test only for the known mutation, not a full genetic evaluation.
- If strong FH but unable to test family member with cancer (not alive or unavailable to be tested) then do full genetic evaluation. A strong FH includes:
  ◦ Two primary breast cancers in a single close relative (first-, second-, and third-degree relatives).

○ Two breast cancer primaries on same side of family with at least 1 diagnosis occurring in a patient <50 y.
○ Ovarian cancer or male breast cancer at any age.
- Start screening 10 y prior to diagnosis of the youngest family member but not before age 30.
–Screen patients with breast, ovarian, pancreas, and prostate cancer who have one of the following conditions (NCCN):
- A known mutation in a cancer susceptibility gene within a family.
- Early age onset of breast cancer (<50 y).
- Triple negative (ER-PR-, HER2-) breast cancer diagnosed in <60-y-old.
- An individual of Ashkenazi Jewish descent with breast, ovarian, or pancreatic cancer at any age.
- Test all women with ovarian cancer (epithelial and nonmucinous) at any age for *BRCA1* and *2* mutations.

Prevention: Women, High Risk

Recommendations from

> NCCN 2023, USPSTF 2019

–If a woman is at high risk secondary to a strong FH or very early onset of breast or ovarian cancer, offer genetic counseling.
–Risk-reducing agents for high-risk patients: (NCCN)
- Discuss relative and absolute risk reducing with tamoxifen, raloxifene, or aromatase inhibitors.
- Treatment with tamoxifen for 5 y reduced breast CA risk by 40%–50%. (*Ann Intern Med.* 2013;159:698–718). Meta-analysis shows RR = 2.4 (95% confidence interval [CI], 1.5–4.0) for endometrial CA and 1.9 (95% CI, 1.4–2.6) for venous thromboembolic events.
- Raloxifene has similar effect and risk as tamoxifen, except no reduction in noninvasive tumor and no increased risk of endometrial CA or cataracts. (*Lancet.* 2013;381:1827)
- Aromatase inhibitor use as a prevention of breast cancer will reduce the risk of developing breast cancer by 3%–5% (*Lancet.* 2014;383:1041). Harmful effects include decreased bone mineral density and increased risk of fracture, hot flashes, increased falls, decreased cognitive function, fibromyalgia, and carpal tunnel syndrome but no life-threatening side effects.
–Contraindications to tamoxifen or raloxifene: history of deep vein thrombosis, pulmonary embolus, thrombotic stroke, transient ischemic attack, or known inherited clotting trait.
–Contraindications to tamoxifen, raloxifene, and aromatase inhibitors: current pregnancy or pregnancy potential without effective nonhormonal method of contraception. Common and serious adverse effects of tamoxifen, raloxifene, or aromatase inhibitors with emphasis on age-dependent risks.
–Risk-reducing surgery for high-risk patients (NCCN):
- Consider risk-reducing mastectomy only in women with a genetic mutation conferring a high risk for breast cancer, a compelling FH, or possibly with prior thoracic radiation therapy at <30 y of age.

- Reduces risk of breast cancer as much as 90%.
- Approximately 6% of high-risk women undergoing bilateral mastectomies were dissatisfied with their decision after 10 y. Regrets about mastectomy were less common among women who opted not to have breast reconstruction.
- If no compelling FH of breast cancer, the value of risk-reducing mastectomy in women with deleterious mutations in other genes associated with a 2-fold or greater risk for breast cancer (based on large epidemiologic studies) is unknown.
- Prophylactic salpingo-oophorectomy in *BRCA*-positive women decreases breast cancer incidence by up to 50%. Perform in *BRCA1* patients at 35 y of age and in *BRCA2* patients at >40 y.

–For women aged ≥35 y at increased risk for breast cancer and low risk for medication effects, prescribe tamoxifen, raloxifene, or aromatase inhibitors. Of these, only tamoxifen is used in premenopausal women. (USPSTF)

–No single risk tool is endorsed, but NCI Breast Cancer Risk Assessment Tool (bcrisktool.cancer.gov) and Breast Cancer Surveillance Consortium Risk Calculator (https://www.bcsc-research.org/index.php/tools) are noted to be modeled after US populations. (USPSTF)

–A 5-y risk of >3% may be considered "high risk." (USPSTF)

–Do not use these medications if risk is not increased. (USPSTF)

Sources
–*NCCN Guidelines Version 1: Breast Cancer Risk Reduction.* 2019. www.nccn.org
–*JAMA.* 2019;322:857.

CERVICAL CANCER

Screening: Women

Recommendations from

> ACOG 2021, ACS 2020, USPSTF 2018

–Do not screen patients older than 65 y who have had adequate prior screening with negative results (2 consecutive, negative primary human papillomavirus [HPV] tests, or 2 negative cotests, or 3 negative cytology tests within the past 10 y, with the most recent test occurring within the past 3–5 y).

–Do not screen those without a cervix and without a history of CIN2 or more severe diagnosis in the past 25 y.

Guidelines Alert 17–3	
GUIDELINES DISCORDANT: SCREENING FOR CERVICAL CANCER, AGE < 25 AT AVERAGE RISK	
Recommendations from:	**Guidance**
ACS	Do not screen
USPSTF, ACOG	Screen with cytology alone every 3 y in women aged 21–29

Applying to Clinical Practice
- Historically, guidelines have recommended screening at age 21 or onset of sexual activity.
- In the era of HPV vaccines <1% of cervical cancer occurs before age 25.
- Many abnormalities in this age group will regress spontaneously, and the patient-centered cost of more coloposcopies and biopsies, along with the attendant anxiety, does not bring an obvious mortality benefit.
- ACOG notes that access to HPV vaccine and hrHPV testing is not universal, and that raising the screening age to 25 may harm marginalized communities.
- Consider barriers to access in the local community when determining which screening age to adopt.

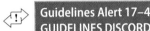

Guidelines Alert 17–4
GUIDELINES DISCORDANT: SCREENING FOR CERVICAL CANCER, AGE 25–65 AT AVERAGE RISK

Recommendations from:	Guidance
ACS	Screen with primary HPV test alone every 5 y
	Alternatively, consider screening with HPV and cytology "cotesting" every 5 y or cytology alone every 3 y
USPSTF, ACOG	Women aged 30–65 y: screen with cytology alone every 3 y, every 5 y with hrHPV testing alone, or every 5 y with cotesting

Applying to Clinical Practice
- HPV vaccination may be reducing the prevalence of cervical cancer.
- Cotesting vs. hrHPV alone: more precancerous lesions identified, more follow-up testing and cost, uncertain impact on outcomes.
- Stand-alone high-risk HPV testing may not be available in every practice setting.

Practice Pearls

- The United States is in a transition period moving from cytology to HPV testing, but cytology will continue to play a role in the near future, either alone or as part of cotesting, as practice patterns and access to primary HPV testing continue to evolve. (*CA Cancer J Clin.* 2020;70:321–346)
- Cervical CA is causally related to infection with HPV (almost all cases are caused by persistent infection with either HPV-16 or HPV-18 genotypes).
- Immunocompromised women (organ transplantation, chemotherapy, chronic steroid therapy, or HIV) should be tested twice during the first year after initiating screening and annually thereafter. (*CA Cancer J Clin.* 2011;61:8) (*Ann Intern Med.* 2011;155:698)
- Women aged <30 y with a history of cervical CA or in utero exposure to diethylstilbestrol (DES) should indefinitely continue average-risk screening protocol.
- HPV vaccination of young women is now widely recommended. The vaccine is effective at preventing invasive cervical cancer, especially when given before age 17. (*N Engl J Med.* 2020;383(14):1340–1348)

- Long-term use of oral contraceptives may increase the risk of cervical CA in women who test positive for cervical HPV DNA. (*Lancet.* 2002;359:1085)
- Smoking increases risk of cervical CA 4-fold. (*Am J Epidemiol.* 1990;131:945)
- *Benefits:* based on solid evidence, regular screening of appropriate women with the Pap test reduces mortality from cervical CA. Screening is effective when started at age 21.
- *Harms:* based on solid evidence, regular screening with the Pap test leads to additional diagnostic procedures and treatment for low-grade squamous intraepithelial lesions (LSILs), with uncertain long-term consequences on fertility and pregnancy. Harms are greatest for younger women, who have a higher prevalence of LSILs. LSILs often regress without treatment. False-positives in postmenopausal women are a result of mucosal atrophy. (NCI 2008)
- In a study of 43,000 women aged 29–61 with both HPV DNA and cervical cytology, cotesting every 5 y found that the cumulative incidence of cervical cancer in women negative for both tests at baseline was 0.01% at 9 y and 0.07% after 14 y. (*BMJ.* 2016;355:4924)
- The risk of developing invasive cervical CA is 3–10 times greater in women who have not been screened. (*CA Cancer J Clin.* 2017;67:106)

Sources
–http://www.cancer.org
–http://www.survivorshipguidelines.org
–*CA Cancer J Clin.* 2020:1–26.
–*N Engl J Med.* 2013;369:2324.
–https://www.uspreventiveservicestaskforce.org/Page/Document/RecommendationStatementFinal/cervical-cancer-screening2. 2018.
–https://www.acog.org/clinical/clinical-guidance/practice-advisory/articles/2021/04/updated-cervical-cancer-screening-guidelines

Screening: Women with HIV

Recommendations from

➤ CDC 2015

–Screen sexually active women with HIV at first visit and at least annually thereafter. Refer to Table 17–1 for details.

Prevention: Women and Girls

Recommendations from

➤ ACOG 2021, ACS 2020, USPSTF 2018

–Screen for and treat high-grade precancerous cervical lesions to prevent the progression to cervical cancer.
–Vaccinate girls and boys routinely with the HPV vaccine.

TABLE 17–1 CERVICAL CANCER SCREENING RECOMMENDATIONS

	American Cancer Society (ACS) 2020, American College of Obstetricians and Gynecologists (ACOG) 2021	US Preventive Services Task Force (USPSTF) 2018
When to start screening[a]	Age 25. Do not screen <25 y regardless of the age of onset of sexual activity or other risk factors	Age 21. Do not screen patients < 21 y[b]
Statement about annual screening	Women of any age should not be screened annually by any screening method	Individuals and clinicians can use the annual Pap test screening visit as an opportunity to discuss other health problems and preventive measures. Individuals, clinicians, and health systems should seek effective ways to facilitate the receipt of recommended preventive services at intervals that are beneficial to the patient. Efforts also should be made to ensure that individuals are able to seek care for additional health concerns as they present
Cytology (conventional or liquid based)[c]		
21–29 y of age	Not recommended <25 y	Every 3 y
30–65 y of age	Every 3 y[d]	Every 3 y (A recommendation)
HPV cotest (cytology + HPV test administered together)		
21–29 y of age	Start at age 25 y, primary HPV[e] test alone every 5 y (preferred) Cotesting every 5 y or cytology alone every 3 y are acceptable options	Recommend against HPV cotesting in women aged < 30 y
30–65 y of age	Primary HPV test alone every 5 y (preferred) Cotesting every 5 y or cytology alone every 3 y are acceptable options	For women who want to extend their screening interval, HPV cotesting every 5 y is an option

TABLE 17–1   CERVICAL CANCER SCREENING RECOMMENDATIONS *(continued)*

Primary hrHPV testing[f] (as an alternative to cotesting or cytology alone)[g]	For women aged 25–65 primary HPV testing every 5 y is the preferred screening strategy[h, i]	Every 5 y for women 30–65 y of age
When to stop screening	Individuals with a cervix who are >65 y, no history of CIN2+ within the past 25 y, and who have documented negative prior screening	Aged >65 y with adequate screening history[j] and are not otherwise at high risk for cervical cancer[k]
When to screen after age 65 y	Aged >65 y without documentation of prior screening should continue screening until criteria for cessation are met as noted above	Women aged >65 y who have never been screened, do not meet the criteria for adequate prior screening, or for whom the adequacy of prior screening cannot be accurately accessed or documented[l] Routine screening[m] should continue for at least 20 y after spontaneous regression or appropriate management of a high-grade precancerous lesion, even if this extends screening past age 65 y. Certain considerations may support screening in women aged >65 y who are otherwise considered high risk (such as women with a high-grade precancerous lesion or cervical cancer, women with in utero exposure to diethylstilbestrol, or women who are immunocompromised)
Screening posthysterectomy	Individuals without a cervix and without a history of CIN2 or a more severe diagnosis in the past 25 y or cervical cancer ever should not be screened	Recommend against screening in women who have had a hysterectomy (with removal of the cervix)[n]
Screening among those immunized with HPV vaccine	Women at any age with a history of HPV vaccination should be screened according to the age-specific recommendations for the general population	The possibility that vaccination might reduce the need for screening with cytology alone or in combination with HPV testing is not established. Given these uncertainties, women should continue to be screened regardless of vaccination status

TABLE 17–1   CERVICAL CANCER SCREENING RECOMMENDATIONS (continued)

HPV = human papillomavirus; CIN = cervical intraepithelial neoplasia; AIS = adenocarcinoma in situ; hrHPV = high-risk HPV.

[a]These recommendations do not address special, high-risk populations who may need more intensive or alternative screening. These special populations include women with a history of CIN2, CIN3, or cervical cancer, women who were exposed in utero to diethylstilbestrol, women who are infected with HIV, or women who are immunocompromised (such as those who have received solid organ transplants).

[b]Since cervical cancer is believed to be caused by sexually transmissible HPV infections, women who have not had sexual exposures (eg, virgins) are likely at low risk. Women aged >21 y who have not engaged in sexual intercourse may not need a Pap test depending on circumstances. The decision should be made at the discretion of the women and her physician. Women who have had sex with women are still at risk for cervical cancer. Ten to fifteen percent of woman aged 21–24 y in the United States report no vaginal intercourse (Saraiya M, Martinez G, Glaser K, et al. Obstet Gynecol. 2009;114(6):1213–1219. doi:10.1097/AOG.0b013e3181be3db4). Providers should also be aware of instances in which patients may have experienced nonconsensual sex.

[c]Conventional cytology and liquid-based cytology are equivalent regarding screening guidelines, and no distinction should be made by test when recommending next screening.

[d]There is insufficient evidence to support longer intervals in women aged 30–65 y, even with a screening history of negative cytology results.

[e]All ACOG references to HPV testing are for high-risk HPV testing only. Tests for low-risk HPV should not be performed.

[f]Primary hrHPV testing is defined as a stand-alone test for cervical cancer screening without concomitant cytology testing. It may be followed by other tests (like a Pap) for triage. This test specifically identifies HPV-16 and HPV-18, while concurrently detecting 12 other types of high-risk HPVs.

[g]Because of equivalent or superior effectiveness, primary hrHPV screening can be considered as an alternative to current US cytology-based cervical cancer screening methods. Cytology alone and cotesting remain the screening options specifically recommended in major guidelines.

[h]More experience and data analysis pertaining to the primary hrHPV screening will permit a more formal ACS evaluation.

[i]Primary hrHPV screening should begin 3 y after the last negative cytology and should not be performed only 1 or 2 y after a negative cytology result at 23–24 y of age.

[j]Adequate negative prior screening results are defined as 2 consecutive, negative primary HPV tests, or 2 negative cotests, or 3 negative cytology tests within the past 10 y, with the most recent test occurring within the past 3–5 y, depending on the test used.

[k]Once screening is discontinued, it should not resume for any reason, even if a woman reports having a new sexual partner.

[l]Women older than 65 y who have never been screened, women with limited access to care, women of color and women from countries where screening is not available may be less likely to meet the criteria for adequate prior screening.

[m]Routine screening is defined as screening every 5 y using cotesting (preferred) or every 3 y using cytology alone (acceptable).

[n]Unless the hysterectomy was done as a treatment for cervical precancer or cancer.

Practice Pearl

- Minimize risk factor exposure:
  - HPV infection[1]: abstinence from sexual activity; condom, and/or spermicide use (RR, 0.4), HPV vaccination per CDC schedule.
  - HPV-16/HPV-18 vaccination[2]: reduces incidence and persistent infections with efficacy of 91.6% (95% CI, 64.5–98.0) and 100% (95% CI, 45–100), respectively; duration of efficacy is not yet known; impact on long-term cervical CA rates is also unknown but likely to be significant. Two doses of vaccine if 9- to 14-y-old, 3 doses if 15- to 26-y-old. Shared decision-making for those aged 27–45 but strong focus on preteen vaccination due to minimal public health benefit at later ages. (*Lancet*. 2009;374:1975) (*N Engl J Med*. 2015;372:711, 775) (ACIP 2020). Also, will likely decrease the risk of other HPV-driven malignancies (oropharynx and anal CA).
  - Cigarette smoke (active or passive): increased risk of high-grade cervical intraepithelial neoplasia (CIN) or invasive cancer 2- to 3-fold among HPV-infected women.

[1] Methods to minimize risk of HPV infection include abstinence from sexual activity and the use of barrier contraceptives and/or spermicidal gel during sexual intercourse.

[2] On June 8, 2006, the US Food and Drug Administration announced approval of Gardasil, the first vaccine developed to prevent cervical CA, precancerous genital lesions, and genital warts caused by HPV types 6, 11, 16, and 18. The vaccine is approved for use in women age 9–26 y (http://www.fda.gov). A bivalent vaccine, Cervarix, is also Food and Drug Administration-approved with activity against HPV subtypes 16 and 18. (*N Engl J Med*. 2006;354:1109–1112)

- High parity: HPV-infected women with 7 or more full-term pregnancies have a 4-fold increased risk of squamous cell CA of the cervix compared with nulliparous women.
- Long-term use of oral contraceptives (>5 y): increases risk by 3-fold. Longer use related to even higher risk.

Sources

–https://www.uspreventiveservicestaskforce.org/Page/Document/RecommendationStatement Final/cervical-cancer-screening2. 2018.

–http://www.cancer.org

–https://www.acog.org/clinical/clinical-guidance/practice-advisory/articles/2021/04/ updated-cervical-cancer-screening-guidelines

CERVICAL CANCER, ABNORMAL PAP

Prevention: Women with Abnormal Cervical Cancer Screening Studies

Recommendations from

> **ASCCP 2019**

–Manage abnormal results by assessing the risk of CIN3 or higher grade lesion.

–Intervene if immediate CIN3+ risk is >4%.
  - 60%–100%: expedited treatment.[1]
  - 25%–59%: expedited treatment or colposcopy.
  - 4%–24%: colposcopy.

–If immediate CIN3+ risk <4%, choose surveillance interval based on 5-y CIN3+ risk.
  - >0.55%: return in 1 y.
  - 0.15%–0.54%: return in 3 y.
  - <0.15%: return in 5 y for routine screening interval.

–Follow-up intervals or treatment pathways are determined by Pap and HPV results as well as recent history (Tables 17–2 and 17–3).

–When performing colposcopy, obtain 2–4 targeted biopsies of acetowhite lesions.

–Obtain endocervical sample if unable to visualize the entire lesion or squamocolumnar junction.

–If low-risk (cytology < LSIL, no HPV-16/18, and no anomalies on colposcopy), do not obtain random nontargeted biopsies.

–If colposcopy with biopsy shows CIN1 or less, return in 1 y for Pap. Subsequent intervals described in Table 17–4.

–If colposcopy with biopsy shows CIN2, CIN3, AIS, or cancer, proceed to treatment.

Sources

–*J Low Genit Tract Dis.* 2020;24:102–131. https://pubmed.ncbi.nlm.nih.gov/32243307/

–*J Low Genit Tract Dis.* 2017;21:230–234. https://pubmed.ncbi.nlm.nih.gov/28953111/

---

[1] Expedited treatment: start therapy without obtaining colposcopic biopsy.

TABLE 17–2 RESPONSES TO ABNORMAL SCREENING RESULTS, PATIENTS AGED 25–65 WITHOUT PRIOR ANOMALIES[a]

Pap	HPV	Most Recent	Next Step
NILM[b]	Neg	None, HPV–, or Cotest–	Return 5 y
NILM	Pos or 16–/18+	None, HPV–, or Cotest–	Return 1 y
NILM	16+	HPV– or Cotest–	Return 1 y
NILM	16+	None	Colposcopy
LSIL[c]	Neg	Cotest–	Return 3 y
LSIL	Neg	None or HPV–	Return 1 y
LSIL	16–/18+	None, HPV–, or Cotest–	Return 1 y
LSIL	16+	None, HPV–, or Cotest–	Colposcopy
LSIL	Pos	None	Colposcopy
LSIL	Pos	HPV– or Cotest–	Return 1 y
High grade	16+ or 16–/18+	HPV– or Cotest–	Colposcopy
HSIL[d]+	Neg	HPV– or Cotest–	Colposcopy
HSIL+	Pos	HPV– or Cotest–	Treat[e] or Colposcopy
HSIL+	Neg, Pos, or 16–/18+	None	Treat or Colposcopy
HSIL+	16+	None	Treat
ASC-US[f]	Neg	None, HPV–, or Cotest–	Return 3 y
ASC-US	16+	None, HPV–, or Cotest–	Colposcopy
ASC-US	Pos	None	Colposcopy
ASC-US	Pos	HPV– or Cotest–	Return 1 y
ASC-US	16–/18+	None, HPV–, or Cotest–	Return 1 y
ASC-H[g]	Neg	None, HPV–, or Cotest–	Return 1 y
ASC-H	Pos or 16+	None	Treatment or Colposcopy
ASC-H	Pos	HPV– or Cotest-	Colposcopy
ASC-H	16–/18+	None	Colposcopy
AGC[h]	Neg	None, HPV–, or Cotest–	Return 1 y
AGC	Pos, 16+ or 16–/18+	None	Treatment or Colposcopy
AGC	Pos	HPV– or Cotest–	Colposcopy

[a]Abnormal screening results at https://cervixca.nlm.nih.gov/RiskTables/, accessed October 9, 2020.
[b]Negative for intraepithelial lesion or malignancy.
[c]Low-grade squamous intraepithelial lesion.
[d]High-grade squamous intraepithelial lesion.
[e]"Treat" refers to expedited treatment, proceeding to therapy without first obtaining a colposcopic biopsy.
[f]Atypical squamous cells of undetermined significance.
[g]Atypical squamous cells cannot exclude high-grade squamous intraepithelial lesion.
[h]Atypical glandular cells.

TABLE 17–3   RESPONSES TO ABNORMAL SCREENING RESULTS, PATIENTS AGED 25–65 WITH PRIOR ANOMALIES[a]

Pap	HPV	Most Recent	Prior 2	Next Step
NILM	Neg	HPV–/ASC-US		Return 5 y
NILM	Neg	NPV–/LSIL		Return 3 y
NILM	Neg	Cotest–	HPV+/NILM	Return 3 y
NILM	Neg	HPV+/NILM		Return 1 y
NILM	Pos	HPV– or Cotest–	HPV+/NILM	Return 1 y
NILM	Pos	HPV–/ASCUS or HPV–/LSIL		Return 1 y
NILM	16–/18+	HPV+/NILM		Return 1 y
NILM	Pos or 16+	HPV+/NILM		Colposcopy
LSIL	Neg	HPV–/ASC-US, HPV–/LSIL, or HPV+/NILM		Return 1 y
LSIL	Pos	HPV–/ASC-US		Return 1 y
LSIL	Pos	HPV–/ASC-US, HPV–/LSIL, or HPV+/NILM		Colposcopy
LSIL	16–/18+	HPV+/NILM		Return 1 y
LSIL	16+	HPV+/NILM		Colposcopy
High grade	Pos	HPV– or Cotest–	HPV+/NILM	Colposcopy
High grade	16–/18+ or 16+	HPV+/NILM		Treat or colposcopy
HSIL+	Neg	HPV–/LSIL		Return 5 y
HSIL+	Neg	HPV–/ASC-US		Colposcopy
HSIL+	Neg	HPV+/NILM		Treat or colposcopy
HSIL+	Pos	HPV–/ASC-US, HPV–/LSIL, or HPV+/NILM		Treat or colposcopy
ASC-US	Neg	HPV–/ASC-US, HPV–/LSIL, or HPV+/NILM		Return 1 y
ASC-US	Pos	HPV–/ASC-US		Return 1 y
ASC-US	Pos, 16–/18+, or 16+	HPV–/LSIL or HPV+NILM		Colposcopy
ASC-US, LSIL	Pos	HPV– or Cotest–	HPV+/NILM	Return 1 y
ASC-H	Neg	HPV–/LSIL		Return 5 y
ASC-H	Neg	HPV–/ASC-US		Colposcopy
ASC-H	Pos	HPV–/ASC-US or HPV+/NILM		Colposcopy
ASC-H	Pos	HPV–/LSIL		Treat or colposcopy
AGC	Neg	HPV–/ASC-US or HPV–/LSIL		Return 5 y
AGC	Neg	HPV+/NILM		Colposcopy
AGC	Pos	HPV–/ASC-US or HPV–/LSIL		Return 5 y
AGC	Pos	HPV+/NILM		Treat or colposcopy

[a]Surveillance following results not requiring immediate colposcopic referral, https://cervixca.nlm.nih.gov/RiskTables/, accessed October 9, 2020.

TABLE 17–4   MANAGEMENT OF RETURN CYTOLOGY AND HPV AFTER CIN < 2 COLPOSCOPY[a]

Initial Abnormality	Prior Postcolpo Result	Current Pap	Current HPV	Next Step
Low grade	None or HPV–	ALL	Neg	Return 3 y
Low grade	HPV– ×2	ALL	Neg	Return 5 y
Low grade	None	ASC-US/LSIL	Neg or Pos	Return 1 y
Low grade	Cotest–	ASC-US/LSIL	Neg	Return 3 y
Low grade	Cotest–	ASC-US/LSIL	Pos	Return 1 y
Low grade	HPV–/ASC-US/LSIL	ASC-US/LSIL	Neg	Return 1 y
Low grade	None or Cotest–	High grade	Neg or Pos	Colposcopy
Low grade	None or Cotest– or HPV–/ASC-US/LSIL	NILM	Neg	Return 3 y
Low grade	None or Cotest–	NILM	Pos	Return 1 y
Low grade	Cotest– ×2	NILM	Neg	Return 5 y
High grade		ALL	Neg	Return 1 y
High grade	HPV– (×1 or ×2)	ALL	Neg	Return 3 y
High grade		ASC-US/LSIL	Neg	Return 1 y
High grade		ASC-US/LSIL	Pos	Colposcopy
High grade	Cotest–	ASC-US/LSIL	Neg	Return 3 y
High grade	Cotest–	ASC-US/LSIL	Pos	Return 1 y
High grade		High grade	Neg	Colposcopy
High grade		High grade	Pos	Treat or colposcopy
High grade		NILM	Neg	Return 3 y
High grade		NILM	Pos	Colposcopy
High grade	Cotest– (×1 or ×2)	NILM	Neg	Return 3 y
High grade	Cotest–	NILM	Pos	Return 1 y

[a]Surveillance visit following colposcopy/biopsy finding less than CIN-2 (no treatment), https://cervixca.nlm.nih.gov/RiskTables/, accessed October 9, 2020.

ENDOMETRIAL CANCER

Screening: Women

Recommendations from

➢ ACS 2008

  –Do not screen postmenopausal women routinely.

  –Inform women about risks and symptoms of endometrial CA and strongly encourage them to report any unexpected bleeding or spotting. This is especially important for women with an increased risk of endometrial CA (history of unopposed estrogen therapy, tamoxifen therapy, late menopause, nulliparity, infertility or failure to ovulate, obesity, diabetes, or hypertension).

Practice Pearls

- *Benefits:* there is inadequate evidence that screening with endometrial sampling or TVU decreases mortality. *Harms:* based on solid evidence, screening with TVU will result in unnecessary additional exams because of low specificity. Based on solid evidence, endometrial biopsy may result in discomfort, bleeding, infection, and, rarely, uterine perforation. (NCI 2008)
- Presence of atypical glandular cells on Pap test from postmenopausal (age > 40 y) women not taking exogenous hormones is abnormal and requires further evaluation (TVU and endometrial biopsy). Pap test is not sensitive for endometrial screening.
- Endometrial thickness of <4 mm on TVU is associated with low risk of endometrial CA. (*Am J Obstet Gynecol.* 2001;184:70)
- Most cases of endometrial CA are diagnosed as a result of symptoms reported by patients (uterine bleeding), and a high proportion of these cases are diagnosed at an early stage and have high rates of cure. Type II endometrial CA accounts for 15% of patients. Histology is serous or clear cell. Five-year survival is 55% vs. 85% for endometrial Type I cancer. (NCI 2008) (*Lancet.* 2016;387:1094)
- Tamoxifen use for 5 y raises the risk of endometrial CA 2- to 3-fold, but CAs are low stage, low grade, with high cure rates. (*J Natl Cancer Inst.* 1998;90:1371)
- In 2022, there will be an estimated 65,950 new cases of endometrial cancer diagnosed with 12,550 deaths. The mean age at diagnosis is 60 y.

Source
–http://www.cancer.org

Prevention: Women

Recommendations from

➤ ACS 2008

–Evidence-based guidelines do not address prevention of endometrial cancer in average-risk women.

Practice Pearls

- Unopposed estrogen: a significant risk factor for the development of uterine cancer. Unopposed estrogen use in postmenopausal women for 5 or more years more than doubled the risk of endometrial CA compared to women who did not use estrogen. Other significant events from unopposed estrogen use include stroke (39% relative increase) and pulmonary embolus (34% relative increase). (*Lancet.* 2005;365:1543) (*JAMA.* 2004;291:1701)
- Combined estrogen and progesterone: use of oral contraceptives for 4 y reduces the risk of endometrial CA by 56%; 8 y, by 67%; and 12 y, by 72%, but will increase risk of breast cancer by 26%.
- Obesity: risk increases 1.59-fold for each 5 kg/m^2 change in body mass, but there is insufficient evidence to conclude that weight loss decreases incidence of endometrial cancer.

- Exercise: regular exercise (2 h/wk) with 38%–48% decrease in risk.
- Tamoxifen: use for >2 y has a 2.3- to 7.5-fold increased risk of endometrial CA (usually stage I—95% cure rate with surgery).
- Parity: nulliparous women have a 35% increased risk of endometrial CA. Breastfeeding also reduces risk.
- Endometrial hyperplasia and atypia: 50% go on to develop uterine cancer. Most often occurs in women over 50-y-old. (*Gynecol.* 1995;5:233)

Source
–http://www.cancer.org

INTIMATE PARTNER VIOLENCE

Screening: Women

Recommendations from

➤ USPSTF 2018
–Screen all women of reproductive age for intimate partner violence.
–If positive, offer ongoing support services.

Practice Pearl

- The HARK, HITS/E-HITS, PVS, and WAST are validated screening tools.

Source
–USPSTF. *JAMA.* 2018;320(16):1678-1687.

OVARIAN CANCER

Screening: Women

Recommendations from

➤ USPSTF 2018, ACOG 2017, ACS 2017, ACR 2010, AAFP 2017, NICE 2023, ACR 2023
–Do not routinely screen asymptomatic women at average risk.[1]
–Beware of symptoms of ovarian CA that can be present in early-stage disease (abdominal, pelvic, and back pain; bloating and change in bowel habits; urinary symptoms). (*Ann Intern Med.* 2012;157:900–904) (*J Clin Oncol.* 2005;23:7919) (*Ann Intern Med.* 2012;156:182)

---

[1] Lifetime risk of ovarian CA in a woman with no affected relatives is 1 in 70. If 1 first-degree relative has ovarian CA, lifetime risk is 5%. If 2 or more first-degree relatives have ovarian CA, lifetime risk is 7%. Women with 2 or more family members affected by ovarian cancer have a 3% chance of having a hereditary ovarian CA syndrome. If *BRCA1* mutation, lifetime risk of ovarian CA is 45%–50%; if *BRCA2* mutation, lifetime risk is 15%–20%. Lynch syndrome = 8%–10% lifetime risk of ovarian CA.

Practice Pearls

- Transvaginal ultrasound and CA-125 are useful to evaluate signs and symptoms of ovarian cancer.
- Risk factors: age > 60 y; low parity; personal history of endometrial, colon, or breast CA; FH of ovarian CA; and hereditary breast/ovarian CA syndrome. Use of oral contraceptives for 5 y decreases the risk of ovarian CA by 50%. (*JAMA.* 2004;291:2705)
- *Benefits:* there is inadequate evidence to determine whether routine screening for ovarian CA with serum markers such as CA-125 levels, TVU, or pelvic examinations would result in a decrease in mortality from ovarian CA.
- *Harms:* problems have been lack of specificity (positive predictive value) and need for invasive procedures to make a diagnosis. Based on solid evidence, routine screening for ovarian CA would result in many diagnostic laparoscopies and laparotomies for each ovarian CA found. (NCI 2008) (*JAMA.* 2011;305:2295)
- In addition, cancers found by screening have not consistently been found to be lower stage. (*Lancet Oncol.* 2009;10:327)
- A large United Kingdom trial assessing multimodal screening strategy (annual CA-125, risk of ovarian CA algorithm, TVU) vs. annual ultrasound vs. usual care: >200,000 women recruited (age 50–74) found no mortality reduction at average of 16 y F/U. (*Lancet.* 2021;397(10290):2182–2193)
- If a woman is newly diagnosed with ovarian cancer, she should be tested for *BRCA1* or *2* at any age—if positive, family members should be tested for that specific gene mutation and undergo genetic counseling.

Sources
  –*JAMA.* 2018;319(6):588–594.
  –*Obstet Gynecol.* 2017;130(3):e146–e149.
  –*CA Cancer J Clin.* 2017;67(2):100–121.
  –*Ultrasound Q.* 2010;26(4):219–223.
  –https://www.aafp.org/patient-care/clinical-recommendations/all/ovarian-cancer.html
  –Overview | Ovarian cancer: recognition and initial management | Guidance | NICE.

Screening: Women, High Risk Family History[1]

Recommendations from

> USPSTF 2013, NCCN 20122, ACOG 2017, NICE 2023
  –Do not routinely screen.
  –Refer for genetic counseling and evaluation for *BRCA* testing.

Practice Pearl

- Screening with CA-125, TVU, and pelvic exam has not been shown to improve survival rate.

---

[1] USPSTF recommends against routine referral for genetic counseling or routine *BRCA* testing of women whose family history is not associated with increased risk for deleterious mutation in *BRCA1* or *2* genes.

Sources
   –NCCN guideline version 1.2022. https://www.nccn.org
   –*Obstet Gynecol.* 2017;130:e110–126.
   –http://www.ahrq.gov/clinic/uspstf/uspsbrgen.htm

Prevention: Women, Known or Suspected *BRCA1* or *2* Mutations

Recommendations from

➤ ACOG 2009, NCCN 2022

   –Encourage patient to undergo risk-reducing salpingo-oophorectomy (RRSO) between age 35 and 40 and upon completion of childbearing.
   –If patient opts against risk-reducing salpingo-oophorectomy, consider screening with CA-125 and TVU at age 30–35 y.

Sources
   –NCCN guideline version 1.2022. https://www.nccn.org
   –http://www.ahrq.gov/clinic/uspstf/uspsbrgen.htm

Prevention

   –Evidence-based guidelines do not address prevention of ovarian cancer in average-risk women.

Practice Pearls

- Risk factors for ovarian cancer:
  - Postmenopausal use of unopposed estrogen replacement will lead to a 3.2-fold increased risk of ovarian cancer after >20 y of use.
  - Talc exposure and use of fertility drugs have inadequate data to show increased risk of ovarian cancer—remains controversial.
  - Obesity and height: elevated BMI including during adolescence associated with increased mortality from ovarian cancer. (*J Natl Cancer Inst.* 2003;95:1244). Taller women with higher risk of ovarian cancer. RR of ovarian cancer per 5 cm increase in height is 1.07.
- Approaches to reduce risk:
  - Oral contraceptives: 5%–10% reduction in ovarian cancer per year of use, up to 80% maximum risk reduction. Increased risk of deep venous thrombosis with oral contraceptive pill. The risk amounts to about 3 events per 10,000 women per year; increased breast CA risk among long-term oral contraceptive pill users of about 1 extra case per 100,000 women per year.
  - Tubal ligation decreases the risk of ovarian cancer (30% reduction).
  - Breastfeeding associated with an 8% decrease in ovarian cancer with every 5 mo of breastfeeding.

OVARIAN CANCER FOLLOW-UP CARE

Management: Women Treated Successfully for Ovarian Cancer (Stages I–IV)

Recommendations from

➤ NCCN 2020

   –Office visits every 2–4 mo for 2 y, then 3–6 mo for 3 y, then annually after 5 y.

–Physical exam including pelvic exam and measurement of CA-125 with each visit.

–Refer for genetic risk evaluation if not previously done.

–Chest/abdominal/pelvic CT, MRI, PET-CT, or PET as clinically indicated due to symptoms or rising CA-125.

Practice Pearls

- All patients with ovarian cancer should be screened for *BRCA1* and *2* mutations. Ovarian cancer will develop in 10% of patients with Lynch syndrome.
- Around 22,000 new cases of ovarian cancer are reported in the United States, with approximately 14,000 deaths; 5-y survival is related to stage:
  - Stage I: 92.6% alive at 5 y.
  - Stage II: 74.8%.
  - Stage III–IV: 30.2%.
- Seventy percent of patients receive an initial diagnosis of advanced ovarian cancer, usually stage III.
- Relapsed ovarian cancer is rarely curable, but sequential treatments and intraperitoneal chemotherapy have extended survival to 50–60 mo.

Sources

–https://www.nccn.org/professionals/physician_gls/pdf/ovarian/pdf

–https://www.journalofclinicalpathways.com/overview-updated-nccn-guidelines-ovarian-cancer

PELVIC EXAMINATIONS

Screening: Women

Recommendations from

> AAFP 2017, ACP 2014, USPSTF 2017, ACOG 2012

Guidelines Alert 17–5
GUIDELINES DISCORDANT: WHETHER TO PERFORM ROUTINE SCREENING PELVIC EXAMS IN ASYMPTOMATIC PATIENTS

Recommendations from:	Guidance
AAFP, ACP	Do not perform routine screening pelvic examinations
USPSTF	Insufficient evidence to recommend for or against
ACOG	Screen all women age 21+ with annual pelvic exam

Applying to Clinical Practice
- Tradition and patient or physician experience may support an annual exam.
- Outcome data do not support, though they also do not clearly refute the exam.
- Potential harms associated with screening include overdiagnosis, fear/anxiety/embarrassment, discomfort, and additional diagnostic procedures.
- Potential benefits include early detection of anomalies, normalization of an area of the body that is taboo for some, and increased clinician experience with an examination for when it is necessary diagnostically.

Practice Pearl

- Pelvic examination remains a necessary component of evaluation for many complaints.

Sources
–AAFP. *Clinical Recommendation: Screening Pelvic Exam.* 2017.
–*Ann Intern Med.* 2014;161(1):67–72.
–*JAMA.* 2017;317(9):947–953.
–*Obstet Gynecol.* 2012;120:421–424.

PELVIC FLOOR DYSFUNCTION

Prevention: Women

Recommendations from

> NICE 2022

–Raise awareness of pelvic floor dysfunction and educate patients.
–Modifiable risk factors include:
- BMI > 25.
- Smoking.
- Lack of exercise.
- Constipation.
- Diabetes.

–Nonmodifiable risk factors include:
- Age (risk increases with increasing age).
- Family history of urinary incontinence, overactive bladder, or fecal incontinence.
- Gynecological cancer and any treatments.
- Gynecological surgery (such as a hysterectomy).
- Fibromyalgia.
- Chronic respiratory disease and cough (chronic cough may increase the risk of fecal incontinence and flatus incontinence).
- Related to pregnancy: delivery after age 30, prior childbirth before current pregnancy.
- Related to labor: assisted vaginal birth (forceps or vacuum), occiput posterior birth position, second stage >1 h, anal sphincter injury.

–Prevent pelvic floor dysfunction by encouraging:
- Physical activity and healthy diet.
- Weight loss (if BMI > 30), smoking cessation, managing constipation, managing diabetes.
- Pelvic floor muscle training throughout patient's life.
- Pelvic floor muscle training during and after pregnancy.
- Three-month program of supervised training from week 20 of pregnancy if patient has first-degree relative with pelvic floor dysfunction OR patient had assisted vaginal birth, anal sphincter injury, or if baby's position is occiput posterior.

Source
  –NICE. *Pelvic Floor Dysfunction: Prevention and Non-Surgical Management.* 2022.

Management: Women

Recommendations from

➢ **NICE 2022**

–Recommend physical activity and healthy diet.

–Recommend weight loss (if BMI > 30), stopping smoking, managing constipation, managing diabetes.

–Recommend formal physical training.

–Offer bladder retraining.

–Consider intravaginal devices for urinary incontinence.

–Consider pessaries for symptomatic pelvic organ prolapse.

–Do not offer vaginal diazepam.

–Discuss psychological impact.

Source
  –NICE. *Pelvic Floor Dysfunction: Prevention and Non-Surgical Management.* 2022.

PELVIC PAIN, CHRONIC

Management: Women

Recommendations from

➢ **ACOG 2020**

Evaluation

–Include in the initial evaluation a thorough history and physical exam. Focus the history on chronology, triggers, treatments of pain, prior medical, surgical, and obstetric history, and psychosocial factors. Focus examination on abdominal and pelvic neuromusculoskeletal system. Palpate the lower back, sacroiliac joints, pubic symphysis, abdomen, and genitalia.

–Beyond the reproductive system, consider interstitial cystitis, irritable bowel syndrome, diverticulitis, and comorbid mood disorders.

Therapies

–Consider referral to pelvic floor physical therapy, sex therapy, and/or cognitive behavioral therapy when there is pelvic pain with dyspareunia.

–Prescribe serotonin-norepinephrine reuptake inhibitors (ie, duloxetine) if there is a neuropathic component to pain.

–Avoid opioid therapies.

–Consider referral to pain specialists.

–Consider acupuncture and yoga for pain relief.

–Do not routinely refer for laparoscopic lysis of abdominal adhesions.

Source
–*Obstet Gynecol.* 2020;135(3):e98–e109.

PELVIC PAIN, ACUTE

Management: Women

Recommendations from

➤ ACR 2023

Evaluation

–Premenopausal patients with acute pelvic pain. To image or not to image?
–Consider hemorrhagic ovarian cysts, pelvic inflammatory disease, ovarian torsion, ectopic pregnancy, spontaneous abortion, labor, and placental abruption.
–Beyond gynecologic system, must also consider appendicitis, IBD, infectious enteritis, diverticulitis, urinary tract calculi, pyelonephritis, and pelvic thrombophlebitis.

Imaging Considerations During Pregnancy

–US duplex doppler is the safest modality during pregnancy.
–MRI without contrast during pregnancy is also considered relatively safe.
–Caution with MRI with contrast as gadolinium-chelate molecules are excreted into amniotic fluid.
–Avoid radiation with CT scans.

Source
–Bhosale PR, Javitt MC, Atri M, et al. ACR Appropriateness Criteria® acute pelvic pain in the reproductive age group. *Ultrasound Q.* 2016;32(2):108–115.

VAGINITIS

Management: Women

Recommendations from

➤ ACOG 2020

–Assess with a complete history, physical exam of the vulva, and vagina and clinical testing of the discharge.
–See Table 17–5 for a guide to the clinical diagnosis of the most common etiologies.
–Treat bacterial vaginosis with metronidazole (oral or intravaginal) or intravaginal clindamycin.
–Treat trichomoniasis with oral metronidazole.
–Do not treat vaginitis without first performing an examination.

Practice Pearls

- Recommended dosing for bacterial vaginosis:
  - Metronidazole 500 mg PO BID ×7 d
  - Metronidazole 0.75% gel 1 applicator (5 g) intravaginally ×5 d
  - Clindamycin 2% cream 1 applicator (5 g) intravaginally ×7 d
- Recommended dosing for trichomoniasis: metronidazole 2 g PO ×1 or divided doses on same day.

TABLE 17–5 CLINICAL DIAGNOSIS OF VAGINITIS

Clinical Findings	Normal Discharge	Bacterial Vaginosis	Trichomoniasis	Vulvovaginal Candidiasis
Discharge	White, creamy, or clear	Thin, watery, white-gray; fishy odor	Yellow-green, frothy; odor	Normal or thick, white, curd-like
Other symptoms	None	None	None, or pruritus, irritation, dysuria	Pruritus, burning, dyspareunia, dysuria
Exam	Discharge adherent to walls	Discharge	Discharge; erythema and petechiae of vagina +/− cervix	Discharge; erythema and edema if severe
Microscopy	Mature squamous cells, rare PMNs Mostly lactobacilli	Clue cells (>20%) Positive KOH whiff test No PMNs Decreased/absent lactobacilli; increase cocci and small curved rods	Motile trichomonads Many PMNs Whiff test variable Bacilli and cocci	Branching/budding pseudohyphae (10×), spores (40×) on KOH prep. Rare PMNs Lactobacilli

Source
  –Obstet Gynecol. 2020;135(1):e1–e17.

VULVAR SKIN DISORDERS

Management: Women

Recommendations from

> **ACOG 2020**

–Consider in the differential diagnosis contact dermatitis, lichen simplex chronicus, lichen sclerosus, and lichen planus among other possible etiologies.

–Acute vulvar pruritus: rule out infectious causes (BV, trichomoniasis, candidiasis, molluscum, scabies) using exam and analysis including vaginal pH, saline and KOH preps, amine test, and consider fungal culture or evaluate for noninfectious conditions if the initial analysis is unrevealing.

–Chronic vulvar pruritus: consider dermatoses such as atopic dermatitis, contact dermatitis, lichen simplex chronicus, lichen sclerosus, psoriasis, neoplasia, and other systemic diseases. Biopsy if diagnosis is not immediately apparent, if concern for neoplasia, or if diagnosis is uncertain after treatment.

–Vulvar pain with pruritus: likely to be either lichen planus or genitourinary syndrome of menopause.

–Vulvar pain without pruritus: evaluate for other etiologies, then consider diagnosis of vulvodynia.

–Contact dermatitis: treat with avoidance of offending agents and education about proper vulvar care (avoid irritants, use mild soaps, cleanse vulva with water only, pat dry gently, emollient use, cotton/unscented/fragrance free menstrual pads, adequate lubrication for intercourse). Consider topical corticosteroid (once-twice daily until lesions heal) and oral antipruritics (antihistamines) as needed.

–Lichen simplex chronicus: treat with education about vulvar care and a medium- or high-potency corticosteroid.

–Lichen sclerosus: treat initially with medium- or high-potency corticosteroid (expert-recommended regimen: clobetasol 0.05% ointment qHS ×4 wk, then alternate nights ×4 wk, then twice weekly ×4 wk). Biopsy if persistent lesions or new growths. Transition to maintenance therapy with twice-weekly medium- or high-potency steroid to improve symptom control, adhesions and scarring, and vulvar cancer.

–Lichen planus: treat with high-potency steroid (twice daily initially, then taper). Consider topical calcineurin inhibitors if steroids fail.

Source
–*Obstet Gynecol.* 2020;136(1):e1–e14.

PREMENSTRUAL DISORDERS

Management: Women

Recommendations from

➤ ACOG 2023

–Recommend routine moderate exercise to help manage physical and affective premenstrual symptoms.

–Use NSAIDs for management of premenstrual pain symptoms.

–Use combined oral contraception for general premenstrual symptoms.

–Use SSRIs and cognitive behavioral therapy for affective symptoms.

–Consider gonadotropin-releasing hormone agonists with adjunctive combined hormonal add-back therapy for adults with severe, refractory premenstrual symptoms.

–Recommend calcium supplementation of 1000–1200 mg per day in adults and adequate calcium intake in to help adolescents manage physical and affective premenstrual symptoms.

–Reserve surgical management for adults with severe premenstrual symptoms only when medical management has failed.

Practice Pearls

- Up to 90% of reproductive-aged women report at least 1 premenstrual symptom, 20%–30% meet PNS criteria, 2%–5% report severe and disabling symptoms meeting diagnostic criteria for PMDD.
- Individuals with PMDD experience on average 3000 symptomatic days (3.8 y) worth of disabling days within their reproductive years.

- Premenstrual disorders are a diagnosis of exclusion. Requires thorough history and physical. Diagnosis based on retrospective patient report of symptoms. Recommend prospective symptom monitoring with journal, calendar, symptom logging.
- Premenstrual disorders are difficult to diagnose in adolescence as this is a period of emotional lability, wide emotional and mood variation, and lack of research in this age group.
- Important to provide patient education about premenstrual symptoms as well as self-coping strategies so patients know what to expect and how to holistically help their bodies.

Source

–Management of premenstrual disorders: ACOG clinical practice guideline No. 7. *Obstet Gynecol.* 2023;142(6):1516–1533. doi:10.1097/AOG.00-00000000005426

OLDER ADULTS

CARE DEPENDENCY

Screening: Older Adults

Recommendations from

> WHO 2019

–Screen older adults for declines in intrinsic capacity: cognitive decline, mobility limitations, malnutrition, visual impairment, hearing loss, and depressive symptoms. (Refer to appendix "WHO ICOPE Screening Tool" in Chapter 19.)

–Further evaluate and pursue care pathways for potential limitations.

Prevention: Older Adults

Recommendations from

> WHO 2019

–Mobility:

• If abnormal chair rise test (cannot rise from chair 5 times in 14 s without using arms), perform Short Physical Performance Battery.[1]

• If SPPB score is normal or mildly limited, consider a multimodal exercise program such as Vivifrail.[2]

• Optimize polypharmacy, osteoarthritis, osteoporosis, frailty, and pain.

–Environment: assess fall risk in physical environment, adapt home for fall prevention, consider assistive device, and identify safe space for walking.

–Nutrition: overcome barriers to good nutrition, encourage family and social dining, and arrange assistance with preparation of food.

–Vision: optimize hypertension, diabetes, and steroid use. Adapt home with lighting and contrasting colors to prevent falls and remove hazards from walking path.

---

[1] http://hdcs.fullerton.edu/csa/research/documents/sppbinstructions_scoresheet.pdf
[2] http://www.vivifrail.com/resources

–Hearing: if abnormal audiology, provide hearing age or refer to hearing specialist if severe or atypical (ear pain, drainage, dizziness, otitis media, unilateral). Provide emotional support and auditory aids for phone and doorbell.

–Depression: if depressive symptoms, offer cognitive behavioral therapy, multimodal exercise, and mindfulness practice. If significant depression, consider specialized care. Optimize polypharmacy, anemia, malnutrition, thyroid disease, and pain. Strengthen social support, minimize stressors, promote daily activities, and work against loneliness.

Source

–WHO. *Integrated Care for Older People (ICOPE): Guidance for Person-Centered Assessment and Pathways in Primary Care.* Geneva: World Health Recommendations from: 2019 (WHO/FWC/ALC/19.1).

DEMENTIA

Screening: Older Adults

Recommendations from

> USPSTF 2020, CTFPHC 2019, AAN 2021, ACR 2020

Guidelines Alert 18–1	
GUIDELINES DISCORDANT: ROUTINE SCREENING FOR COGNITIVE IMPAIRMENT	
Recommendations from:	**Guidance**
USPSTF	Insufficient evidence to recommend for or against routine screening for cognitive impairment or dementia
CTFPHC	Do not screen asymptomatic adults for cognitive impairment
AAN/Alzheimer Association	Assess for cognitive impairment only when a patient or close contact voices concern about memory or impaired cognition. Use a validated assessment tool. Do not dismiss the concern as normal aging.

Applying to Clinical Practice
• No guidelines support the routine screening of asymptomatic patients.
• When evaluating symptoms of potential cognitive impairment, use a standardized tool.

Practice Pearls

• False-positive rate for screening is high, and treatment interventions do not show consistent benefits.
• Early recognition of cognitive impairment allows clinicians to anticipate problems that patients may have in understanding and adhering to recommended therapy and help patients and their caregivers anticipate and plan for future problems related to progressive cognitive decline.
• Of patients with mild cognitive impairment (MCI), 6%–25% annually progress to dementia or Alzheimer disease.

- Good evidence supports use of MME, Memory Impairment Screen, and neuropsychological batteries.
- To meet Medicare Annual Wellness Visit requirement of screening for cognitive impairment, use a validated screening instrument rather than subjective report of memory concerns.
- Monitor MCI over time and recommend exercise.

Sources
–*Neurology*. 2018;90:126–135.
–*CMAJ*. 2016;188(1):37–46. http://www.cmaj.ca/content/188/1/37
–*JAMA*. 2020;323(8):757–763.

Prevention: Older Adults

Recommendations from

> ### WHO 2019

–Evaluate with tools such as Mini-Cog,[1] Montreal cognitive assessment,[2] mini-mental state examination,[3] or general practitioner assessment of cognition.[4]
–Optimize malnutrition, delirium, polypharmacy, cerebrovascular disease, and depressive symptoms.
–Prevent further decline with multimodal exercise and cognitive stimulation.
–Optimize smoking cessation, hypertension, and diabetes.
–Environment: assess need for social care, provide personal care and support with activities of daily living, give advice to maintain independent toileting, assess for caregiver burden, develop social care and support plan.
–Recommend physical activity to adults with normal cognition and with MCI.
–Recommend the Mediterranean diet to adults with normal cognition or MCI.
–Pursue tobacco cessation.
–If harmful alcohol use, pursue reduction in use.
–Manage hypertension and diabetes according to existing guidelines.
–Do not recommend vitamin B, E, polyunsaturated fatty acids, or multicomplex supplementation to prevent cognitive decline.
–There are insufficient data to recommend:
  - For or against social activity, but it has other connections to good health so should be encouraged.
  - Antidepressant medications to preserve cognition, though they may be otherwise indicated to treat depression.
  - Hearing aids to preserve cognition, though they may be otherwise indicated.

---

[1] http://mini-cog.com/wp-content/uploads/2015/12/Universal-Mini-Cog-Form-011916.pdf
[2] https://www.mocatest.org
[3] https://www.parinc.com/products/pkey/237
[4] http://gpcog.com.au/index/downloads

Practice Pearl

- The following may be considered, albeit with low- or very low-quality evidence:
    - Cognitive training for older adults with normal cognition or MCI.
    - Interventions for obesity midlife.
    - Manage dyslipidemia.

Sources

–WHO. *Risk Reduction of Cognitive Decline and Dementia: WHO Guidelines*. Geneva: World Health Organization; 2019.

–WHO. *Integrated Care for Older People (ICOPE): Guidance for Person-Centered Assessment and Pathways in Primary Care*. Geneva: World Health Organization; 2019 (WHO/FWC/ALC/19.1).

Management: Older Adults, Alzheimer Disease

Recommendations from

> ### NICE 2019, American Geriatric Society 2015

–At initial assessment take a history including cognitive, behavioral, and psychological symptoms and impact on daily life. Discuss advanced care planning early and ongoing.

–Consider donepezil, galantamine, and rivastigmine for mild-to-moderate Alzheimer disease.

–Consider memantine for moderate Alzheimer disease in patients who cannot tolerate acetylcholinesterase inhibitors, or in severe Alzheimer disease.

–Offer occupational therapy, group reminiscence therapy, and group cognitive stimulation in mild-to-moderate dementia.

–Do not offer ginseng, vitamin E supplements, acupuncture, or herbal formulations to treat dementia. Do not offer cognitive training to treat mild-to-moderate Alzheimer disease or interpersonal therapy to treat cognitive symptoms of mild-to-moderate disease.

–Antipsychotics: do not use as first line. Only use if acute agitations/hallucinations/delusions are causing severe stress or patient at risk of harm to self or others. Use the lowest effective dose and revisit need every 6 wk.

Practice Pearls

- Common adverse effects of acetylcholinesterase inhibitors include diarrhea, nausea, vomiting, muscle cramps, bradycardia, and insomnia.
- Common adverse effects of memantine are dizziness, headache, constipation, somnolence, and hypertension.
- Reassess the efficacy of the pharmacologic intervention. If the desired clinical effect (eg, stabilization of cognition) is not perceived by 12 wk or so, discontinue the medication. (AGS 2015)
- Ineffective medications include statins, NSAID, ginkgo, and omega-3 fatty acids. (AAFP 2017)
- Antipsychotics have limited and inconsistent benefit while posing risks including increased fall, strokes, mortality, oversedation, and cognitive worsening.
- Do *not* use feeding tubes for older adults with advanced dementia. Careful hand-feedings and tube-feedings have identical outcomes of death, aspiration pneumonia, functional status, and patient comfort. In addition, tube-feeding is associated with agitation, increased use of physical and chemical restraints, and worsening pressure ulcers. (*J Am Geriatr Soc.* 2014;62(8))

Source

–*NICE Guidance: Dementia: Assessment, Management and Support for People Living with Dementia and Their Carers.* NICE Guideline (NG97); 2019. www.nice.org.uk/guidance/qs184

Management: Older Adults, non-Alzheimer Dementia

Recommendations from

➤ NICE 2019

–Offer donepezil or rivastigmine in patients with mild-to-moderate dementia with Lewy bodies. Consider galantamine if donepezil/rivastigmine is not tolerated.

–Consider memantine for patient with Lewy bodies if AChE inhibitors are not tolerated or are contraindicated.

–Only consider AChE inhibitors or memantine for people with vascular dementia if they have suspected comorbid Alzheimer dementia, Parkinson disease dementia, or dementia with Lewy bodies.

–AChE inhibitors and memantine are not recommended for patients with frontotemporal dementia or cognitive impairment caused by multiple sclerosis.

Source

–*NICE Guidance: Dementia: Assessment, Management and Support for People Living with Dementia and Their Carers.* NICE Guideline (NG97); 2019. www.nice.org.uk/guidance/qs184

DRIVING RISK

Prevention : Older Adults

Recommendations from

➤ AAN 2019

–Assess patients with dementia for the following characteristics that place them at increased risk for unsafe driving (Clinical Dementia Rating Scale):

- Caregiver's assessment that the patient's driving ability is marginal or unsafe.
- History of traffic citations and motor vehicle collisions.
- Self-reported situational avoidance.
- Reduced driving mileage (<60 miles/wk).
- Mini-Mental Status Exam score ≤ 24.
- Aggression or impulsivity.
- Alcohol, medications, sleep disorders, visual impairment, motor impairment.

Sources

–*Neurology.* 2010;74(16):1316; Reaffirmed 2022.
–https://www.aan.com/Guidelines/home/GuidelineDetail/396

FALLS IN OLDER ADULTS

Screening: Older Adults

Recommendations from

> NICE 2020, AGS 2010, NFPCG/Public Health England 2017

–In persons > 65, ask yearly about falls.

Sources

–NICE. *Falls in Older People: Assessing Risk and Prevention.* 2013, published 2020.

–2010 AGS/BGS Clinical Practice Guideline: Prevention of Falls in Older Persons. http://www.americangeriatrics.org/files/documents/health_care_pros/Falls.Summary.Guide.pdf

–*Public Health England/National Falls Prevention Coordination Group.* 2017. Falls and Fracture Consensus Statement, Supporting Commissioning for Prevention.

Prevention: Older Adults

Recommendations from

> USPSTF 2018, Cochrane Database of Systematic Reviews 2012

–Do not give vitamin D supplementation to community-dwelling older adults for fall prevention who do not have vitamin D deficiency or osteoporosis.

–Recommend vitamin D supplementation to older adults in care facilities. This reduces the rate of falls by 37%.

–Recommend home-hazard modification (eg, adding nonslip tape to rugs and steps, provision of grab bars, etc.) for all homes of persons aged >65 y.

–Recommend exercise interventions to prevent falls including group and home-based programs as well as balance and strength training.

–Selectively offer a multifactorial assessment and management approach in community-dwelling older adults at increased risk for falls.

–Pursue cataract surgery if indicated, foot wear assessment with customized insoles and foot/ankle exercises in people with disabling foot pain, and pacemaker if carotid sinus hypersensitivity.

Practice Pearls

- Falls are the leading cause of fatal and nonfatal injuries among persons aged >65 y.
- A review and modification of chronic medications, including psychotropic medications, is important although not proven to reduce falls. Please refer to appendix "Vulnerable Seniors: Preventing Adverse Drug Events" in Chapter 19 for Beers List of potentially problematic medications.
- Public Health England (2017): older adults should aim for at least 150 min of moderate activity or 75 min of vigorous activity per week. Strength/balance training is recommended at least 2 d/wk. Extended sedentary periods should be minimized.

- Persons aged ≥65 y that are admitted to hospital should have a multifactorial assessment for fall risk.
- Individuals are at increased risk if they report at least 2 falls in the previous year, or 1 fall with injury. Risk factors: intrinsic: lower-extremity weakness, poor grip strength, balance disorders, functional and cognitive impairment, visual deficits. Extrinsic: polypharmacy (≥4 prescription medications), environment (poor lighting, loose carpets, lack of bathroom safety equipment).
- A fall prevention clinic appears to reduce the number of falls among the elderly. (*Am J Phys Med Rehabil*. 2006;85:882)
- Effective exercise interventions include supervised individual and group classes and physical therapy.
- Multifactorial interventions include initial assessment of modifiable fall risk factors (balance, vision, postural blood pressure, gait, medication, environment, cognition, psychological health) and interventions (nurses, clinicians, physical/occupational therapy, dietitian/nutritionist, CBT, education, medication management, urinary incontinence management, environmental modification, social/community resources, referral to specialist "ophthalmologist, neurologist, etc.").
- All who report a single fall should be observed as they stand up from a chair without using their arms, walk several paces, and return (see "Functional Assessment Screening in Older Adults," Chapter 19). Those demonstrating no difficulty or unsteadiness need no further assessment. Those who have difficulty or demonstrate unsteadiness, have ≥1 fall, or present for medical attention after a fall should have a fall evaluation.
- Free "Tip Sheet" for patients from AGS: http://www.healthinaging.org/public_education/falls_tips.php.
- Of US adults aged ≥65 y, 15.9% fell in the preceding 3 mo; of these, 31.3% sustained an injury that resulted in a doctor visit or restricted activity for at least 1 d. (*MMWR Morb Mortal Wkly Rep.* 2008;57(9):225)

Sources

–USPSTF. *Falls Prevention in Older Adults: Counseling and Preventive Medication.* 2018.
–Cochrane Collaborative. *Interventions for Preventing Falls in Older People in Care Facilities and Hospitals.* 2012; 2018.
–Public Health England. *Falls and Fracture Consensus Statement: Supporting Commissioning for Prevention.* 2012; 2017.

FAMILY VIOLENCE AND ABUSE

Screening: Older Adults

Recommendations from

> USPSTF 2018

–Insufficient evidence to recommend for or against routine screening of all older or vulnerable adults for abuse and neglect.

Practice Pearls

- All clinicians should be aware of physical and behavioral signs and symptoms associated with abuse and neglect, including burns, bruises, and repeated suspect trauma.
- CDC publishes a toolkit of assessment instruments: https://www.cdc.gov/violenceprevention/pdf/ipv/ipvandsvscreening.pdf

Source

–Screening for intimate partner violence, elder abuse, and abuse of vulnerable adults. *JAMA.* 2018;320(16):1678–1787.

HEARING LOSS

Screening: Older Adults

Recommendations from

➢ USPSTF 2021, UK NSC 2021, AAO-HNS 2024

Guidelines Alert 18–2 GUIDELINES DISCORDANT: SCREENING FOR HEARING LOSS IN ASYMPTOMATIC ADULTS AGED >50 Y	
Recommendations from:	**Recommendation**
USPSTF	Insufficient evidence to recommend for or against screening for hearing loss
UK NSC	Do not screen routinely
AAO-HNS	Screen all patients aged ≥ 50 y

Applying to Clinical Practice
- Refer for an audiology evaluation if patient or loved one has concern for hearing loss.
- Screening modalities range from clinical tests such as whispered voice to single questions (ie, "do you have difficulty hearing?") to formal questionnaires (ie, HHIE-S[a]); their accuracy is inconsistent.
- There is a significant preventable burden, including impairment of activities of daily living, and few potential harms, so a general screening strategy may be reasonable despite the absence of definitive evidence of benefit.

[a]https://www.uspreventiveservicestaskforce.org/Home/GetFileByID/231

Practice Pearl

- Increasing age is the most important risk factor for hearing loss.

Sources

–Screening for hearing loss in older adults. *JAMA.* 2021;325(12):1196–1201. doi:10.1001/jama.2021.2566
–https://view-health-screening-recommendations.service.gov.uk/hearing-loss-adult/
–*Audiol Today.* 2006;18(5):1–44.
–*Otolaryngology.* 2024;170(S2):S1–S54.

Management: Older Adults

Recommendations from

➤ NICE 2023, AAO-HNS 2024

–When a patient expresses concern, assess hearing difficulties, manage earwax, and refer adults for audiology assessments.

–Refer immediately for:

- Acquired unilateral hearing loss with ipsilateral altered sensation or facial droop.
- Otalgia and otorrhea in immunocompromised patients who have not responded to treatment within 72 h.

–Order MRI of internal auditory canal when there is hearing loss with localizing signs/symptoms (ie, facial nerve weakness) that suggest vestibular schwannoma or cerebellopontine angle lesion.

–Offer hearing aids, especially when hearing loss affects communication and/or environmental awareness.

–Counsel regarding strategies for communication partners (AAO-HNS):

- Face the person you are talking to on the same level (sitting vs. standing) in good lighting.
- Do not talk as you walk away or from another room.
- Speak clearly, slowly, distinctly, but naturally.
- Get the person's attention before starting to talk. This gives the listener a chance to focus attention.
- When communicating complicated information, avoid complex sentences.
- Keep your hands away from your face while talking.
- Minimize extraneous noise (TV, water running, other sound sources).
- If the message is not understood, rephrase rather than repeating.
- If time, date, or medication information is being provided, have the individual repeat the instructions.
- Provide important information and instructions in writing.
- Speakers should take turns speaking and not speak over each other.

–Reassess hearing at least every 3 y. (AAO-HNS)

Sources
–www.nice.org.uk/guidance/ng98
–*Otolaryngology.* 2024;170(S2):S1–S54.

HIP FRACTURES

Management: Older Adults

Recommendations from

➤ AAOS 2021

–Use preoperative pain control in patients with hip fractures including nerve blocks.
–Perform hip fracture surgery within 24–48 h of admission.

–Use VTE prophylaxis.

–Do not delay hip fracture surgery for patients on antiplatelet drugs.

–Perform operative fixation for nondisplaced femoral neck fractures.

–Arrange intensive physical therapy postdischarge to improve functional outcomes.

–Evaluate all patients who have sustained a hip fracture for osteoporosis.

–Do not routinely use traction preoperatively.

–Use a blood transfusion threshold of no higher than 8 g/dL. Consider tranexamic acid to reduce blood loss and need for transfusion.

Source

–https://www.aaos.org/hipfxcpg

HORMONE REPLACEMENT THERAPY TO PREVENT CHRONIC CONDITIONS

Prevention: Women, Postmenopausal

Recommendations from

> USPSTF 2022

–Do not use combined estrogen and progestin to prevent chronic conditions, including osteoporosis, coronary artery disease, breast cancer, and cognitive impairment.

–If history of hysterectomy, do not use estrogen to prevent chronic conditions, including osteoporosis, coronary artery disease, breast cancer, and cognitive impairment.

Source

–*JAMA.* 2017;318(22):2224–2233.

Practice Pearls

- This recommendation does not apply to women under the age of 50 y who have undergone a surgical menopause and require estrogen for hot flashes and vasomotor symptoms.
- The results of studies including the WHI and the Heart and Estrogen/Progestin Replacement Study reveal that hormone therapy (HT) reduces osteoporotic fractures; however, HT may lead to an increased risk of breast CA, stroke, cholecystitis, dementia, and venous thromboembolism, so the net benefit from HT is not favorable. HT does not decrease the risk of coronary artery disease or all-cause mortality.

Source

–*JAMA.* 2022;328(17):1740–1746. doi:10.1001/jama.2022.18625

OSTEOPOROSIS

Screening: Older Adults

Recommendations from

> USPSTF 2018, ACOG 2021, NAMS 2021, AACE 2020, BHOF 2022, Endocrine Society 2012, CTF 2023

–Screen for osteoporosis when indicated by age, sex, and risk factors.

Guidelines Alert 18-3	
GUIDELINES DISCORDANT: SCREENING STRATEGIES FOR OSTEOPOROSIS IN OLDER WOMEN	
Recommendations from:	**Guidance**
USPSTF, AACE, Endocrine Society, ACOG, NAMS, BHOF	For women aged ≥65 y, or younger women (age 50+) at increased risk,[a] measure bone mineral density using dual-energy X-ray absorptiometry (DXA) of the hip and lumbar spine and use it to calculate fracture risk
CTF	For women aged ≥65y, assess risk first using Fragility Fracture Decision Aid. If risk is sufficient to consider preventive medication, assess bone mineral density and recalculate the fracture risk

Applying to Clinical Practice
- Begin to consider osteoporosis risk factors at age 50 and screen early for high-risk patients.
- Screen most women when they reach age 65 unless low clinical risk.
- Canadian Fragility Fracture Decision Aid: https://frax.canadiantaskforce.ca/

[a]Several tools are available to assess osteoporosis risk: the Simple Calculated Osteoporosis Risk Estimation (SCORE), Osteoporosis Risk Assessment Instrument (ORAI), Osteoporosis Index of Risk (OSIRIS), and the Osteoporosis Self-Assessment Tool (OST).

Guidelines Alert 18–4	
GUIDELINES DISCORDANT: WHETHER TO SCREEN OLDER MEN FOR OSTEOPOROSIS	
Recommendations from:	**Guidance**
USPSTF	Insufficient evidence to recommend for or against routine osteoporosis screening
BHOF, ACPM, Endocrine Society	Age ≥ 70 y: screen routinely using bone mineral density (BMD) Age 50–69: consider screening men with risk factors
CTF	Age ≥ 70y, assess first using Fragility Fracture Decision Aid. Assess bone mineral density if moderate risk of fracture. Age 50–69: consider screening men with risk factors.

Applying to Clinical Practice
- Men over 70 or with predisposing conditions may be offered the opportunity for screening.

Practice Pearls

- USPSTF specifically defines "increased risk" as having a fracture risk equivalent to that of a 65-y-old White woman.
- The optimal screening interval is unclear, but should not be more frequent than every 2 y.
- ACOG: if FRAX score does not suggest treatment, DXA should be repeated every 15 y if T-score ≥ 1.5, every 5 y if T-score is −1.5 to −1.99, and annually if T-score is −2.0 to −2.49.
- Ten-year risk for osteoporotic fractures can be calculated for individuals by using the FRAX tool. (http://www.shef.ac.uk/FRAX/)
- Quantitative ultrasonography of the calcaneus predicts fractures of the femoral neck, hip, and spine as effectively as does DXA. May be used in reduced resource settings.
- The criteria for treatment of osteoporosis rely on DXA measurements.

Sources

–Screening for osteoporosis to prevent fractures. *JAMA*. 2018;318(24):2521–2531.

–*Osteoporosis*. Washington, DC: ACOG; 2012 (ACOG practice bulletin; no. 129).

–*Menopause*. 2021;28(9):973.

–*Endocr Pract*. 2020;26(suppl 1).

–*Osteoporos Int*. 2014;25(10):2359–2381.

–Osteoporosis in men: an Endocrine Society Clinical Practice Guideline. *J Clin Endocrinol Metab*. 2012;97(6):1802–1822.

–*JAMA*. 2018;319(15):1592–1599.

–*Osteoporos Int*. 2022;33:2049–2102.

–*CMAJ*. 2023;195:E639–E649.

Prevention: Older Adults

Recommendations from

➤ USPSTF 2018, ACPM 2009, ACOG 2021, NAMS 2021, AACE 2020, BHOF 2022, Endocrine Society 2012

–Screen for osteoporosis in women aged 65+ according to guidelines and intervene when indicated (see section "Osteoporosis" in this chapter for intervention guidelines).

Guidelines Alert 18–5 **GUIDELINES DISCORDANT: CALCIUM AND VITAMIN D SUPPLEMENTATION FOR PREVENTION OF OSTEOPOROTIC FRACTURES**	
Recommendations from:	**Guidance**
USPSTF	Insufficient evidence to recommend for or against routine vitamin D and/or calcium supplementation (though doses ≤400 IU vitamin D and ≤1000 mg calcium are definitively ineffective)
BHOF	Ensure intake of ≥1200 mg/d calcium after age 50 (or, ≥1000 mg/d for men aged 50–70) Monitor vitamin D levels and supplement as needed to maintain level 30–50 ng/mL

Applying to Clinical Practice
- Adequately powered studies are not available to determine whether a benefit exists to supplementing with calcium or vitamin D in the general population.
- Patients with osteoporosis should ensure adequate calcium and vitamin D intake per the BHOF guidance.
- Those without do not require supplementation unless vitamin D deficient or other comorbidities that would require it (ie, hyperparathyroidism).
- There is probably a small benefit to supplementing calcium and vitamin D in older adults undergoing long-term hospitalization or institutionalization.

Practice Pearls

- There is insufficient evidence for vitamin D and calcium supplementation for anyone for the primary prevention of fractures.
- These recommendations do not apply to individuals with history of osteoporotic fractures, increased risk for fall, diagnosis of osteoporosis, or vitamin D deficiency.

Sources

–Screening for osteoporosis to prevent fractures. *JAMA*. 2018;318(24):2521–2531.

–*Osteoporosis*. Washington, DC: ACOG; 2012 (ACOG practice bulletin; no. 129).

–*Menopause*. 2021;28(9):973.

–*Endocr Pract*. 2020;26(suppl 1).

–*Osteoporos Int*. 2014;25(10):2359–2381.

–Osteoporosis in men: an Endocrine Society Clinical Practice Guideline. *J Clin Endocrinol Metab*. 2012;97(6):1802–1822.

–*JAMA*. 2018;319(15):1592–1599.

–*Osteoporos Int*. 2022;33:2049–2102.

Management: Older Adults

Recommendations from

➤ BHOF 2022, ACOG 2022, ACP 2023, AACE 2020

Evaluation

–Diagnosis of osteoporosis is by fracture in adulthood or T-score (−2.5 or below), even if subsequent DXA T-score is above −2.5.

–To detect subclinical vertebral fractures, perform vertebral fracture imaging (X-ray or DXA vertebral fracture assessment) in the following:
- Women aged 65 y and older if T-score is less than or equal to −1.0 at the femoral neck.
- Women aged 70 y or older and men aged 80 y or older if T-score is less than or equal to −1.0 at the lumbar spine, total hip, or femoral neck.
- Men aged 70–79 y if T-score is less than or equal to −1.5 at the lumbar spine, total hip, or femoral neck.
- Postmenopausal women and men aged ≥50 y with the following specific risk factors: fracture(s) during adulthood (any cause), history height loss of ≥1.5 inches, prospective height loss of ≥0.8 inches, recent or ongoing long-term glucocorticoid treatment, diagnosis of hyperparathyroidism.

–Rule out secondary causes of bone loss, osteoporosis, and/or fractures.

Therapies

–Identify and address modifiable risk factors associated with falls, such as sedating medications, polypharmacy, hypotension, gait or vision disorders, and out-of-date prescription glasses.

–Counsel on smoking cessation and avoidance of excessive alcohol intake.

–Counsel on balance training, muscle-strengthening exercise, safe movement strategies to reduce falls and prevent fracture(s).

–In community-dwelling patients, refer for home fall hazard evaluation and remediation.

–Consider initiating pharmacologic treatment in postmenopausal women and men ≥ 50 y of age who have the following:
- Primary fracture prevention:
  - ○ T-score −2.5 or greater at the femoral neck, total hip, lumbar spine, 33% radius (some uncertainty with data) by DXA.
  - ○ Low bone mass (osteopenia: T-score between −1.0 and −2.5) at the femoral neck or total hip by DXA with a 10-y hip fracture risk ≥ 3% or a 10-y major osteoporosis-related fracture risk ≥ 20% based on the US-adapted FRAX model.
- Secondary fracture prevention:
  - ○ Fracture of the hip or vertebra regardless of BMD.
  - ○ Fracture of proximal humerus, pelvis, or distal forearm in persons with low bone mass (osteopenia: T-score between −1.0 and −2.5).

–Initiate antiresorptive therapy following discontinuation of denosumab, teriparatide, abaloparatide, or romosozumab.

–Current FDA-approved pharmacologic options for osteoporosis:
- Bisphosphonates (alendronate, ibandronate, risedronate, zoledronic acid). Prefer oral agents, with IV option available for those that cannot tolerate PO or have contraindications.
- Estrogen-related therapy (ET/HT, raloxifene-conjugated estrogens/bazedoxifene). Consider for postmenopausal patients at increased risk for fracture and breast cancer who have low venous thromboembolism risk and no vasomotor symptoms. (ACOG)
- Parathyroid hormone analogs (teriparatide, abaloparatide). Use for high-risk individuals with fracture or whose bone density worsens on bisphosphonates; limit use to 2 y and follow with another agent (bisphosphonate or RANK-ligand inhibitor). Daily injectable.
- RANK-ligand inhibitor (denosumab). Second-line option for high-risk individuals and individuals with fracture, who cannot use bisphosphonates, or who prefer the q6 mo in-office dosing.
- Sclerostin inhibitor (romosozumab). Consider use up to 1 y in women with very high fracture risk, low cardiovascular disease risk, who have not had success with other treatments.
- Calcitonin salmon.

Surveillance

–Investigate any broken bone in adulthood as suspicious for osteoporosis, regardless of cause.

–Measure height annually without shoes. Record history of falls.

–Consider repeating DEXA q1–3 y during treatment until findings are stable. (ACOG)

–Consider discontinuation of bisphosphonates to allow a drug holiday for low-to-moderate risk patients who are stable after 5 y of treatment with intravenous zoledronic acid. Consider longer treatment of up to 10 y for oral bisphosphonates or up to 6 y for intravenous zoledronic acid for patients at high risk for fracture.

Sources

–ACP. *Pharmacologic Treatment of Primary Osteoporosis or Low Bone Mass to Prevent Fractures in Adults: A Living Clinical Guideline from the American College of Physicians.* 2023.

–ACOG. *Clinical Practice Guideline: Management of Postmenopausal Osteoporosis.* 2022.

–AACE; Camacho PM, et al. American Association of Clinical Endocrinologist American College of Endocrinology Clinical Practice guidelines for the diagnosis and treatment of postmenopausal osteoporosis. *Endocr Pract.* 2020.

–The clinician's guide to prevention and treatment of osteoporosis. The Bone Health and Osteoporosis Foundation (BHOF) formerly NOF. *Osteopor Int.* 2022.

PALLIATIVE CARE

Management: Dying Adults

Recommendations from

> NICE 2017, NCCN 2020

–Care of the dying patient should be aligned with the patient's goals and wishes and cultural values.

–Give patients and people important to them opportunities to discuss, develop, and review an individualized care plan.

–Symptom management should address physical, emotional, social, and spiritual needs.

–Determine who should be the surrogate decision maker if they cannot make their own decisions.

–Establish if the patient has a preferred care setting.

–Medical management of symptoms:

• Pain is typically managed with opioids (see Table 18–1 for further ideas).

• Breathlessness can be managed with opioids or benzodiazepines +/– oxygen (if on chronic opiates, increase O_2 by 25%). Nonpharmacologic therapies include fans, cooler temperatures, stress management, relaxation therapy, and physical comfort measures.

• Manage nausea with dopamine antagonists or 5-HT_3 antagonists. May add benzodiazepines especially with anxiety component. If vertiginous components, add anticholinergics or antihistamines. Identify cause of nausea and treat that part of emetic pathway. Haloperidol, metoclopramide, and dexamethasone are options if nausea is refractory.

• Anxiety can be managed with benzodiazepines.

• Reduce or eliminate delirium causing agents such as steroids, anticholinergics, or benzodiazepines. Manage with antipsychotics.

• Manage secretions by reducing fluids (IV or PO), repositioning patient, and using pharmacologic agents such as scopolamine, atropine, or glycopyrrolate.

Practice Pearl

• Recognize and treat opioid-induced neurotoxicity, including myoclonus and hyperalgesia.

Sources

–NICE. 2015 Guideline; *Quality Standard. Care of Dying Adults in the Last Days of Life.* 2017.

–NCCN Guidelines Version 2. 2020 Palliative Care.

–WHO's cancer pain ladder for adults. who.int/cancer/palliative/painladder

TABLE 18–1 PALLIATIVE AND END-OF-LIFE CARE: PAIN MANAGEMENT	
Principles of Analgesic Use	
By the mouth	The oral route is the preferred route for analgesics, including morphine
By the clock	Persistent pain requires round-the-clock treatment to prevent further pain. As-needed (PRN) dosing is irrational and inhumane; it requires patients to experience pain before becoming eligible for relief. Relief is accomplished with long-acting delayed-release preparations (fentanyl patch, slow-release morphine, or oxycodone)
By the WHO ladder	If a maximum dose of medication fails to adequately relieve pain, move up the ladder, not laterally to a different drug in the same efficiency group. Severe pain requires immediate use of an opioid recommended for controlling severe pain, without progressing sequentially through Steps 1 and 2. When using a long-acting opioid, the dose for breakthrough pain should be 10% of the 24-h opioid dose (ie, if a patient is on 100 mg/d of an extended-release morphine preparation, their breakthrough dose is 10 mg of morphine or equivalent every 1–2 h until pain relief is achieved). Refer to appendix "WHO Pain Relief Ladder" in Chapter 19
Individualize treatment	The right dose of an analgesic is the dose that relieves pain with acceptable side effects for a specific patient
Monitor	Monitoring is required to ensure the benefits of treatment are maximized while adverse effects are minimized
Use adjuvant drugs	For example, a nonsteroidal anti-inflammatory drug (NSAID) is often helpful in controlling bone pain. Nonopioid analgesics, such as NSAIDs or acetaminophen, can be used at any step of the ladder. Adjuvant medications also can be used at any step to enhance pain relief or counteract the adverse effects of medications. Neuropathic pain should be treated with gabapentin, duloxetine, nortriptyline, or pregabalin. Moderate- to high-dose dexamethasone is effective as an adjunct to opioids in a pain crisis situation

Source: Adapted from *Pocket Guide to Hospice/Palliative Medicine.*

VISUAL IMPAIRMENT, GLAUCOMA, OR CATARACT

Screening: Older Adults

Recommendations from

➢ USPSTF 2022, ICSI 2014, AAO 2020

Guidelines Alert 18–6	
GUIDELINES DISCORDANT: WHETHER TO SCREEN FOR VISUAL IMPAIRMENT	
Recommendations from:	**Guidance**
USPSTF	Insufficient evidence to recommend for or against visual acuity screening or glaucoma screening in older adults

ICSI	Age ≥ 65 y: test vision objectively (Snellen chart)
AAO	Age ≥ 65 y: examination by an ophthalmologist every 1–2 y

Applying to Clinical Practice
• Evaluate vision when concerns are raised by patient or loved one.

Practice Pearls

- Adults with no signs or risk factors for eye disease should have a baseline comprehensive eye exam at age 40. Those with no signs or risk factors aged 40–54 should be examined by an ophthalmologist every 2–4 y, then every 1–3 y at age 55–64.
- Increase frequency for adults at risk for glaucoma (Black and Latino persons).
- Smoking is a risk factor for many ocular diseases—recommend smoking cessation.

Sources

–*JAMA*. doi:10.1001/jama.2022.7015

–ICSI. *Preventive Services for Adults*. 20th ed. 2014.

–AAO Policy Statement. *Frequency of Ocular Examinations*. 2020.

APPENDICES

ESTIMATE OF 10-Y CARDIAC RISK FOR MEN

ESTIMATE OF 10-Y CARDIAC RISK FOR MEN[a]					
Age (y)		**Points**			
20–34		−9			
35–39		−4			
40–44		0			
45–49		3			
50–54		6			
55–59		8			
60–64		10			
65–69		11			
70–74		12			
75–79		13			
Total Cholesterol	**Points**				
	Age 20–39	**Age 40–49**	**Age 50–59**	**Age 60–69**	**Age 70–79**
<160	0	0	0	0	0
160–199	4	3	2	1	0
200–239	7	5	3	1	0
240–279	9	6	4	2	1
≥280	11	8	5	3	1
Nonsmoker	0	0	0	0	0
Smoker	8	5	3	1	1
High-Density Lipoprotein (mg/dL)	**Points**				
≥60		−1			

ESTIMATE OF 10-Y CARDIAC RISK FOR MEN[a] (Continued)					
50–59		0			
40–49		1			
<40		2			
Systolic Blood Pressure (mmHg)		**If Untreated**		**If Treated**	
<120		0		0	
120–129		0		1	
130–139		1		2	
140–159		1		2	
≥160		2		3	
Point Total	**10-y Risk %**	**Point Total**	**10-y Risk %**		
<0	<1	9	5		
0	1	10	6		
1	1	11	8		
Age (y)		**Points**			
2	1	12	10		
3	1	13	12		
4	1	14	16		
5	2	15	20		
6	2	16	25		
7	3	≥17	≥30	**10-y Risk** _____ **%**	
8	4				

[a]Framingham point scores.

Source: U.S. Department of Health and Human Services, Public Health Service, National Institutes of Health, National Heart, Lung, and Blood Institute. NIH Publication No. 01-3305, 2001. https://www.nhlbi.nih.gov/files/docs/guidelines/atglance.pdf

ESTIMATE OF 10-Y CARDIAC RISK FOR WOMEN

ESTIMATE OF 10-Y CARDIAC RISK FOR WOMEN[a]					
Age (y)		**Points**			
20–34		−7			
35–39		−3			
40–44		0			
45–49		3			
50–54		6			
55–59		8			
60–64		10			
65–69		12			
70–74		14			
75–79		16			
Total Cholesterol		**Points**			
	Age 20–39	**Age 40–49**	**Age 50–59**	**Age 60–69**	**Age 70–79**
<160	0	0	0	0	0
160–199	4	3	2	1	1
200–239	8	6	4	2	1
240–279	11	8	5	3	2
≥280	13	10	7	4	2
Nonsmoker	0	0	0	0	0
Smoker	9	7	4	2	1
High-Density Lipoprotein (mg/dL)		**Points**			
≥60		−1			
50–59		0			
40–49		1			
<40		2			
Systolic Blood Pressure (mmHg)		**If Untreated**		**If Treated**	
<120		0		0	
120–129		1		3	
130–139		2		4	
140–159		3		5	
≥160		4		6	

ESTIMATE OF 10-Y CARDIAC RISK FOR WOMEN[a] *(Continued)*

Point Total	10-y Risk %	Point Total	10-y Risk %		
<9	<1	17	5		
9	1	18	6		
10	1	19	8		
11	1	20	11		
12	1	21	14		
13	2	22	17		
14	2	23	22		
15	3	24	27	**10-y Risk_____%**	
16	4	≥25	≥30		

[a]Framingham point scores.

Source: U.S. Department of Health and Human Services, Public Health Service, National Institutes of Health, National Heart, Lung, and Blood Institute. NIH Publication No. 01-3305, 2001. https://www.nhlbi.nih.gov/files/docs/guidelines/atglance.pdf

BODY MASS INDEX (BMI) CONVERSION TABLE

BODY MASS INDEX (BMI) CONVERSION TABLE			
Height in Inches (cm)	BMI 25	BMI 27	BMI 30
	Body weight in pounds (kg)		
58 (147.32)	119 (53.98)	129 (58.51)	143 (64.86)
59 (149.86)	124 (56.25)	133 (60.33)	148 (67.13)
60 (152.40)	128 (58.06)	138 (62.60)	153 (69.40)
61 (154.94)	132 (59.87)	143 (64.86)	158 (71.67)
62 (157.48)	136 (61.69)	147 (66.68)	164 (74.39)
63 (160.02)	141 (63.96)	152 (68.95)	169 (76.66)
64 (162.56)	145 (65.77)	157 (71.22)	174 (78.93)
65 (165.10)	150 (68.04)	162 (73.48)	180 (81.65)
66 (167.64)	155 (70.31)	167 (75.75)	186 (84.37)
67 (170.18)	159 (72.12)	172 (78.02)	191 (86.64)
68 (172.72)	164 (74.39)	177 (80.29)	197 (89.36)
69 (175.26)	169 (76.66)	182 (82.56)	203 (92.08)
70 (177.80)	174 (78.93)	188 (85.28)	207 (93.90)
71 (180.34)	179 (81.19)	193 (87.54)	215 (97.52)
72 (182.88)	184 (83.46)	199 (90.27)	221 (100.25)
73 (185.42)	189 (85.73)	204 (92.53)	227 (102.97)
74 (187.96)	194 (88.00)	210 (95.26)	233 (105.69)
75 (190.50)	200 (90.72)	216 (97.98)	240 (108.86)
76 (193.04)	205 (92.99)	221 (100.25)	246 (111.59)
Metric conversion formula = weight (kg)/height (m²)		Nonmetric conversion formula = [weight (lb)/height (in.²)] × 704.5	
Example of BMI calculation: A person who weighs 78.93 kg and is 177 cm tall has a BMI of 25: Weight (78.93 kg)/height (1.77 m²) = 25		Example of BMI calculation: A person who weighs 164 lb and is 68 in. (or 5'8") tall has a BMI of 25: [weight (164 lb)/height (68 in.²)] × 704.5 = 25	
BMI categories: Underweight = <18.5 Normal weight = 18.5–24.9 Overweight = 25–29.9 Obesity = ≥30			

Source: Adapted from NHLBI Obesity Guidelines in Adults. http://www.nhlbi.nih.gov/guidelines/obesity/bmi_tbl.htm, accessed October 13, 2011. BMI online calculator. http://www.nhlbisupport.com/bmi/bmicalc.htm, accessed October 13, 2011.

FUNCTIONAL ASSESSMENT SCREENING IN OLDER ADULTS

FUNCTIONAL ASSESSMENT SCREENING IN OLDER ADULTS			
Target Area	**Assessment Procedure**	**Abnormal Result**	**Suggested Intervention**
Vision	Inquire about vision changes, Snellen chart testing	Presence of vision changes; inability to read >20/40	Refer to ophthalmologist
Hearing	Whisper a short, easily answered question such as "What is your name?" in each ear while the examiner's face is out of direct view Use audioscope set at 40 dB; test using 1000 and 2000 Hz Brief hearing loss screener	Inability to answer question Inability to hear 1000 or 2000 Hz in both ears or inability to hear frequencies in either ear Brief hearing loss screen score ≥ 3	Examine auditory canals for cerumen and clean if necessary. Repeat test; if still abnormal in either ear, refer for audiometry and possible prosthesis
Balance and gait	Observe the patient after instructing as follows: "Rise from your chair, walk 10 ft, return, and sit down" Check orthostatic blood pressure and heart rate	Inability to complete task in 15 s	Performance-Oriented Mobility Assessment (POMA). Consider referral for physical therapy
Continence of urine	Ask, "Do you ever lose your urine and get wet?" If yes, then ask, "Have you lost urine on at least 6 separate days?"	"Yes" to both questions	Ascertain frequency and amount. Search for remediable causes, including local irritations, polyuric states, and medications. Consider urologic referral
Nutrition	Ask, "Without trying, have you lost 10 lb or more in the last 6 mo?" Weigh the patient. Measure height	"Yes" or weight is below acceptable range for height	Do appropriate medical evaluation
Mental status	Instruct as follows: "I am going to name three objects (pencil, truck, and book). I will ask you to repeat their names now and then again a few minutes from now"	Inability to recall all three objects after 1 min	Administer Folstein Mini-Mental State Examination. If score is <24, search for causes of cognitive impairment. Ascertain onset, duration, and fluctuation of overt symptoms. Review medications. Assess consciousness and affect. Do appropriate laboratory tests

FUNCTIONAL ASSESSMENT SCREENING IN OLDER ADULTS (Continued)

Depression	Ask, "Do you often feel sad or depressed?" or "How are your spirits?"	"Yes" or "Not very good, I guess"	Administer Geriatric Depression Scale or PHQ-9. If positive, check for antihypertensive, psychotropic, or other pertinent medications. Consider appropriate pharmacologic or psychiatric treatment
ADL-IADL[a]	Ask, "Can you get out of bed yourself?" "Can you dress yourself?" "Can you make your own meals?" "Can you do your own shopping?"	"No" to any question	Corroborate responses with patient's appearance; question family members if accuracy is uncertain. Determine reasons for the inability (motivation compared with physical limitation). Institute appropriate medical, social, or environmental interventions
Home environment	Ask, "Do you have trouble with stairs inside or outside of your home?" Ask about potential hazards inside the home with bathtubs, rugs, or lighting	"Yes"	Evaluate home safety and institute appropriate countermeasures
Social support	Ask, "Who would be able to help you in case of illness or emergency?"	–	List identified persons in the medical record. Become familiar with available resources for older adults in the community
Pain	Inquire about pain	Presence of pain	Pain inventory
Dentition	Oral examination	Poor dentition	Dentistry referral
Falls	Inquire about falls in past year and difficulty with walking or balance	Presence of falls or gait/balance problems	Falls evaluation

[a]Activities of Daily Living–Instrumental Activities of Daily Living.
Source: Modified from Fleming KC et al. Practical functional assessment of elderly persons: a primary-care approach. Mayo Clin Proc. 1995;70(9):890–910.

GERIATRIC DEPRESSION SCALE

GERIATRIC DEPRESSION SCALE	
Choose the best answer for how you felt over the past week	
1. Are you basically satisfied with your life?	Yes/No
2. Have you dropped many of your activities and interests?	Yes/No
3. Do you feel that your life is empty?	Yes/No
4. Do you often get bored?	Yes/No
5. Are you hopeful about the future?	Yes/No
6. Are you bothered by thoughts you can't get out of your head?	Yes/No
7. Are you in good spirits most of the time?	Yes/No
8. Are you afraid that something bad is going to happen to you?	Yes/No
9. Do you feel happy most of the time?	Yes/No
10. Do you often feel helpless?	Yes/No
11. Do you often get restless and fidgety?	Yes/No
12. Do you prefer to stay at home, rather than going out and doing new things?	Yes/No
13. Do you frequently worry about the future?	Yes/No
14. Do you feel you have more problems with memory than most?	Yes/No
15. Do you think it is wonderful to be alive now?	Yes/No
16. Do you often feel downhearted and blue?	Yes/No
17. Do you feel pretty worthless the way you are now?	Yes/No
18. Do you worry a lot about the past?	Yes/No
19. Do you find life very exciting?	Yes/No
20. Is it hard for you to get started on new projects?	Yes/No
21. Do you feel full of energy?	Yes/No
22. Do you feel that your situation is hopeless?	Yes/No
23. Do you think that most people are better off than you are?	Yes/No
24. Do you frequently get upset over little things?	Yes/No
25. Do you frequently feel like crying?	Yes/No
26. Do you have trouble concentrating?	Yes/No
27. Do you enjoy getting up in the morning?	Yes/No
28. Do you prefer to avoid social gatherings?	Yes/No
29. Is it easy for you to make decisions?	Yes/No
30. Is your mind as clear as it used to be?	Yes/No

One point for each is response suggestive of depression. (Specifically, "no" responses to questions 1, 5, 7, 9, 15, 19, 21, 27, 29, and 30, and "yes" responses to the remaining questions are suggestive of depression.)

A score of ≥15 yields a sensitivity of 80% and a specificity of 100%, as a screening test for geriatric depression. *Clin Gerontol*. 1982;1:37.

Source: Reproduced with permission from Yesavage JA et al. Development and validation of a geriatric depression screening scale: a preliminary report. *J Psychiatr Res*. 1982–1983;17:37.

IMMUNIZATION SCHEDULE

CDC VACCINE SCHEDULES FOR CHILDREN AND ADOLESCENTS

TABLE 1   RECOMMENDED CHILD AND ADOLESCENT IMMUNIZATION SCHEDULE FOR AGES 18 Y OR YOUNGER, UNITED STATES, 2024

Vaccines and Other Immunizing Agents in the Child and Adolescent Immunization Schedule*

Monoclonal antibody	Abbreviation(s)	Trade name(s)
Respiratory syncytial virus monoclonal antibody (Nirsevimab)	RSV-mAb	Beyfortus™

Vaccine	Abbreviation(s)	Trade name(s)
COVID-19	1vCOV-mRNA	Comirnaty*/Pfizer-BioNTech COVID-19 Vaccine Spikevax*/Moderna COVID-19 Vaccine
	1vCOV-aPS	Novavax COVID-19 Vaccine
Dengue vaccine	DEN4CYD	Dengvaxia*
Diphtheria, tetanus, and acellular pertussis vaccine	DTaP	Daptacel* Infanrix*
Haemophilus influenzae type b vaccine	Hib (PRP-T)	ActHIB* Hiberix*
	Hib (PRP-OMP)	PedvaxHIB*
Hepatitis A vaccine	HepA	Havrix* Vaqta*
Hepatitis B vaccine	HepB	Engerix-B* Recombivax HB*
Human papillomavirus vaccine	HPV	Gardasil 9*
Influenza vaccine (inactivated)	IIV4	Multiple
Influenza vaccine (live, attenuated)	LAIV4	FluMist* Quadrivalent
Measles, mumps, and rubella vaccine	MMR	M-M-R II* Priorix*
Meningococcal serogroups A, C, W, Y vaccine	MenACWY-CRM	Menveo*
	MenACWY-TT	MenQuadfi*
Meningococcal serogroup B vaccine	MenB-4C	Bexsero*
	MenB-FHbp	Trumenba*
Meningococcal serogroup A, B, C, W, Y vaccine	MenACWY-TT/MenB-FHbp	Penbraya™
Mpox vaccine	Mpox	Jynneos*
Pneumococcal conjugate vaccine	PCV15	Vaxneuvance™
	PCV20	Prevnar 20*
Pneumococcal polysaccharide vaccine	PPSV23	Pneumovax 23*
Poliovirus vaccine (inactivated)	IPV	Ipol*
Respiratory syncytial virus vaccine	RSV	Abrysvo™
Rotavirus vaccine	RV1	Rotarix*
	RV5	RotaTeq*
Tetanus, diphtheria, and acellular pertussis vaccine	Tdap	Adacel* Boostrix*
Tetanus and diphtheria vaccine	Td	Tenivac* Tdvax™
Varicella vaccine	VAR	Varivax*

Combination vaccines (use combination vaccines instead of separate injections when appropriate)		
DTaP, hepatitis B, and inactivated poliovirus vaccine	DTaP-HepB-IPV	Pediarix*
DTaP, inactivated poliovirus, and *Haemophilus influenzae* type b vaccine	DTaP-IPV/Hib	Pentacel*
DTaP and inactivated poliovirus vaccine	DTaP-IPV	Kinrix* Quadracel*
DTaP, inactivated poliovirus, *Haemophilus influenzae* type b, and hepatitis B vaccine	DTaP-IPV-Hib-HepB	Vaxelis*
Measles, mumps, rubella, and varicella vaccine	MMRV	ProQuad*

*Administer recommended vaccines if immunization history is incomplete or unknown. Do not restart or add doses to vaccine series for extended intervals between doses. When a vaccine is not administered at the recommended age, administer at a subsequent visit. The use of trade names is for identification purposes only and does not imply endorsement by the ACIP or CDC.

06/27/2024

How to use the child and adolescent immunization schedule

1 Determine recommended vaccine by age **(Table 1)**

2 Determine recommended interval for catch-up vaccination **(Table 2)**

3 Assess need for additional recommended vaccines by medical condition or other indication **(Table 3)**

4 Review vaccine types, frequencies, intervals, and considerations for special situations **(Notes)**

5 Review contraindications and precautions for vaccine types **(Appendix)**

6 Review new or updated ACIP guidance **(Addendum)**

Recommended by the Advisory Committee on Immunization Practices (www.cdc.gov/vaccines/acip) and approved by the Centers for Disease Control and Prevention (www.cdc.gov), American Academy of Pediatrics (www.aap.org), American Academy of Family Physicians (www.aafp.org), American College of Obstetricians and Gynecologists (www.acog.org), American College of Nurse-Midwives (www.midwife.org), American Academy of Physician Associates (www.aapa.org), and National Association of Pediatric Nurse Practitioners (www.napnap.org).

Report

* Suspected cases of reportable vaccine-preventable diseases or outbreaks to your state or local health department
* Clinically significant adverse events to the Vaccine Adverse Event Reporting System (VAERS) at www.vaers.hhs.gov or 800-822-7967

Questions or comments

Contact www.cdc.gov/cdc-info or 800-CDC-INFO (800-232-4636), in English or Spanish, 8 a.m.–8 p.m. ET, Monday through Friday, excluding holidays

 Download the CDC Vaccine Schedules app for providers at www.cdc.gov/vaccines/schedules/hcp/schedule-app.html

Helpful information

* Complete Advisory Committee on Immunization Practices (ACIP) recommendations: www.cdc.gov/vaccines/hcp/acip-recs/index.html
* ACIP Shared Clinical Decision-Making Recommendations: www.cdc.gov/vaccines/acip/acip-scdm-faqs.html
* *General Best Practice Guidelines for Immunization* (including contraindications and precautions): www.cdc.gov/vaccines/hcp/acip-recs/general-recs/index.html
* Vaccine information statements: www.cdc.gov/vaccines/hcp/vis/index.html
* Manual for the Surveillance of Vaccine-Preventable Diseases (including case identification and outbreak response): www.cdc.gov/vaccines/pubs/surv-manual

Scan QR code for access to online schedule

 CDC

U.S. Department of Health and Human Services Centers for Disease Control and Prevention

CS310020-D

These recommendations must be read with the notes that follow. For those who fall behind or start late, provide catch-up vaccination at the earliest opportunity as indicated by the green bars. To determine minimum intervals between doses, see the catch-up schedule (Table 2).

Vaccine and other immunizing agents	Birth	1 mo	2 mos	4 mos	6 mos	9 mos	12 mos	15 mos	18 mos	19–23 mos	2–3 yrs	4–6 yrs	7–10 yrs	11–12 yrs	13–15 yrs	16 yrs	17–18 yrs
Respiratory syncytial virus (RSV-mAb [Nirsevimab])	1 dose depending on maternal RSV vaccination status, See Notes				1 dose (8 through 19 months), See Notes												
Hepatitis B (HepB)	1st dose	◄— 2nd dose —►			◄——————— 3rd dose ———————►												
Rotavirus (RV): RV1 (2-dose series), RV5 (3-dose series)			1st dose	2nd dose	See Notes												
Diphtheria, tetanus, acellular pertussis (DTaP <7 yrs)			1st dose	2nd dose	3rd dose		◄——— 4th dose ———►					5th dose					
Haemophilus influenzae type b (Hib)			1st dose	2nd dose	See Notes		3rd or 4th dose, See Notes										
Pneumococcal conjugate (PCV15, PCV20)			1st dose	2nd dose	3rd dose		◄——— 4th dose ———►										
Inactivated poliovirus (IPV <18 yrs)			1st dose	2nd dose		◄——————— 3rd dose ———————►						4th dose					See Notes
COVID-19 (1vCOV-mRNA, 1vCOV-aPS)					1 or more doses of updated (2023–2024 Formula) vaccine (See Notes)												
Influenza (IIV4)					Annual vaccination 1 or 2 doses									Annual vaccination 1 dose only			
or Influenza (LAIV4)											Annual vaccination 1 or 2 doses		**or**	Annual vaccination 1 dose only			
Measles, mumps, rubella (MMR)					See Notes		◄——— 1st dose ———►					2nd dose					
Varicella (VAR)							◄——— 1st dose ———►					2nd dose					
Hepatitis A (HepA)					See Notes		2-dose series, See Notes										
Tetanus, diphtheria, acellular pertussis (Tdap ≥7 yrs)														1 dose			
Human papillomavirus (HPV)														See Notes			
Meningococcal (MenACWY-CRM ≥2 mos, MenACWY-TT ≥2years)					See Notes									1st dose		2nd dose	
Meningococcal B (MenB-4C, MenB-FHbp)															See Notes		
Respiratory syncytial virus vaccine (RSV [Abrysvo])														Seasonal administration during pregnancy, See Notes			
Dengue (DEN4CYD; 9-16 yrs)														Seropositive in endemic dengue areas (See Notes)			
Mpox																	

Range of recommended ages for all children   Range of recommended ages for catch-up vaccination   Range of recommended ages for certain high-risk groups   Recommended vaccination can begin in this age group   Recommended vaccination based on shared clinical decision-making   No recommendation/ not applicable

https://www.cdc.gov/vaccines/schedules/downloads/child/0-18yrs-child-combined-schedule.pdf

TABLE 2 RECOMMENDED CATCH-UP IMMUNIZATION SCHEDULE FOR CHILDREN AND ADOLESCENTS WHO START LATE OR WHO ARE MORE THAN 1 MO BEHIND, UNITED STATES, 2024

The table below provides catch-up schedules and minimum intervals between doses for children whose vaccinations have been delayed. A vaccine series does not need to be restarted, regardless of the time that has elapsed between doses. Use the section appropriate for the child's age. **Always use this table in conjunction with Table 1 and the Notes that follow.**

Vaccine	Minimum Age for Dose 1	Minimum Interval Between Doses			
		Dose 1 to Dose 2	Dose 2 to Dose 3	Dose 3 to Dose 4	Dose 4 to Dose 5
Children age 4 months through 6 years					
Hepatitis B	Birth	4 weeks	**8 weeks and at least 16 weeks after first dose** minimum age for the final dose is 24 weeks		
Rotavirus	6 weeks Maximum age for first dose is 14 weeks, 6 days.	4 weeks	4 weeks maximum age for final dose is 8 months, 0 days.		
Diphtheria, tetanus, and acellular pertussis	6 weeks	4 weeks	4 weeks	6 months	**6 months** A fifth dose is not necessary if the fourth dose was administered at age 4 years or older and at least 6 months after dose 3
Haemophilus influenzae type b	6 weeks	**No further doses needed** if first dose was administered at age 15 months or older. **4 weeks** if first dose was administered before the 1st birthday. **8 weeks (as final dose)** if first dose was administered at age 12 through 14 months.	**No further doses needed** if previous dose was administered at age 15 months or older **4 weeks** if current age is younger than 12 months and first dose was administered at younger than age 7 months and at least 1 previous dose was PRP-T (ActHIB®, Pentacel®, Hiberix®, Vaxelis®) or unknown **8 weeks and age 12 through 59 months (as final dose)** if current age is younger than 12 months and first dose was administered at age 7 through 11 months; OR if current age is 12 through 59 months and first dose was administered before the 1st birthday and second dose was administered at younger than 15 months; OR if both doses were PedvaxHIB® and were administered before the 1st birthday	**8 weeks (as final dose)** This dose only necessary for children age 12 through 59 months who received 3 doses before the 1st birthday.	
Pneumococcal conjugate	6 weeks	**No further doses needed** for healthy children if first dose was administered at age 24 months or older **4 weeks** if first dose was administered before the 1st birthday **8 weeks (as final dose for healthy children)** if first dose was administered at the 1st birthday or after	**No further doses needed** for healthy children if previous dose was administered at age 24 months or older **4 weeks** if current age is younger than 12 months and previous dose was administered at <7 months old **8 weeks (as final dose for healthy children)** if previous dose was administered between 7–11 months (wait until at least 12 months old); OR if current age is 12 months or older and at least 1 dose was administered before age 12 months	**8 weeks (as final dose)** This dose is only necessary for children age 12 through 59 months regardless of risk, or age 60 through 71 months with any risk, who received 3 doses before age 12 months.	
Inactivated poliovirus	6 weeks	4 weeks	**4 weeks** if current age is <4 years **6 months (as final dose)** if current age is 4 years or older	6 months (minimum age 4 years for final dose)	
Measles, mumps, rubella	12 months	4 weeks			
Varicella	12 months	3 months			
Hepatitis A	12 months	6 months			
Meningococcal ACWY	2 months MenACWY-CRM 2 years MenACWY-TT	8 weeks	See Notes	See Notes	
Children and adolescents age 7 through 18 years					
Meningococcal ACWY	Not applicable (N/A)	8 weeks			
Tetanus, diphtheria; tetanus, diphtheria, and acellular pertussis	7 years	4 weeks	**4 weeks** if first dose of DTaP/DT was administered before the 1st birthday **6 months (as final dose)** if first dose of DTaP/DT or Tdap/Td was administered at or after the 1st birthday	**6 months** if first dose of DTaP/DT was administered before the 1st birthday	
Human papillomavirus	9 years	Routine dosing intervals are recommended.			
Hepatitis A	N/A	6 months			
Hepatitis B	N/A	4 weeks	**8 weeks and at least 16 weeks after first dose**		
Inactivated poliovirus	N/A	4 weeks	**6 months** A fourth dose is not necessary if the third dose was administered at age 4 years or older and at least 6 months after the previous dose.	A fourth dose of IPV is indicated if all previous doses were administered at <4 years OR if the third dose was administered <6 months after the second dose.	
Measles, mumps, rubella	N/A	4 weeks			
Varicella	N/A	3 months if younger than age 13 years. 4 weeks if age 13 years or older			
Dengue	9 years	6 months	6 months		

TABLE 3 RECOMMENDED CHILD AND ADOLESCENT IMMUNIZATION SCHEDULE BY MEDICAL INDICATIONS, UNITED STATES, 2024

Always use this table in conjunction with Table 1 and the Notes that follow. Medical conditions are often not mutually exclusive. If multiple conditions are present, refer to guidance in all relevant columns. See Notes for medical conditions not listed.

Vaccine and other immunizing agents	Pregnancy	Immunocompromised (excluding HIV infection)	HIV infection CD4 percentage and count[a] <15% or <200mm	HIV infection CD4 percentage and count[a] ≥15% and ≥200mm	CSF leak or cochlear implant	Asplenia or persistent complement deficiencies	Heart disease or chronic lung disease	Kidney failure, End-stage renal disease or on Dialysis	Chronic liver disease	Diabetes
RSV-mAb (nirsevimab)		2nd RSV season	1 dose depending on maternal RSV vaccination status, See Notes							
Hepatitis B										
Rotavirus		SCID[b]								
DTaP/Tdap	DTaP / Tdap: 1 dose each pregnancy									
Hib		HSCT: 3 doses	See Notes			See Notes				
Pneumococcal										
IPV			See Notes							
COVID-19		See Notes								
IIV4										
LAIV4							Asthma, wheezing: 2–4 years[c]			
MMR	*									
VAR	*									
Hepatitis A										
HPV	*	3 dose series, See Notes								
MenACWY										
MenB										
RSV (Abrysvo)	Seasonal administration, See Notes						2nd RSV season for chronic lung disease (See Notes)	1 dose depending on maternal RSV vaccination status, See Notes		
Dengue										
Mpox	See Notes									

Legend

- Recommended for all age-eligible children who lack documentation of a complete vaccination series
- Recommended for all children, but is recommended for some children based on increased risk for or severe outcomes from disease
- Recommended for all age-eligible children, and additional doses may be necessary based on medical condition or other indications. See Notes.
- Precaution: Might be indicated if benefit of protection outweighs risk of adverse reaction
- Contraindicated or not recommended *Vaccinate after pregnancy, if indicated
- No Guidance/ Not Applicable

a. For additional information regarding HIV laboratory parameters and use of live vaccines, see the General Best Practice Guidelines for Immunization, "Altered Immunocompetence," at www.cdc.gov/vaccines/hcp/acip-recs/general-recs/immunocompetence.html and Table 4-1 (footnote J) at www.cdc.gov/vaccines/hcp/acip-recs/general-recs/contraindications.html.

b. Severe Combined Immunodeficiency

c. LAIV4 contraindicated for children 2–4 years of age with asthma or wheezing during the preceding 12 months

Notes | Recommended Child and Adolescent Immunization Schedule for Ages 18 Years or Younger, United States, 2024

For vaccination recommendations for persons ages 19 years or older, see the Recommended Adult Immunization Schedule, 2024.

Additional information

- For calculating intervals between doses, 4 weeks = 28 days. Intervals of ≥4 months are determined by calendar months.
- Within a number range (e.g., 12–18), a dash (–) should be read as "through."
- Vaccine doses administered ≤4 days before the minimum age or interval are considered valid. Doses of any vaccine administered ≥5 days earlier than the minimum age or minimum interval should not be counted as valid and should be repeated as age appropriate. **The repeat dose should be spaced after the invalid dose by the recommended minimum interval.** For further details, see Table 3-2, Recommended and minimum ages and intervals between vaccine doses, in *General Best Practice Guidelines for Immunization* at www.cdc.gov/vaccines/hcp/acip-recs/general-recs/timing.html.
- Information on travel vaccination requirements and recommendations is available at www.cdc.gov/travel/.
- For vaccination of persons with immunodeficiencies, see Table 8-1, Vaccination of persons with primary and secondary immunodeficiencies, in *General Best Practice Guidelines for Immunization* at www.cdc.gov/vaccines/hcp/acip-recs/general-recs/immunocompetence.html, and Immunization in Special Clinical Circumstances (In: Kimberlin DW, Barnett ED, Lynfield Ruth, Sawyer MH, eds. Red Book: 2021–2024 Report of the Committee on Infectious Diseases. 32nd ed. Itasca, IL: American Academy of Pediatrics; 2021:72–86).
- For information about vaccination in the setting of a vaccine-preventable disease outbreak, contact your state or local health department.
- The National Vaccine Injury Compensation Program (VICP) is a no-fault alternative to the traditional legal system for resolving vaccine injury claims. All vaccines included in the child and adolescent vaccine schedule are covered by VICP except dengue, PPSV23, RSV, Mpox and COVID-19 vaccines. Mpox and COVID-19 vaccines are covered by the Countermeasures Injury Compensation Program (CICP). For more information, see www.hrsa.gov/vaccinecompensation or www.hrsa.gov/cicp.

COVID-19 vaccination

(minimum age: 6 months [Moderna and Pfizer-BioNTech COVID-19 vaccines], 12 years [Novavax COVID-19 Vaccine])

Routine vaccination

Age 6 months–4 years

- **Unvaccinated:**
  - 2-dose series of updated (2023–2024 Formula) Moderna at 0, 4-8 weeks
  - 3-dose series of updated (2023–2024 Formula) Pfizer-BioNTech at 0, 3-8, 11-16 weeks
- **Previously vaccinated* with 1 dose of any Moderna:** 1 dose of updated (2023–2024 Formula) Moderna 4-8 weeks after the most recent dose.
- **Previously vaccinated* with 2 or more doses of any Moderna:** 1 dose of updated (2023–2024 Formula) Moderna at least 8 weeks after the most recent dose.
- **Previously vaccinated* with 1 dose of any Pfizer-BioNTech:** 2-dose series of updated (2023–2024 Formula) Pfizer-BioNTech at 0, 8 weeks (minimum interval between previous Pfizer-BioNTech and dose 1:3-8 weeks).
- **Previously vaccinated* with 2 or more doses of any Pfizer-BioNTech:** 1 dose of updated (2023–2024 Formula) Pfizer-BioNTech at least 8 weeks after the most recent dose.

Age 5–11 years

- **Unvaccinated:** 1 dose of updated (2023–2024 Formula) Moderna or Pfizer-BioNTech vaccine.
- **Previously vaccinated* with 1 or more doses of Moderna or Pfizer-BioNTech:** 1 dose of updated (2023–2024 Formula) Moderna or Pfizer-BioNTech at least 8 weeks after the most recent dose.

Age 12–18 years

- **Unvaccinated:**
  - 1 dose of updated (2023–2024 Formula) Moderna or Pfizer-BioNTech vaccine
  - 2-dose series of updated (2023–2024 Formula) Novavax at 0, 3-8 weeks
- **Previously vaccinated* with any COVID-19 vaccine(s):** 1 dose of any updated (2023–2024 Formula) COVID-19 vaccine at least 8 weeks after the most recent dose.

Special situations

Persons who are moderately or severely immunocompromised**

Age 6 months–4 years

- **Unvaccinated:**
  - 3-dose series of updated (2023–2024 Formula) Moderna at 0, 4, 8 weeks
  - 3-dose series of updated (2023–2024 Formula) Pfizer-BioNTech at 0, 3, 11 weeks.
- **Previously vaccinated* with 1 dose of any Moderna:** 2-dose series of updated (2023–2024 Formula) Moderna at 0, 4 weeks (minimum interval between previous Moderna and dose 1: 4 weeks).
- **Previously vaccinated* with 2 doses of any Moderna:** 1 dose of updated (2023–2024 Formula) Moderna at least 4 weeks after the most recent dose.
- **Previously vaccinated* with 3 or more doses of any Moderna:** 1 dose of updated (2023–2024 Formula) Moderna at least 8 weeks after the most recent dose.
- **Previously vaccinated* with 1 dose of any Pfizer-BioNTech:** 2-dose series of updated (2023–2024 Formula) Pfizer-BioNTech at 0, 8 weeks (minimum interval between previous Pfizer-BioNTech and dose 1: 3 weeks).
- **Previously vaccinated* with 2 or more doses of any Pfizer-BioNTech:** 1 dose of updated (2023–2024 Formula) Pfizer-BioNTech at least 8 weeks after the most recent dose.

Age 5–11 years

- **Unvaccinated:**
  - 3-dose series of updated (2023–2024 Formula) Moderna at 0, 4, 8 weeks
  - 3-dose series updated (2023–2024 Formula) Pfizer-BioNTech at 0, 3, 7 weeks.
- **Previously vaccinated* with 1 dose of any Moderna:** 2-dose series of updated (2023–2024 Formula) Moderna at 0, 4 weeks (minimum interval between previous Moderna and dose 1: 4 weeks).
- **Previously vaccinated* with 2 doses of any Moderna:** 1 dose of updated (2023–2024 Formula) Moderna at least 4 weeks after the most recent dose.
- **Previously vaccinated* with 1 dose of any Pfizer-BioNTech:** 2-dose series of updated (2023–2024 Formula) Pfizer-BioNTech at 0, 4 weeks (minimum interval between previous Pfizer-BioNTech and dose 1: 3 weeks).
- **Previously vaccinated* with 2 doses of any Pfizer-BioNTech:** 1 dose of 2023–2024 Pfizer-BioNTech at least 4 weeks after the most recent dose.

Notes

Recommended Child and Adolescent Immunization Schedule for Ages 18 Years or Younger, United States, 2024

Current COVID-19 schedule and dosage formulation available at www.cdc.gov/covidschedule. For more information on Emergency Use Authorization (EUA) indications for COVID-19 vaccines, see www.fda.gov/emergency-preparedness-and-response/coronavirus-disease-2019-covid-19/covid-19-vaccines

*Note: Previously vaccinated is defined as having received any Original monovalent or bivalent COVID-19 vaccine (Janssen, Moderna, Novavax, Pfizer-BioNTech) prior to the updated 2023–2024 formulation.

**Note: Persons who are moderately or severely immunocompromised have the option to receive one additional dose of updated (2023–2024 Formula) COVID-19 vaccine at least 2 months following the last recommended updated (2023–2024 Formula) COVID-19 vaccine dose. Further additional updated (2023–2024 Formula) COVID-19 vaccine dose(s) may be administered, informed by the clinical judgement of a healthcare provider and personal preference and circumstances. Any further additional doses should be administered at least 2 months after the last updated (2023–2024 Formula) COVID-19 vaccine dose. Moderately or severely immunocompromised children 6 months–4 years of age should receive homologous updated (2023–2024 Formula) mRNA vaccine dose(s) if they receive additional doses.

Dengue vaccination
(minimum age: 9 years)

Routine vaccination

- Age 9–16 years living in areas with endemic dengue **AND** have laboratory confirmation of previous dengue infection
  - 3-dose series administered at 0, 6, and 12 months
- Endemic areas include Puerto Rico, American Samoa, US Virgin Islands, Federated States of Micronesia, Republic of Marshall Islands, and the Republic of Palau. For updated guidance on dengue endemic areas and pre-vaccination laboratory testing see www.cdc.gov/mmwr/volumes/70/rr/rr7006a1.htm?s_cid=rr7006a1_w and www.cdc.gov/dengue/vaccine/hcp/index.html
- Dengue vaccine should not be administered to children traveling to or visiting endemic dengue areas.

Diphtheria, tetanus, and pertussis (DTaP) vaccination (minimum age: 6 weeks [4 years for Kinrix® or Quadracel®])

Routine vaccination

- 5-dose series (3-dose primary series at age 2, 4, and 6 months, followed by a booster doses at ages 15–18 months and 4–6 years

- **Prospectively:** Dose 4 may be administered as early as age 12 months if at least 6 months have elapsed since dose 3.
- **Retrospectively:** A 4th dose that was inadvertently administered as early as age 12 months may be counted if at least 4 months have elapsed since dose 3.

Catch-up vaccination

- Dose 5 is not necessary if dose 4 was administered at age 4 years or older and at least 6 months after dose 3.
- For other catch-up guidance, see Table 2.

Special situations

- **Wound management** in children less than age 7 years with history of 3 or more doses of tetanus-toxoid-containing vaccine: For all wounds except clean and minor wounds, administer DTaP if more than 5 years since last dose of tetanus-toxoid-containing vaccine. For detailed information, see www.cdc.gov/mmwr/volumes/67/rr/rr6702a1.htm.

Haemophilus influenzae type b vaccination
(minimum age: 6 weeks)

Routine vaccination

- **ActHIB®, Hiberix®, Pentacel®, or Vaxelis®:** 4-dose series (3-dose primary series at age 2, 4, and 6 months, followed by a booster dose* at age 12–15 months)
  - *Vaxelis® is not recommended for use as a booster dose. A different Hib-containing vaccine should be used for the booster dose.
- **PedvaxHIB®:** 3-dose series (2-dose primary series at age 2 and 4 months, followed by a booster dose at age 12–15 months)

Catch-up vaccination

- **Dose 1 at age 7–11 months:** Administer dose 2 at least 4 weeks later and dose 3 (final dose) at age12–15 months or 8 weeks after dose 2 (whichever is later).
- **Dose 1 at age 12–14 months:** Administer dose 2 (final dose) at least 8 weeks after dose 1.
- **Dose 1 before age 12 months and dose 2 before age 15 months:** Administer dose 3 (final dose) at least 8 weeks after dose 2.
- **2 doses of PedvaxHIB® before age 12 months:** Administer dose 3 (final dose) at age12–59 months and at least 8 weeks after dose 2.
- **1 dose administered at age 15 months or older:** No further doses needed
- **Unvaccinated at age 15–59 months:** Administer 1 dose.

- **Previously vaccinated* with 3 or more doses of any Moderna or Pfizer-BioNTech:** 1 dose of updated (2023–2024 Formula) Moderna or Pfizer-BioNTech at least 8 weeks after the most recent dose.

Age 12–18 years

- **Unvaccinated:**
  - 3-dose series of updated (2023–2024 Formula) Moderna at 0, 4, 8 weeks
  - 3-dose series of updated (2023–2024 Formula) Pfizer-BioNTech at 0, 3, 7 weeks
  - 2-dose series of updated (2023–2024 Formula) Novavax at 0, 3 weeks
- **Previously vaccinated* with 1 dose of any Moderna:** 2-dose series of updated (2023–2024 Formula) Moderna at 0, 4 weeks (minimum interval between previous Moderna dose and dose 1: 4 weeks).
- **Previously vaccinated* with 2 doses of any Moderna:** 1 dose of updated (2023–2024 Formula) Moderna at least 4 weeks after the most recent dose.
- **Previously vaccinated* with 1 dose of any Pfizer-BioNTech:** 2-dose series of updated (2023–2024 Formula) Pfizer-BioNTech at 0, 4 weeks (minimum interval between previous Pfizer-BioNTech dose and dose 1: 3 weeks).
- **Previously vaccinated* with 2 doses of any Pfizer-BioNTech:** 1 dose of updated (2023–2024 Formula) Pfizer-BioNTech at least 4 weeks after the most recent dose.
- **Previously vaccinated* with 3 or more doses of any Moderna or Pfizer-BioNTech:** 1 dose of any updated (2023–2024 Formula) COVID-19 vaccine at least 8 weeks after the most recent dose.
- **Previously vaccinated* with 1 or more doses of Janssen or Novavax or with or without dose(s) of any Original monovalent or bivalent COVID-19 vaccine:** 1 dose of any updated (2023–2024 Formula) COVID-19 vaccine at least 8 weeks after the most recent dose.

There is no preferential recommendation for the use of one COVID-19 vaccine over another when more than one recommended age-appropriate vaccine is available.

Administer an age-appropriate COVID-19 vaccine product for each dose. For information about transition from age 4 years to age 5 years or age 11 years to age 12 years during COVID-19 vaccination series, see Tables 1 and 2 at www.cdc.gov/vaccines/covid-19/clinical-considerations/interim-considerations-us.html#covid-vaccines.

Notes — Recommended Child and Adolescent Immunization Schedule for Ages 18 Years or Younger, United States, 2024

- **Previously unvaccinated children age 60 months or older who are not considered high risk:** Do not require catch-up vaccination

For other catch-up guidance, see Table 2. Vaxelis* can be used for catch-up vaccination in children less than age 5 years. Follow the catch-up schedule even if Vaxelis* is used for one or more doses. For detailed information on use of Vaxelis* see www.cdc.gov/mmwr/volumes/69/wr/mm6905a5.htm.

Special situations

Chemotherapy or radiation treatment:
Age 12–59 months
- Unvaccinated or only 1 dose before age 12 months: 2 doses, 8 weeks apart
- 2 or more doses before age 12 months: 1 dose at least 8 weeks after previous dose

Doses administered within 14 days of starting therapy or during therapy should be repeated at least 3 months after therapy completion.

Hematopoietic stem cell transplant (HSCT):
- 3-dose series 4 weeks apart starting 6 to 12 months after successful transplant, regardless of Hib vaccination history

Anatomic or functional asplenia (including sickle cell disease):
Age 12–59 months
- Unvaccinated or only 1 dose before age 12 months: 2 doses, 8 weeks apart
- 2 or more doses before age 12 months: 1 dose at least 8 weeks after previous dose

Unvaccinated persons age 5 years or older*
- 1 dose

Elective splenectomy:
Unvaccinated persons age 15 months or older*
- 1 dose (preferably at least 14 days before procedure)

HIV infection:
Age 12–59 months
- Unvaccinated or only 1 dose before age 12 months: 2 doses, 8 weeks apart
- 2 or more doses before age 12 months: 1 dose at least 8 weeks after previous dose

Unvaccinated persons age 5–18 years*
- 1 dose

Immunoglobulin deficiency, early component complement deficiency:
Age 12–59 months
- Unvaccinated or only 1 dose before age 12 months: 2 doses, 8 weeks apart
- 2 or more doses before age 12 months: 1 dose at least 8 weeks after previous dose

Unvaccinated = Less than routine series (through age 14 months) OR no doses (age 15 months or older)

Hepatitis A vaccination
(minimum age: 12 months for routine vaccination)

Routine vaccination
- 2-dose series (minimum interval: 6 months) at age 12–23 months

Catch-up vaccination
- Unvaccinated persons through age 18 years should complete a 2-dose series (minimum interval: 6 months).
- Persons who previously received 1 dose at age 12 months or older should receive dose 2 at least 6 months after dose 1.
- Adolescents age 18 years or older may receive the combined HepA and HepB vaccine, Twinrix*, as a 3-dose series (0, 1, and 6 months) or 4-dose series (3 doses at 0, 7, and 21–30 days, followed by a booster dose at 12 months).

International travel
- Persons traveling to or working in countries with high or intermediate endemic hepatitis A (www.cdc.gov/travel/):
- **Infants age 6–11 months:** 1 dose before departure; revaccinate with 2 doses (separated by at least 6 months) between age 12–23 months.
- **Unvaccinated age 12 months or older:** Administer dose 1 as soon as travel is considered.

Hepatitis B vaccination
(minimum age: birth)

Routine vaccination
- 3-dose series at age 0, 1–2, 6–18 months (**use monovalent HepB vaccine for doses administered before age 6 weeks**)
- Birth weight ≥2,000 grams: 1 dose within 24 hours of birth if medically stable
- Birth weight <2,000 grams: 1 dose at chronological age 1 month or hospital discharge (whichever is earlier and if weight is still <2,000 grams).
- Infants who did not receive a birth dose should begin the series as soon as possible (see Table 2 for minimum intervals).
- Administration of 4 doses is permitted when a combination vaccine containing HepB is used after the birth dose.
- **Minimum intervals (see Table 2):** when 4 doses are administered, substitute "dose 4" for "dose 3" in these calculations

- **Final (3rd or 4th) dose:** age 6–18 months (**minimum age 24 weeks**)

- **Mother is HBsAg-positive**
- **Birth dose (monovalent HepB vaccine only):** administer **HepB vaccine and hepatitis B immune globulin (HBIG)** (in separate limbs) within 12 hours of birth, regardless of birth weight.
- **Birth weight <2000 grams:** administer 3 additional doses of HepB vaccine beginning at age 1 month (total of 4 doses)
- **Final (3rd or 4th) dose:** administer at age 6 months (**minimum age 24 weeks**)
- Test for HBsAg and anti-HBs at age 9–12 months. If HepB series is delayed, test 1–2 months after final dose. Do not test before age 9 months.

- **Mother is HBsAg-unknown**

If other evidence suggestive of maternal hepatitis B infection exists (e.g., presence of HBV DNA, HBeAg-positive, or mother known to have chronic hepatitis B infection), manage infant as if mother is HBsAg-positive
- **Birth dose (monovalent HepB vaccine only):**
- Birth weight ≥2,000 grams: administer **HepB vaccine** within 12 hours of birth. Determine mother's HBsAg status as soon as possible. If mother is determined to be HBsAg-positive, administer **HBIG** as soon as possible (in separate limb), but no later than 7 days of age.
- Birth weight <2,000 grams: administer **HepB vaccine** and **HBIG** (in separate limbs) within 12 hours of birth. Administer 3 additional doses of **HepB vaccine** beginning at age 1 month (total of 4 doses)
- **Final (3rd or 4th) dose:** administer at age 6 months (**minimum age 24 weeks**)
- If mother is determined to be HBsAg-positive or if status remains unknown, test for HBsAg and anti-HBs at age 9–12 months. If HepB series is delayed, test 1–2 months after final dose. Do not test before age 9 months.

Catch-up vaccination
- Unvaccinated persons should complete a 3-dose series at 0, 1–2, 6 months. See Table 2 for minimum intervals
- Adolescents age 11–15 years may use an alternative 2-dose schedule with at least 4 months between doses (adult formulation **Recombivax HB*** only).
- Adolescents age 18 years may receive:
- **Heplisav-B*:** 2-dose series at least 4 weeks apart
- **PreHevbrio*:** 3-dose series at 0, 1, and 6 months
- Combined HepA and HepB vaccine, **Twinrix*:** 3-dose series (0, 1, and 6 months) or 4-dose series (3 doses at 0, 7, and 21–30 days, followed by a booster dose at 12 months).

Notes   Recommended Child and Adolescent Immunization Schedule for Ages 18 Years or Younger, United States, 2024

Special situations

- Revaccination is not generally recommended for persons with a normal immune status who were vaccinated as infants, children, adolescents, or adults.
- **Post-vaccination serology testing and revaccination** (if anti-HBs <10mIU/mL) is recommended for certain populations, including:
  - Infants born to HBsAg-positive mothers
  - Persons who are predialysis or on maintenance dialysis
  - Other immunocompromised persons
- For detailed revaccination recommendations, see www.cdc. gov/vaccines/hcp/acip-recs/vacc-specific/hepb.html.

Note: HepLisav-B and PreHevbrio are not recommended in pregnancy due to lack of safety data in pregnant persons

Human papillomavirus vaccination
(minimum age: 9 years)

Routine and catch-up vaccination

- HPV vaccination routinely recommended at **age 11–12 years** (can start at **age 9 years**) and catch-up HPV vaccination recommended for all persons through age 18 years if not adequately vaccinated
- 2- or 3-dose series depending on age at initial vaccination:
  - **Age 9–14 years at initial vaccination:** 2-dose series at 0, 6–12 months (minimum interval: 5 months; repeat dose if administered too soon)
  - **Age 15 years or older at initial vaccination:** 3-dose series at 0, 1–2 months, 6 months (minimum intervals: dose 1 to dose 2: 4 weeks / dose 2 to dose 3: 12 weeks / dose 1 to dose 3: 5 months; repeat dose if administered too soon)
- No additional dose recommended when any HPV vaccine series **of any valency** has been completed using recommended dosing intervals.

Special situations

- **Immunocompromising conditions, including HIV infection:** 3-dose series, even for those who initiate vaccination at age 9 through 14 years.
- **History of sexual abuse or assault:** Start at age 9 years
- **Pregnancy:** Pregnancy testing not needed before vaccination; HPV vaccination not recommended until after pregnancy; no intervention needed if vaccinated while pregnant

Influenza vaccination
(minimum age: 6 months [IIV], 2 years [LAIV4], 18 years [recombinant influenza vaccine, RIV4])

Routine vaccination

- Use any influenza vaccine appropriate for age and health status annually.
  - **Age 6 months–8 years** who have received **fewer than** 2 influenza vaccine doses before July 1, 2023, or whose influenza vaccination history is unknown: 2 doses, separated by at least 4 weeks. Administer dose 2 even if the child turns 9 years between receipt of dose 1 and dose 2.
  - **Age 6 months–8 years** who have received **at least 2** influenza vaccine doses before July 1, 2023: 1 dose
  - **Age 9 years or older:** 1 dose
- For the 2023–2024 season, see www.cdc.gov/mmwr/ volumes/72/rr/rr7202a1.htm.
- For the 2024–25 season, see the 2024–25 ACIP influenza vaccine recommendations.

Special situations

- **Close contacts (e.g., household contacts) of severely immunosuppressed persons who require a protected environment:** should not receive LAIV4. If LAIV4 is given, they should avoid contact with for such immunosuppressed persons for 7 days after vaccination.

Note: Persons with an egg allergy can receive any influenza vaccine (egg-based and non-egg-based) appropriate for age and health status.

Measles, mumps, and rubella vaccination
(minimum age: 12 months for routine vaccination)

Routine vaccination

- 2-dose series at age 12–15 months, age 4–6 years
- MMR or MMRV* may be administered

Note: For dose 1 in children age 12–47 months, it is recommended to administer MMR and varicella vaccines separately. MMRV* may be used if parents or caregivers express a preference.

Catch-up vaccination

- Unvaccinated children and adolescents: 2-dose series at least 4 weeks apart*
- The maximum age for use of MMRV* is 12 years.

Special situations

- **International travel**
  - **Infants age 6–11 months:** 1 dose before departure; revaccinate with 2-dose series at age 12–15 months (12 months for children in high-risk areas) and dose 2 as early as 4 weeks later.*
  - **Unvaccinated children age 12 months or older:** 2-dose series at least 4 weeks apart before departure*
- In mumps outbreak settings, for information about additional doses of MMR (including 3rd dose of MMR), see www.cdc.gov/mmwr/volumes/67/wr/mm6701a7.htm

*Note: If MMRV is used, the minimum interval between MMRV doses is 3 months

Meningococcal serogroup A,C,W,Y vaccination
(minimum age: 2 months [MenACWY-CRM, Menveo], 2 years [MenACWY-TT, MenQuadfi], 10 years [MenACWY-TT/MenB-FHbp, Penbraya])

Routine vaccination

- 2-dose series at age 11–12 years; 16 years

Catch-up vaccination

- Age 13–15 years: 1 dose now and booster at age 16–18 years (minimum interval: 8 weeks)
- Age 16–18 years: 1 dose

Special situations

Anatomic or functional asplenia (including sickle cell disease), HIV infection, persistent complement component deficiency, complement inhibitor (e.g., eculizumab, ravulizumab) use:

- **Menveo****
  - Dose 1 at age 2 months: 4-dose series (additional 3 doses at age 4, 6, and 12 months)
  - Dose 1 at age 3–6 months: 3- or 4-dose series (dose 2 [and dose 3 if applicable] at least 8 weeks after previous dose until a dose is received at age 7 months or older, followed by an additional dose at least 12 weeks later and after age 12 months)
  - Dose 1 at age 7–23 months: 2-dose series (dose 2 at least 12 weeks after dose 1 and after age 12 months)
  - Dose 1 at age 24 months or older: 2-dose series at least 8 weeks apart
- **MenQuadfi***
  - Dose 1 at age 24 months or older: 2-dose series at least 8 weeks apart

| Notes |

Recommended Child and Adolescent Immunization Schedule for Ages 18 Years or Younger, United States, 2024

Travel to countries with hyperendemic or epidemic meningococcal disease, including countries in the African meningitis belt or during the Hajj (www.cdc.gov/travel/):

• Children less than age 24 months:

– **Menveo** (age 2–23 months)**

· Dose 1 at age 2 months: 4-dose series (additional 3 doses at age 4, 6, and 12 months)

· Dose 1 at age 3–6 months: 3- or 4-dose series (dose 2 [and dose 3 if applicable] at least 8 weeks after previous dose until a dose is received at age 7 months or older, followed by an additional dose at least 12 weeks later and after age 12 months)

· Dose 1 at age 7–23 months: 2-dose series (dose 2 at least 12 weeks after dose 1 and after age 12 months)

• Children age 2 years or older: 1 dose Menveo** or MenQuadfi®

First-year college students who live in residential housing (if not previously vaccinated at age 16 years or older) or military recruits:

• 1 dose Menveo** or MenQuadfi®

Adolescent vaccination of children who received MenACWY prior to age 10 years:

• **Children for whom boosters are recommended** because of an ongoing increased risk of meningococcal disease (e.g., those with complement component deficiency, HIV, or asplenia): Follow the booster schedule for persons at increased risk.

• **Children for whom boosters are not recommended** (e.g., a healthy child who received a single dose for travel to a country where meningococcal disease is endemic): Administer MenACWY according to the recommended adolescent schedule with dose 1 at age 11–12 years and dose 2 at age 16 years.

*Menveo has two formulations: lyophilized and liquid. The liquid formulation should not be used before age 10 years. See www.cdc.gov/vaccines/vpd/mening/downloads/menveo-single-vial-presentation.pdf

Note: For MenACWY **booster dose recommendations** for groups listed under "Special situations" and in an outbreak setting and additional meningococcal vaccination information, see www.cdc.gov/mmwr/volumes/69/rr/rr6909a1.htm

Children age 10 years or older may receive a single dose of Penbraya™ as an alternative to separate administration of MenACWY and MenB when both vaccines would be given on the same clinic day (see "Meningococcal serogroup B vaccination" section below for more information).

Meningococcal serogroup B vaccination

(minimum age: 10 years [MenB-4C, Bexsero®; MenB-FHbp, Trumenba®; MenACWY-TT/MenB-FHbp, Penbraya™])

Shared clinical decision-making

• **Adolescents not at increased risk** age 16–23 years (preferred age 16–18 years) based on shared clinical decision-making:

– **Bexsero®:** 2-dose series at least 1 month apart

– **Trumenba®:** 2-dose series at least 6 months apart (if dose 2 is administered earlier than 6 months, administer a 3rd dose at least 4 months after dose 2)

For additional information on shared clinical decision-making for MenB, see www.cdc.gov/vaccines/hcp/admin/downloads/isd-job-aid-scdm-mening-b-shared-clinical-decision-making.pdf

Special situations

Anatomic or functional asplenia (including sickle cell disease), persistent complement component deficiency, complement inhibitor (e.g., eculizumab, ravulizumab) use:

• **Bexsero®:** 2-dose series at least 1 month apart

• **Trumenba®:** 3-dose series at 0, 1–2, 6 months (if dose 2 was administered at least 6 months after dose 1, dose 3 not needed; if dose 3 is administered earlier than 4 months after dose 2, a 4th dose should be administered at least 4 months after dose 3)

Note: Bexsero® and Trumenba® are not interchangeable; the same product should be used for all doses in a series.

For MenB **booster dose recommendations** for groups listed under "Special situations" and in an outbreak setting and additional meningococcal vaccination information, see www.cdc.gov/mmwr/volumes/69/rr/rr6909a1.htm

Children age 10 years or older may receive a dose of Penbraya™ as an alternative to separate administration of MenACWY and MenB when both vaccines would be given on the same clinic day. For age-eligible children not at increased risk, if Penbraya™ is used for dose 1 MenB, MenB-FHbp (Trumenba) should be administered for dose 2 MenB. For age-eligible children at increased risk of meningococcal disease, Penbraya™ may be used for additional MenACWY and MenB doses (including booster doses) if both would be given on the same clinic day **and** at least 6 months have elapsed since most recent Penbraya™ dose.

Mpox vaccination

(minimum age: 18 years [Jynneos®])

Special situations

• **Age 18 years and at risk for Mpox infection:** 2-dose series, 28 days apart.

Risk factors for Mpox infection include:

– Persons who are gay, bisexual, and other MSM, transgender or nonbinary people who in the past 6 months have had:

· A new diagnosis of at least 1 sexually transmitted disease

· More than 1 sex partner

· Sex at a commercial sex venue

· Sex in association with a large public event in a geographic area where Mpox transmission is occurring

– Persons who are sexual partners of the persons described above

– Persons who anticipate experiencing any of the situations described above

• **Pregnancy:** There is currently no ACIP recommendation for Jynneos use in pregnancy due to lack of safety data in pregnant persons. Pregnant persons with any risk factor described above may receive Jynneos.

For detailed information, see: www.cdc.gov/vaccines/acip/meetings/downloads/slides-2023-10-25-26/04-MPOX-Rao-508.pdf

Pneumococcal vaccination

(minimum age: 6 weeks [PCV15], [PCV 20]; 2 years [PPSV23])

Routine vaccination with PCV

• 4-dose series at 2, 4, 6, 12–15 months

Catch-up vaccination with PCV

• Healthy children ages 2–4 years with any incomplete* PCV series: 1 dose PCV

• For other catch-up guidance, see Table 2.

Note: For children **without** risk conditions, PCV20 is not indicated if they have received 4 doses of PCV13 or PCV15 or another age appropriate complete PCV series.

Notes

Recommended Child and Adolescent Immunization Schedule for Ages 18 Years or Younger, United States, 2024

Special situations

Children and adolescents with cerebrospinal fluid leak; chronic heart disease; chronic kidney disease (excluding maintenance dialysis and nephrotic syndrome); chronic liver disease; chronic lung disease (including moderate persistent or severe persistent asthma); cochlear implant; or diabetes mellitus:

Age 2–5 years

- Any incomplete* PCV series with:
  - 3 PCV doses: 1 dose PCV (at least 8 weeks after the most recent PCV dose)
  - Less than 3 PCV doses: 2 doses PCV (at least 8 weeks after the most recent dose and administered at least 8 weeks apart)
- Completed recommended PCV series but have not received PPSV23
  - Previously received at least 1 dose of PCV20: no further PCV or PPSV23 doses needed
  - Not previously received PCV20: administer 1 dose PCV20 OR 1 dose PPSV23 administer at least 8 weeks after the most recent PCV dose.**

Age 6–18 years

- Not previously received any dose of PCV13, PCV15, or PCV20: administer 1 dose of PCV15 or PCV20. If PCV15 is used and no previous receipt of PPSV23, administer 1 dose of PPSV23 at least 8 weeks after the PCV15 dose.**
- Received PCV before age 6 years but have not received PPSV23
  - Previously received at least 1 dose of PCV20: no further PCV or PPSV23 doses needed
  - Not previously received PCV20: 1 dose PCV20 OR 1 dose PPSV23 administer at least 8 weeks after the most recent PCV dose.
- Received PCV13 only at or after age 6 years: administer 1 dose PCV20 OR 1 dose PPSV23 at least 8 weeks after the most recent PCV13 dose.
- Received 1 dose PCV13 and 1 dose PPSV23 at or after age 6 years: no further doses of any PCV or PPSV23 indicated.

Children and adolescents on maintenance dialysis, or with immunocompromising conditions such as nephrotic syndrome; congenital or acquired asplenia or splenic dysfunction; congenital or acquired immunodeficiencies; diseases and conditions treated with immunosuppressive drugs or radiation therapy, including malignant neoplasms, leukemias, lymphomas, Hodgkin disease, and solid organ transplant; HIV infection; or sickle cell disease or other hemoglobinopathies:

Age 2–5 years

- Any incomplete* PCV series:
  - 3 PCV doses: 1 dose PCV (at least 8 weeks after the most recent PCV dose)
  - Less than 3 PCV doses: 2 doses PCV (at least 8 weeks after the most recent dose and administered at least 8 weeks apart)
- Completed recommended PCV series but have not received PPSV23
  - Previously received at least 1 dose of PCV20: no further PCV or PPSV23 doses needed
  - Not previously received PCV20: administer 1 dose PCV20 OR 1 dose PPSV23 at least 8 weeks after the most recent PCV dose. If PPSV23 is used, administer either PCV20 or dose 2 PPSV23 at least 5 years after dose 1 PPSV23.

Age 6–18 years

- Not previously received any dose of PCV13, PCV15, or PCV20: administer 1 dose of PCV15 or 1 dose of PCV20. If PCV15 is used and no previous receipt of PPSV23, administer 1 dose of PPSV23 at least 8 weeks after the PCV15 dose.**
- Received PCV before age 6 years but have not received PPSV23
  - Previously received at least 1 dose of PCV20: no additional dose of PCV or PPSV23
  - Not previously received PCV20: administer 1 dose PCV20 OR 1 dose PPSV23 at least 8 weeks after the most recent PCV dose. If PPSV23 is used, administer either PCV20 or dose 2 PPSV23 at least 5 years after dose 1 PPSV23.
- Received PCV13 only at or after age 6 years: administer 1 dose PCV20 OR 1 dose PPSV23 at least 8 weeks after the most recent PCV13 dose. If PPSV23 is used, administer 1 dose of PCV20 or dose 2 PPSV23 at least 5 years after dose 1 PPSV23.
- Received 1 dose PCV13 and 1 dose PPSV23 at or after age 6 years: administer 1 dose of PCV20 OR 1 dose PPSV23 at least 8 weeks after the most recent PCV13 dose and at least 5 years after dose 1 PPSV23.

*Incomplete series = Not having received all doses in either the recommended series or an age-appropriate catch-up series. See Table 2 in ACIP pneumococcal recommendations at stacks.cdc.gov/view/cdc/133252

**When both PCV15 and PPSV23 are indicated, administer all doses of PCV15 first. PCV15 and PPSV23 should not be administered during the same visit.

For guidance on determining which pneumococcal vaccines a patient needs and when, please refer to the mobile app, which can be downloaded here: www.cdc.gov/vaccines/vpd/pneumo/hcp/pneumoapp.html

Poliovirus vaccination
(minimum age: 6 weeks)

Routine vaccination

- 4-dose series at ages 2, 4, 6–18 months, 4–6 years; administer the final dose on or after age 4 years and at least 6 months after the previous dose.
- 4 or more doses of IPV can be administered before age 4 years when a combination vaccine containing IPV is used. However, a dose is still recommended on or after age 4 years and at least 6 months after the previous dose.

Catch-up vaccination

- In the first 6 months of life, use minimum ages and intervals only for travel to a polio-endemic region or during an outbreak.
- **Adolescents age 18 years known or suspected to be unvaccinated or incompletely vaccinated:** administer remaining doses (1, 2, or 3 IPV doses) to complete a 3-dose primary series.* Unless there are specific reasons to believe they were not vaccinated, most persons aged 18 years or older born and raised in the United States can assume they were vaccinated against polio as children.

Series containing oral poliovirus vaccine (OPV), either mixed OPV-IPV or OPV-only series:

- Total number of doses needed to complete the series is the same as that recommended for the U.S. IPV schedule. See www.cdc.gov/mmwr/volumes/66/wr/mm6601a6.htm?s_%20cid=mm6601a6_w.
- Only trivalent OPV (tOPV) counts toward the U.S. vaccination requirements.
  - Doses of OPV administered before April 1, 2016, should be counted (unless specifically noted as administered during a campaign).
  - Doses of OPV administered on or after April 1, 2016, should not be counted.
- For guidance to assess doses documented as "OPV," see www.cdc.gov/mmwr/volumes/66/wr/mm6606a7.htm?s_cid=mm6606a7_w.
- For other catch-up guidance, see Table 2.

Notes — Recommended Child and Adolescent Immunization Schedule for Ages 18 Years or Younger, United States, 2024

Special situations

- **Adolescents aged 18 years at increased risk of exposure to poliovirus and completed primary series*:** may administer one lifetime IPV booster

*Note: Complete primary series consist of at least 3 doses of IPV or trivalent oral poliovirus vaccine (tOPV) in any combination.

For detailed information, see: www.cdc.gov/vaccines/vpd/polio/hcp/recommendations.html

Respiratory syncytial virus immunization
(minimum age: birth [Nirsevimab, RSV-mAb (Beyfortus™])

Routine immunization

- **Infants born October – March in most of the continental United States***

- Mother did not receive RSV vaccine OR mother's RSV vaccination status is unknown: administer 1 dose nirsevimab within 1 week of birth in hospital or outpatient setting
- Mother received RSV vaccine **less than 14 days** prior to delivery: administer 1 dose nirsevimab within 1 week of birth in hospital or outpatient setting
- Mother received RSV vaccine **at least 14 days** prior to delivery: nirsevimab may be considered but can be considered in rare circumstances at the discretion of healthcare providers (see special populations and situations at www.cdc.gov/vaccines/vpd/rsv/hcp/child-faqs.html)

- **Infants born April–September in most of the continental United States***

- Mother did not receive RSV vaccine OR mother's RSV vaccination status is unknown: administer 1 dose nirsevimab shortly before start of RSV season*
- Mother received RSV vaccine **less than 14 days** prior to delivery: administer 1 dose nirsevimab shortly before start of RSV season*
- Mother received RSV vaccine **at least 14 days** prior to delivery: nirsevimab not needed but can be considered in rare circumstances at the discretion of healthcare providers(see special populations and situations at www.cdc.gov/vaccines/vpd/rsv/hcp/child-faqs.html)

Infants with prolonged birth hospitalization** (e.g., for prematurity) discharged October through March should be immunized shortly before or promptly after discharge.

Special situations

- **Ages 8–19 months with chronic lung disease of prematurity requiring medical support (e.g., chronic corticosteroid therapy, diuretic therapy, or supplemental oxygen) any time during the 6-month period before the start of the second RSV season; severe immunocompromise; cystic fibrosis with either weight for length <10th percentile or manifestation of severe lung disease (e.g., previous hospitalization for pulmonary exacerbation in the first year of life or abnormalities on chest imaging that persist when stable)**:**

- 1 dose nirsevimab shortly before start of second RSV season*

- **Ages 8–19 months who are American Indian or Alaska Native:**

- 1 dose nirsevimab shortly before start of second RSV season*

- **Age-eligible and undergoing cardiac surgery with cardiopulmonary bypass**:** 1 additional dose of nirsevimab after surgery. For additional details see special populations and situations at www.cdc.gov/vaccines/vpd/rsv/hcp/child-faqs.html

*Note: While the timing of the onset and duration of RSV season may vary, nirsevimab may be administered October through March in most of the continental United States. Providers in jurisdictions with RSV seasonality that differs from most of the continental United States (e.g., Alaska, jurisdiction with tropical climate) should follow guidance from public health authorities (e.g., CDC, health departments) or regional medical centers on timing of administration based on local RSV seasonality. Although optimal timing of administration is just before the start of the RSV season, nirsevimab may also be administered during the RSV season to infants and children who are age-eligible.

**Note: Nirsevimab can be administered to children who are eligible to receive palivizumab. Children who have received nirsevimab should not receive palivizumab for the same RSV season.

For further guidance, see www.cdc.gov/mmwr/volumes/72/wr/mm7234a4.htm and www.cdc.gov/vaccines/vpd/rsv/hcp/child-faqs.html

Respiratory syncytial virus vaccination
(RSV [Abrysvo™])

Routine vaccination

- **Pregnant at 32 weeks 0 days through 36 weeks and 6 days gestation from September through January in most of the continental United States*:** 1 dose RSV vaccine (Abrysvo™). Administer RSV vaccine regardless of previous RSV infection.

- Either maternal RSV vaccination or infant immunization with nirsevimab (RSV monoclonal antibody) is recommended to prevent respiratory syncytial virus lower respiratory tract infection in infants.

- **All other pregnant persons:** RSV vaccine not recommended.

There is currently no ACIP recommendation for RSV vaccination in subsequent pregnancies. No data are available to inform whether additional doses are needed in later pregnancies.

*Note: Providers in jurisdictions with RSV seasonality that differs from most of the continental United States (e.g., Alaska, jurisdiction with tropical climate) should follow guidance from public health authorities (e.g., CDC, health departments) or regional medical centers on timing of administration based on local RSV seasonality.

Rotavirus vaccination
(minimum age: 6 weeks)

Routine vaccination

- **Rotarix*:** 2-dose series at age 2 and 4 months
- **RotaTeq*:** 3-dose series at age 2, 4, and 6 months
- If any dose in the series is either **RotaTeq*** or unknown, default to 3-dose series.

Catch-up vaccination

- Do not start the series on or after age 15 weeks, 0 days.
- The maximum age for the final dose is 8 months, 0 days.
- For other catch-up guidance, see Table 2.

Detailed Vaccine Recommendations, Children and Adolescents, United States, 2024

Notes — Recommended Child and Adolescent Immunization Schedule for Ages 18 Years or Younger, United States, 2024

Tetanus, diphtheria, and pertussis (Tdap) vaccination

(minimum age: 11 years for routine vaccination, 7 years for catch-up vaccination)

Routine vaccination

- **Age 11–12 years:** 1 dose Tdap (adolescent booster)
- **Pregnancy:** 1 dose Tdap during each pregnancy, preferably in early part of gestational weeks 27–36.

Note: Tdap may be administered regardless of the interval since the last tetanus- and diphtheria-toxoid-containing vaccine.

Catch-up vaccination

- **Age 13–18 years who have not received Tdap:** 1 dose Tdap (adolescent booster)
- **Age 7–18 years not fully vaccinated* with DTaP:** 1 dose Tdap as part of the catch-up series (preferably the first dose); if additional doses are needed, use Td or Tdap.
- **Tdap administered at age 7–10 years:**
  - **Age 7–9 years** who receive Tdap should receive the adolescent Tdap booster dose at age 11–12 years.
  - **Age 10 years** who receive Tdap do not need the adolescent Tdap booster dose at age 11–12 years.
- **DTaP inadvertently administered on or after age 7 years:**
  - **Age 7–9 years:** DTaP may count as part of catch-up series. Administer adolescent Tdap booster dose at age 11–12 years.
  - **Age 10–18 years:** Count dose of DTaP as the adolescent Tdap booster dose.
- For other catch-up guidance, see Table 2.

Special situations

- **Wound management** in persons age 7 years or older with history of 3 or more doses of tetanus-toxoid-containing vaccine: For clean and minor wounds, administer Tdap or Td if more than 10 years since last dose of tetanus-toxoid-containing vaccine; for all other wounds, administer Tdap or Td if more than 5 years since last dose of tetanus-toxoid-containing vaccine. Tdap is preferred for persons age 11 years or older who have not previously received Tdap or whose Tdap history is unknown. If a tetanus-toxoid-containing vaccine is indicated for a pregnant adolescent, use Tdap.
- For detailed information, see www.cdc.gov/mmwr/volumes/69/wr/mm6903a5.htm

*Fully vaccinated = 5 valid doses of DTaP OR 4 valid doses of DTaP if dose 4 was administered at age 4 years or older

Varicella vaccination

(minimum age: 12 months)

Routine vaccination

- 2-dose series at age 12–15 months, 4–6 years
- VAR or MMRV may be administered*
- Dose 2 may be administered as early as 3 months after dose 1 (a dose inadvertently administered after at least 4 weeks may be counted as valid)

*Note:** For dose 1 in children age 12–47 months, it is recommended to administer MMR and varicella vaccines separately. MMRV may be used if parents or caregivers express a preference.

Catch-up vaccination

- Ensure persons age 7–18 years without evidence of immunity (see MMWR at www.cdc.gov/mmwr/pdf/rr/rr5604.pdf) have a 2-dose series:
  - **Age 7–12 years:** Routine interval: 3 months (a dose inadvertently administered after at least 4 weeks may be counted as valid)
  - **Age 13 years and older:** Routine interval: 4–8 weeks (minimum interval: 4 weeks)
  - The maximum age for use of MMRV is 12 years.

Appendix

Recommended Child and Adolescent Immunization Schedule for Ages 18 Years or Younger, United States, 2024

Guide to Contraindications and Precautions to Commonly Used Vaccines

Adapted from Table 4-1 in Advisory Committee on Immunization Practices (ACIP) General Best Practice Guidelines for Immunization: Contraindication and Precautions, Prevention and Control of Seasonal Influenza with Vaccines: Recommendations of the Advisory Committee on Immunization Practices—United States, 2023–24 Influenza Season | MMWR (cdc.gov), Contraindications and Precautions for COVID-19 Vaccination, and Contraindications and Precautions for JYNNEOS Vaccination

Vaccines and other Immunizing Agents	Contraindicated or Not Recommended[1]	Precautions[2]
COVID-19 mRNA vaccines [Pfizer-BioNTech, Moderna]	• Severe allergic reaction (e.g., anaphylaxis) after a previous dose or to a component of an mRNA COVID-19 vaccine[4]	• Diagnosed non-severe allergy (e.g., urticaria beyond the injection site) to a component of an mRNA COVID-19 vaccine[4] or non-severe, immediate (onset less than 4 hours) allergic reaction after administration of a previous dose of an mRNA COVID-19 vaccine • Myocarditis or pericarditis within 3 weeks after a dose of any COVID-19 vaccine • Multisystem inflammatory syndrome in children (MIS-C) or multisystem inflammatory syndrome in adults (MIS-A) • Moderate or severe acute illness, with or without fever
COVID-19 protein subunit vaccine [Novavax]	• Severe allergic reaction (e.g., anaphylaxis) after a previous dose or to a component of a Novavax COVID-19 vaccine[4]	• Diagnosed non-severe allergy (e.g., urticaria beyond the injection site) to a component of Novavax COVID-19 vaccine[4], or non-severe, immediate (onset less than 4 hours) allergic reaction after administration of a previous dose of a Novavax COVID-19 vaccine • Myocarditis or pericarditis within 3 weeks after a dose of any COVID-19 vaccine • Multisystem inflammatory syndrome in children (MIS-C) or multisystem inflammatory syndrome in adults (MIS-A) • Moderate or severe acute illness, with or without fever
Influenza, egg-based, inactivated injectable (IIV4)	• Severe allergic reaction (e.g., anaphylaxis) after previous dose of any influenza vaccine (i.e., any egg-based IIV, ccIIV, RIV, or LAIV of any valency) • Severe allergic reaction (e.g., anaphylaxis) to any vaccine component[3] (excluding egg)	• Guillain-Barré syndrome (GBS) within 6 weeks after a previous dose of any type of influenza vaccine • Moderate or severe acute illness with or without fever
Influenza, cell culture-based inactivated injectable (ccIIV4) [Flucelvax Quadrivalent]	• Severe allergic reaction (e.g., anaphylaxis) to any ccIIV of any valency, or to any component[3] of ccIIV4	• Guillain-Barré syndrome (GBS) within 6 weeks after a previous dose of any type of influenza vaccine • Persons with a history of severe allergic reaction (e.g., anaphylaxis) after a previous dose of any egg-based IIV, RIV, or LAIV of any valency. If using ccIIV4, administer in medical setting under supervision of health care provider who can recognize and manage severe allergic reactions. May consult an allergist. • Moderate or severe acute illness with or without fever
Influenza, recombinant injectable (RIV4) [Flublok Quadrivalent]	• Severe allergic reaction (e.g., anaphylaxis) to any RIV of any valency, or to any component[3] of RIV4	• Guillain-Barré syndrome (GBS) within 6 weeks after a previous dose of any type of influenza vaccine • Persons with a history of severe allergic reaction (e.g., anaphylaxis) after a previous dose of any egg-based IIV, ccIIV, or LAIV of any valency. If using RIV4, administer in medical setting under supervision of health care provider who can recognize and manage severe allergic reactions. May consult an allergist. • Moderate or severe acute illness with or without fever
Influenza, live attenuated (LAIV4) [Flumist Quadrivalent]	• Severe allergic reaction (e.g., anaphylaxis) after previous dose of any influenza vaccine (i.e., any egg-based IIV, ccIIV, RIV, or LAIV of any valency) • Severe allergic reaction (e.g., anaphylaxis) to any vaccine component[3] (excluding egg) • Children age 2–4 years with a history of asthma or wheezing • Anatomic or functional asplenia • Immunocompromised due to any cause including, but not limited to, medications and HIV infection • Close contacts or caregivers of severely immunosuppressed persons who require a protected environment • Pregnancy • Cochlear implant • Active communication between the cerebrospinal fluid (CSF) and the oropharynx, nasopharynx, nose, ear or any other cranial CSF leak • Children and adolescents receiving aspirin or salicylate-containing medications • Received influenza antiviral medications oseltamivir or zanamivir within the previous 48 hours, peramivir within the previous 5 days, or baloxavir within the previous 17 days	• Guillain-Barré syndrome (GBS) within 6 weeks after a previous dose of any type of influenza vaccine • Asthma in persons age 5 years old or older • Persons with underlying medical conditions other than those listed under contraindications that might predispose to complications after wild-type influenza virus infection, e.g., chronic pulmonary, cardiovascular (except isolated hypertension), renal, hepatic, neurologic, hematologic, or metabolic disorders (including diabetes mellitus) • Moderate or severe acute illness with or without fever

1. When a contraindication is present, a vaccine should **NOT** be administered. Kroger A, Bahta L, Hunter P. ACIP General Best Practice Guidelines for Immunization.
2. When a precaution is present, vaccination should generally be deferred but might be indicated if the benefit of protection from the vaccine outweighs the risk for an adverse reaction. Kroger A, Bahta L, Hunter P. ACIP General Best Practice Guidelines for Immunization.
3. Vaccination providers should check FDA-approved prescribing information for the most complete and updated information, including contraindications, warnings, and precautions. See Package inserts for U.S.-licensed vaccines.
4. See package inserts and FDA EUA fact sheets for a full list of vaccine ingredients. mRNA COVID-19 vaccines contain polyethylene glycol (PEG).

Appendix

Recommended Child and Adolescent Immunization Schedule for Ages 18 Years or Younger, United States, 2024

Vaccines and other Immunizing Agents	Contraindicated or Not Recommended[1]	Precautions[2]
Dengue (DEN4CYD)	• Severe allergic reaction (e.g., anaphylaxis) after a previous dose or to a vaccine component[3] • Severe immunodeficiency (e.g., hematologic and solid tumors, receipt of chemotherapy, congenital immunodeficiency, long-term immunosuppressive therapy or patients with HIV infection who are severely immunocompromised) • Lack of laboratory confirmation of a previous Dengue infection	• Pregnancy • HIV infection without evidence of severe immunosuppression • Moderate or severe acute illness with or without fever
Diphtheria, tetanus, pertussis (DTaP)	• Severe allergic reaction (e.g., anaphylaxis) after a previous dose or to a vaccine component[3] • For DTaP only: Encephalopathy (e.g., coma, decreased level of consciousness, prolonged seizures) not attributable to another identifiable cause within 7 days of administration of previous dose of DTP or DTaP	• Guillain-Barré syndrome (GBS) within 6 weeks after previous dose of tetanus-toxoid–containing vaccine • History of Arthus-type hypersensitivity reactions after a previous dose of diphtheria-toxoid–containing or tetanus-toxoid–containing vaccine; defer vaccination until at least 10 years have elapsed since the last tetanus-toxoid–containing vaccine • For DTaP only: Progressive neurologic disorder, including infantile spasms, uncontrolled epilepsy, progressive encephalopathy; defer DTaP until neurologic status clarified and stabilized • Moderate or severe acute illness with or without fever
Haemophilus influenzae type b (Hib)	• Severe allergic reaction (e.g., anaphylaxis) after a previous dose or to a vaccine component[3] • Less than age 6 weeks	• Moderate or severe acute illness with or without fever
Hepatitis A (HepA)	• Severe allergic reaction (e.g., anaphylaxis) after a previous dose or to a vaccine component[3] including neomycin	• Moderate or severe acute illness with or without fever
Hepatitis B (HepB)	• Severe allergic reaction (e.g., anaphylaxis) after a previous dose or to a vaccine component[3] including yeast *Pregnancy: Heplisav-B and PreHevbrio are not recommended due to lack of safety data in pregnant persons. Use other hepatitis B vaccines if HepB is indicated[4].*	• Moderate or severe acute illness with or without fever
Hepatitis A-Hepatitis B vaccine (HepA-HepB) [Twinrix]	• Severe allergic reaction (e.g., anaphylaxis) after a previous dose or to a vaccine component[3] including neomycin and yeast	• Moderate or severe acute illness with or without fever
Human papillomavirus (HPV)	• Severe allergic reaction (e.g., anaphylaxis) after a previous dose or to a vaccine component[3] *Pregnancy: HPV vaccination not recommended.*	• Moderate or severe acute illness with or without fever
Measles, mumps, rubella (MMR) Measles, mumps, rubella, and varicella (MMRV)	• Severe allergic reaction (e.g., anaphylaxis) after a previous dose or to a vaccine component[3] • Severe immunodeficiency (e.g., hematologic and solid tumors, receipt of chemotherapy, congenital immunodeficiency, long-term immunosuppressive therapy or patients with HIV infection who are severely immunocompromised) • Pregnancy • Family history of altered immunocompetence, unless verified clinically or by laboratory testing as immunocompetent	• Recent (≤11 months) receipt of antibody-containing blood product (specific interval depends on product) • History of thrombocytopenia or thrombocytopenic purpura • Need for tuberculin skin testing or interferon-gamma release assay (IGRA) testing • Moderate or severe acute illness with or without fever • For MMRV only: Personal or family history (i.e., sibling or parent) history of seizures of any etiology
Meningococcal ACWY (MenACWY) MenACWY-CRM (Menveo) MenACWY-TT (MenQuadfi)	• Severe allergic reaction (e.g., anaphylaxis) after a previous dose or to a vaccine component[3] • For Men ACWY-CRM only: severe allergic reaction to any diphtheria toxoid—or CRM197—containing vaccine • For MenACWY-TT only: severe allergic reaction to a tetanus toxoid-containing vaccine	• For MenACWY-CRM only: Preterm birth if less than age 9 months • Moderate or severe acute illness with or without fever
Meningococcal B (MenB) MenB-4C (Bexsero) MenB-FHbp (Trumenba)	• Severe allergic reaction (e.g., anaphylaxis) after a previous dose or to a vaccine component[3]	• Pregnancy • For MenB-4C only: Latex sensitivity • Moderate or severe acute illness with or without fever
Meningococcal ABCWY (MenACWY-TT/MenB-FHbp) [Penbraya]	• Severe allergic reaction (e.g., anaphylaxis) after a previous dose or to a vaccine component[3] • Severe allergic reaction to a tetanus toxoid-containing vaccine	• Moderate or severe acute illness, with or without fever
Mpox (Jynneos)	• Severe allergic reaction (e.g., anaphylaxis) after a previous dose or to a vaccine component[3]	• Moderate or severe acute illness with or without fever
Pneumococcal conjugate (PCV)	• Severe allergic reaction (e.g., anaphylaxis) after a previous dose or to a vaccine component[3] • Severe allergic reaction (e.g., anaphylaxis) to any diphtheria-toxoid-containing vaccine or its component[3]	• Moderate or severe acute illness with or without fever
Pneumococcal polysaccharide (PPSV23)	• Severe allergic reaction (e.g., anaphylaxis) after a previous dose or to a vaccine component[3]	• Moderate or severe acute illness with or without fever
Poliovirus vaccine, inactivated (IPV)	• Severe allergic reaction (e.g., anaphylaxis) after a previous dose or to a vaccine component[3]	• Pregnancy • Moderate or severe acute illness with or without fever
RSV monoclonal antibody (RSV-mAb)	• Severe allergic reaction (e.g., anaphylaxis) after a previous dose or to a vaccine component[3]	• Moderate or severe acute illness with or without fever
Respiratory syncytial virus vaccine (RSV)	• Severe allergic reaction (e.g., anaphylaxis) after a previous dose or to a vaccine component[3]	• Moderate or severe acute illness with or without fever
Rotavirus (RV) RV1 [Rotarix] RV5 [RotaTeq]	• Severe allergic reaction (e.g., anaphylaxis) after a previous dose or to a vaccine component[3] • Severe combined immunodeficiency (SCID) • History of intussusception	• Altered immunocompetence other than SCID • Chronic gastrointestinal disease • RV1 only: Spina bifida or bladder exstrophy • Moderate or severe acute illness with or without fever
Tetanus, diphtheria, and acellular pertussis (Tdap) Tetanus, diphtheria (Td)	• Severe allergic reaction (e.g., anaphylaxis) after a previous dose or to a vaccine component[3] • For Tdap only: Encephalopathy (e.g., coma, decreased level of consciousness, prolonged seizures) not attributable to another identifiable cause within 7 days of administration of previous dose of DTP, DTaP, or Tdap	• Guillain-Barré syndrome (GBS) within 6 weeks after a previous dose of tetanus-toxoid–containing vaccine • History of Arthus-type hypersensitivity reactions after a previous dose of diphtheria-toxoid–containing or tetanus-toxoid–containing vaccine; defer vaccination until at least 10 years have elapsed since the last tetanus-toxoid–containing vaccine • For Tdap only: Progressive or unstable neurological disorder, uncontrolled seizures, or progressive encephalopathy until a treatment regimen has been established and the condition has stabilized • Moderate or severe acute illness with or without fever
Varicella (VAR)	• Severe allergic reaction (e.g., anaphylaxis) after a previous dose or to a vaccine component[3] • Severe immunodeficiency (e.g., hematologic and solid tumors, receipt of chemotherapy, congenital immunodeficiency, long-term immunosuppressive therapy or patients with HIV infection who are severely immunocompromised) • Pregnancy • Family history of altered immunocompetence, unless verified clinically or by laboratory testing as immunocompetent	• Recent (≤11 months) receipt of antibody-containing blood product (specific interval depends on product) • Receipt of specific antiviral drugs (acyclovir, famciclovir, or valacyclovir) 24 hours before vaccination (avoid use of these antiviral drugs for 14 days after vaccination) • Use of aspirin or aspirin-containing products • Moderate or severe acute illness with or without fever • If using MMRV, see MMR/MMRV for additional precautions

1. When a contraindication is present, a vaccine should NOT be administered. When a precaution is present, vaccination should generally be deferred but might be indicated if the benefit of protection from the vaccine outweighs the risk for an adverse reaction. Kroger A, Bahta L, Hunter P. ACIP General Best Practice Guidelines for Immunization. www.cdc.gov/vaccines/hcp/acip-recs/general-recs/contraindications.html
2. When a precaution is present, vaccination should generally be deferred but might be indicated if the benefit of protection from the vaccine outweighs the risk for an adverse reaction. Kroger A, Bahta L, Hunter P. ACIP General Best Practice Guidelines for Immunization. www.cdc.gov/vaccines/hcp/acip-recs/general-recs/contraindications.html
3. Vaccination providers should check FDA-approved prescribing information for the most complete and updated information, including contraindications, warnings, and precautions. Package inserts for U.S.-licensed vaccines are available at www.fda.gov/vaccines-blood-biologics/approved-products/vaccines-licensed-use-united-states.
4. For information on the pregnancy exposure registries for persons who were inadvertently vaccinated with Heplisav-B or PreHevbrio while pregnant, please visit heplisavbpregnancyregistry.com or www.prehevbrio.com/#safety.
5. Full prescribing information for BEYFORTUS (nirsevimab-alip) www.accessdata.fda.gov/drugsatfda_docs/label/2023/761328s000lbl.pdf

Addendum

Recommended Child and Adolescent Immunization Schedule for Ages 18 Years or Younger, United States, 2024

In addition to the recommendations presented in the previous sections of this immunization schedule, ACIP has approved the following recommendations by majority vote since October 26, 2023. The following recommendations have been adopted by the CDC Director and are now official. Links are provided if these recommendations have been published in *Morbidity and Mortality Weekly Report (MMWR)*.

Vaccines	Recommendations	Effective Date of Recommendation*
COVID-19 (Moderna, Pfizer-BioNTech, Novavax)	• ACIP recommends 2024-2025 COVID-19 vaccines as authorized or approved by FDA in persons ≥6 months of age.	June 27, 2024
Influenza	• ACIP reaffirms the recommendation for routine annual influenza vaccination of all persons aged ≥6 months who do not have contraindications. • ACIP recommends high–dose inactivated (HD–IIV3) and adjuvanted inactivated (aIIV3) influenza vaccines as acceptable options for influenza vaccination of solid organ transplant recipients aged 18 through 64 years who are on immunosuppressive medication regimens, without a preference over other age-appropriate IIV3s or RIV3.	June 27, 2024
Vaxelis (DTaP-IPV-Hib-HepB)	• ACIP recommends DTaP-IPV-Hib-HepB (Vaxelis®) should be included with PRP-OMP (PedvaxHIB®) in the preferential recommendation for American Indian and Alaska Native Infants based on the *Haemophilus influenzae* type b (Hib) component.	June 26, 2024

*The effective date is the date when the CDC director adopted the recommendation and when the ACIP recommendation became official.

Source: https://www.cdc.gov/vaccines/schedules/hcp/imz/child-adolescent.html

CDC VACCINE SCHEDULES FOR ADULTS

TABLE 4   RECOMMENDED ADULT IMMUNIZATION SCHEDULE FOR AGES 19 Y OR OLDER, UNITED STATES, 2024

Vaccines in the Adult Immunization Schedule*

Vaccine	Abbreviation(s)	Trade name(s)
COVID-19 vaccine	1vCOV-mRNA	Comirnaty®/Pfizer-BioNTech COVID-19 Vaccine Spikevax®/Moderna COVID-19 Vaccine
	1vCOV-aPS	Novavax COVID-19 Vaccine
Haemophilus influenzae type b vaccine	Hib	ActHIB® Hiberix® PedvaxHIB®
Hepatitis A vaccine	HepA	Havrix® Vaqta®
Hepatitis A and hepatitis B vaccine	HepA-HepB	Twinrix®
Hepatitis B vaccine	HepB	Engerix-B® Heplisav-B® PreHevbrio® Recombivax HB®
Human papillomavirus vaccine	HPV	Gardasil 9®
Influenza vaccine (inactivated)	IIV4	Many brands
Influenza vaccine (live, attenuated)	LAIV4	FluMist® Quadrivalent
Influenza vaccine (recombinant)	RIV4	Flublok® Quadrivalent
Measles, mumps, and rubella vaccine	MMR	M-M-R II® Priorix®
Meningococcal serogroups A, C, W, Y vaccine	MenACWY-CRM MenACWY-TT	Menveo® MenQuadfi®
Meningococcal serogroup B vaccine	MenB-4C MenB-FHbp	Bexsero® Trumenba®
Meningococcal serogroup A, B, C, W, Y vaccine	MenACWY-TT/ MenB-FHbp	Penbraya™
Mpox vaccine	Mpox	Jynneos®
Pneumococcal conjugate vaccine	PCV15 PCV20	Vaxneuvance™ Prevnar 20™
Pneumococcal polysaccharide vaccine	PPSV23	Pneumovax 23®
Poliovirus vaccine	IPV	Ipol®
Respiratory syncytial virus vaccine	RSV	Arexvy® Abrysvo™
Tetanus and diphtheria toxoids	Td	Tenivac® Tdvax™
Tetanus and diphtheria toxoids and acellular pertussis vaccine	Tdap	Adacel® Boostrix®
Varicella vaccine	VAR	Varivax®
Zoster vaccine, recombinant	RZV	Shingrix

*Administer recommended vaccines if vaccination history is incomplete or unknown. Do not restart or add doses to vaccine series if there are extended intervals between doses. The use of trade names is for identification purposes only and does not imply endorsement by the ACIP or CDC.

6/27/2024

How to use the adult immunization schedule

1 Determine recommended vaccinations by age **(Table 1)**

2 Assess need for additional recommended vaccinations by medical condition or other indication **(Table 2)**

3 Review vaccine types, dosing frequencies and intervals, and considerations for special situations **(Notes)**

4 Review contraindications and precautions for vaccine types **(Appendix)**

5 Review new or updated ACIP guidance **(Addendum)**

Recommended by the Advisory Committee on Immunization Practices (www.cdc.gov/vaccines/acip) and approved by the Centers for Disease Control and Prevention (www.cdc.gov), American College of Physicians (www.acponline.org), American Academy of Family Physicians (www.aafp.org), American College of Obstetricians and Gynecologists (www.acog.org), American College of Nurse-Midwives (www.midwife.org), American Academy of Physician Associates (www.aapa.org), American Pharmacists Association (www.pharmacist.com), and Society for Healthcare Epidemiology of America (www.shea-online.org).

Report
- Suspected cases of reportable vaccine-preventable diseases or outbreaks to the local or state health department
- Clinically significant adverse events to the Vaccine Adverse Event Reporting System at www.vaers.hhs.gov or 800-822-7967

Questions or comments
Contact www.cdc.gov/cdc-info or 800-CDC-INFO (800-232-4636), in English or Spanish, 8 a.m.–8 p.m. ET, Monday through Friday, excluding holidays.

 Download the CDC Vaccine Schedules app for providers at www.cdc.gov/vaccines/schedules/hcp/schedule-app.html.

Helpful information
- Complete Advisory Committee on Immunization Practices (ACIP) recommendations: www.cdc.gov/vaccines/hcp/acip-recs/index.html
- ACIP Shared Clinical Decision-Making Recommendations: www.cdc.gov/vaccines/acip/acip-scdm-faqs.html
- *General Best Practice Guidelines for Immunization* www.cdc.gov/vaccines/hcp/acip-recs/general-recs/index.html
- Vaccine information statements: www.cdc.gov/vaccines/hcp/vis/index.html
- Manual for the Surveillance of Vaccine-Preventable Diseases (including case identification and outbreak response): www.cdc.gov/vaccines/pubs/surv-manual

U.S. Department of Health and Human Services
Centers for Disease Control and Prevention

Scan QR code for access to online schedule

CS310021-D

Vaccine	19–26 years	27–49 years	50–64 years	≥65 years
COVID-19	1 or more doses of updated (2023–2024 Formula) vaccine (See Notes)			
Influenza inactivated (IIV4) or **Influenza recombinant (RIV4)** **or**	1 dose annually **or**			
Influenza live, attenuated (LAIV4)	1 dose annually			
Respiratory Syncytial Virus (RSV)	Seasonal administration during pregnancy. See Notes.			≥60 years
Tetanus, diphtheria, pertussis (Tdap or Td)	1 dose Tdap each pregnancy; 1 dose Td/Tdap for wound management (see notes)			
	1 dose Tdap, then Td or Tdap booster every 10 years			
Measles, mumps, rubella (MMR)	1 or 2 doses depending on indication (if born in 1957 or later)			For healthcare personnel, see notes
Varicella (VAR)	2 doses (if born in 1980 or later)		2 doses	
Zoster recombinant (RZV)	2 doses for immunocompromising conditions (see notes)		2 doses	
Human papillomavirus (HPV)	2 or 3 doses depending on age at initial vaccination or condition	27 through 45 years		
Pneumococcal (PCV15, PCV20, PPSV23)				See Notes
				See Notes
Hepatitis A (HepA)	2, 3, or 4 doses depending on vaccine			
Hepatitis B (HepB)	2, 3, or 4 doses depending on vaccine or condition			
Meningococcal A, C, W, Y (MenACWY)	1 or 2 doses depending on indication, see notes for booster recommendations			
Meningococcal B (MenB)	19 through 23 years	2 or 3 doses depending on vaccine and indication, see notes for booster recommendations		
***Haemophilus influenzae* type b (Hib)**	1 or 3 doses depending on indication			
Mpox				

Recommended vaccination for adults who meet age requirement, lack documentation of vaccination, or lack evidence of immunity	Recommended vaccination for adults with an additional risk factor or another indication	Recommended vaccination based on shared clinical decision-making	No recommendation/ Not applicable

TABLE 5 RECOMMENDED ADULT IMMUNIZATION SCHEDULE BY MEDICAL CONDITION OR OTHER INDICATION, UNITED STATES, 2024

Always use this table in conjunction with Table 1 and the Notes that follow. Medical conditions or indications are often not mutually exclusive. If multiple medical conditions or indications are present, refer to guidance in all relevant columns. See Notes for medical conditions or indications not listed.

VACCINE	Pregnancy	Immunocompromised (excluding HIV infection)	HIV infection CD4 percentage and count <15% or <200mm³	HIV infection CD4 percentage and count ≥15% and ≥200mm³	Men who have sex with men	Asplenia, complement deficiency	Heart or lung disease	Kidney failure, End-stage renal disease or on dialysis	Chronic liver disease; alcoholism*	Diabetes	Healthcare Personnel[b]
COVID-19		See Notes									
IIV4 or RIV4											
LAIV4	Seasonal administration. See Notes				1 dose annually if age 19–49 years				1 dose annually if age 19–49 years		
RSV		See Notes			1 dose annually			See Notes			
Tdap or Td	Tdap: 1 dose each pregnancy					1 dose Tdap, then Td or Tdap booster every 10 years					
MMR	*			See Notes							
VAR	*			See Notes							
RZV		See Notes									
HPV	*	3 dose series if indicated									
Pneumococcal											
HepA											
Hep B	See Notes							Age ≥ 60 years			
MenACWY											
MenB											
Hib		HSCT: 3 doses[c]				Asplenia: 1 dose					
Mpox	See Notes				See Notes						See Notes

Legend:

- Recommended for all adults who lack documentation of vaccination, OR lack evidence of immunity
- Not recommended for all adults, but recommended for some adults based on either age OR increased risk for or severe outcomes from disease
- Recommended based on shared clinical decision-making
- Recommended for all adults, and additional doses may be necessary based on medical condition or other indications. See Notes.
- Precaution: Might be indicated if benefit of protection outweighs risk of adverse reaction
- Contraindicated or not recommended *vaccinate after pregnancy, if indicated
- No Guidance/ Not Applicable

a. Precaution for LAIV4 does not apply to alcoholism.   b. See notes for influenza; hepatitis B; measles, mumps, and rubella; and varicella vaccinations.   c. Hematopoietic stem cell transplant.

Notes | Recommended Adult Immunization Schedule for Ages 19 Years or Older, United States, 2024

For vaccination recommendations for persons ages 18 years or younger, see the Recommended Child and Adolescent Immunization Schedule, 2024: www.cdc.gov/vaccines/schedules/hcp/child-adolescent.html

Additional Information

- For calculating intervals between doses, 4 weeks = 28 days. Intervals of ≥4 months are determined by calendar months.
- Within a number range (e.g., 12–18), a dash (–) should be read as "through."
- Vaccine doses administered ≤4 days before the minimum age or interval are considered valid. Doses of any vaccine administered ≥5 days earlier than the minimum age or minimum interval should not be counted as valid and should be repeated. **The repeat dose should be spaced after the invalid dose by the recommended minimum interval.** For further details, see Table 3-2, Recommended and minimum ages and intervals between vaccine doses, in *General Best Practice Guidelines for Immunization* at www.cdc.gov/vaccines/hcp/acip-recs/general-recs/timing.html.
- Information on travel vaccination requirements and recommendations is available at www.cdc.gov/travel/.
- For vaccination of persons with immunodeficiencies, see Table 8-1, Vaccination of persons with primary and secondary immunodeficiencies, in *General Best Practice Guidelines for Immunization* at www.cdc.gov/vaccines/hcp/acip-recs/general-recs/immunocompetence.html
- For information about vaccination in the setting of a vaccine-preventable disease outbreak, contact your state or local health department.
- The National Vaccine Injury Compensation Program (VICP) is a no-fault alternative to the traditional legal system for resolving vaccine injury claims. All vaccines included in the adult immunization schedule except PPSV23, RSV, RZV, Mpox, and COVID-19 vaccines are covered by the National Vaccine Injury Compensation Program (VICP). Mpox and COVID-19 vaccines are covered by the Countermeasures Injury Compensation Program (CICP). For more information, see www.hrsa.gov/vaccinecompensation or www.hrsa.gov/cicp.

COVID-19 vaccination

Routine vaccination

Age 19 years or older

- **Unvaccinated:**
  - 1 dose of updated (2023–2024 Formula) Moderna or Pfizer-BioNTech vaccine
  - 2-dose series of updated (2023–2024 Formula) Novavax at 0, 3–8 weeks
- **Previously vaccinated* with 1 or more doses of any COVID-19 vaccine:** 1 dose of any updated (2023–2024 Formula) COVID-19 vaccine administered at least 8 weeks after the most recent COVID-19 vaccine dose.

Special situations

Persons who are moderately or severely immunocompromised**

- **Unvaccinated:**
  - 3-dose series of updated (2023–2024 Formula) Moderna at 0, 4, 8 weeks
  - 3-dose series of updated (2023–2024 Formula) Pfizer-BioNTech at 0, 3, 7 weeks
  - 2-dose series of updated (2023–2024 Formula) Novavax at 0, 3 weeks
- **Previously vaccinated* with 1 dose of any Moderna:** 2-dose series of updated (2023–2024 Formula) Moderna at 0, 4 weeks (minimum interval between previous Moderna dose and dose 1: 4 weeks)
- **Previously vaccinated* with 2 doses of any Moderna:** 1 dose of updated (2023–2024 Formula) Moderna at least 4 weeks after most recent dose.
- **Previously vaccinated* with 1 dose of any Pfizer-BioNTech:** 2-dose series of updated (2023–2024 Formula) Pfizer-BioNTech at 0, 4 weeks (minimum interval between previous Pfizer-BioNTech dose and dose 1: 3 weeks).
- **Previously vaccinated* with 2 doses of any Pfizer-BioNTech:** 1 dose of updated (2023–2024 Formula) Pfizer-BioNTech at least 4 weeks after most recent dose.

- **Previously vaccinated* with 3 or more doses of any Moderna or Pfizer-BioNTech:** 1 dose of any updated (2023–2024 Formula) COVID-19 vaccine at least 8 weeks after the most recent dose.
- **Previously vaccinated* with 1 or more doses of Janssen or Novavax with or without dose(s) of any Original monovalent or bivalent COVID-19 vaccine:** 1 dose of any updated (2023–2024 Formula) of COVID-19 vaccine at least 8 weeks after the most recent dose.

There is no preferential recommendation for the use of one COVID-19 vaccine over another when more than one recommended age-appropriate vaccine is available.

Current COVID-19 vaccine information available at www.cdc.gov/covidschedule. For information on Emergency Use Authorization (EUA) indications for COVID-19 vaccines, see www.fda.gov/emergency-preparedness-and-response/coronavirus-disease-2019-covid-19/covid-19-vaccines.

*Note: Previously vaccinated is defined as having received any Original monovalent or bivalent COVID-19 vaccine (Janssen, Moderna, Novavax, Pfizer-BioNTech) prior to the updated 2023–2024 formulation.

**Note: Persons who are moderately or severely immunocompromised have the option to receive one additional dose of updated (2023–2024 Formula) COVID-19 vaccine at least 2 months following the last recommended updated (2023–2024 Formula) COVID-19 vaccine dose. Further additional updated (2023–2024 Formula) COVID-19 vaccine dose(s) may be administered, informed by the clinical judgement of a healthcare provider and personal preference and circumstances. Any further additional doses should be administered at least 2 months after the last updated (2023–2024 Formula) COVID-19 vaccine dose.

Notes Recommended Adult Immunization Schedule for Ages 19 Years or Older, United States, 2024

Haemophilus influenzae type b vaccination

Special situations

- **Anatomical or functional asplenia (including sickle cell disease):** 1 dose if previously did not receive Hib vaccine; if elective splenectomy, 1 dose preferably at least 14 days before splenectomy.
- **Hematopoietic stem cell transplant (HSCT):** 3-dose series 4 weeks apart starting 6–12 months after successful transplant, regardless of Hib vaccination history.

Hepatitis A vaccination

Routine vaccination

- **Any person who is not fully vaccinated and requests vaccination** (identification of risk factor not required): 2-dose series HepA (Havrix 6–12 months apart or Vaqta 6–18 months apart [minimum interval: 6 months]) or 3-dose series HepA-HepB (Twinrix at 0, 1, 6 months [minimum intervals: dose 1 to dose 2: 4 weeks / dose 2 to dose 3: 5 months])

Special situations

- **Any person who is not fully vaccinated and who is at risk for hepatitis A virus infection:** 2-dose series HepA or 3-dose series HepA-HepB as above. Risk factors for hepatitis A virus infection include:
  - **Chronic liver disease** (e.g., persons with hepatitis B, hepatitis C, cirrhosis, fatty liver disease, alcoholic liver disease, autoimmune hepatitis, alanine aminotransferase [ALT] or aspartate aminotransferase [AST] level greater than twice the upper limit of normal)
  - **HIV infection**
  - **Men who have sex with men**
  - **Injection or noninjection drug use**
  - **Persons experiencing homelessness**
  - **Work with hepatitis A virus** in research laboratory or with nonhuman primates with hepatitis A virus infection

- **Travel in countries with high or intermediate endemic hepatitis A** (HepA-HepB [Twinrix] may be administered on an accelerated schedule of 3 doses at 0, 7, and 21–30 days, followed by a booster dose at 12 months)
- **Close, personal contact with international adoptee** (e.g., household or regular babysitting) in first 60 days after arrival from country with high or intermediate endemic hepatitis A (administer dose 1 as soon as adoption is planned, at least 2 weeks before adoptee's arrival)
- **Pregnancy** if at risk for infection or severe outcome from infection during pregnancy
- **Settings for exposure,** including health care settings targeting services to injection or noninjection drug users or group homes and nonresidential day care facilities for developmentally disabled persons (individual risk factor screening not required)

Hepatitis B vaccination

Routine vaccination

- **Age 19 through 59 years:** complete a 2- or 3- or 4-dose series
- 2-dose series only applies when 2 doses of Heplisav-B* are used at least 4 weeks apart
- 3-dose series Engerix-B, PreHevbrio* or Recombivax HB at 0, 1, 6 months [minimum intervals: dose 1 to dose 2: 4 weeks / dose 2 to dose 3: 8 weeks / dose 1 to dose 3: 16 weeks)]
- 3-dose series HepA-HepB (Twinrix at 0, 1, 6 months [minimum intervals: dose 1 to dose 2: 4 weeks / dose 2 to dose 3: 5 months])
- 4-dose series HepA-HepB (Twinrix) accelerated schedule of 3 doses at 0, 7, and 21–30 days, followed by a booster dose at 12 months

*Note: Heplisav-B and PreHevbrio are not recommended in pregnancy due to lack of safety data in pregnant persons.

- **Travel in countries with high or intermediate endemic hepatitis B** virus infection **may** receive a HepB vaccine series.
- **Age 60 years or older with** known risk factors for hepatitis B virus infection **should** receive a HepB vaccine series.
- **Any adult age 60 years of age or older** who requests HepB vaccination should receive a HepB vaccine series.
- **Risk factors for hepatitis B virus infection include:**
  - **Chronic liver disease** e.g., persons with hepatitis C, cirrhosis, fatty liver disease, alcoholic liver disease, autoimmune hepatitis, alanine aminotransferase (ALT) or aspartate aminotransferase (AST) level greater than twice the upper limit of normal
  - **HIV infection**
  - **Sexual exposure risk** e.g., sex partners of hepatitis B surface antigen (HBsAg)-positive persons, sexually active persons not in mutually monogamous relationships, persons seeking evaluation or treatment for a sexually transmitted infection, men who have sex with men
  - **Current or recent injection drug use**
  - **Percutaneous or mucosal risk for exposure to blood** e.g., household contacts of HBsAg-positive persons, residents and staff of facilities for developmentally disabled persons, health care and public safety personnel with reasonably anticipated risk for exposure to blood or blood-contaminated body fluids; persons on maintenance dialysis (including in-center or home hemodialysis and peritoneal dialysis), persons who are predialysis, and patients with diabetes*
  - **Incarceration**
  - **Travel in countries with high or intermediate endemic hepatitis B**

*Age 60 years or older with diabetes: Based on shared clinical decision making, 2-, 3-, or 4-dose series as above.

- **Age 60 years or older without** known risk factors for hepatitis B virus infection **may** receive a HepB vaccine series.

Notes   Recommended Adult Immunization Schedule for Ages 19 Years or Older, United States, 2024

Special situations

- **Patients on dialysis:** complete a 3- or 4-dose series
  - 3-dose series Recombivax HB at 0, 1, 6 months (Note: Use Dialysis Formulation 1 mL = 40 mcg)
  - 4-dose series Engerix-B at 0, 1, 2, and 6 months (Note: Use 2 mL dose instead of the normal adult dose of 1 mL)

Human papillomavirus vaccination

Routine vaccination

- **All persons up through age 26 years:** 2- or 3-dose series depending on age at initial vaccination or condition
  - **Age 9–14 years at initial vaccination and received 1 dose or 2 doses less than 5 months apart:** 1 additional dose
  - **Age 9–14 years at initial vaccination and received 2 doses at least 5 months apart:** HPV vaccination series complete, no additional dose needed
  - **Age 15 years or older at initial vaccination:** 3-dose series at 0, 1–2 months, 6 months (minimum intervals: dose 1 to dose 2: 4 weeks / dose 2 to dose 3: 12 weeks / dose 1 to dose 3: 5 months; repeat dose if administered too soon)
- No additional dose recommended when any HPV vaccine series of any valency has been completed using the recommended dosing intervals.

Shared clinical decision-making

- **Adults age 27–45 years:** Based on shared clinical decision-making, complete a 2-dose series (if initiated age 9–14 years) or 3-dose series (if initiated ≥15 years)

For additional information on shared clinical decision-making for HPV; see www.cdc.gov/vaccines/hcp/admin/downloads/isd-job-aid-scdm-hpv-shared-clinical-decision-making-hpv.pdf

Special situations

- **Age ranges recommended above for routine and catch-up vaccination or shared clinical decision-making also apply in special situations**
  - **Immunocompromising conditions, including HIV infection:** 3-dose series, even for those who initiate vaccination at age 9 through 14 years.
  - **Pregnancy:** Pregnancy testing is not needed before vaccination. HPV vaccination is not recommended until after pregnancy. No intervention needed if inadvertently vaccinated while pregnant.

Influenza vaccination

Routine vaccination

- **Age 19 years or older:** 1 dose any influenza vaccine appropriate for age and health status annually.
- **Age 65 years or older:** Any one of quadrivalent high-dose inactivated influenza vaccine (HD-IIV4), quadrivalent recombinant influenza vaccine (RIV4), or quadrivalent adjuvanted inactivated influenza vaccine (aIIV4) is preferred. If none of these three vaccines are available, then any other age-appropriate influenza vaccine should be used.
- For the 2023–2024 season, see www.cdc.gov/mmwr/volumes/72/rr/rr7202a1.htm
- For the 2024–2025 season, see the 2024–2025 ACIP influenza vaccine recommendations.

Special situations

- **Close contacts (e.g., caregivers, healthcare workers) of severely immunosuppressed persons who require a protected environment:** should not receive LAIV4. If LAIV4 is given, they should avoid contact with/caring for such immunosuppressed persons for 7 days after vaccination.

Note: Persons with an egg allergy can receive any influenza vaccine (egg-based and non-egg based) appropriate for age and health status.

Measles, mumps, and rubella vaccination

Routine vaccination

- **No evidence of immunity to measles, mumps, or rubella:** 1 dose
  - **Evidence of immunity:** Born before 1957 (except for health care personnel, see below), documentation of receipt of MMR vaccine, laboratory evidence of immunity or disease (diagnosis of disease without laboratory confirmation is not evidence of immunity)

Special situations

- **Pregnancy with no evidence of immunity to rubella:** MMR contraindicated during pregnancy; after pregnancy (before discharge from health care facility), 1 dose
- **Nonpregnant persons of childbearing age with no evidence of immunity to rubella:** 1 dose
- **HIV infection with CD4 percentages ≥15% and CD4 count ≥200 cells/mm³ for at least 6 months and no evidence of immunity to measles, mumps, or rubella:** 2-dose series at least 4 weeks apart; MMR contraindicated for HIV infection with CD4 percentage <15% or CD4 count <200 cells/mm³
- **Severe immunocompromising conditions:** MMR contraindicated
- **Students in postsecondary educational institutions, international travelers, and household or close, personal contacts of immunocompromised persons with no evidence of immunity to measles, mumps, or rubella:** 2-dose series at least 4 weeks apart if previously did not receive any doses of MMR or 1 dose if previously received 1 dose MMR
- **In mumps outbreak settings,** for information about additional doses of MMR (including 3rd dose of MMR), see www.cdc.gov/mmwr/volumes/67/wr/mm6701a7.htm

Notes — Recommended Adult Immunization Schedule for Ages 19 Years or Older, United States, 2024

- **Health care personnel:**
  - **Born before 1957 with no evidence of immunity to measles, mumps, or rubella:** Consider 2-dose series at least 4 weeks apart for protection against measles or mumps or 1 dose for protection against rubella
  - **Born in 1957 or later with no evidence of immunity to measles, mumps, or rubella:** 2-dose series at least 4 weeks apart for protection against measles or mumps or at least 1 dose for protection against rubella

Meningococcal vaccination

Special situations for MenACWY

- **Anatomical or functional asplenia (including sickle cell disease), HIV infection, persistent complement component deficiency, complement inhibitor (e.g., eculizumab, ravulizumab) use:** 2-dose series MenACWY (Menveo or MenQuadfi) at least 8 weeks apart and revaccinate every 5 years if risk remains
- **Travel in countries with hyperendemic or epidemic meningococcal disease, or microbiologists routinely exposed to *Neisseria meningitidis*:** 1 dose MenACWY (Menveo or MenQuadfi) and revaccinate every 5 years if risk remains
- **First-year college students who live in residential housing (if not previously vaccinated at age 16 years or older) or military recruits:** 1 dose MenACWY (Menveo or MenQuadfi)
- For MenACWY **booster dose recommendations** for groups listed under "Special situations" and in an outbreak setting (e.g., in community or organizational settings, or among men who have sex with men) and additional meningococcal vaccination information, see www.cdc.gov/mmwr/volumes/69/rr/rr6909a1.htm

Shared clinical decision-making for MenB

- **Adolescents and young adults age 16–23 years (age 16–18 years preferred) not at increased risk for meningococcal disease:** Based on shared clinical decision-making, 2-dose series MenB-4C (Bexsero) at least 1 month apart or 2-dose series MenB-FHbp (Trumenba) at 0, 6 months (if dose 2 was administered less than 6 months after dose 1, administer dose 3 at least 4 months after dose 2); MenB-4C and MenB-FHbp are not interchangeable (use same product for all doses in series).

For additional information on shared clinical decision-making for MenB, see www.cdc.gov/vaccines/hcp/admin/downloads/isd-job-aid-scdm-mening-b-shared-clinical-decision-making.pdf

Special situations for MenB

- **Anatomical or functional asplenia (including sickle cell disease), persistent complement component deficiency, complement inhibitor (e.g., eculizumab, ravulizumab) use, or microbiologists routinely exposed to *Neisseria meningitidis*:** 2-dose primary series MenB-4C (Bexsero) at least 1 month apart or 3-dose primary series MenB-FHbp (Trumenba) at 0, 1–2, 6 months (if dose 2 was administered at least 6 months after dose 1, dose 3 not needed; if dose 3 is administered earlier than 4 months after dose 2, a fourth dose should be administered at least 4 months after dose 3); MenB-4C and MenB-FHbp are not interchangeable (use same product for all doses in series); 1 dose MenB booster 1 year after primary series and revaccinate every 2–3 years if risk remains.
- **Pregnancy:** Delay MenB until after pregnancy unless at increased risk and vaccination benefits outweigh potential risks.

- For MenB **booster dose recommendations** for groups listed under "Special situations" and in an outbreak setting (e.g., in community or organizational settings and among men who have sex with men) and additional meningococcal vaccination information, see www.cdc.gov/mmwr/volumes/69/rr/rr6909a1.htm

Note: MenB vaccines may be administered simultaneously with MenACWY vaccines if indicated, but at a different anatomic site, if feasible.

Adults may receive a single dose of Penbraya as an alternative to separate administration of MenACWY and MenB when both vaccines would be given on the same clinic day. For adults not at increased risk, if Penbraya is used for dose 1 MenB, MenB-FHbp (Trumenba) should be administered for dose 2 MenB. For adults at increased risk of meningococcal disease, Penbraya may be used for additional MenACWY and MenB doses (including booster doses) if both would be given on the same clinic day **and** at least 6 months have elapsed since most recent Penbraya dose.

Mpox vaccination

Special situations

- **Any person at risk for Mpox infection:** 2-dose series, 28 days apart.

  Risk factors for Mpox infection include:
  - Persons who are gay, bisexual, and other MSM, transgender or nonbinary people who in the past 6 months have had:
    - A new diagnosis of at least 1 sexually transmitted disease
    - More than 1 sex partner
  - Sex at a commercial sex venue
  - Sex in association with a large public event in a geographic area where Mpox transmission is occurring
  - Persons who are sexual partners of the persons described above
  - Persons who anticipate experiencing any of the situations described above

Notes — Recommended Adult Immunization Schedule for Ages 19 Years or Older, United States, 2024

• **Pregnancy:** There is currently no ACIP recommendation for Jynneos use in pregnancy due to lack of safety data in pregnant persons. Pregnant persons with any risk factor described above may receive Jynneos.

• **Healthcare personnel:** Except in rare circumstances (e.g. no available personal protective equipment), healthcare personnel who do not have any of the sexual risk factors described above should not receive Jynneos.

For detailed information, see: www.cdc.gov/vaccines/acip/meetings/downloads/slides-2023-10-25-26/04-MPOX-Rao-508.pdf

Pneumococcal vaccination

Routine vaccination

• **Age 65 years or older who have:**

- **Not previously received a dose of PCV13, PCV15, or PCV20 or whose previous vaccination history is unknown:** 1 dose PCV15 OR 1 dose PCV20.
  - If PCV15 is used, administer 1 dose PPSV23 at least 1 year after the PCV15 dose (may use minimum interval of 8 weeks for adults with an immunocompromising condition,* cochlear implant, or cerebrospinal fluid leak).
- **Previously received only PCV7:** follow the recommendation above.
- **Previously received only PCV13:** 1 dose PCV20 OR 1 dose PPSV23.
  - If PCV20 is selected, administer at least 1 year after the last PCV13 dose.
  - If PPSV23 is selected, administer at least 1 year after the last PCV13 dose (may use minimum interval of 8 weeks for adults with an immunocompromising condition,* cochlear implant, or cerebrospinal fluid leak).
- **Previously received only PPSV23:** 1 dose PCV15 OR 1 dose PCV20. Administer either PCV15 or PCV20 at least 1 year after the last PPSV23 dose.
  - If PCV15 is used, no additional PPSV23 doses are recommended.
- **Previously received both PCV13 and PPSV23 but NO PPSV23 was received at age 65 years or older:** 1 dose PCV20 OR 1 dose PPSV23.
  - If PCV20 is selected, administer at least 5 years after the last pneumococcal vaccine dose.
  - If PPSV23 is selected, see dosing schedule at www.cdc.gov/vaccines/vpd/pneumo/downloads/pneumo-vaccine-timing.pdf.
- **Previously received both PCV13 and PPSV23, AND PPSV23 was received at age 65 years or older:** Based on shared clinical decision-making, 1 dose of PCV20 at least 5 years after the last pneumococcal vaccine dose.

• For guidance on determining which pneumococcal vaccines a patient needs and when, please refer to the mobile app, which can be downloaded here: www.cdc.gov/vaccines/vpd/pneumo/hcp/pneumoapp.html.

Special situations

• **Age 19–64 years with certain underlying medical conditions or other risk factors** who have:**

- **Not previously received a PCV13, PCV15, or PCV20 or whose previous vaccination history is unknown:** 1 dose PCV15 OR 1 dose PCV20.
  - If PCV15 is used, administer 1 dose PPSV23 at least 1 year after the PCV15 dose (may use minimum interval of 8 weeks for adults with an immunocompromising condition,* cochlear implant, or cerebrospinal fluid leak).
- **Previously received only PCV7:** follow the recommendation above.
- **Previously received only PCV13:** 1 dose PCV20 OR 1 dose PPSV23.
  - If PCV20 is selected, administer at least 1 year after the PCV13 dose.
  - If PPSV23 is selected, see dosing schedule at www.cdc.gov/vaccines/vpd/pneumo/downloads/pneumo-vaccine-timing.pdf
- **Previously received only PPSV23:** 1 dose PCV15 OR 1 dose PCV20. Administer either PCV15 or PCV20 at least 1 year after the last PPSV23 dose.
  - If PCV15 is used, no additional PPSV23 doses are recommended.
- **Previously received PCV13 and 1 dose of PPSV23:** 1 dose PCV20 OR 1 dose PPSV23.
  - If PCV20 is selected, administer at least 5 years after the last pneumococcal vaccine dose.
  - If PPSV23 is selected, see dosing schedule at www.cdc.gov/vaccines/vpd/pneumo/downloads/pneumo-vaccine-timing.pdf

• For guidance on determining which pneumococcal vaccines a patient needs and when, please refer to the mobile app which can be downloaded here: www.cdc.gov/vaccines/vpd/pneumo/hcp/pneumoapp.html

*Note: Immunocompromising conditions include chronic renal failure, nephrotic syndrome, immunodeficiencies, iatrogenic immunosuppression, generalized malignancy, HIV infection, Hodgkin disease, leukemia, lymphoma, multiple myeloma, solid organ transplant, congenital or acquired asplenia, or sickle cell disease or other hemoglobinopathies.

**Note: Underlying medical conditions or other risk factors include alcoholism, chronic heart/liver/lung disease, chronic renal failure, cigarette smoking, cochlear implant, congenital or acquired asplenia, CSF leak, diabetes mellitus, generalized malignancy, HIV infection, Hodgkin disease, immunodeficiencies, iatrogenic immunosuppression, leukemia, lymphoma, multiple myeloma, nephrotic syndrome, solid organ transplant, or sickle cell disease or other hemoglobinopathies.

Poliovirus vaccination

Routine vaccination

• **Adults known or suspected to be unvaccinated or incompletely vaccinated:** administer remaining doses (1, 2, or 3 IPV doses) to complete a 3-dose primary series.* Unless there are specific reasons to believe they were not vaccinated, most adults who were born and raised in the United States can assume they were vaccinated against polio as children.

Notes   Recommended Adult Immunization Schedule for Ages 19 Years or Older, United States, 2024

Special situations

- **Adults at increased risk of exposure to poliovirus who completed primary series***: may administer one lifetime IPV booster

  *Note: Complete primary series consists of at least 3 doses of IPV or trivalent oral poliovirus vaccine (tOPV) in any combination.

  For detailed information, see: www.cdc.gov/vaccines/vpd/polio/hcp/recommendations.html

Respiratory syncytial virus vaccination

Routine vaccination

- **Pregnant at 32 weeks 0 days through 36 weeks and 6 days gestation from September through January in most of the continental United States***: 1 dose RSV vaccine (Abrysvo™). Administer RSV vaccine regardless of previous RSV infection.

  - Either maternal RSV vaccination or infant immunization with nirsevimab (RSV monoclonal antibody) is recommended to prevent respiratory syncytial virus lower respiratory tract infection in infants.

- **All other pregnant persons:** RSV vaccine not recommended

  There is currently no ACIP recommendation for RSV vaccination in subsequent pregnancies. No data are available to inform whether additional doses are needed in later pregnancies.

Special situations

- **Age 60 years or older:** Based on shared clinical decision-making, 1 dose RSV vaccine (Arexvy® or Abrysvo™). Persons most likely to benefit from vaccination are those considered to be at increased risk for severe RSV disease.** For additional information on shared clinical decision-making for RSV in older adults, see www.cdc.gov/vaccines/vpd/rsv/downloads/provider-job-aid-for-older-adults-508.pdf

  For further guidance, see www.cdc.gov/mmwr/volumes/72/wr/mm7229a4.htm

*Note: Providers in jurisdictions with RSV seasonality that differs from most of the continental United States (e.g., Alaska, jurisdiction with tropical climate) should follow guidance from public health authorities (e.g., CDC, health departments) or regional medical centers on timing of administration based on local RSV seasonality. Refer to the 2024 Child and Adolescent Immunization Schedule for considerations regarding nirsevimab administration to infants.

**Note: Adults age 60 years or older who are at increased risk for severe RSV disease include those with chronic medical conditions such as lung diseases (e.g., chronic obstructive pulmonary disease, asthma), cardiovascular diseases (e.g., congestive heart failure, coronary artery disease), neurologic or neuromuscular conditions, kidney disorders, liver disorders, hematologic disorders, diabetes mellitus, and moderate or severe immune compromise (either attributable to a medical condition or receipt of immunosuppressive medications or treatment); those who are considered to be frail; those of advanced age; those who reside in nursing homes or other long-term care facilities; and those with other underlying medical conditions or factors that a health care provider determines might increase the risk of severe respiratory disease.

Tetanus, diphtheria, and pertussis vaccination

Routine vaccination

- **Previously did not receive Tdap at or after age 11 years*:** 1 dose Tdap, then Td or Tdap every 10 years

Special situations

- **Previously did not receive primary vaccination series for tetanus, diphtheria, or pertussis:** 1 dose Tdap followed by 1 dose Td or Tdap at least 4 weeks later, and a third dose of Td or Tdap 6–12 months later (Tdap is preferred as first dose and can be substituted for any Td dose), Td or Tdap every 10 years thereafter.

- **Pregnancy:** 1 dose Tdap during each pregnancy, preferably in early part of gestational weeks 27–36.

- **Wound management:** Persons with 3 or more doses of tetanus-toxoid-containing vaccine: For clean and minor wounds, administer Tdap or Td if more than 10 years since last dose of tetanus-toxoid-containing vaccine; for all other wounds, administer Tdap or Td if more than 5 years since last dose of tetanus-toxoid-containing vaccine. Tdap is preferred for persons who have not previously received Tdap or whose Tdap history is unknown. If a tetanus-toxoid-containing vaccine is indicated for a pregnant woman, use Tdap. For detailed information, see www.cdc.gov/mmwr/volumes/69/wr/mm6903a5.htm

*Note: Tdap administered at age 10 years may be counted as the adolescent dose recommended at age 11–12 years

Varicella vaccination

Routine vaccination

- **No evidence of immunity to varicella:** 2-dose series 4–8 weeks apart if previously did not receive varicella-containing vaccine (VAR or MMRV [measles-mumps-rubella-varicella vaccine] for children); if previously received 1 dose varicella-containing vaccine, 1 dose at least 4 weeks after first dose.

  - **Evidence of immunity:** U.S.-born before 1980 (except for pregnant persons and health care personnel [see below]), documentation of 2 doses varicella-containing vaccine at least 4 weeks apart, diagnosis or verification of history of varicella or herpes zoster by a health care provider, laboratory evidence of immunity or disease.

Special situations

- **Pregnancy with no evidence of immunity to varicella:** VAR contraindicated during pregnancy; after pregnancy (before discharge from health care facility), 1 dose if previously received 1 dose varicella-containing vaccine or dose 1 of 2-dose series (dose 2: 4–8 weeks later) if previously did not receive any varicella-containing vaccine, regardless of whether U.S.-born before 1980.

Notes — Recommended Adult Immunization Schedule for Ages 19 Years or Older, United States, 2024

- **Health care personnel with no evidence of immunity to varicella:** 1 dose if previously received 1 dose varicella-containing vaccine; 2-dose series 4–8 weeks apart if previously did not receive any varicella-containing vaccine, regardless of whether U.S.-born before 1980.

- **HIV infection with CD4 percentages ≥15% and CD4 count ≥200 cells/mm³ with no evidence of immunity:** Vaccination may be considered (2 doses 3 months apart); VAR contraindicated for HIV infection with CD4 percentage <15% or CD4 count <200 cells/mm³

- **Severe immunocompromising conditions:** VAR contraindicated.

- **Immunocompromising conditions (including persons with HIV regardless of CD4 count)**:** 2-dose series recombinant zoster vaccine (RZV, Shingrix) 2–6 months apart (minimum interval: 4 weeks; repeat dose if administered too soon). For detailed information, see www.cdc.gov/shingles/vaccination/immunocompromised-adults.html

**Note: If there is no documented history of varicella, varicella vaccination, or herpes zoster, providers should refer to the clinical considerations for use of RZV in immunocompromised adults aged ≥19 years and the ACIP varicella vaccine recommendations for further guidance: www.cdc.gov/mmwr/volumes/71/wr/mm7103a2.htm

Zoster vaccination

Routine vaccination

- **Age 50 years or older*:** 2-dose series recombinant zoster vaccine (RZV, Shingrix) 2–6 months apart (minimum interval: 4 weeks; repeat dose if administered too soon), regardless of previous herpes zoster or history of zoster vaccine live (ZVL, Zostavax) vaccination.

*Note: Serologic evidence of prior varicella is not necessary for zoster vaccination. However, if serologic evidence of varicella susceptibility becomes available, providers should follow ACIP guidelines for varicella vaccination first. RZV is not indicated for the prevention of varicella, and there are limited data on the use of RZV in persons without a history of varicella or varicella vaccination.

Special situations

- **Pregnancy:** There is currently no ACIP recommendation for RZV use in pregnancy. Consider delaying RZV until after pregnancy.

Appendix   Recommended Adult Immunization Schedule for Ages 19 Years or Older, United States, 2024

Contraindications and Precautions to Commonly Used Vaccines

Adapted from Table 4-1 in Advisory Committee on Immunization Practices (ACIP) General Best Practice Guidelines for Immunization: *Contraindication and Precautions.* Prevention and Control of Seasonal Influenza with Vaccines: Recommendations of the Advisory Committee on Immunization Practices—United States, 2023–24 Influenza Season | MMWR (cdc.gov), Contraindications and Precautions for COVID-19 Vaccination, and Contraindications and Precautions for Jynneos Vaccination

Vaccines and Other Immunizing Agents	Contraindicated or Not Recommended[1]	Precautions[2]
COVID-19 mRNA vaccines [Pfizer-BioNTech, Moderna]	• Severe allergic reaction (e.g., anaphylaxis) after a previous dose or to a component of an mRNA COVID-19 vaccine[4]	• Diagnosed non-severe allergy (e.g., urticaria beyond the injection site) to a component of an mRNA COVID-19 vaccine[4]; or non-severe, immediate (onset less than 4 hours) allergic reaction after administration of a previous dose of an mRNA COVID-19 vaccine • Myocarditis or pericarditis within 3 weeks after a dose of any COVID-19 vaccine • Multisystem inflammatory syndrome in children (MIS-C) or multisystem inflammatory syndrome in adults (MIS-A) • Moderate or severe acute illness, with or without fever
COVID-19 protein subunit vaccine [Novavax]	• Severe allergic reaction (e.g., anaphylaxis) after a previous dose or to a component of a Novavax COVID-19 vaccine[4]	• Diagnosed non-severe allergy (e.g., urticaria beyond the injection site) to a component of Novavax COVID-19 vaccine[4]; or non-severe, immediate (onset less than 4 hours) allergic reaction after administration of a previous dose of a Novavax COVID-19 vaccine • Myocarditis or pericarditis within 3 weeks after a dose of any COVID-19 vaccine • Multisystem inflammatory syndrome in children (MIS-C) or multisystem inflammatory syndrome in adults (MIS-A) • Moderate or severe acute illness, with or without fever
Influenza, egg-based, inactivated injectable (IIV4)	• Severe allergic reaction (e.g., anaphylaxis) after previous dose of any influenza vaccine (i.e., any egg-based IIV, ccIIV, RIV, or LAIV of any valency) • Severe allergic reaction (e.g., anaphylaxis) to any vaccine component[3] (excluding egg)	• Guillain-Barré syndrome (GBS) within 6 weeks after a previous dose of any type of influenza vaccine • Moderate or severe acute illness with or without fever
Influenza, cell culture-based inactivated injectable (ccIIV4) [Flucelvax Quadrivalent]	• Severe allergic reaction (e.g., anaphylaxis) to any ccIIV of any valency, or to any component[3] of ccIIV4	• Guillain-Barré syndrome (GBS) within 6 weeks after a previous dose of any type of influenza vaccine • Persons with a history of severe allergic reaction (e.g., anaphylaxis) after a previous dose of any egg-based IIV, RIV, or LAIV of any valency. If using ccIIV4, administer in medical setting under supervision of health care provider who can recognize and manage severe allergic reactions. May consult an allergist. • Moderate or severe acute illness with or without fever
Influenza, recombinant injectable (RIV4) [Flublok Quadrivalent]	• Severe allergic reaction (e.g., anaphylaxis) to any RIV of any valency, or to any component[3] of RIV4	• Guillain-Barré syndrome (GBS) within 6 weeks after a previous dose of any type of influenza vaccine • Persons with a history of severe allergic reaction (e.g., anaphylaxis) after a previous dose of any egg-based IIV, ccIIV, or LAIV of any valency. If using RIV4, administer in medical setting under supervision of health care provider who can recognize and manage severe allergic reactions. May consult an allergist. • Moderate or severe acute illness with or without fever
Influenza, live attenuated (LAIV4) [Flumist Quadrivalent]	• Severe allergic reaction (e.g., anaphylaxis) after previous dose of any influenza vaccine (i.e., any egg-based IIV, ccIIV, RIV, or LAIV of any valency) • Severe allergic reaction (e.g., anaphylaxis) to any vaccine component[3] (excluding egg) • Anatomic or functional asplenia • Immunocompromised due to any cause including, but not limited to, medications and HIV infection • Close contacts or caregivers of severely immunosuppressed persons who require a protected environment • Pregnancy • Cochlear implant • Active communication between the cerebrospinal fluid (CSF) and the oropharynx, nasopharynx, nose, ear, or any other cranial CSF leak • Received influenza antiviral medications oseltamivir or zanamivir within the previous 48 hours, peramivir within the previous 5 days, or baloxavir within the previous 17 days.	• Guillain-Barré syndrome (GBS) within 6 weeks after a previous dose of any type of influenza vaccine • Asthma in persons aged 5 years or older • Persons with underlying medical conditions (other than those listed under contraindications) that might predispose to complications after wild-type influenza virus infection (e.g., chronic pulmonary, cardiovascular (except isolated hypertension), renal, hepatic, neurologic, hematologic, or metabolic disorders (including diabetes mellitus)) • Moderate or severe acute illness with or without fever

1. When a contraindication is present, a vaccine should NOT be administered. Kroger A, Bahta L, Hunter P. ACIP General Best Practice Guidelines for Immunization.
2. When a precaution is present, vaccination should generally be deferred but might be indicated if the benefit of protection from the vaccine outweighs the risk for an adverse reaction. Kroger A, Bahta L, Hunter P. ACIP General Best Practice Guidelines for Immunization.
3. Vaccination providers should check FDA-approved prescribing information for the most complete and updated information, including contraindications, warnings, and precautions. See Package inserts for U.S.-licensed vaccines.
4. See package inserts and FDA EUA fact sheets for a full list of vaccine ingredients. mRNA COVID-19 vaccines contain polyethylene glycol (PEG).

Appendix — Recommended Adult Immunization Schedule for Ages 19 Years or Older, United States, 2024

Vaccine	Contraindicated or Not Recommended[1]	Precautions[2]
Haemophilus influenzae type b (Hib)	• Severe allergic reaction (e.g., anaphylaxis) after a previous dose or to a vaccine component[3]	• Moderate or severe acute illness with or without fever
Hepatitis A (HepA)	• Severe allergic reaction (e.g., anaphylaxis) after a previous dose or to a vaccine component[3] including neomycin	• Moderate or severe acute illness with or without fever
Hepatitis B (HepB)	• Severe allergic reaction (e.g., anaphylaxis) after a previous dose or to a vaccine component[3] including yeast • Pregnancy: Heplisav-B and PreHevbrio are not recommended due to lack of safety data in pregnant persons. Use other hepatitis B vaccines if HepB is indicated[4]	• Moderate or severe acute illness with or without fever
Hepatitis A-Hepatitis B vaccine (HepA-HepB) [Twinrix]	• Severe allergic reaction (e.g., anaphylaxis) after a previous dose or to a vaccine component[3] including neomycin and yeast	• Moderate or severe acute illness with or without fever
Human papillomavirus (HPV)	• Severe allergic reaction (e.g., anaphylaxis) after a previous dose or to a vaccine component[3] • Pregnancy: HPV vaccination not recommended	• Moderate or severe acute illness with or without fever
Measles, mumps, rubella (MMR)	• Severe allergic reaction (e.g., anaphylaxis) after a previous dose or to a vaccine component[3] • Severe immunodeficiency (e.g., hematologic and solid tumors, receipt of chemotherapy, congenital immunodeficiency, long-term immunosuppressive therapy or patients with HIV infection who are severely immunocompromised) • Pregnancy • Family history of altered immunocompetence, unless verified clinically or by laboratory testing as immunocompetent	• Recent (≤11 months) receipt of antibody-containing blood product (specific interval depends on product) • History of thrombocytopenia or thrombocytopenic purpura • Need for tuberculin skin testing or interferon-gamma release assay (IGRA) testing • Moderate or severe acute illness with or without fever
Meningococcal ACWY (MenACWY) (MenACWY-CRM) [Menveo] (MenACWY-TT) [MenQuadfi]	• Severe allergic reaction (e.g., anaphylaxis) after a previous dose or to a vaccine component[3] • For MenACWY-CRM only: severe allergic reaction to any diphtheria toxoid– or CRM197-containing vaccine • For MenACWY-TT only: severe allergic reaction to a tetanus toxoid-containing vaccine	• Moderate or severe acute illness with or without fever
Meningococcal B (MenB) MenB-4C [Bexsero] MenB-FHbp [Trumenba]	• Severe allergic reaction (e.g., anaphylaxis) after a previous dose or to a vaccine component[3]	• Pregnancy • For MenB-4C only: Latex sensitivity • Moderate or severe acute illness with or without fever
Meningococcal ABCWY (MenACWY-TT/MenB-FHbp) [Penbraya]	• Severe allergic reaction (e.g., anaphylaxis) after a previous dose or to a vaccine component[3] • Severe allergic reaction to a tetanus toxoid-containing vaccine	• Moderate or severe acute illness, with or without fever
Mpox [Jynneos]	• Severe allergic reaction (e.g., anaphylaxis) after a previous dose or to a vaccine component[3]	• Moderate or severe acute illness, with or without fever
Pneumococcal conjugate (PCV15, PCV20)	• Severe allergic reaction (e.g., anaphylaxis) after a previous dose or to a vaccine component[3] to any diphtheria-toxoid–containing vaccine or to its vaccine component[3]	• Moderate or severe acute illness with or without fever
Pneumococcal polysaccharide (PPSV23)	• Severe allergic reaction (e.g., anaphylaxis) after a previous dose or to a vaccine component[3]	• Moderate or severe acute illness with or without fever
Poliovirus vaccine, inactivated (IPV)	• Severe allergic reaction (e.g., anaphylaxis) after a previous dose or to a vaccine component[3]	• Pregnancy • Moderate or severe acute illness with or without fever
Respiratory syncytial virus vaccine (RSV)	• Severe allergic reaction (e.g., anaphylaxis) after a previous dose or to a vaccine component	• Moderate or severe acute illness with or without fever
Tetanus, diphtheria, and acellular pertussis (Tdap) Tetanus, diphtheria (Td)	• Severe allergic reaction (e.g., anaphylaxis) after a previous dose or to a vaccine component[3] • For Tdap only: Encephalopathy (e.g., coma, decreased level of consciousness, prolonged seizures), not attributable to another identifiable cause, within 7 days of administration of previous dose of DTP, DTaP, or Tdap	• Guillain-Barré syndrome (GBS) within 6 weeks after a previous dose of tetanus-toxoid–containing vaccine • History of Arthus-type hypersensitivity reactions after a previous dose of diphtheria-toxoid–containing or tetanus-toxoid–containing vaccine; defer vaccination until at least 10 years have elapsed since the last tetanus-toxoid–containing vaccine • Moderate or severe acute illness with or without fever • For Tdap only: Progressive or unstable neurological disorder, uncontrolled seizures, or progressive encephalopathy until a treatment regimen has been established and the condition has stabilized • Moderate or severe acute illness with or without fever
Varicella (VAR)	• Severe allergic reaction (e.g., anaphylaxis) after a previous dose or to a vaccine component[3] • Severe immunodeficiency (e.g., hematologic and solid tumors, receipt of chemotherapy, congenital immunodeficiency, long-term immunosuppressive therapy or patients with HIV infection who are severely immunocompromised) • Pregnancy • Family history of altered immunocompetence, unless verified clinically or by laboratory testing as immunocompetent	• Recent (≤11 months) receipt of antibody-containing blood product (specific interval depends on product) • Receipt of specific antiviral drugs (acyclovir, famciclovir, or valacyclovir) 24 hours before vaccination (avoid use of these antiviral drugs for 14 days after vaccination) • Use of aspirin or aspirin-containing products • Moderate or severe acute illness with or without fever
Zoster recombinant vaccine (RZV)	• Severe allergic reaction (e.g., anaphylaxis) after a previous dose or to a vaccine component[4]	• Moderate or severe acute illness with or without fever • Current herpes zoster infection

1. When a contraindication is present, a vaccine should NOT be administered. Kroger A, Bahta L, Hunter P. ACIP General Best Practice Guidelines for Immunization. www.cdc.gov/vaccines/hcp/acip-recs/general-recs/contraindications.html

2. When a precaution is present, vaccination should generally be deferred but might be indicated if the benefit of protection from the vaccine outweighs the risk for an adverse reaction. Kroger A, Bahta L, Hunter P. ACIP General Best Practice Guidelines for Immunization. www.cdc.gov/vaccines/hcp/acip-recs/general-recs/contraindications.html

3. Vaccination providers should check FDA-approved prescribing information for the most complete and updated information, including contraindications, warnings, and precautions. Package inserts for U.S.-licensed vaccines are available at www.fda.gov/vaccines-blood-biologics/approved-products/vaccines-licensed-use-united-states.

4. For information on the pregnancy exposure registries for persons who were inadvertently vaccinated with Heplisav-B or PreHevbrio while pregnant, please visit heplisavbpregnancyregistry.com/ or www.prehevbrio.com/#safety.

Detailed Vaccine Recommendations, Adults, United States, 2024

Addendum   Recommended Adult Immunization Schedule for Ages 19 Years or Older, United States, 2024

In addition to the recommendations presented in the previous sections of this immunization schedule, ACIP has approved the following recommendations by majority vote since October 26, 2023. The following recommendations have been adopted by the CDC Director and are now official. Links are provided if these recommendations have been published in *Morbidity and Mortality Weekly Report (MMWR)*.

Vaccine	Recommendations	Effective Date of Recommendation*
COVID-19	• ACIP recommends persons ≥65 years of age should receive an additional dose of 2023–2024 Formula COVID-19 vaccine. • For detailed information, see: www.cdc.gov/covidschedule	February 28, 2024
COVID-19 (Moderna, Pfizer-BioNTech, Novavax)	• ACIP recommends 2024–2025 COVID-19 vaccines as authorized or approved by FDA in persons ≥6 months of age.	June 27, 2024
Influenza	• ACIP reaffirms the recommendation for routine annual influenza vaccination of all persons aged ≥6 months who do not have contraindications. • ACIP recommends high-dose inactivated (HD-IIV3) and adjuvanted inactivated (aIIV3) influenza vaccines as acceptable options for influenza vaccination of solid organ transplant recipients aged 18 through 64 years who are on immunosuppressive medication regimens, without a preference over other age-appropriate IIV3s or RIV3.	June 27, 2024
Pneumococcal conjugate vaccine	• ACIP recommends PCV21 as an option for adults aged ≥19 years who currently have a recommendation to receive a dose of PCV.	June 27, 2024
Respiratory syncytial virus vaccine (RSV)	• ACIP recommends adults 75 years of age and older receive a single dose of RSV vaccine.[a,b] • ACIP recommends adults 60–74 years of age and older who are at increased risk of severe RSV disease receive a single dose of RSV vaccine.[a,b]	June 26, 2024

[a] RSV vaccination is recommended as a single lifetime dose only. Persons who have already received RSV vaccination are NOT recommended to receive another dose.

[b] These recommendations supplant the current recommendation that adults 60 years of age and older may receive RSV vaccination, using shared clinical decision-making. Adults 60–74 years of age who are not at increased risk of severe RSV disease are NOT recommended to receive RSV vaccination.

[c] CDC will publish Clinical Considerations that describe chronic medical conditions and other risk factors for severe RSV disease for use in this risk-based recommendation.

*The effective date is the date when the CDC director adopted the recommendation and when the ACIP recommendation became official.

Source: https://www.cdc.gov/vaccines/schedules/hcp/imz/adult.html.

MODIFIED CHECKLIST FOR AUTISM IN TODDLERS, REVISED WITH FOLLOW-UP (M-CHAT-R/F)

MODIFIED CHECKLIST FOR AUTISM IN TODDLERS, REVISED WITH FOLLOW-UP (M-CHAT-R/F)

Instructions: Please answer these questions about your child. Keep in mind how your child usually behaves. If you have seen your child do the behavior a few times, but he or she does not usually do it, then please answer no. Please circle YES or NO for every question. Thank you very much!

1.	If you point at something across the room, does your child look at it? (FOR EXAMPLE, if you point at a toy or an animal, does your child look at the toy or animal?)	YES or NO
2.	Have you ever wondered if your child might be deaf?	YES or NO
3.	Does your child play pretend or make-believe? (FOR EXAMPLE, pretend to drink from an empty cup, pretend to talk on a phone, or pretend to feed a doll or stuffed animal)	YES or NO
4.	Does your child like climbing on things? (FOR EXAMPLE, furniture, playground equipment, or stairs)	YES or NO
5.	Does your child make unusual finger movements near his or her eyes? (FOR EXAMPLE, does your child wiggle his or her fingers close to his or her eyes?)	YES or NO
6.	Does your child point with one finger to ask for something or to get help? (FOR EXAMPLE, pointing to a snack or a toy that is out of reach)	YES or NO
7.	Does your child point with one finger to show you something interesting? (FOR EXAMPLE, pointing to an airplane in the sky or a big truck in the road)	YES or NO
8.	Is your child interested in other children? (FOR EXAMPLE, does your child watch other children, smile at them, or go to them?)	YES or NO
9.	Does your child show you things by bringing them to you or holding them up for you to see— not to get help, but just to share? (FOR EXAMPLE, showing you a flower, a stuffed animal, or a toy truck)	YES or NO
10.	Does your child respond when you call his or her name? (FOR EXAMPLE, does he or she look up, talk or babble, or stop what he or she is doing when you call his or her name?)	YES or NO
11.	When you smile at your child, does he or she smile back at you?	YES or NO
12.	Does your child get upset by everyday noises? (FOR EXAMPLE, does your child scream or cry to noise such as a vacuum cleaner or loud music?)	YES or NO
13.	Does your child walk?	YES or NO
14.	Does your child look you in the eye when you are talking to him or her, playing with him or her, or dressing him or her?	YES or NO
15.	Does your child try to copy what you do? (FOR EXAMPLE, wave bye-bye, clap, or make a funny noise when you do)	YES or NO
16.	If you turn your head to look at something, does your child look around to see what you are looking at?	YES or NO
17.	Does your child try to get you to watch him or her? (FOR EXAMPLE, does your child look at you for praise, or say "look" or "watch me"?)	YES or NO

MODIFIED CHECKLIST FOR AUTISM IN TODDLERS, REVISED WITH FOLLOW-UP (M-CHAT-R/F) *(Continued)*	
18. Does your child understand when you tell him or her to do something? (FOR EXAMPLE, if you don't point, can your child understand "put the book on the chair" or "bring me the blanket"?)	YES or NO
19. If something new happens, does your child look at your face to see how you feel about it? (FOR EXAMPLE, if he or she hears a strange or funny noise, or sees a new toy, will he or she look at your face?)	YES or NO
20. Does your child like movement activities? (FOR EXAMPLE, being swung or bounced on your knee)	YES or NO

Scoring: For all items except 2, 5, and 12, "NO" response indicates autism spectrum disorder risk.
Low risk: 0–2; no further action required.
Medium risk: 3–7; administer the follow-up (M-CHAT-R/F); if score remains ≥2, screening is positive.
High risk: ≥8; refer immediately for diagnostic evaluation and early intervention.
Source: Reproduced with permission. © 2009 Diana Robins, Deborah Fein, Marianne Barton. Follow-up questions and additional information can be found at www.mchatscreen.com.

SCREENING INSTRUMENTS: ALCOHOL ABUSE

SENSITIVITY AND SPECIFICITY OF SCREENING TESTS FOR PROBLEM DRINKING

Instrument Name	Screening Questions/Scoring	Threshold Score	Sensitivity/ Specificity (%)	Source
CAGE[a]	1 point each for: – Cutting down – Annoyance from criticism – Guilt – Eye-openers	>1 >2[b] >3	77/58 53/81 29/92	*Am J Psychiatry.* 1974;131:1121 *J Gen Intern Med.* 1998;13:379
AUDIT	See page 718. Available at: https://auditscreen .org/	>4 >5[b] >6	87/70 77/84 66/90	*BMJ.* 1997;314:420 *J Gen Intern Med.* 1998;13:379

[a]The CAGE may be less applicable to binge drinkers (eg, college students), the older adults, and minority populations.
[b]A CAGE score of 2 or an AUDIT score of 5 are generally accepted as "positive" screens.

SCREENING INSTRUMENTS: DEPRESSION			
Instrument Name	**Screening Questions/ Scoring**	**Threshold Score**	**Source**
Beck Depression Inventory (short form)	See page 610	0–4: None or minimal depression 5–7: Mild depression 8–15: Moderate depression >15: Severe depression	*Postgrad Med.* 1972;81
Geriatric Depression Scale	See page 582	≥15: Depression	*J Psychiatr Res.* 1983;17:37
PRIME-MD© (mood questions)	1. During the last month, have you often been bothered by feeling down, depressed, or hopeless? 2. During the last month, have you often been bothered by little interest or pleasure in doing things?	"Yes" to either question[a]	*JAMA.* 1994;272:1749 *J Gen Intern Med.* 1997;12:439
Patient Health Questionnaire (PHQ-9)©	http://www.pfizer.com/phq-9/ See page 721	*Major depressive syndrome:* if answers to #1a or b and ≥5 of #1a–i are at least "More than half the days" (count #1i if present at all) *Other depressive syndrome:* if #1a or b and 2–4 of #1a–i are at least "More than half the days" (count #1i if present at all) 5–9: mild depression 10–14: moderate depression 15–19: moderately severe depression 20–27: severe depression	*JAMA.* 1999;282:1737 *J Gen Intern Med.* 2001;16:606
[a]Sensitivity 86%–96%; specificity 57%–75%.			

SCREENING INSTRUMENTS: DEPRESSION				
PHQ-9 DEPRESSION SCREEN, ENGLISH				
OVER THE PAST 2 WK, HOW OFTEN HAVE YOU BEEN BOTHERED BY ANY OF THE FOLLOWING PROBLEMS?				
	Not at All	**Several Days**	**>Half the Days**	**Nearly Every Day**
a. Little interest or pleasure in doing things	0	1	2	3
b. Feeling down, depressed, or hopeless	0	1	2	3
c. Trouble falling or staying asleep, or sleeping too much	0	1	2	3
d. Feeling tired or having little energy	0	1	2	3
e. Poor appetite or overeating	0	1	2	3
f. Feeling bad about yourself—or that you are a failure or that you have let yourself or your family down	0	1	2	3
g. Trouble concentrating on things, such as reading the newspaper or watching television	0	1	2	3
h. Moving or speaking so slowly that other people could have noticed? Or the opposite—being so fidgety or restless that you have been moving around a lot more than usual?	0	1	2	3
i. Thoughts that you would be better off dead or of hurting yourself in some way	0	1	2	3
For office coding: Total Score	— =	— +	— +	—

Major depressive syndrome: If ≥5 items present scored ≥2 and one of the items is depressed mood (b) or anhedonia (a). If item "i" is present, then this counts, even if score = 1.
Depressive screen positive: If at least one item ≥2 (or item "i" is ≥1).
Source: From Pfizer; *Primary Care Evaluation of Mental Disorders Patient Health Questionnaire (PRIME-MD PHQ)* by Dr. Robert L. et al. 1999.

SCREENING INSTRUMENTS: DEPRESSION
PHQ-9 DEPRESSION SCREEN, SPANISH
DURANTE LAS ÚLTIMAS 2 SEMANAS, ¿CON QUÉ FRECUENCIA LE HAN MOLESTADO LOS SIGUIENTES PROBLEMAS?

	Nunca	Varios dias	>La mitad de los dias	Casi todos los dias
a. Tener poco interés o placer en hacer las cosas	0	1	2	3
b. Sentirse desanimada, deprimida, o sin esperanza	0	1	2	3
c. Con problemas en dormirse o en mantenerse dormida, o en dormir demasiado	0	1	2	3
d. Sentirse cansada o tener poca energía	0	1	2	3
e. Tener poco apetito o comer en exceso	0	1	2	3
f. Sentir falta de amor propio—o qe sea un fracaso o que decepcionara a sí misma o a su familia	0	1	2	3
g. Tener dificultad para concentrarse en cosas tales como leer el periódico o mirar la televisión	0	1	2	3
h. Se mueve o habla tan lentamente que otra gente se podría dar cuenta—o de lo contrario, está tan agitada o inquieta que se mueve mucho más de lo acostumbrado	0	1	2	3
i. Se le han ocurrido pensamientos de que se haría daño de alguna manera	0	1	2	3
For office coding: Total Store	— =	— +	— +	—

Source: From Pfizer; *Primary Care Evaluation of Mental Disorders Patient Health Questionnaire (PRIME-MD PHQ)* by Dr. Robert L. et al. 1999.

SCREENING INSTRUMENTS: DEPRESSION

BECK DEPRESSION INVENTORY, SHORT FORM

Instructions: This is a questionnaire. On the questionnaire are groups of statements. Please read the entire group of statements in each category. Then pick out the one statement in that group that best describes the way you feel today, that is, right now! Circle the number beside the statement you have chosen. If several statements in the group seem to apply equally well, circle each one. Sum all numbers to calculate a score.

Be sure to read all the statements in each group before making your choice.

Sadness
3 I am so sad or unhappy that I can't stand it.
2 I am blue or sad all the time and I can't snap out of it.
1 I feel sad or blue.
0 I do not feel sad.

Pessimism
3 I feel that the future is hopeless and that things cannot improve.
2 I feel I have nothing to look forward to.
1 I feel discouraged about the future.
0 I am not particularly pessimistic or discouraged about the future.

Sense of failure
3 I feel I am a complete failure as a person (parent, husband, wife).
2 As I look back on my life, all I can see is a lot of failures.
1 I feel I have failed more than the average person.
0 I do not feel like a failure.

Social withdrawal
3 I have lost all of my interest in other people and don't care about them at all.
2 I have lost most of my interest in other people and have little feeling for them.
1 I am less interested in other people than I used to be.
0 I have not lost interest in other people.

Indecisiveness
3 I can't make any decisions at all anymore.
2 I have great difficulty in making decisions.
1 I try to put off making decisions.
0 I make decisions about as well as ever.

Self-image change
3 I feel that I am ugly or repulsive looking.
2 I feel that there are permanent changes in my appearance and they make me look unattractive.
1 I am worried that I am looking old or unattractive.
0 I don't feel that I look worse than I used to.

Dissatisfaction
3 I am dissatisfied with everything.
2 I don't get satisfaction out of anything anymore.
1 I don't enjoy things the way I used to.
0 I am not particularly dissatisfied.

Guilt
3 I feel as though I am very bad or worthless.
2 I feel quite guilty.
1 I feel bad or unworthy a good part of the time.
0 I don't feel particularly guilty.

Self-dislike
3 I hate myself.
2 I am disgusted with myself.
1 I am disappointed in myself.
0 I don't feel disappointed in myself.

Self-harm
3 I would kill myself if I had the chance.
2 I have definite plans about committing suicide.
1 I feel I would be better off dead.
0 I don't have any thoughts of harming myself.

Work difficulty
3 I can't do any work at all.
2 I have to push myself very hard to do anything.
1 It takes extra effort to get started at doing something.
0 I can work about as well as before.

Fatigability
3 I get too tired to do anything.
2 I get tired from doing anything.
1 I get tired more easily than I used to.
0 I don't get any more tired than usual.

Anorexia
3 I have no appetite at all anymore.
2 My appetite is much worse now.
1 My appetite is not as good as it used to be.
0 My appetite is no worse than usual.

Source: Reproduced with permission from Beck AT, Beck RW. Screening depressed patients in family practice: a rapid technic. *Postgrad Med.* 1972;52:81–85.

VULNERABLE SENIORS: PREVENTING ADVERSE DRUG EVENTS

For older adults, minimize exposure to potentially inappropriate medications. Below is a summary of the 2015 American Geriatric Society Beers Criteria to prevent adverse drug events in older patients.

SELECTED MEDICATIONS TO AVOID IN OLDER ADULTS

These medications carry risks specific to an older population and should be avoided except in specific situations.

Class of Medications	Reason to Avoid	Exceptions
First-Generation Antihistamines *(ie, diphenhydramine, hydroxyzine, promethazine, etc.)*	Clearance is reduced as age advances; risk of confusion and other anticholinergic effects	Diphenhydramine for acute allergic reaction may be appropriate
Antiparkinsonian agents *(ie, benztropine, trihexyphenidyl)*	More effective agents exist for Parkinson disease	
Antispasmodics *(ie, atropine, belladonna alkaloids, dicyclomine, etc.)*	Risk of confusion and other anticholinergic effects	
Nitrofurantoin	Pulmonary, hepato-, and neurotoxicity with long-term use; safer alternatives exist for UTI ppx	
Alpha-1 blockers, peripheral *(ie, doxazosin, prazosin, terazosin)*	High risk of orthostatic hypotension	
Alpha-1 blockers, central *(ie, clonidine, guanfacine, methyldopa)*	Risk of CNS effect, bradycardia, orthostatic hypotension	Clonidine may be appropriate in some cases as adjunctive agent in refractory HTN
Digoxin	AFib: more effective alternatives exist and mortality may increase Heart failure: Benefit is arguable; mortality may increase	May be appropriate in some cases as adjunctive agent for refractory symptomatic atrial fibrillation or heart failure. If used, avoid doses > 0.125 mg/d
Nifedipine	Risk of hypotension, myocardial ischemia	
Amiodarone	AFib: more toxicity than other agents	May be appropriate for rhythm control if LVH or significant heart failure
Antidepressants with anticholinergic profile *(ie, amitriptyline, nortriptyline, paroxetine)*	Sedating; orthostatic hypotension; anticholinergic effects including confusion	
Antipsychotics, first and second generation	Risk of CVA, cognitive decline	Schizophrenia, bipolar disorder Dementia/delirium: only appropriate if nonpharmacologic options fail and patient threatens significant harm to self or others

VULNERABLE SENIORS: PREVENTING ADVERSE DRUG EVENTS (*Continued*)

For older adults, minimize exposure to potentially inappropriate medications. Below is a summary of the 2015 American Geriatric Society Beers Criteria to prevent adverse drug events in older patients.

SELECTED MEDICATIONS TO AVOID IN OLDER ADULTS

These medications carry risks specific to an older population and should be avoided except in specific situations.

Barbiturates *(ie, phenobarbital, butalbital)*	Risk of overdose at low dosages, dependence, escalating dose due to tolerance	
Benzodiazepines	Increased sensitivity with age, slower metabolism of longer-acting agents. Risk of cognitive impairment, falls, delirium	Seizure disorders, alcohol withdrawal, severe generalized anxiety, anesthesia
Nonbenzodiazepine hypnotics *(ie, zolpidem, zaleplon, eszopiclone)*	Similar to benzodiazepine risk; minimal improvement in sleep	
Androgens *(ie, testosterone, methyltestosterone)*	Cardiac problems; contraindicated in prostate cancer	Lab-verified symptomatic hypogonadism
Estrogen, +/− progestin	Risk of breast and endometrial cancer; no evidence for cardioprotection or cognitive protection in older adults	Vaginal estrogens safe/effective for vaginal dryness
Insulin on a sliding scale	Hypoglycemia risk; no outcome benefit in outpatient or inpatient settings	
Megestrol	Does not improve weight; higher risk of VTE and death	
Sulfonylureas of longer duration *(ie, glyburide, chlorpropamide)*	Severe prolonged hypoglycemia	
Metoclopramide	Extrapyramidal effects	Gastroparesis
Proton pump inhibitors	*Clostridioides difficile* infection; osteopenia/osteoporosis	Short-courses (ie, <8 wk). May be appropriate to treat severe conditions such as erosive esophagitis, Barrett esophagus, or for prevention in high-risk patients (ie, NSAID or corticosteroid use)
NSAIDs *(ie, high-dose aspirin, ibuprofen, naproxen, indomethacin, ketorolac, etc.)*	GI bleed or peptic ulcer disease. Some (ie, indomethacin, ketorolac) carry higher risk of AKI	Only use if alternative treatments are exhausted and patient can take PPI or misoprostol for gastroprotection (which reduces but does not eliminate risk)
Muscle relaxants *(ie, cyclobenzaprine, methocarbamol, carisoprodol)*	Anticholinergic effects, sedation, fracture risk; minimal efficacy	Urinary retention

Source: https://www.ncbi.nlm.nih.gov/pubmed/26446832

WHO INTEGRATED CARE FOR OLDER PEOPLE SCREENING TOOL

TABLE 6 WHO ICOPE SCREENING TOOL		
Priority Conditions Associated with Declines in Intrinsic Capacity	**Tests**	**Assess Fully Any Domain with a Check Box**
Cognitive decline	1. Remember three words: flower, door, rice (for example)	Wrong to either question or does not know
	2. Orientation in time and space: What is the full date today? Where are you now (home, clinic, etc.)?	
	Recalls the three words?	Cannot recall all three words
Limited mobility	Chair rise test: Rise from chair 5 times without using arms. Did the person complete five chair raises in 14 s?	No
Malnutrition	1. Weight loss: Have you unintentionally lost more than 3 kg over the last 3 mo?	Yes
	2. Appetite loss: Have you experienced appetite loss?	Yes
Visual impairment	Do you have any problems with your eyes: difficulties in seeing far, reading, eye diseases or currently under medical treatment (eg, diabetes, high blood pressure)?	Yes
Hearing loss	Hears whispers (whisper test) or	Fail
	Screening audiometry result ≤ 35 dB or	
	Passes automated App-based digits-in-noise test	
Depressive symptoms	Over the past 2 wk, have you been bothered by …	
	– Feeling down, depressed or hopeless?	Yes
	– Little interest or pleasure in doing things?	Yes

Source: Reproduced with permission from *Integrated Care for Older People (ICOPE): Guidance for Person-Centered Assessment and Pathways in Primary Care.* Geneva: World Health Organization; 2019.

WHO PAIN RELIEF LADDER

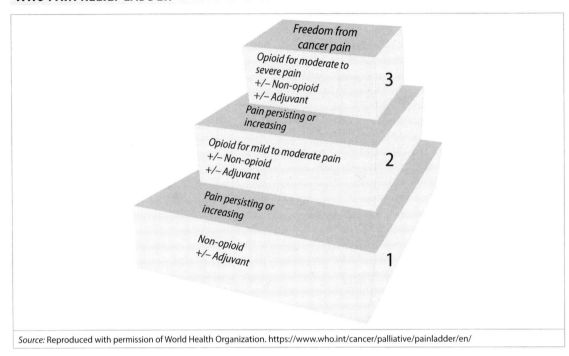

Source: Reproduced with permission of World Health Organization. https://www.who.int/cancer/palliative/painladder/en/

ORGANIZATIONS REFERENCED

PROFESSIONAL SOCIETIES AND GOVERNMENTAL AGENCIES		
Abbreviation	**Full Name**	**Internet Address**
	Bright Futures	http://brightfutures.org
AACE	American Association of Clinical Endocrinologists	http://www.aace.com
AAD	American Academy of Dermatology	http://www.aad.org
AAFP	American Academy of Family Physicians	http://www.aafp.org
AAHPM	American Academy of Hospice and Palliative Medicine	http://www.aahpm.org
AAN	American Academy of Neurology	http://www.aan.com
AAO	American Academy of Ophthalmology	http://www.aao.org
AAO-HNS	American Academy of Otolaryngology—Head and Neck Surgery	http://www.entnet.org
AAOS	American Academy of Orthopedic Surgeons and American Association of Orthopedic Surgeons	http://www.aaos.org
AAP	American Academy of Pediatrics	http://www.aap.org

PROFESSIONAL SOCIETIES AND GOVERNMENTAL AGENCIES *(Continued)*		
Abbreviation	**Full Name**	**Internet Address**
ACC	American College of Cardiology	http://www.acc.org
ACCP	American College of Chest Physicians	http://www.chestnet.org
ACIP	Advisory Committee on Immunization Practices	http://www.cdc.gov/vaccines/acip/index.html
ACOG	American Congress of Obstetricians and Gynecologists	http://www.acog.com
ACP	American College of Physicians	http://www.acponline.org
ACR	American College of Radiology	http://www.acr.org
ACR	American College of Rheumatology	http://www.rheumatology.org
ACS	American Cancer Society	http://www.cancer.org
ACSM	American College of Sports Medicine	http://www.acsm.org
ADA	American Diabetes Association	http://www.diabetes.org
AGA	American Gastroenterological Association	http://www.gastro.org
AGS	American Geriatrics Society	http://www.americangeriatrics.org
AHA	American Heart Association	http://www.americanheart.org
ANA	American Nurses Association	http://www.nursingworld.org
AOA	American Optometric Association	http://www.aoa.org
ARC	International Agency for Research on Cancer	http://screening.iarc.fr
ASA	American Stroke Association	http://www.strokeassociation.org
ASAM	American Society of Addiction Medicine	http://www.asam.org
ASCCP	American Society for Colposcopy and Cervical Pathology	http://www.asccp.org
ASCO	American Society of Clinical Oncology	http://www.asco.org
ASCRS	American Society of Colon and Rectal Surgeons	http://www.fascrs.org
ASGE	American Society for Gastrointestinal Endoscopy	http://asge.org
ASHA	American Speech-Language-Hearing Association	http://www.asha.org
ASN	American Society of Neuroimaging	http://www.asnweb.org
ATA	American Thyroid Association	http://www.thyroid.org
ATS	American Thoracic Society	http://www.thoracic.org
AUA	American Urological Association	http://auanet.org
BASHH	British Association for Sexual Health and HIV	http://www.bashh.org
BGS	British Geriatrics Society	http://www.bgs.org.uk/
BHOF	Bone Health and Osteoporosis Foundation	https://www.bonehealthandosteoporosis.org/

PROFESSIONAL SOCIETIES AND GOVERNMENTAL AGENCIES (*Continued*)		
Abbreviation	**Full Name**	**Internet Address**
BSAC	British Society for Antimicrobial Chemotherapy	http://www.bsac.org.uk
CDC	Centers for Disease Control and Prevention	http://www.cdc.gov
COG	Children's Oncology Group	http://www.childrensoncologygroup.org
CSVS	Canadian Society for Vascular Surgery	http://canadianvascular.ca
CTF	Canadian Task Force on Preventive Health Care	http://canadiantaskforce.ca
EASD	European Association for the Study of Diabetes	http://www.easd.org
EASL	European Association for the Study of the Liver	https://easl.eu
EAU	European Association of Urology	http://www.uroweb.org
ERS	European Respiratory Society	http://ersnet.org
ESC	European Society of Cardiology	http://www.escardio.org
ESH	European Society of Hypertension	http://www.eshonline.org
ICSI	Institute for Clinical Systems Improvement	http://www.icsi.org
IDF	International Diabetes Federation	http://www.idf.org
KDIOG	Kidney Disease Improving Global Outcomes	https://kdigo.org
NAPNAP	National Association of Pediatric Nurse Practitioners	http://www.napnap.org
NCCN	National Comprehensive Cancer Network	http://www.nccn.org/cancer-guidelines.html
NCI	National Cancer Institute	http://www.cancer.gov/cancerinformation
NEI	National Eye Institute	http://www.nei.nih.gov
NGC	National Guideline Clearinghouse	http://www.guidelines.gov
NHLBI	National Heart, Lung, and Blood Institute	http://www.nhlbi.nih.gov
NIAAA	National Institute on Alcohol Abuse and Alcoholism	http://www.niaaa.nih.gov
NICE	National Institute for Health and Clinical Excellence	http://www.nice.org.uk
NIDCR	National Institute of Dental and Craniofacial Research	http://www.nidr.nih.gov
NIHCDC	National Institutes of Health Consensus Development Program	http://www.consensus.nih.gov
NIP	National Immunization Program	http://www.cdc.gov/vaccines
NKF	National Kidney Foundation	http://www.kidney.org
NTSB	National Transportation Safety Board	http://www.ntsb.gov
SCF	Skin Cancer Foundation	http://www.skincancer.org
SFP	Society for Family Planning	https://societyfp.org

PROFESSIONAL SOCIETIES AND GOVERNMENTAL AGENCIES (*Continued*)		
Abbreviation	**Full Name**	**Internet Address**
SGIM	Society of General Internal Medicine	http://www.sgim.org
SKI	Sloan-Kettering Institute	http://www.mskcc.org/mskcc/ html/5804.cfm
SVU	Society for Vascular Ultrasound	http://www.svunet.org
UK-NHS	United Kingdom National Health Service	http://www.nhs.uk
USPSTF	United States Preventive Services Task Force	http://www.ahrq.gov/clinic/ uspstfix.htm
WHO	World Health Organization	http://www.who.int/en

INDEX

Page references followed by "f" denote figures, "t" denote tables, and "n" denote footnotes.